Anatomy and Physiology

Understanding the Human Body

Jones and Bartlett Titles in Biological Science

AIDS: Science and Society, Fourth Edition
Fan/Conner/Villarreal

AIDS: The Biological Basis, Third Edition
Alcamo

Alcamo's Fundamentals of Microbiology, Seventh Edition
Pommerville

Alcamo's Laboratory Fundamentals of Microbiology,
Seventh Edition
Pommerville

Aquatic Entomology
McCafferty/Provonsha

Botany: An Introduction to Plant Biology, Third Edition
Mauseth

The Cancer Book
Cooper

Cell Biology: Organelle Structure and Function
Sadava

Creative Evolution?!
Campbell/Schopf

Defending Evolution: A Guide to the Evolution/Creation
Controversy
Alters

Diversity of Life: The Illustrated Guide to the Five Kingdoms
Margulis/Schwartz/Dolan

DNA Sequencing: Optimizing the Process and Analysis
Kieleczawa

Early Life, Evolution on the Precambrian Earth,
Second Edition
Margulis/Dolan

Electron Microscopy, Second Edition
Bozzola/Russell

Elements of Human Cancer
Cooper

Encounters in Microbiology
Alcamo

Essential Genetics: A Genomic Perspective,
Third Edition
Hartl/Jones

Essential Medical Terminology, Second Edition
Stanfield

Essentials of Molecular Biology, Fourth Edition
Malacinski

Evolution, Third Edition
Strickberger

Experimental Techniques in Bacterial Genetics
Maloy

Exploring the Way Life Works: The Science of Biology
Hoagland/Dodson/Hauck

Genetics, Analysis of Genes and Genomes,
Sixth Edition
Hartl/Jones

Genetics of Populations, Third Edition
Hedrick

Genomic and Molecular Neuro-Oncology
Zhang/Fuller

Guide to Infectious Diseases by Body System
Pommerville

Grant Application Writer's Handbook
Reif-Lehrer

How Cancer Works
Sompayrac

How Pathogenic Viruses Work
Sompayrac

How the Human Genome Works
McConkey

Human Anatomy and Physiology Coloring Workbook and
Study Guide, Second Edition
Anderson/Spitzer

Human Anatomy Flash Cards
Clark

Human Biology, Fifth Edition
Chiras

Human Body Systems: Structure, Function and Environment
Chiras

Human Embryonic Stem Cells: An Introduction to the Science
and Therapeutic Potential
Kiessling/Anderson

Human Genetics: The Molecular Revolution
McConkey

The Illustrated Glossary of Protoctista
Margulis/McKhann/Olendzenski

Introduction to Human Disease, Sixth Edition
Crowley

Introduction to the Biology of Marine Life, Eighth Edition
Sumich/Morrissey

Laboratory and Field Investigations in Marine Life,
Eighth Edition
Sumich/Gordon

Laboratory Research Notebooks
Jones and Bartlett Publishers

A Laboratory Textbook of Anatomy and Physiology, Cat
Version, Eighth Edition
Donnersberger/Lesak Scott

A Laboratory Textbook of Anatomy and Physiology, Fetal Pig
Version
Donnersberger/Lesak Scott

Major Events in the History of Life
Schopf

Medical Genetics: Pearls of Wisdom
Sanger

Microbes and Society: An Introduction to Microbiology
Alcamo

Microbial Genetics, Second Edition
Maloy/Cronan/Freifelder

Microbiology: Pearls of Wisdom
Booth

Missing Links: Evolutionary Concepts and Transitions
Through Time
Martin

Oncogenes, Second Edition
Cooper

100 Years Exploring Life, 1888–1988, The Marine Biological
Laboratory at Woods Hole
Maienschein

Origin and Evolution Of Intelligence
Schopf

Plant Cell Biology: Structure and Function
Gunning/Steer

Plants, Genes, and Crop Biotechnology, Second Edition
Chrispeels/Sadava

Population Biology
Hedrick

Protein Microarrays
Schena

Statistics: Concepts and Applications for Science
LeBlanc

Teaching Biological Evolution in Higher Education
Alters

Vertebrates: A Laboratory Text
Wessels

Anatomy and Physiology

Understanding the Human Body

Robert K. Clark

JONES AND BARTLETT PUBLISHERS

Sudbury, Massachusetts

BOSTON   TORONTO   LONDON   SINGAPORE

World Headquarters

Jones and Bartlett Publishers
40 Tall Pine Drive
Sudbury, MA 01776
978-443-5000
info@jbpub.com
www.jbpub.com

Jones and Bartlett Publishers
Canada
2406 Nikanna Road
Mississauga, ON L5C 2W6
CANADA

Jones and Bartlett Publishers
International
Barb House, Barb Mews
London W6 7PA
UK

Production Credits

Chief Executive Officer: Clayton Jones
Chief Operating Officer: Don W. Jones, Jr.
President, Higher Education and Professional Publishing: Robert W. Holland, Jr.
V.P., Design and Production: Anne Spencer
V.P., Sales and Marketing: William Kane
V.P., Manufacturing and Inventory Control: Therese Bräuer
Executive Editor, Science: Stephen L. Weaver
Managing Editor, Science: Dean W. DeChambeau
Associate Editor, Science: Rebecca Seastrong
Senior Production Editor: Louis C. Bruno, Jr.
Marketing Manager: Matthew Payne
Marketing Associate: Laura M. Kavigian
Text and Cover Design: Anne Spencer
Photo Researcher: Kimberly Potvin
Illustrations: Elizabeth Morales
Printing and Binding: Courier Kendallville
Cover Printing: John Pow Company

About the Cover: A racing scull is propelled through the water by the coordinated action of the oars. Likewise, the contraction of muscle requires the coordinated activities of the proteins present in myofilaments within muscle cells. These molecular activities can be understood by considering rowing technique. In this textbook, this and similar analogies will help you to understand the molecular and cellular processes that occur in the human body.

Library of Congress Cataloging-in-Publication Data

Clark, Robert K., 1958–
    Anatomy and physiology: understanding the human body / Robert K. Clark.
p. cm.
ISBN 0-7637-4816-1 (alk. paper)
1. Human physiology. 2. Human anatomy. 3. Physiology, Pathological. 1. Title.
    QP34.5C537 2004
    612—dc22
                                                      2004051586

Printed in the United States of America
09 08 07 06 05   10 9 8 7 6 5 4 3 2 1

Brief Contents

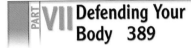

Contents

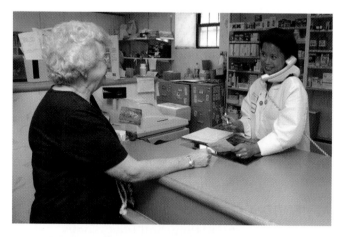

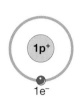
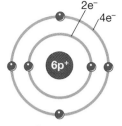
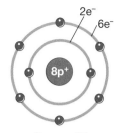

Hydrogen (H) Carbon (C) Oxygen (O)

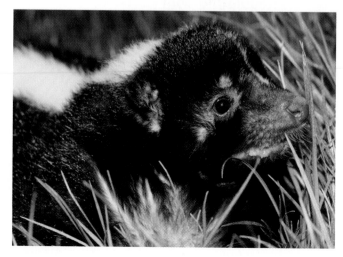

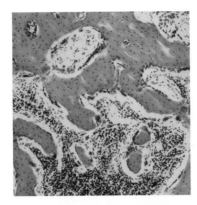
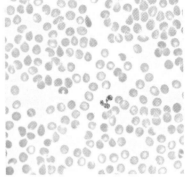

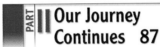

PART II Our Journey Continues 87

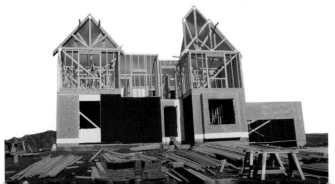

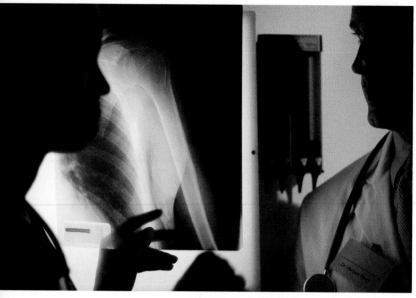

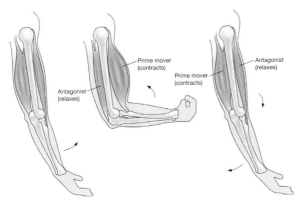

PART III Regulating Your Body   171

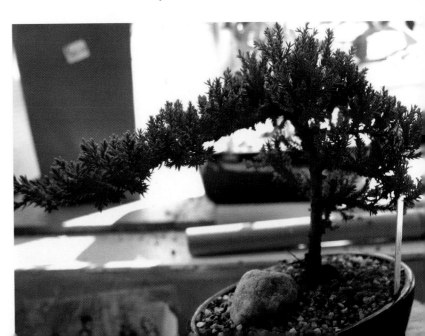

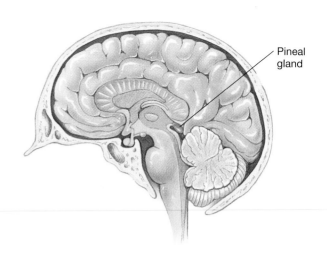

Pineal gland

PART IV Reproducing Your Body   253

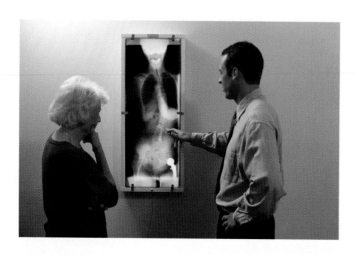

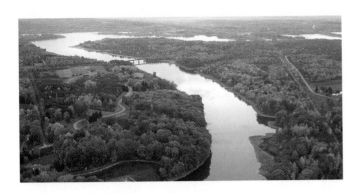

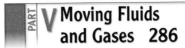

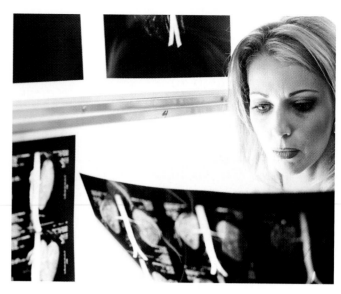

PART VI Management of Nutrients and Wastes 341

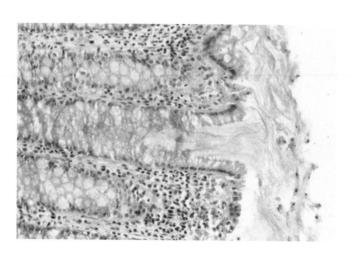

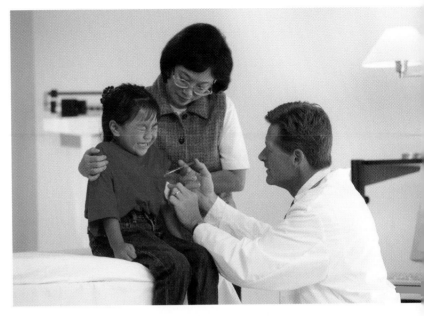

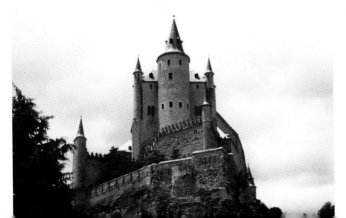

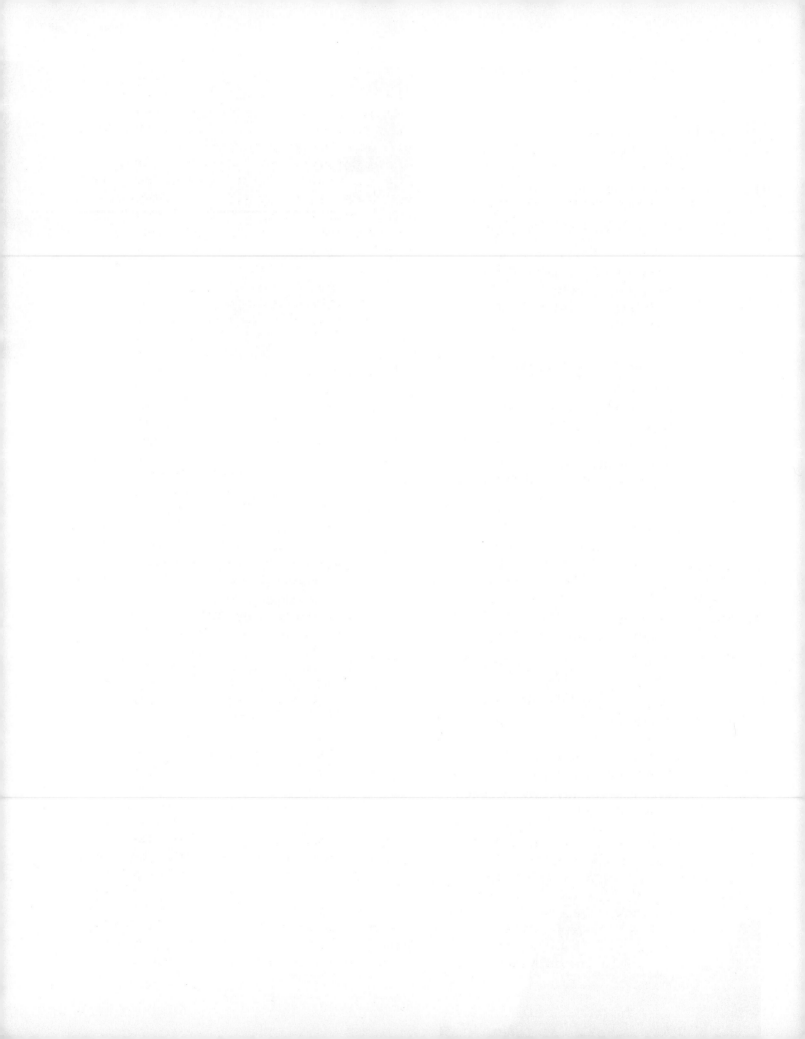

Preface

Anatomy and Physiology: Understanding the Human Body was designed to meet the needs of a diverse group of students. We are living in an era of amazing technological advancements, and those of our health care system are perhaps the most astonishing of all. Those preparing for careers in the allied health sciences, including careers involving direct patient care and the many allied technologies, need to understand the human body in greater detail than ever before. I wrote *Anatomy and Physiology: Understanding the Human Body* at the depth and detail these students require, while not loosing sight of their overriding need for conceptual understanding and critical thinking skills.

Many students preparing for careers outside of the biomedical field also need to understand the human body. The range of disciplines that this is true for increases yearly, but includes such diverse fields as the social sciences, criminal justice, preschool through secondary education, athletics and fitness training and in some cases, the visual and performing arts. This book provides the pedagogic tools these students need to ensure their learning.

Additionally, many people today face difficult decisions about their own health and the health care of their loved-ones. Many of these people recognize that an understanding of the human body enables them to ask the types of questions of their health care providers that help them make informed decisions; decisions they will be comforted by. Increasingly, people enroll in basic biomedical science courses at community colleges for just this reason. This book has been prepared with these people in mind as well. The text was written in a way that will encourage these students to continue reading and stick with their course even if they have not previously been successful in the sciences.

Students who do not have a strong background in the sciences or who may be intimidated by science courses often report that their textbooks are dry, difficult to follow and more than a little daunting. *Anatomy and Physiology: Understanding the Human Body* was written using a conversational style and an informal manner, much the way a friend would explain anatomy and physiology to them. It builds confidence as it teaches.

Much of what we learn in anatomy and physiology requires an understanding of processes at the cellular and molecular level, the very processes that are often the most difficult to grasp. Without this knowledge, the functions of the organ systems become merely words to memorize, or "magical" activities that are beyond comprehension. When students see that they can understand molecular and cellular activities, their interest in their studies increases greatly. This text makes these processes easy to understand because it relates them to objects and activities that students see daily, or can easily imagine. These teaching analogies are clear and simple and sometimes humorous. This increases reader enjoyment, encouraging continued reading and studying. When difficult concepts are presented, the text directly encourages the reader and offers learning strategies, just as many effective educators do in the classroom. This helps to build student confidence and encourages those who might otherwise become frustrated and abandon their studies.

Pedagogical features that aid student success abound. The entire first chapter is aimed at helping students to become effective learners and to develop life-long learning skills. By teaching students how to evaluate the biomedical information they encounter in their daily lives, it also prepares them to be effective at the kind of critical thinking skills our information era requires. Each chapter begins with a *What You Will Learn* feature, a set of goals for that chapter. It presents, as simple statements, the types of information students should expect to learn from their reading of the chapter. A similar, but longer and more detailed feature called *What You Should Know* can be found at the end of each chapter. This too contains information from the chapter in the form of simple statements. An understanding of these statements is one way to assess accomplishment of the goals of the chapter.

Learning outcomes or student success can be further determined by using the questions in the *What Did You Learn?* feature that follows each chapter. Notice that Appendix B contains the answers to the multiple choice questions so students can quickly evaluate their progress.

Although this book primarily presents the normal activities of the body, pathologic processes (disease, injury, and the body's response to these conditions) are presented where it aids understanding of normal activities. This is done in two ways: short descriptions within the text and slightly longer discussions called *Breaching Homeostasis . . . When Things Go Wrong* strategically placed at the end of key chapters. These discussions are not intended as a complete presentation on these conditions but as a starting point from which student understanding can grow. Appendix C helps the instructor to locate the pathologies that are of interest. As students explore these diseases, they should keep in mind the material presented in Chapter 1 on how to find and evaluate biomedical information. This helps them to avoid the pitfalls of the misinformation about diseases that is so abundant today.

The chemistry and cell biology chapters have been kept very simple, just enough to get these students started. Often our students are frustrated early in the course when they have to learn so much material that they don't consider to be "real" anatomy and physiology. Some of the larger concepts (i.e., the details of protein syntheses) are moved further into the text for inclusion after students have gained confidence and interest. Also included is a separate chapter specifically presenting the concept of electrical activity in cells. In this way, students learn the basics of this fascinating but sometimes challenging topic before moving into the specific activities of muscle cells or neurons. Instructors may choose to adopt the order of topics as presented here or to adapt the order of text chapters to follow their own syllabus. The text is flexible enough to instructors to do what works best for their students.

As you examine and use this text, I believe that you will find it distinctly different from others you have tried. I hope you enjoy using *Anatomy and Physiology: Understanding the Human Body.*

Ancillaries

Instructor's Tool Kit CD-ROM   Compatible with Windows and Macintosh platforms, this CD-ROM provides instructors with the following traditional ancillaries.

The Instructor's Manual, provided as a text file, includes goals and objectives suitable to use as handouts and classroom exercises.

The Test Bank is available as text files and as part of the Diploma™ Test Generator software included on the CD. The Test Generator software enables you to choose an appropriate variety of questions, create multiple versions of tests, even administer and grade tests on-line.

The PowerPoint™ Lecture Outline Slides presentation package provides lecture notes and images for each chapter of *Anatomy and Physiology: Understanding the Human Body.* A PowerPoint™ viewer is provided on the CD. Instructors with the Microsoft PowerPoint™ software can customize the outlines, art, and order of presentation.

The Kaleidoscope Media Viewer provides a library of all the art, tables, and photographs in the text to which Jones and Bartlett Publishers holds the copyright or that are in the public domain. The Kaleidoscope Media Viewer uses your browser—Internet Explorer or Netscape Navigator—so you may project images from the text in the classroom, insert images into PowerPoint presentations, or print your own acetates.

Anatomy and Physiology On Line This text's Web site, www.bioscience.jbpub.com/anatomy, provides additional resources to expand the scope of the textbook and make sure students have access to the most up-to-date information in anatomy and physiology. Students can find a variety of study aids in the eLearning area, such as chapter outlines, flash cards, and review questions. Carefully chosen links to relevant Web sites enable students to explore specific topics in anatomy and physiology in more detail. A brief description of each link places the site in context before the student connects to it.

Acknowledgments

I would like to thank the many people who assisted and encouraged me in the preparation of this textbook. The administration and faculty of Cumberland County College in Vineland, New Jersey have been very supportive. Special thanks go to the following members of our college community: President Dr. Kenneth Ender, Vice President of Academic Affairs and Enrollment Services Dr. Thomas Isekenegbe, former Academic Dean Dr. Jack Lobb, and Health and Science Division Chair Ms. Jane Leggieri. I express special thanks to my esteemed humanities colleague, Professor John Adair, who bravely read and red-inked an entire early draft. Thanks also go to Mr. Amar Madineni for his tireless answers to my endless technology questions.

The great people at Jones and Bartlett Publishers who worked hard to convert my manuscript into this text also deserve thanks and congratulations. These include Stephen Weaver, Executive Editor; Dean DeChambeau, Managing Editor; Rebecca Seastrong, Associate Editor; and Anne Spencer, Vice President of Design and Production. Art editor and illustrator Elizabeth Morales has done a remarkable job and was a real joy to work with. Photo researcher Kimberly Potvin deserves special thanks for her willingness to shoot photos even when special courage was required. Senior Production Editor Louis Bruno's impressive organizational skills, positive outlook, and great humor made this project a real pleasure. Special congratulations and thanks go to Lou. Thanks go to copyeditor Ellice Gerber, proofreader Debbie Liehs, indexer Sherri Dietrich, and to the compositor Circle Graphics who did a beautiful job setting the text and art. I would also like to acknowledge the valuable contribution of the anatomy and physiology faculty from across the country, who reviewed this text. Their hard work demonstrates a special dedication to their discipline and improves the teaching done by each of us.

Bert Atsma
  Union County College, New Jersey

Judy Cunningham
  Montgomery County Community College, Pennsylvania

Chaya Gopalan
  St. Louis Community College-Florissant Valley, Missouri

Susan Klarr
  Washtenaw Community College, Michigan

Scott Layton
  Cowley College, Kansas

Stephen Lebsack
  Linn Benton Community College, Oregon

Wendy McCullen-Vermillion
  Columbus State Community College, Ohio

Margaret Ott
  Tyler Junior College, Texas

Cynthia Prentice
  Chemeketa Community College, Oregon

Cynthia Schauer
  Kalamazoo Valley Community College, Michigan

Michael Squires
  Columbus State Community College, Ohio

Jeffery Thompson
  Hudson Valley Community College, New York

Patricia Torrence
  Seattle Central Community College, Washington

Finally, I would like to thank my closest collaborator, Lise Desquenne Clark, V.M.D., Ph.D., for her ongoing support and specifically for her critical reading of the manuscript and extensive work on Chapter 21.

The writing of this textbook was aided, in part, by a sabbatical leave from Cumberland County College, Vineland, New Jersey.

Robert K. Clark
Pilesgrove, New Jersey
January, 2005

About the Author

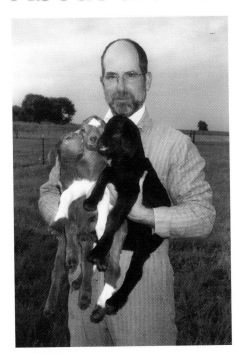

Dr. Clark is an associate professor in the Health and Science Division of Cumberland County College in Vineland, New Jersey, where he teaches Anatomy and Physiology I and II, Human Biology, Pathology, and Genetics and has been awarded the President's Award for Excellence in Leadership, Service and Scholarship. He was named 2001 New Jersey Professor of the Year by the Carnegie Foundation for the Advancement of Teaching.

He earned a Bachelor of Science Degree in Marine Biology from the University of New England and a Ph.D. from Hahnemann University (now part of Drexel University) in Experimental Pathology. His extensive research experience has led to numerous publications in the fields of cancer, stroke, and HIV/AIDS.

Commercial farmers for more than 21 years, Bob and Lise Clark raise specialty produce and goats on their southern New Jersey farm. He is shown here with week-old triplets, the results of the Clark's tinkering with goat coat-color genetics.

Foundations For Understanding The Human Body

Why Must We Learn These Foundations?

We are about to embark on a study of the basic anatomy (form) and physiology (function) of the human body. These disciplines can be highly complex and we will need to develop a common language to understand what happens within the body. Some students approach these topics with a thorough background in the sciences. Others have not yet had the opportunity to develop this science foundation. In the first section of this text, we will work at developing a common level of science literacy. This will allow us to discuss the human body with the language of science and some basic knowledge of science as we move into the disciplines in which we are specifically interested: anatomy and physiology. We will also spend some time learning study skills and examination techniques that may help you to be more successful in your studies. Whether you are reading this book as part of a course or reading on your own to increase your understanding of your body, these techniques may assist you in reaching your goal.

Some students may be tempted to skip over this early information and move right into the chapters dealing with the organs or systems that interest them. That would be a mistake. We can only understand the organs if we understand the cells of which they are composed. We can only understand how these cells work if we have some knowledge of basic chemistry. Without this knowledge, the functions of our organs appear to be magic and beyond our comprehension. Rather than developing an understanding of the body, you would merely memorize a lot of terminology that you would quickly forget. The fact that you are reading this text shows that you have a desire to understand your body. Do not cheat yourself of this understanding by not laying a suitable foundation for it. Please spend some time on the chapters in this section now, and trust that this information will help you to develop the understanding you seek.

1 Foundations For Success

What You Will Learn

- The definitions of anatomy and physiology: what it is that you are about to begin studying.
- Why it is beneficial to study these two disciplines (anatomy and physiology) at the same time.
- How you will benefit from knowing more about your body, whether or not you are planning a career in the health sciences.
- How to develop study habits that will help you to do well in your anatomy and physiology class, as well as in other classes.
- Things you can do to improve your test-taking skills.
- Where you can find useful biomedical information.
- How to evaluate the validity of biomedical information.

1.1 Anatomy and Physiology: What Are We Studying?

You are about to undertake the study of two exciting and related disciplines: anatomy and physiology. These two disciplines are often studied together rather than as separate subjects, at least at the introductory level. The reason for this becomes apparent as we consider what these two terms mean. Anatomy involves the study of the structure of the body, including the naming of the parts of the body, and consideration of how they physically relate to each other. The study of anatomy includes several subdisciplines, such as microscopic anatomy and gross anatomy. Microscopic anatomy, also called histology, involves the study of the structure of the body at the microscopic level. Gross anatomy is the study of the structure of the body at the level you can see with your naked eye. Both of these areas of anatomy are considered in this text.

Physiology is the study of the function of the body. In this discipline one considers how the various components of the body work. Subdivisions of physiology include cell physiology, the study of how cells function; histophysiology, the study of how tissues function; and systemic physiology, the study of the function of the organ systems of the body. All of these are considered in this text.

Why Study Two Disciplines at One Time?

Now that we know what these terms mean, let's consider why we study these topics together. Maybe you know the names of the parts of your automobile. Perhaps you have examined your car's engine and learned the names of its parts. Would this necessarily mean that you know how all of these parts work to make your car move? Not really. To understand how your car moves, you would have to know how these parts work, what their functions are, and how these functions relate to one another. Knowing the names of the parts of your car would mean you have an understanding of its anatomy. Knowing the functions of these parts would mean you have an understanding of your car's physiology. If you were to simply study the names and locations of the parts of your car, you would develop a vocabulary and some knowledge of how your car is put together, but your knowledge would be incomplete. It would also make for a rather dry study. If you were to try to learn how your car works without knowing the names and locations of the parts, you would have a very difficult task indeed. Form and function are so tightly linked that we cannot understand function without some knowledge of form.

These issues also apply to the human body. A study of anatomy alone requires much memorization, but does not allow one the satisfaction that comes from actually understanding the body. Physiology cannot be learned without some knowledge of basic anatomy. For these reasons, we will study these two disciplines together.

How This Material May Benefit You

Anatomy and physiology, the form and function of the human body, are two of the most fascinating disciplines we can study. If you are preparing for a career in one of the medical disciplines, this information is of obvious benefit to you; it is at the core of almost every branch of the medical sciences. Regardless of individual academic or career goals, this material is of benefit to all. Despite the great diversity of cultures, interests, and talents, all people have bodies that are structurally very similar and function in similar ways. When we study anatomy and physiology, we are studying ourselves and those around us.

At some point in time, each of us will become ill or injured. We also observe aging in those we care about and the changes associated with that process. A basic understanding of the human body enables us to better comprehend what is happening to ourselves and to those around us during times of difficulty. Even if we do not enter the health-care professions, this information enables us to communicate more effectively with those who are our health-care providers.

Finally, the vast amount of material we can study about the body allows us to exercise our minds in ways that increase our ability to study other disciplines. It also allows us, in some ways, to see the natural world and our place in it with greater clarity. In a word, we are all greatly improved by this understanding.

1.2 How to Succeed in Your Study of Anatomy and Physiology

Relax, You Can Succeed!

As you begin this study, you may have some anxiety about the difficulty of this material. Perhaps science is "just not your thing." Relax! I have some pointers that may help you learn this material.

Despite your fears, the simple truth is that most of the concepts you will learn in anatomy and physiology are not especially difficult to understand. Most, in fact, are quite easy, and others can be understood with a little effort. One difficulty lies in the fact that there is so much information to learn. You must endeavor to study every day, even on days that your class does not meet, to be sure you do not fall behind. In some ways, it is as much the amount of material as the individual concepts that lead to difficulty. Further, as you proceed with your study, you will find that the information presented later on builds upon the information you learned earlier in the course. So you cannot afford to fall behind; it will make learning the later material more difficult.

Conversely, some of the early material will not be completely clear to you until you learn the later material. It is much like building a jigsaw puzzle. When you put the first few pieces in place, you cannot see the picture, so you are not clear on what you are building. Later on, as more pieces are in place, the picture becomes apparent and the work with which you began, which seemed difficult at the time, now seems quite simple. The problem is that if you make mistakes in the early work, the picture can never become clear. The situation is the same with anatomy and physiology. Early in your study, you will not have enough pieces in place to see the big picture. You will sometimes study material that will be difficult to relate to the whole body. Don't despair. Instead, work hard to understand that material. Later on you will see the role it plays in developing your understanding of the body. Do not skip material because you don't understand its role or because you find it difficult or uninteresting. You will need it later on, and by then it may be too late to learn it. If you are using this book as a text for a course, the following tips may help you achieve a good grade.

■ Tips for Successful Studying

1. Before each lecture, read the material in the text that will be covered (**FIGURE 1.1**). Even if you don't fully understand it, you will at least become familiar with the terms. This will help you to get the most out of each lecture. If your instructor does not assign specific reading, look in the text for the material covered in the previous lecture and begin your reading there. In this way, you will generally be able to figure out what will be covered in each lecture before that lecture. You may even want to take notes in outline form during your initial reading.

2. Take careful notes during each lecture. Develop "shorthand" for common terms that will enable you to write quickly and accurately.

3. Study your notes after each lecture, preferably on the same day that you heard the lecture. This will allow you to recall what was said during the lecture and fill in any gaps that may be present in your notes.

4. As you study your notes, follow along in your textbook. This will help you to correlate what you learned in your pre-lecture reading of the text with what you learned in the lecture. By comparing your textbook illustrations and explanations with those of your lecturer, you will develop a deeper understanding of the material.

5. Write brief notes that relate the text material to your lecture notes in the margins of your textbook. This will reinforce the information that was presented in lecture, information that your instructor deems most important.

6. Develop and practice these good study habits whether you find the material easy or difficult. Good study habits will lead to a deeper understanding and increased retention.

7. If possible, keep your textbooks after your courses end. In this way, you will build a library that you can refer back to in the future to refresh your memory of what you learned. Being able to look back at the very text you studied with the margin notes you wrote will enable you to recall rapidly what you studied.

■ Tips for Successful Examinations

As you begin studying for and taking exams, these tips may help you to achieve a better grade (**FIGURE 1.2**).

In the weeks before the exam:

1. About 2 weeks before each examination, you must begin to prepare for that exam, in addition to continuing your routine daily studying.

2. Begin exam preparation by developing a schedule that allows ample time to cover all the material that will be on that examination. Have the timeline of that schedule end the day before the examination.

3. Work in a study group or with classmates only if it proves productive. Study groups can be very effective if they remain focused on the work at hand. Often, however, they become social occasions that result in much wasted study time.

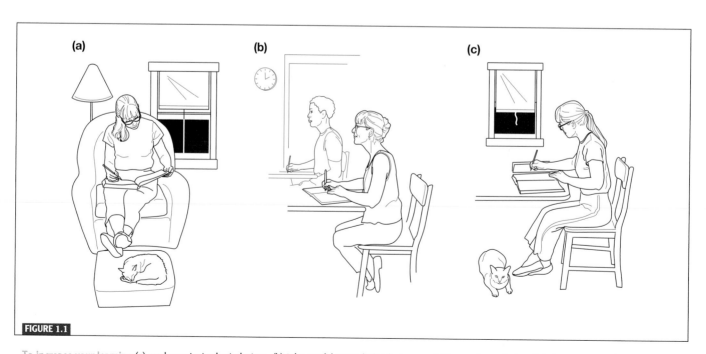

(a)   **(b)**   **(c)**

FIGURE 1.1

To increase your learning (a) read your text prior to lecture, (b) take careful notes during lecture, and (c) reread your text and study your notes after lecture.

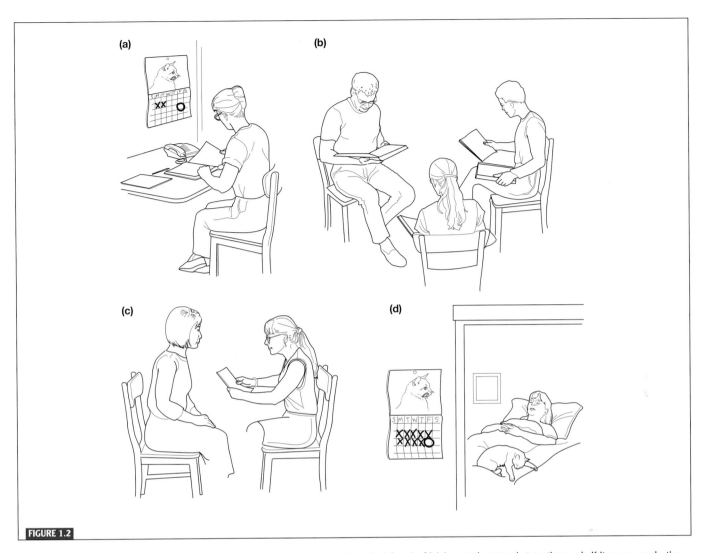

To improve your performance on examinations (a) prepare a study schedule and stick to it, (b) join a study group, but continue only if it proves productive, (c) go to your instructor with specific questions about topics you do not understand, and (d) always get a good night's sleep on the night before the exam.

4. If certain topics are confusing to you, write down specific questions and go to your instructor or teaching assistant during their office hours. It is very important to write down your questions in advance; otherwise, you might forget what to ask while you are with your instructor. This also shows your instructor that you are a serious student who is trying hard to master this subject.

5. On the night before the exam, do not study very late or "pull an all-nighter." This will lead to exhaustion and ultimately cost you more points than it will add. Instead, complete your studying at a reasonable hour and get a good night's sleep.

On the day of the exam:

1. On the day of the exam, look over the material, if possible, but do not study right up to the time of the exam. It is better to take a little time to relax and collect your thoughts right before the exam.

2. Do not arrive at the exam room early. Some of your classmates will be in the room and hallway before the exam. Many of these classmates may not have studied as well as you have. You may overhear them questioning each other and sharing incorrect answers. This may confuse you or lower your confidence level. Confidence is very important during an exam; do not let your classmates reduce your confidence.

3. Do not arrive late for an exam. It shows disrespect for your classmates and your instructor.

4. Make sure all electronic communication equipment (cell phones, pagers, etc.) is shut off before the exam. There are few things more annoying than a phone going off during an exam. It disrupts your concentration and that of your classmates. Also be sure to

go to the restroom before entering the classroom. You may be in there for some time.

5. If at all possible, bring nothing with you to an exam that you do not need for that exam (**FIGURE 1.3**). Often students will bring book bags, athletic gear, articles of clothing, and enough other stuff to be traveling for a month. They assemble this stuff around their desks like mighty fortresses and proceed to take their exams in cramped discomfort. This reduces their ability to concentrate. Bring only what you need but be sure to bring whatever writing implements the exam format requires.

As you take the exam:

1. When your instructor passes out the exam, you may find that your heart begins to race, your rate of breathing increases, and you begin to sweat. These signs of anxiety indicate that your sympathetic nervous system is becoming active (to be explained in Chapter 12). Try to control your anxiety before you begin. Briefly turn the exam face down, close your eyes, and make yourself relax. The exam is only a simple list of questions. It cannot leap off of the desk and attack you. Begin once your respiration and heart rate return to normal.

2. Proceed through the exam one question at a time. When you come to a question you can't answer, mark that question and take a moment to relax before proceeding. Make sure your sympathetic nervous system is under control and then proceed carefully. Make a mental note, however, to watch for informa-

tion that will help you to answer that unanswered question. In each question, the exam gives away a piece of information. Often a later question will give away a piece of information needed to answer a question that gave you difficulty.

3. If you are taking an essay or short answer exam, reread each question and answer after you have completed your answer to make sure you have actually answered what is being asked. Sometimes a student will write an answer that is factually correct, but does not answer the question being asked. This can cost you points.

4. Once you have completed the exam, go back and answer any questions you may have skipped. Then you have a decision to make. Some students can go back through an exam (especially a multiple choice exam), identify incorrect answers, and change them to correct ones. If you are this type of student, go back through the exam and make whatever corrections are necessary. Other students tend to change right answers into wrong ones. If you are that type of student, turn in your exam. Do not rob yourself of those points.

5. If your instructor allows you to leave the room when you complete your exam, do not congregate with your classmates directly outside the exam room to discuss the exam and how you performed on it. This is very distracting to the students who are still taking the exam. Show respect for those students by leaving the area quietly. Meet with those who have finished the exam at a site well away from the classroom.

A main point to remember while studying anatomy and physiology is that you are studying fascinating disci-

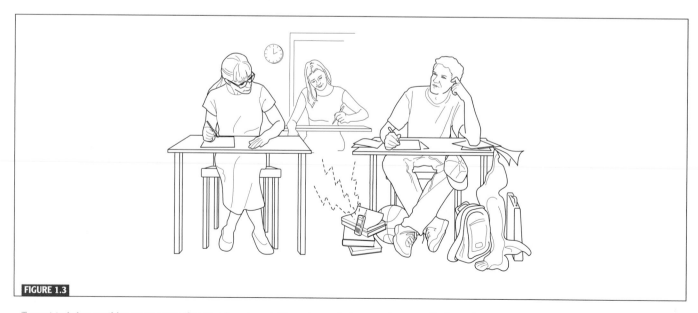

FIGURE 1.3

Try not to bring anything to an exam that you do not need. Always turn cell phones and pagers off prior to class or exams.

plines, and if you concentrate more on really understanding and enjoying the information, and less on how to achieve a good grade, you will most likely gain a solid understanding of the human body, a deep appreciation of its intricacies, and even have some fun in the process. In doing this, you will achieve the grade you desire. Best wishes for success in your endeavor!

1.3 Reliable Sources of Biomedical Information: Where You Can Find Them

Wherever we turn today, we are bombarded with biomedical information. The television and radio are constantly touting new studies, indicating what we must do to live longer, healthier lives. Many of these studies seem to contradict one another. So, how can we decide who to rely on for information about our health?

■ Finding and Evaluating Biomedical Information

It is important to remember that the information you receive from the popular media (newspapers, television, radio, and general interest magazines) is primarily meant to attract an audience and keep it listening or reading. It is not intended to present the details of a medical study in a way that allows a full examination of the science behind it. That is the role of reputable scientific journals. To assure the quality of the work being published in a scientific journal, many of the best journals use a peer-review process. Here's how it works.

■ The Peer-Review Process

When a team of scientists (very little scientific work is done by one individual) decides they have completed a meaningful piece of research, they seek to publish it in a scientific journal. This is the primary way that scientists communicate their results to others in their field. This communication is necessary; without it there would be no point in conducting scientific research.

They will choose a journal that reports on the discipline of their study and submit a written article to that journal. The article will include the rationale behind their study, information on related published studies, the precise methods used in their study, their results, and a discussion or interpretation of the implications and limitations of their results. The journal editor will distribute this article for review to two or three competent scientists working in the same field. These reviewers, or referees, will read the article very carefully and, based on their knowledge of the discipline, judge the quality of the work that is being presented.

They will determine if the basic rationale of the study is valid and whether the reported experiments were actually able to answer the questions posed by the study. They will judge whether there are any serious flaws in the methods used in the study, flaws that would render the results achieved invalid or unreliable. They will determine whether the authors' discussion of how their study fits into the current knowledge in their field is thorough and accurate. They will also point out any additional weaknesses not reported by the authors.

The reviewers then make their recommendations to the journal editor. They may find no fault with the study and recommend that it be published as submitted, or, as more frequently happens, they may request that changes be made before publication. They may request some simple rewriting, additional data (figures, tables, and so on), or changes to the language of the conclusions that have been drawn from the study. They may also request that additional experiments be performed. Sometimes this request can be quite extensive. Alternatively, they may recommend that the paper not be accepted for publication.

The editor then communicates this information to the authors of the study and lets the authors know his or her decision regarding publication. The scientists then will take whatever steps must be taken to make their study ready for publication. This process may take some time, but ultimately it results in journals that are reliable sources of information.

The popular media, including Internet Web pages, do not go through this process. One must, therefore, look with a certain amount of skepticism on what is reported. Even when the media report on studies published in reviewed journals, they are presenting only an interpretation of what was reported in those studies.

To assure the validity of biomedical information, you should always consider the source. If it is not a peer-reviewed journal, try to find the primary source and determine whether it was subjected to peer-review. If not, you should be cautious in your acceptance of the information presented. If it was peer-reviewed, it is a good idea to read the article carefully and examine the manner in which the work was reported. Was it a definitive study or a preliminary study meant to inform other scientists of their short-term findings? Are their conclusions the same as those the popular media claimed were made? Is the size of their study large enough to apply their findings to a larger population? Do the results of other laboratories agree with their results? Do their results make sense, based on what we know of that particular biological system?

A good library is often your best source of this information. Librarians are usually very helpful if you show that you are seriously seeking reliable information. If they do not have what you need, often they will help you to obtain it.

The Internet is a good source of information, but only if you are very careful to consider the origin of information posted there. You will at times find that the person or institution posting the Web page has a particular point of view to promote, or they may actually know less about a subject than you do. Many medical libraries and peer-reviewed biomedical journals now provide their resources online. If you are unable to find them, I am sure your college librarians and information technologists will be happy to assist you.

By critically evaluating any medical information you encounter, you will become better informed and more knowledgeable. Best wishes in your search for knowledge!

What You Should Know

1. Anatomy is the study of the structure or form of the body.

2. Physiology is the study of the function of the body.

3. By studying anatomy and physiology together, we gain a more complete understanding of the body; neither discipline can be fully understood without some knowledge of the other.

4. Reading before the lecture, taking good notes during the lecture, and studying your notes and book together after the lecture as part of your daily studying technique will enable you to do well in this course and in other courses.

5. Developing and sticking to a timetable as part of your test-preparation strategy will improve your grades.

6. Preparing for examinations includes meeting with your instructor to discuss topics you do not understand; being well prepared for these meetings will bring the best results.

7. Focusing your attention, relaxing, and being comfortable during examinations will improve your grades.

8. The most reliable biomedical information can be found in peer-reviewed journals.

9. You must fully evaluate any scientific study you read before accepting the conclusions contained in that study and before drawing any firm conclusions yourself.

10. Librarians are experts in locating information and are there to help you use their resources.

What Did You Learn?

Multiple choice questions: choose the best answer.

1. If someone wants to know the name of the bone that extends from their hip to their knee, they should study:
   a. Physiology
   b. Pathology
   c. Anatomy
   d. Geography

2. If someone wants to learn how their kidneys produce urine, they should study:
   a. Physiology
   b. Pathology
   c. Anatomy
   d. Geography

3. When should you read your textbook?
   a. Prior to each lecture, you should read the material to be covered in that lecture.

   b. After each lecture, you should read the material that was covered in that lecture.

   c. Both of the above. You should read before and after the lecture.

   d. Neither of the above. It is best not to read your book at all.

4. What should you do with your textbook after you have finished with a course?
   a. Sell it to someone else.
   b. Throw it away.
   c. Burn it in an approved fireplace or incinerator.
   d. Keep it as a permanent addition to your library.

5. If, after studying your book and notes, you do not understand something covered in class, you should:
   a. Forget about it. It probably is not important anyway.
   b. Promptly make an appointment to see your instructor.

What Did You Learn? (continued)

    c. Wait to see how you do on the exam.

    d. Ask your cat about it.

6. You should show up in the classroom for examinations:

    a. One hour ahead of the exam.

    b. Exactly on time.

    c. Twenty minutes late.

    d. Only if you feel like it.

7. When taking an examination, it is best to bring:

    a. Anything you could conceivably want or need within the next week.

    b. Lunch, supper, and a few snacks.

    c. Three changes of clothing and lots of sporting goods.

    d. Only the few things you need to take the examination: writing implements and an eraser if you are using a pencil.

8. Study groups are:

    a. Always a good idea.

    b. A good chance to party.

    c. Useful only if they are productively focused on the subject being studied.

    d. Never a good idea.

9. When your instructor passes out your examination you should:

    a. Take a moment to relax and gather your thoughts.

    b. Begin answering questions as fast as you can.

    c. Start chatting with your neighbor.

    d. Ask to go to the restroom.

10. Which of the following is the most reliable source of biomedical information?

    a. Television reports.

    b. Popular magazines.

    c. General Web pages.

    d. Peer-reviewed scientific journals.

Short answer questions: answer briefly and in your own words.

1. Describe the types of information you should expect to learn in an anatomy and physiology course.

2. How can knowledge of anatomy and physiology benefit you?

3. Define the terms *histology* and *gross anatomy*.

4. Indicate four things you can do to make your studying more successful.

5. Indicate five things you can do to improve your examination scores.

6. Write out a plan indicating the approaches you will use as you study anatomy and physiology. Be specific in writing strategies and schedules that fit your routine and that you will actually use.

7. In a fashion magazine, you read about a new diet that the article claims was developed by doctors and will help you lose weight and live longer. Should you immediately go on that diet? Please explain and justify your answer. How will you explore the subject to determine whether that diet is right for you? Be specific in your answers.

8. Describe the peer-review process for the publication of scientific studies. Explain how the peer-review process can be beneficial. Can you think of ways in which this process might be detrimental?

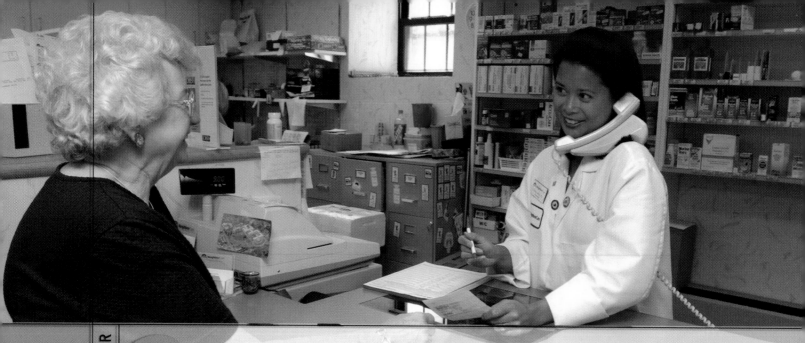

2 Developing a Comon Chemical Language

What You Will Learn

- Why knowledge of chemistry is necessary for an understanding of biology.
- What an atom is, what a molecule is, and the composition of each.
- The types of chemical bonds and how they work.
- What makes a molecule "organic."
- The types of carbohydrates, how to recognize a carbohydrate, and what functions carbohydrates serve.
- The role of lipids in our bodies and how to recognize lipids.
- What a protein is and why proteins are important to us.
- How amino acids join together to form proteins.
- The structure of nucleic acids and the functions they fulfill.
- Why water is important for our health.
- The concept of solvents, solutes, and solutions.
- How we distinguish acids, bases, and salts, and what the pH scale indicates.

2.1 Why Is Knowledge of Chemistry Necessary?

O.K., so you signed up for a course in Human Anatomy and Physiology (or at least you are beginning to read on these topics). What's with the chemistry? Isn't that a different subject altogether? The simple answer to those questions is no, not really. We are, in fact, large sacks of chemicals reacting in various ways that allow us to function, that is to say, live. How can we understand the body if we don't know any chemistry?

That does not mean that this chapter will serve as a mini chemistry course. In fact, what you have here is a biologist's view of chemistry. Many chemists would shudder at some of the things you will read here because of the simplified explanations I will give. The truth of the matter is that I am only trying to develop a simple understanding of some chemical concepts and a common language with which we can discuss those topics. Don't let your eyes glaze over and say that you have never understood chemistry. You will find this a simple introduction to the chemistry you need to understand your body. That said, let's begin with atoms and molecules.

2.2 Atoms and Molecules

What actually is an atom? An atom is the smallest unit of matter that can enter into a chemical reaction. Atoms are the basic units of elements. The "stuff" our world is made up of is all "chemicals," and the building blocks of chemicals are called elements; we now recognize 92 different naturally occurring elements in our world and several manmade ones. However, the smallest amount of one element you could have would be one atom of that element.

Each atom consists of a nucleus with electrons in orbit around that nucleus (**FIGURE 2.1**). It is sort of a mini-solar system, with the nucleus representing the sun and the electrons representing the planets. The nucleus is composed of positively charged particles called protons and noncharged particles called neutrons. The number of protons in the nucleus is the atom's "atomic number." This number is specific for each element. This means that the number of protons in the nucleus determines the element for a specific atom. For example, if an atom has an atomic number of one (one proton in its nucleus), it must be hydrogen. That is what makes it hydrogen. If its atomic number is six (six protons in its nucleus), it is carbon. An atomic number of eight (eight protons in the nucleus) indicates oxygen. See how simple that is? The number of protons in the nucleus specifies the element for which the atom is a unit.

Now, how about the electrons? They orbit the nucleus like planets orbit the sun. How many electrons are there for each atom? We have already learned that the electrons are negatively charged and the protons are positively charged. They carry an equal amount of charge, but one is positive and the other is negative. So, if we have an equal number of electrons and protons, we should have no charge, right? That is often the case. If we had an atom with an atomic number of eight (that would be oxygen), it would have eight protons in its nucleus and the nucleus would have a charge of positive eight. If that nucleus had eight electrons circling it, with their eight negative charges, the atom would have no charge at all. The eight negative charges would cancel out the eight positive charges. If that was how this always worked, we could end our discussion here and move on to other topics. That, however, is not the whole story.

Electrons move around the nucleus at specific distances from the nucleus. It is as if they are in tracks going around the nucleus. These tracks are called electron shells or energy levels. These energy levels can carry specific numbers of electrons. The first energy level (closest to the nucleus) can carry two electrons. The second energy level can carry eight electrons. The third can also carry eight, but under certain circumstances it can carry 18. In all there can be up to seven energy levels, depending on the number of electrons present. Are you getting a little confused? Let's go to a carnival for a short break.

■ Electron Energy Levels: Like a Trip to a Carnival

O.K., here we are at the carnival. There is a great roller coaster we can ride. Notice how the cars of this ride are set up (**FIGURE 2.2**). The first car can hold only two people. Other cars can be attached to this one. The second and third cars can each hold eight people. The carnival is not very busy today (it's raining a little). The roller coaster operator wants to make money with this ride, so he does not like to send cars around empty. If only one person shows up to ride the roller coaster, he will make that person wait until a second person shows up. He can then send the first car around full (it can hold two people). If more people show up, he will attach a second car to the first one and also try to get that one full. What happens if three people show up for a ride (Figure 2.2a)? He will fill up the first car (two people), but he will not want to send the second car around with only one person in it. Since he has only one potential rider and would need seven more to fill it (which he's unlikely to get in this rain), he will convince that person to go to another ride (the merry-go-round is always a good choice). He, in effect, gives that rider away.

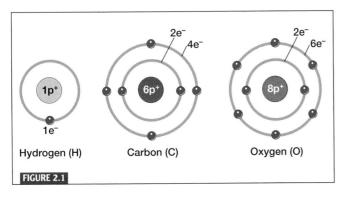

FIGURE 2.1

Examples of three atoms. Note that p+ indicates protons and e− indicates electrons. Neutrons are not shown but are present in the nucleus.

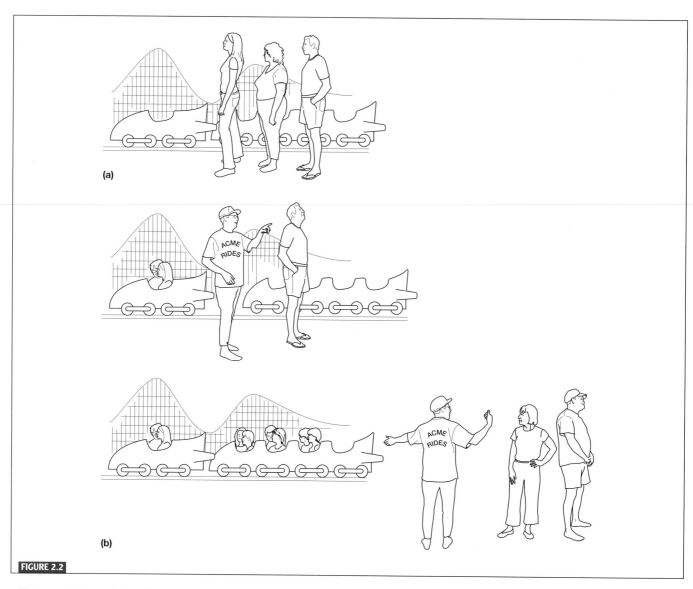

(a)

(b)

FIGURE 2.2

Electrons orbiting nuclei are like people at a carnival ride. Notice that the first car can hold two people (a). When three people want to ride, the operator encourages the third person to try a different ride as he does not want to run a second car for one person. If, instead, the second car is nearly full (b), he tries to find one or two more people to fill it up.

What would have happened instead if he had eight people show up (Figure 2.2b)? He would put two in the first car, then six in the second car. That leaves two empty seats. He wants to make money with this ride, and empty seats don't pay. What's he to do? He tries to attract riders away from the other rides to fill those two seats (face it, the merry-go-round can be a little dull anyway).

What does this have to do with atoms and electrons, you ask? Atoms are just like that ride, and electrons are like the passengers (**FIGURE 2.3**). If an atom has an atomic number of two (helium), it would have two protons in the nucleus; if it has two electrons (no charge, two positive plus two negative), they would both be in the first energy level, and that level would be full. If an atom has an atomic number of eight (oxygen), it would have eight

protons in the nucleus, and its eight electrons would be distributed into two energy levels. The first energy level would have two electrons, so it would be full. The second energy level would have the remaining six electrons, leaving room for two more. This atom would try to fill these two spaces. It is an electron acceptor, seeking two electrons to fill its outer shell. If it could gain two electrons, its numbers of protons and electrons would no longer be equal. It would have two more electrons than protons, giving it a net charge of negative two. Here's one more example. If an atom has an atomic number of 11 (sodium), it has 11 protons in its nucleus and the electrons would be distributed as follows: two in the first energy level, eight in the second energy level, and one in the third energy level. We know that the third

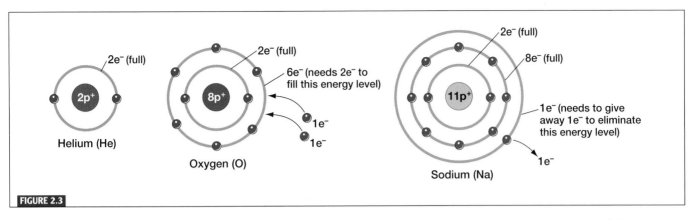

FIGURE 2.3

Helium has one full energy level and, therefore, does not gain or lose any electrons. Oxygen must gain two electrons to fill its outer energy level. Sodium loses one electron to eliminate its outer energy level.

energy level needs eight electrons to be full. That means it needs either to get rid of one or take on seven more. It would get rid of one, acting as an electron donor. This would result in a net charge of one positive (11 protons but only 10 electrons).

This tells us a couple of things. First of all, atoms can have charges. Any charged atom or group of atoms is called an ion. That is the definition of the term *ion*, an atom or group of atoms that is charged. Second, we have learned that the charges can be positive or negative. A positively charged ion is a cation; a negatively charged ion is an anion. If you have trouble remembering which is which (such as, you knew it the night before the exam, but during the exam it gets confusing), just remember you like cats, don't you? (If you don't, you should; they're great.) You feel positively about cats! The positive ion is the cation. If you don't like cats (get to know some, you will), remember that your textbook author feels positively about cats. (More on cats later. I love cats!) One other way of remembering this is to think of cation as being spelled ca+ion.

The next thing we have already learned is that atoms have the ability to either gain or lose electrons, and they do this in specific ways. If they have an outer energy level that is less than half full, they will usually give away or share the electrons in that shell. If their outer energy level is half full or more, but not completely full, they will usually try to gain electrons to fill it. Just remember the carnival ride operator and passengers. The same principle applies. The number of electrons that an atom wants either to gain or lose is referred to as its combining capacity or valence. For example, carbon has an atomic number of six (six protons in the nucleus: two electrons in the first energy level and four in the second energy level). Its second energy level is half full. It will try to gain four electrons to fill that second energy level. It has a valence (combining capacity) of four.

2.3 Chemical Bonds: How We Are Held Together

■ And Now for a Bonding Experience

Atoms are all right, but kind of small and simple. Think of them as bricks. Bricks are O.K. in their own way, but basically kind of dull unless you can stick them together. It is in sticking bricks together that we can create something of use. The same is true of atoms. We combine atoms together to make molecules. Molecules are chemical structures made of atoms. Molecules come in various sizes and forms that we will learn about soon, but first we must consider how we stick atoms together.

Chemical bonds are the links that join atoms. There are three major types in which we are interested: ionic bonds, covalent bonds, and hydrogen bonds.

■ Ionic Bonds: Like Magnetic Toys

Ionic bonds involve bonds between ions. That should be easy to remember. Think about the charges of the ions as we consider this analogy. Have you ever played around with magnets? Magnets are sometimes sold in various shapes as children's toys, but they can be very instructive. Maybe you have seen the magnetic toys that are shaped like elephants? They are neat little toys that stick together, the trunk of one elephant sticking to the tail of the next. If you try to stick them head to head or tail to tail, they repel each other instead. That is because magnets have a positive end and a negative end, and opposites attract. The negative end of a magnet is attracted to the positive end of another magnet, but not to the negative end of that magnet. Ions work similarly. A cation (think, is that positive or negative?) is attracted to an anion. Remember, opposites attract. The bond that forms between them is an ionic bond (**FIGURE 2.4**).

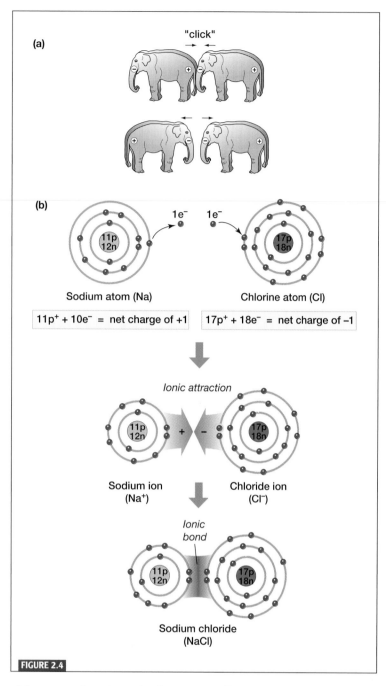

(a)

"click"

(b)

1e⁻   1e⁻

Sodium atom (Na)

Chlorine atom (Cl)

$11p^+ + 10e^- = $ net charge of $+1$ $17p^+ + 18e^- = $ net charge of -1

Ionic attraction

Sodium ion
(Na⁺)

Chloride ion
(Cl⁻)

Ionic bond

Sodium chloride
(NaCl)

FIGURE 2.4

Like magnets, ions of opposite charges attract. This is how ionic bonds are formed.

An example of this is sodium chloride, also known as table salt. Sodium (atomic number of 11) has two electrons in its first energy level, eight in its second, and one in its third. The one electron in the third energy level is given away; therefore, sodium has a positive charge and a valence of one. Chloride has an atomic number of 17. It, therefore, has 17 protons in its nucleus: two electrons in its first energy level, eight in its second, and seven in its third. It picks up one more to fill its third energy level, resulting in a valence of one, and a net negative charge. The negative charge of the chloride and the positive charge of the sodium attract each other, and you end up with something to sprinkle on your french fries.

■ Covalent Bonds: Shared Riches

Not all of the atoms we need to stick together can be joined with ionic bonds. Some of them simply are not ions. Covalent bonds are another type of bond we can use. Covalent bonds are more stable (stronger) than ionic bonds and are quite common in our bodies' chemical composition.

Imagine that you and I have just picked some apples for a local farmer. He agreed to pay us 50 cents each for this work (either he's cheap or there weren't many apples). When it was time to pay us, he had no change, only a dollar bill. We didn't mind, however, as we were walking to town to spend our hard earned money together anyway. Who gets to carry the money? Well, since you think I might run away with it, and I think you might run away with it, we compromise. I carry it half of the time and you carry it half of the time. Half of the time I am satisfied; half of the time you are satisfied (**FIGURE 2.5a**).

Now let's think again about atoms. If we consider two hydrogen atoms (atomic number of one), each has one proton in its nucleus and one electron in its first energy level. Each hydrogen atom can be either an electron donor and give away its one electron, or an electron acceptor and take on one electron to complete its first energy level. Remember that the number of electrons an atom needs to either accept or donate to satisfy its outer energy level is called its combining capacity or valence. In this case, hydrogen has a combining capacity of one, indicating that each atom of hydrogen is capable of making one bond. Two hydrogen atoms will form a covalent bond (bind to each other covalently) by sharing their electrons with each other. Half of the time both electrons will be in the first energy level surrounding one nucleus (in our previous analogy, it is holding the dollar bill); half of the time both electrons are in the first energy level of the other nucleus (then it is holding the dollar bill). When both electrons are orbiting one nucleus, no electrons are orbiting the other nucleus. These two atoms of hydrogen are bound together in a covalent bond by this sharing of electrons (Figure 2.5b).

What would happen in our story if you performed 75 percent of the work and I did only 25 percent of the work? Well, obviously, 75 cents of our dollar belongs to you and only 25 cents of our dollar is mine. As we walk to town, I only get to carry the dollar one fourth of the time; you get to hold it three quarters of the time. It is the only fair way to do it.

Now, how about our atoms? Might a situation exist in which the electrons are not shared equally? That must

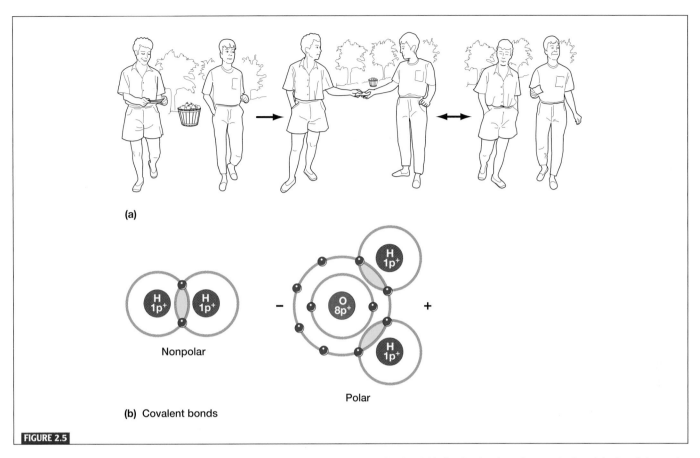

(a)

Nonpolar

Polar

(b) Covalent bonds

FIGURE 2.5

Just like two people sharing money (a), two atoms sharing electrons stick together in a covalent bond (b). Covalent bonds can be nonpolar (equal sharing of electrons) or polar (unequal sharing).

be the case, or I would not be giving you this big explanation of it! Oxygen has an atomic number of eight. It has eight protons in its nucleus: two electrons in its first energy level and six in its second energy level. This gives it a valence (combining capacity) of two. It needs two electrons to fill its outer energy level. It can make two covalent bonds and it does, one each with two hydrogen atoms. Remember that hydrogen atoms have a valence of one. When two hydrogen atoms bind covalently to one oxygen atom, the electrons are shared unequally. The two shared electrons spend more time orbiting the oxygen nucleus and less time orbiting each of the hydrogen nuclei. This results in the oxygen portion of our molecule (remember that a molecule is composed of atoms bound together) being more negative than the hydrogen portion of our molecule. Our molecule, therefore, has a region that is relatively more negative and a region that is relatively more positive. We refer to this as a polar covalent bond. A covalent bond in which the electrons are equally shared is a nonpolar covalent bond. A polar covalent bond results in a polar molecule, a molecule with two poles, like the north pole and the south pole; one is negative and one is positive. What is this molecule in our example anyway? The fact that it has

two hydrogen atoms and one oxygen atom means we can write its formula as H_2O, which you will recognize as water. Water is a polar molecule. More on water later.

■ Hydrogen Bonds: The Serving Line at the Banquet

Have you ever stood in the food line at a banquet that should be a simple straight line, but instead is bunched up into a distorted shape because someone near the front of the line is talking to someone further back in the line? They won't leave their position in the line to talk to each other, but they pull the line into a nonlinear shape by their attraction to each other. It can get pretty annoying to the other people in the line and completely confuse the procession to the food.

A similar situation can happen in molecules. Hydrogen atoms bound either to one oxygen atom or one nitrogen atom in a large molecule may be weakly attracted to an oxygen or nitrogen atom elsewhere in the molecule. This is referred to as a hydrogen bond; although very weak, the hydrogen bond may distort the shape of the molecule. You can imagine how a large molecule containing many hydrogen bonds could have a very complex

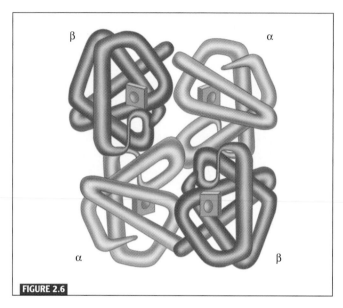

FIGURE 2.6

Molecules such as hemoglobin (shown) can have complex three-dimensional shapes.

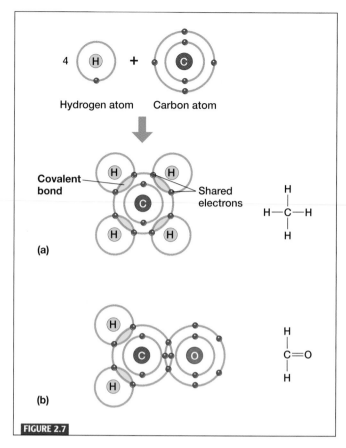

(a)

(b)

FIGURE 2.7

Due to their valence of four, carbon atoms make four covalent bonds (a), but these may include double bonds (b).

shape (**FIGURE 2.6**). Hydrogen bonds and other similar forces that shape molecules are called electrostatic interactions and are important in giving large molecules the three-dimensional shape necessary for them to be functional.

2.4 Organic Compounds

■ What's with All the Carbon?

As "Bones" would have told Captain Kirk (any *Star Trek* fans out there?), we are carbon-based life forms. Big deal, you say? Yes, indeed, it is a big deal. The molecules that make up your body are largely composed of carbon. We refer to the chemistry of these carbon-containing molecules as organic chemistry. They are organic molecules. So how about a little background on carbon?

Carbon's atomic number is six. It has six protons in its nucleus: two electrons in its first energy level and four in its second energy level. It needs four electrons to complete its second energy level. It, therefore, has a valence of four and will normally make four bonds within a molecule. These bonds may be made with four individual atoms, one bond each. These bonds may be made with fewer than four other atoms if double bonds are involved. A double bond occurs when two bonds rather than one are formed between two atoms. In either case, carbon atoms will always form four bonds due to their valence of four (**FIGURE 2.7**). The stability that is built into carbon-containing molecules by these four bonds per carbon atom allows us to build some very large, complex molecules. A number of different categories of organic molecules are found in our bodies. We will cover the basics of each here.

■ Carbohydrates: Energy, Identification, and More

The carbohydrate molecules of our bodies are a large and diverse group of molecules carrying out a number of important functions. These functions include providing a ready source of fuel and a way to store that fuel. They, in fact, form our most readily available source of energy. They also serve as markers on the surfaces of our cells, allowing our cells to identify themselves and communicate with each other. As such they allow our immune systems to identify invaders that need to be eliminated and play an important role in the processes used to eliminate invading microorganisms, neoplastic (cancer) cells, and, unfortunately, grafted organs. They also form components of other important molecules, such as the nucleic acids that make up our DNA (more on that shortly).

Carbon, hydrogen, and oxygen atoms are combined into small ring-shaped molecules called monosaccharides or simple sugars. These are our smallest carbohydrates and serve as the building blocks of larger carbohydrates. An easy way to identify carbohydrates is to count the number of hydrogen and oxygen atoms in a molecule. While many molecules contain hydrogen and oxygen, in carbohydrates the ratio of hydrogen atoms to oxygen atoms is always two to one. (Doesn't that look like an exam question waiting to happen!)

Based on the number of carbon atoms they contain, monosaccharides can be classified into the categories listed in **TABLE 2.1**. Glucose (**FIGURE 2.8a**), an important form of energy for our bodies, is a hexose, or six-carbon monosaccharide. Deoxyribose (Figure 2.8b) is used in making our genetic material and is a pentose, or five-carbon monosaccharide. Note that our 2:1 hydrogen to oxygen ratio does not apply when carbohydrates are combined with other types of molecules. It also does not apply to deoxyribose, which is a ribose monosaccharide minus one oxygen (hence *deoxy-*).

Monosaccharides can be joined together into chains. Two monosaccharides joined together become a disaccharide. Sucrose, table sugar, is an example of a disaccharide. Figure 2.8c shows two monosaccharides being joined together into the disaccharide sucrose. Notice how the chemical reaction that creates the covalent bond between the two monosaccharides results in the liberation of a hydrogen atom from one monosaccharide and the liberation of a hydroxyl group (a hydrogen atom bound to an oxygen atom) from the other group. What do these two released entities form when they bind to each other? If you answered water, you have been paying attention. We call this type of reaction dehydration synthesis because the synthesis of the disaccharide, the product of the reaction, resulted in the liberation of a molecule of water. This is a very common type of reaction in your body.

If we use additional dehydration synthesis reactions to add more monosaccharides to this chain, we will produce a polysaccharide. Glycogen is one example of a polysaccharide (Figure 2.8d). Glycogen is produced by joining together many glucose monosaccharides into large branching chains. This is how the cells of your body store glucose, an important fuel, for future use. We can reverse the dehydration synthesis reaction to release monosaccharides from a polysaccharide. This is impor-

tant if we are to be able to remove glucose from storage. Since we liberated a molecule of water in our dehydration synthesis reaction, doesn't it make sense that we would need to use that molecule of water if we were to reverse that reaction? This reaction is called hydrolysis, which means splitting with water (*-lysis* means to split, *hydro-* refers to water). Notice how that was also depicted in Figure 2.8c. Dehydration synthesis is one form of an anabolic reaction, one that results in the formation of more complex substances. Hydrolysis is a catabolic reaction, one that results in the destruction or breakdown of complex substances. You can keep these terms straight by remembering that cats (as in catabolic) do not create anything, but can be destructive.

We will learn more about carbohydrates in later chapters of this book.

■ Lipids: Everybody's Favorite

The group of organic molecules called lipids includes fats, phospholipids, steroids, prostaglandins, and other important compounds. Like the carbohydrates, these also contain carbon, hydrogen, and oxygen; however, the ratio of hydrogen to oxygen we observed in carbohydrates does not hold true here. There is generally less oxygen in lipids than there is in carbohydrates. You already know one major feature of most lipids. After a greasy meal (take your pick: how about a nice greasy pepperoni pizza?), if you put the dirty dishes into a sink of water but do not have dish detergent in the water, will the dishes rinse clean? You know they won't. In fact, the grease (a lipid) will not disperse into the water but will stick together. More about why this happens later, but for now let's say that lipids are not water soluble.

Let's consider a few examples of lipids now. How about fats? We live in a very fat-conscious society. Everyone knows that "fats are bad for you," but is that really true? Would we be better off without any fat? Actually fats, or triglycerides to be specific, carry out a number of very important functions in our bodies. They provide thermal and shock insulation. This thermal insulation helps you to maintain the proper internal temperature despite changes in the outside temperature. The insulation against shock or trauma that fats provide allows you to sit for an extended period while reading this book without damaging other tissues. Fats also allow us to store energy in a very dense form. In fact, fats are our bodies' most dense form of stored energy, although we do waste some if it as we use this energy (it's not as efficient as carbohydrates). One good feature of this form of stored energy is that fats, like many lipids, are hydrophobic (repel water). Otherwise, as you store energy, you would also retain water. The next time someone

Table 2.1	Names of Monosaccharides
Monosaccharide	**Number of Carbon Atoms**
Triose	Three
Tetrose	Four
Pentose	Five
Hexose	Six
Heptose	Seven

Monosaccharide = one saccharide or simple sugar. Disaccharide = two monosaccharides bound together. Polysaccharide = many monosaccharides bound together.

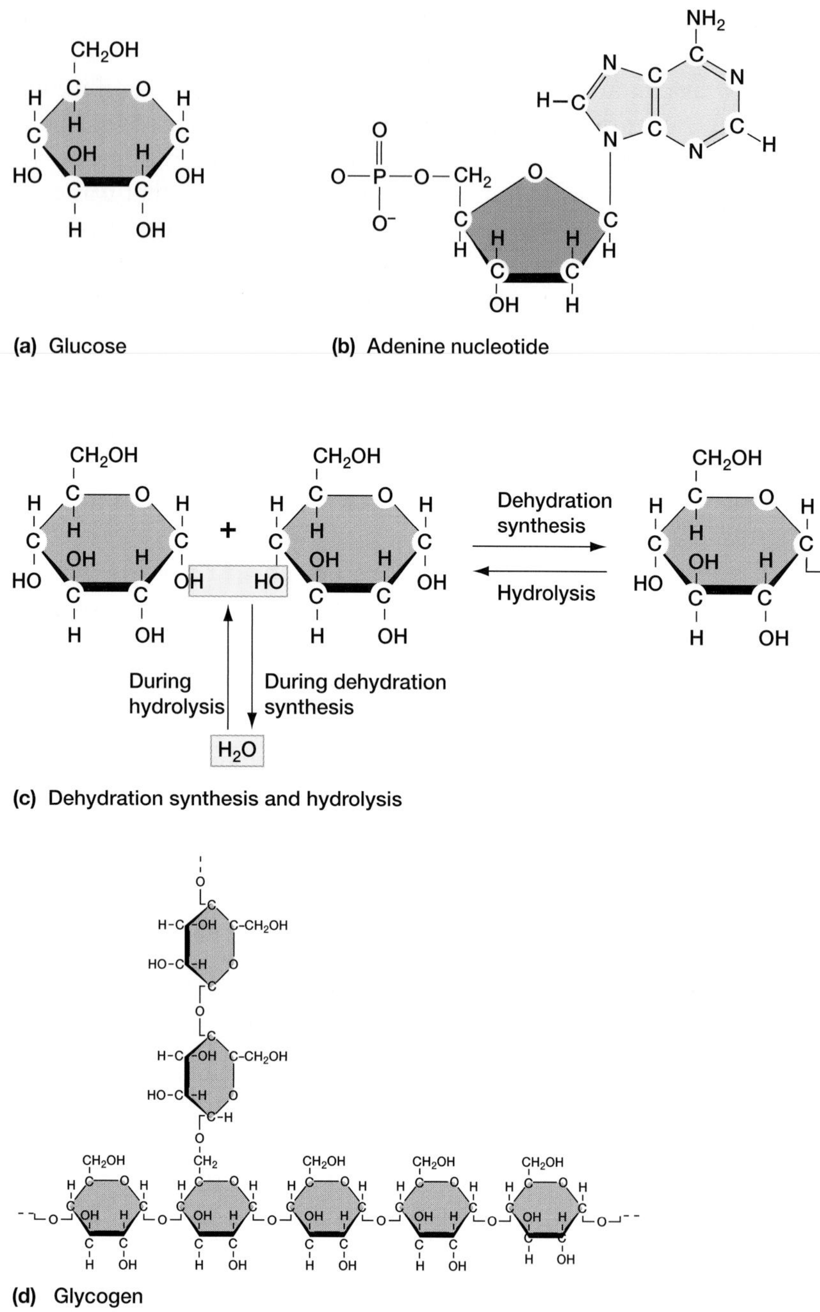

(a) Glucose

(b) Adenine nucleotide

(c) Dehydration synthesis and hydrolysis

(d) Glycogen

FIGURE 2.8

Examples of carbohydrates. Note dehydration synthesis and hydrolysis (c).

notices you have put on a little weight, simply tell them that you are storing up a little energy for later use.

Triglycerides are composed of one molecule of glycerol combined with three molecules of fatty acids (**FIGURE 2.9**). These fatty acids are each chains of carbon, hydrogen, and oxygen. The fatty acids are bound to the glycerol through dehydration synthesis and removed through hydrolysis.

If you think about your dietary fats for a moment, you will recall that some fats are called saturated fats, while others are monosaturated (more accurately monounsaturated) or polyunsaturated fats. The "saturation" refers to the amount of hydrogen in the fatty acid side chains. If every location that can hold a hydrogen atom actually has one, the fat is "saturated." Keep in mind that carbon has a valence of four, so it needs four bonds to be satisfied. If the carbons in the chain have two bonds linking them within the chain (to two other carbons), they also have two available bonds to hold onto hydrogen. If all of the carbons in the chain have done that, the fat is saturated.

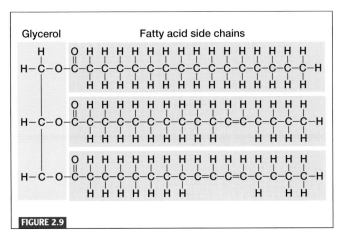

FIGURE 2.9

A triglyceride. Examine the fatty acid side chains. The top side chain demonstrates a saturated fat, the middle side chain demonstrates a monounsaturated fat, and the bottom side chain demonstrates a polyunsaturated fat.

If, at one location, a double bond forms between two carbons, two hydrogens (one from each of the involved carbons) must be released. This would be a monounsaturated fat. Mono means one; this fat has a double bond in one location. If this is repeated at other locations, it is a polyunsaturated fat. See Figure 2.9 for clarity.

Steroids are lipids composed of four carbon-containing rings that serve as hormones (**FIGURE 2.10a**). Hormones are molecules that travel from the endocrine glands that produce them to cells throughout the body. Their role is to carry messages from those glands to specific cells, regulating the activities of those cells. We will learn the details of these activities in Chapter 13. For

(a) Estradiol

(b) PGE₁

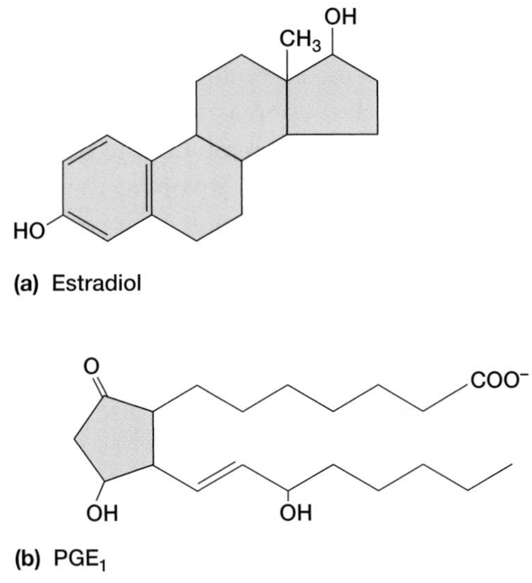

FIGURE 2.10

Examples of lipids. A steroid (a) and a prostaglandin (b). A form of 'chemical shorthand' has been used here. A carbon is present in each place the line changes direction. Every carbon is assumed to hold the number of hydrogens necessary to satisfy its valence of four.

now, be aware that steroids such as testosterone, cortisone, and progesterone are important lipids with a distinctive four-ring structure.

Previously, I noted that prostaglandins are forms of lipids. They are one member of a class of lipid molecules called eicosanoids. Prostaglandins are important molecules for local intercellular signaling. Prostaglandins are 20-carbon fatty acid chains that are folded in the middle to form a five-carbon ring (Figure 2.10b). They are important in activities as diverse as temperature regulation, control of bleeding, inflammation, perception of pain, and childbirth. Aspirin exerts its many effects by inhibiting the synthesis of prostaglandins.

We should briefly think of membrane lipids here. Some lipids are modified to have a hydrophobic moiety (part) and a hydrophilic moiety. The term *hydrophobic* implies water-repelling, the term *hydrophilic* implies water-loving. When both characteristics are present in one molecule, it is said to be *amphipathic*. Some amphipathic lipids form membranes when placed in water. We will learn about these in our next chapter.

■ Proteins: Of First Importance

How important are proteins? Their name (in Greek) means "being of the first importance." To understand the body, we must understand the cells. To understand the cells, we must understand proteins. It's that simple. Let's begin.

Beginning with Amino Acids

Just as we learned that polysaccharides are formed by linking monosaccharides together, we will now learn that proteins are composed of amino acids linked together. We must, therefore, start our discussion of proteins by considering amino acids. Several amino acids are shown in **FIGURE 2.11**. Notice that they all contain the following features: a central carbon, a hydrogen atom, an amino group, a carboxyl group, and one of 20 distinctive side chains. Bear with me for a moment; it's not as complicated as it sounds.

First, let's consider the central carbon. We know that carbon has a valence of four; therefore, this carbon must have four bonds associated with it. One bond is to a hydrogen atom. The next bond is to an amino group. An amino group is simply made up of nitrogen and hydrogen, either NH_2 or NH_3^+. The next bond is to a carboxyl group. This is composed of either one carbon and two oxygens (COO^-) or one carbon, two oxygens, and a hydrogen ($COOH$). Finally, we have the side chain. There are 20 different amino acids used in the proteins of our bodies (**TABLE 2.2**). It is the differences between these side chains that determine which amino acid is which. Some amino acids have very simple side chains; others are more

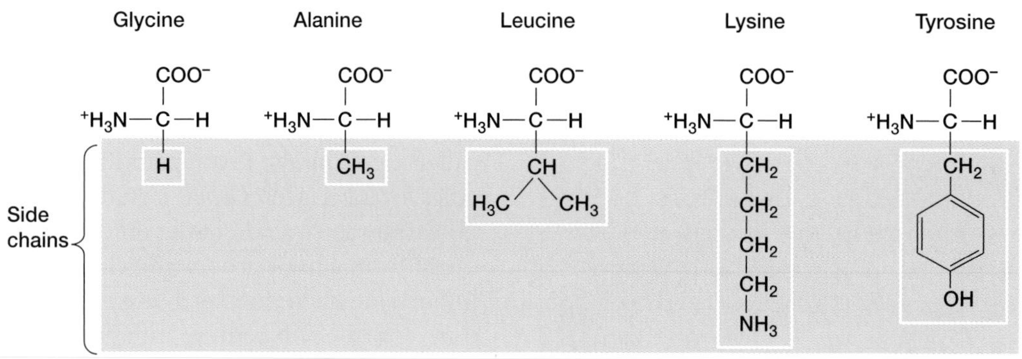

FIGURE 2.11

Examples of amino acids. Only their side chains differ.

complex. Several amino acids are shown in Figure 2.11 with their side chains highlighted for comparison.

Amino Acids: A Different Sort of Alphabet

So, what do we do with amino acids? We combine them into chains using dehydration synthesis. These chains of amino acids are proteins. We can combine the letters of our alphabet to form words, and it is the letters we

Table 2.2 Our Bodies' Amino Acids and Their Abbreviations

Amino Acid	Abbreviation
Alanine	Ala
Arginine	Arg
Asparagine	Asn
Aspartic Acid	Asp
Cysteine	Cys
Glutamine	Gln
Glutamic Acid	Glu
Glycine	Gly
Histidine	His
Isoleucine	Ile
Leucine	Leu
Lysine	Lys
Methionine	Met
Phenylalanine	Phe
Proline	Pro
Serine	Ser
Threonine	Thr
Tryptophan	Trp
Tyrosine	Tyr
Valine	Val

choose that determine which words we create. The same is true of proteins. The amino acids in the chain are selected to form specific proteins. A different group of amino acids would result in a different protein. Due to the characteristics of the side chains present in the amino acids, the resulting chains often have complex three-dimensional shapes. These shapes enable proteins to perform complex functions. A couple of examples of proteins are shown in **FIGURE 2.12**.

Proteins: What They Can Do for You

Proteins are very interesting molecules. We will spend quite a bit of time discussing their roles in other sections of this book. For now, be aware that they have many diverse and important functions. Their potential to assume many complex three-dimensional shapes provides proteins with this functional diversity. Enzymes are one category of protein. Enzymes serve as molecular machines that cause specific chemical reactions to occur in locations and at rates for which these reactions are needed. These reactions may be catabolic, involving the breakdown of complex molecules, or anabolic, involving the synthesis of new molecules. Because of the molecular contractile machinery made of protein, your muscles are able to contract, allowing you to have posture, to move, to breathe, and to pump your blood. Proteins transport oxygen in your blood; they provide structure within your cells and to your bones and other tissues. They are also important for communication throughout your body in your endocrine and nervous systems. Your immune system relies heavily on proteins for your defense. In short, you can expect to read quite a lot about proteins in the upcoming chapters.

■ Nucleic Acids: Why All the Excitement?

Due to recent developments in genetic engineering, the nucleic acids deoxyribonucleic acid (DNA) and ribo-

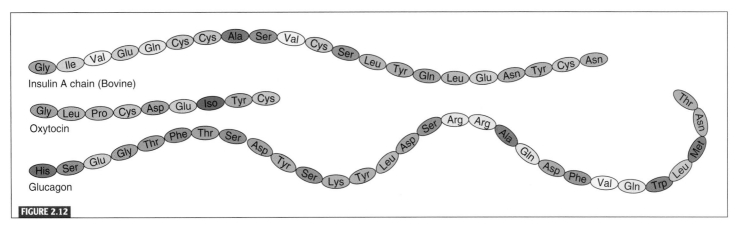

FIGURE 2.12

Examples of proteins. Only their amino acid sequence is shown; this is not their actual shape.

nucleic acid (RNA) have become of major interest to many people. But what actually is a nucleic acid? Nucleic acids are chains of smaller molecules called nucleotides. Each nucleotide is composed of a nitrogenous base, a pentose sugar, and one or more phosphate groups; these are made of carbon, oxygen, hydrogen, nitrogen, and phosphorous. Nitrogenous bases are ring-shaped structures containing carbon, hydrogen, oxygen, and nitrogen. DNA uses four different nitrogenous bases: adenine, thymine, cytosine, and guanine. RNA also uses four different nitrogenous bases: adenine, uracil, cytosine, and guanine. You will notice that uracil does not appear in DNA and thymine does not appear in RNA. The pentose sugar ribose is used in RNA, while the pentose sugar deoxyribose is used in DNA, giving these nucleic acids their names. You will recall that pentose sugars are monosaccharides containing five carbon atoms. The only difference between these two sugars is that ribose contains a hydroxyl group (OH) in a location where deoxyribose contains a hydrogen atom (H). Phosphate groups are composed of an atom of phosphorous and three or four oxygen atoms. Nucleic acids and their components are shown in **FIGURE 2.13a**. Note that DNA is generally present as a two-stranded structure: two chains of nucleotides covalently bound side by side into a ladder-like structure. Note also that this ladder-like double chain is twisted into a spiral resembling a spring (Figure 2.13a).

In proteins, the order of amino acids determines the characteristics of a given protein, including its identity. A similar situation exists in nucleic acids. The order of nucleotides in the nucleic acid has meaning. The order of the nucleotides in our DNA is our bodies' blueprint for the production of proteins. This information is copied into RNA nucleotides as one of the steps leading to protein synthesis. The structure of nucleic acids and the fascinating ways in which they function are presented in much more detail in Chapter 14. Keep this topic in mind as you read the intervening chapters and Chapter 14's discussion will greatly increase your understanding.

ATP: Fuel for Our Cells

Adenosine triphosphate (ATP) is another important nucleotide; it is used as the main form of energy for the molecular processes in the cells of our bodies. It is depicted in Figure 2.13b. Our cells need energy to carry out their many vital processes. They need energy in the same way you need energy to heat your home, run your automobile, or light the lamp you are using to read this book. Simply stated, energy is required to make chemical bonds and is released whenever a bond is broken. That principle is the basis for the use of ATP as a form of energy. The bonds that link the three phosphate groups to the main portion of the molecule are a form of stored energy. As shown in the figure, ATP (adenosine _tri_phosphate) has three phosphate groups bound to it. The "tri" in this name indicates three phosphates. When the bond between the second and third phosphate is broken, energy is released along with the phosphate group. It is this energy that our cells use for other purposes. In doing this, they convert ATP into adenosine _di_phosphate (ADP). As the term _di_ indicates, there are two remaining phosphates in this molecule.

This ends our brief introduction to the organic molecules. We will now spend some time thinking about the main substance that makes up our bodies. What is that substance? Water! We have already learned a little about water; now let's expand on that knowledge.

2.5 Inorganic Compounds

■ Water: Its Importance to Us

Water is a great substance and is very important in our bodies. You know a lot about how water is useful and

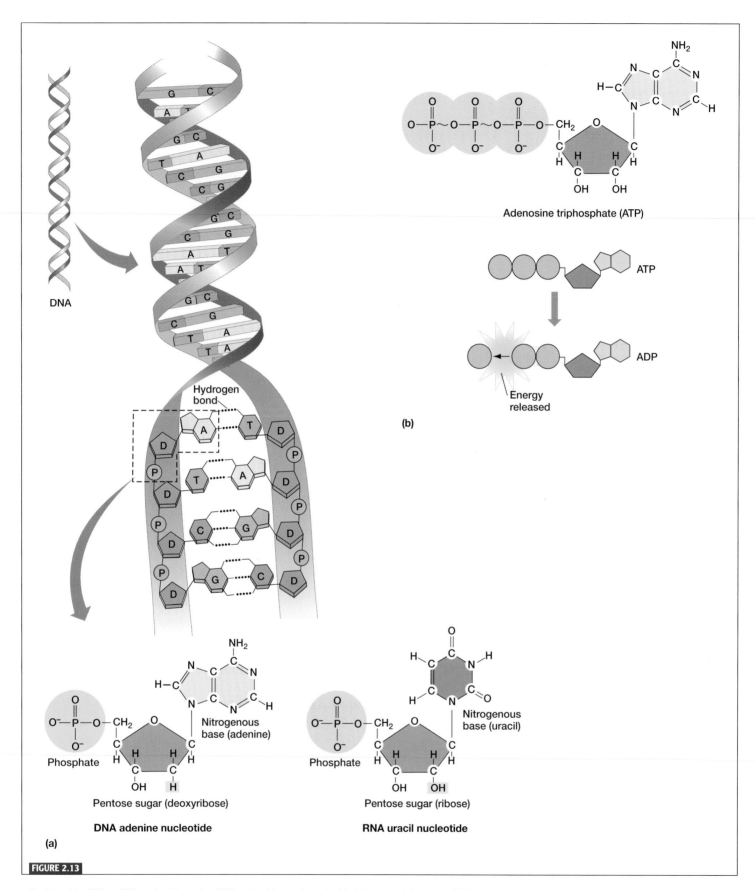

FIGURE 2.13

Nucleic acids, DNA, a DNA nucleotide, and an RNA nucleotide are shown in (a). Adenosine triphosphate (ATP) is shown in (b).

how water acts in the environment. We need to think about how the characteristics of water help us to live. If you were to decide to make a cup of tea right now and were to put a kettle of water on the stove to heat, would it heat instantly? No. You would have to wait for its temperature to rise. The same is true if you were to put water into the freezer to make ice. It would take a while to freeze. Water maintains its temperature for some time; it takes time for it to heat or cool. Similarly, your body takes time to heat or cool, partly due to the high water content of your body. As water evaporates, changing from a liquid to a gas, it absorbs heat. This is important in cooling your body. We will learn more about this concept later.

Have you ever watched a fast river flowing by, perhaps after heavy rains? If you have, you may have noticed that the water was not clear. It had a brownish color from the dirt and other materials it was carrying. Water is an effective suspending medium (**FIGURE 2.14a**). It has the ability to carry materials along as it moves. This too is important in your body.

The Universal Solvent?

You are aware that many substances will dissolve if placed in water. Substances such as table salt and table sugar dissolve readily in water (Figure 2.14b). For this reason, water is referred to as the "universal solvent." It is not actually a universal solvent, as many substances do not dissolve in it. We can be glad of that; one good rainstorm and there would be nothing left! The substances that dissolve in water are generally held together by ionic bonds. Water is a polar molecule, with one end that is more positive and one end that is more negative due to the polar covalent bond that holds it together. Substances that can break down into ions, that is to say, ionize or dissociate into a cation and an anion, often do so in water; their cations are drawn to the negative end of the water molecules, and their anions are drawn to the positive end of the water molecule. Remember, opposite charges attract. This results in their dissolving. If we were to allow the water molecules to evaporate, these other molecules would reform.

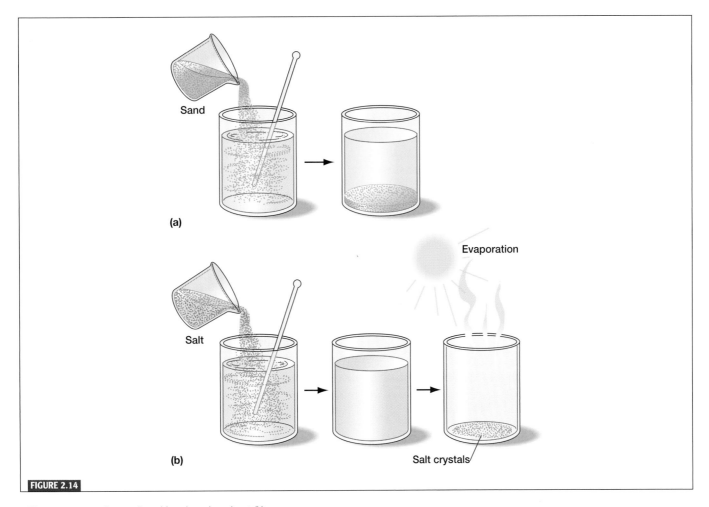

Sand

(a)

Evaporation

Salt

Salt crystals

(b)

FIGURE 2.14

Water as a suspending medium (a) and a polar solvent (b).

We need some language to allow us to consider that process. If a liquid has the ability to dissolve something, that liquid is a solvent. Water is a polar solvent due to its polar nature. Examples of nonpolar solvents include paint thinner and gasoline. Have you ever noticed that substances that will dissolve in paint thinner (oil-based paint, for example) will not dissolve in water? Some substances dissolve in nonpolar solvents; others dissolve in polar solvents. The fact that something can dissolve in the liquid makes the liquid a solvent.

How about the substance that is being dissolved? That substance is called a solute. If we dissolve table sugar in water, the water is the solvent and the table sugar is the solute. The combination of the two is a solution. The more solute there is in the solution, the more concentrated the solution. Have you ever noticed that only a certain amount of salt or sugar can dissolve in water? When we reach a point where no more solute can dissolve, we have a saturated solution. If we continue to add solute, we will build up nondissolved solute and have a supersaturated solution.

■ Acids, Bases, and Salts Made Easy

The ability of water to dissolve substances in this way is very important in our bodies. We have already learned that water is made up of two hydrogens and one oxygen, and that the symbol for it is H_2O. Hydrogen can exist as a cation (positively charged atom) by giving away its one electron. If you take one hydrogen ion away from water and leave its electron behind, you are left with a hydrogen atom and an oxygen atom bound together, possessing one extra electron. This gives them a negative charge; hence, this combination is an anion. This breaking of the water molecule into two ions, a hydrogen cation and a hydroxyl anion, is referred to as dissociation and can happen to many molecules. In **TABLE 2.3**, notice the ions that are formed as a number of molecules dissociate.

Table 2.3 Several Molecules and Their Ions

Molecule	Cation	Anion
NaCl	Na^+	Cl^-
$CaCl_2$	Ca^{++}	$2Cl^-$
$MgCl_2$	Mg^{++}	$2Cl^-$
HCl	H^+	CL^-
H_2CO_3	H^+	HCO_3^-
$NaHCO_3$	Na^+	HCO_3^-
NaOH	Na^+	OH^-
KOH	K^+	OH^-

Let's think about some simple definitions. A salt is a molecule that dissociates into a cation that is not hydrogen and an anion that is not a hydroxyl. An acid is a molecule that dissociates into the cation hydrogen plus some anion that is not a hydroxyl. A base is a molecule that dissociates into some cation that is not hydrogen and an anion that is a hydroxyl. A molecule that binds a hydrogen ion in an aqueous (water) solution is also a base; it leaves behind a hydroxyl anion from water.

Now think about the one remaining possibility. If a molecule dissociates into a cation that is hydrogen and an anion that is a hydroxyl, it must be _____. Think for just a minute. Since the cation is hydrogen and the anion is a hydroxyl, it must be water. There, with that simple bit of information, we now know the definitions of a salt, an acid, and a base. When we add a salt to water, it dissolves. This leaves us with a cation and an anion. Neither one is what actually makes up the water (the water is a hydrogen cation and a hydroxyl anion). If we add a base to water, it dissociates leaving some cation other than hydrogen (sodium, for example) and an anion that is a hydroxyl. In effect, the water now has more hydroxyls than hydrogens. That is the definition of a basic solution. Basic solutions are also referred to as alkaline. If instead we add an acid to water, it dissociates into the cation hydrogen and any anion other than a hydroxyl. The water then has excess hydrogen ions, making this an acidic solution. A strong acid or base is merely one that dissociates (ionizes) readily (more completely), adding a lot of either hydrogen or hydroxyl ions to the solution. A weak acid or base is less apt to dissociate (it dissociates less completely); hence, it adds fewer of these ions.

Our cells take advantage of this fact by using buffer systems to regulate acid-base balance. Buffer systems are used when a strong acid or a strong base (again, "strong" indicates that it dissociates completely) is added to a fluid in the body. The buffer system works to replace a strong acid with a weak acid, and a strong base with either a weak base or a salt. This results in less dissociation of these ions; hence, less hydrogen or hydroxyl ions are running about. Buffers are explained in detail in Chapter 17. For now, be aware that buffers limit the impact of strong acids or bases on fluids within our bodies.

Let's look again at Table 2.3. Based on your knowledge of what the molecules shown dissociate into, can you now identify the salts, acids, and bases? If you are able to do this, good for you. If you can't, read over the definitions for a salt, an acid, and a base and try again. Think carefully. Look at each ion and you will figure it out.

pH: A Balancing Act

Don't we need a way to determine how acidic or how basic any solution is? We do that through the use of the pH scale. Don't worry; this is not complicated. Doesn't every consumer product we buy today say something about pH? Think about it; there's pH balanced mouthwash, deodorant, shampoo, and so on. It is getting out of control! So, let's consider the way pH relates to how acidic or basic a solution is.

If we are to consider how acidic or basic an aqueous solution is (aqueous simply inferring that the solvent is water), we must decide what we will measure and what units of measure we will use. Since we are interested in the balance of hydrogen ions to hydroxide ions (H^+ to OH^-), we could measure either ion. Too many H^+ ions is the same as too few OH^- ions and indicates an acidic solution. Too few H^+ ions is the same as too many OH^- ions and indicates that the solution is basic. The hydrogen ion is most commonly used, and that is to what the pH scale refers. So, we will look at the concentration of hydrogen ions. We now need a unit of measure.

Molarity is one way of quantifying the amount of a substance in a solution. It is based on the concept that each molecule has a molecular weight. The molecular weight is equivalent to the atomic weights of all atoms in the molecule. Atomic weights are determined by adding the number of protons and the number of neutrons in any atom. For instance, sodium has 11 protons and 12 neutrons; hence, it has an atomic weight of 23. Chloride has 17 protons and 18 neutrons; hence, it has an atomic weight of 35. The molecular weight of sodium chloride is 23 plus 35, or 58. We use this information in a measurement of concentration called molarity in the following way. A 1 molar solution is one that contains 1 mole of the solute in 1 liter of water. One mole is equivalent to the molecular weight of that molecule expressed in grams. So, 1 mole of sodium chloride is 58 grams. If we put this in 1 liter of water, we have a 1 molar solution. If we put in twice that amount, we have a 2 molar solution. If we put in half that amount, we have a 0.5 molar solution.

The pH scale is based on the molarity of the hydrogen ions in the solution. It is expressed as the negative log of the hydrogen concentration. This sounds so complicated that even I am lost. It's not at all that complicated; bear with me for a few more minutes. A pH of seven indicates a 10^{-7} molar concentration of hydrogen ions. This means we have a 0.0000001 molar solution (10^{-7} indicates seven decimal places). Pretty weak, huh? At that concentration, we have as many H^+ ions as OH^- ions. This is a neutral pH, neither acidic nor basic. If instead, we have a pH of six, we have a 10^{-6} molar concentration of hydrogen ions. That indicates we have a 0.000001M solution of hydrogen ions. Since 0.000001 is greater than 0.0000001, we have more hydrogen, hence the solution is acidic. See how it works? You try one. What does a pH of four indicate? Think a minute. A pH of four indicates a 10^{-4} or 0.0001 molar solution. This is a lot bigger than 0.0000001; hence, it is much more acidic. For each unit we move on the pH scale, we have moved one decimal place, meaning our solution is 10 times more acidic (or less acidic if we move the other way). Let's try again. What does a pH of eight indicate? It indicates a molar concentration of 10^{-8} or 0.00000001; hence, less hydrogen ions than neutral. This indicates that we have an over abundance of hydroxide ions and, therefore, have a basic solution. A pH of 12 indicates a 10^{-12} molar solution, or one that is much more basic.

That's basically all there is to pH. Look at **FIGURE 2.15** for further explanation, and read this over again if it is still unclear. The examples and questions at the back of this chapter may help you to get the hang of it.

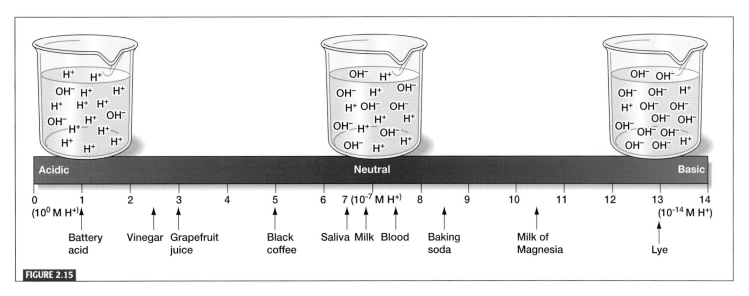

FIGURE 2.15

The pH scale.

Congratulations, you have now finished our section on chemistry. Use the "What You Should Know" and "What Did You Learn?" sections that follow to make sure you are ready to go on. Do not go on until you are sure you have mastered this information, as you will certainly need it later on. If you are somewhat confident, but need to see it in use to really get it, you are right where you need to be. The rest of this book will provide you with lots of examples and applications of this material. Continue working hard and you will do well.

What You Should Know

1. The human body is a large collection of chemicals gathered together in an organized fashion.
2. Some knowledge of the interactions between these chemicals is necessary to the development of an understanding of the body.
3. An atom is the smallest unit of matter that can enter into a chemical reaction.
4. An atom is the smallest unit of an element.
5. Atoms are made up of a nucleus of protons and neutrons, surrounded by orbiting electrons.
6. Electrons orbit nuclei in specific energy levels or shells.
7. Molecules are made by combining atoms.
8. Ionic bonds, covalent bonds, and hydrogen bonds are used to combine atoms, and each type of bond differs in the attractive force that holds it together.
9. Organic molecules are molecules largely composed of carbon.
10. Carbohydrates are composed of carbon, hydrogen, and oxygen, with a 2:1 ratio between hydrogen and oxygen.
11. The simplest form of carbohydrate is the monosaccharide, ringed structures containing three to seven carbon atoms.
12. Carbohydrates serve as a major energy source in our bodies; they are one component of our DNA and they are important in interactions between cells.
13. Dehydration synthesis and hydrolysis are two types of chemical reactions that involve water.
14. Like carbohydrates, lipids also contain carbon, hydrogen, and oxygen, but the hydrogen to oxygen ratio is altered; there is generally less oxygen (relative to hydrogen) in lipids than in carbohydrates.
15. Lipids are insoluble in water and maybe hydrophobic or amphipathic.
16. Triglycerides contain one glycerol and three fatty acid side chains.
17. Prostaglandins and steroids are lipid molecules that are important in intercellular signaling.
18. Proteins are chains of amino acids.
19. Amino acids are composed of a central carbon, a hydrogen, an amino group, a carboxyl group, and a distinctive side chain.
20. The side chain present in an amino acid determines the identity of that amino acid.
21. We use 20 different amino acids in the synthesis of proteins in our bodies.
22. Proteins have many important functions; they serve as hormones, enzymes, carriers of other molecules, and structural components.
23. Nucleic acids are chains of nucleotides.
24. Nucleotides are each composed of a nitrogenous base, a pentose sugar, and one or more phosphate groups.
25. DNA is made up of adenine, thymine, cytosine, and guanine deoxyribonucleotides; RNA is made up of adenine, uracil, cytosine, and guanine riboniucleotides.
26. ATP is a nucleotide that serves as the main form of fuel to power our molecular machinery.
27. Water is a polar molecule that heats and cools slowly, absorbs heat as it changes from a liquid to a gas, serves as a good suspending medium, and is a polar solvent.
28. A solvent plus one or more solutes equals a solution.
29. Acids are molecules that ionize to the cation hydrogen and any anion other than a hydroxyl.
30. Bases are molecules that ionize to the hydroxyl anion and any cation other than hydrogen, or molecules that bind a hydrogen cation, leaving behind a hydroxyl anion.
31. Salts are molecules that ionize to any cation other than hydrogen and any anion other than a hydroxyl.
32. The pH scale is based on the molarity of the hydrogen ions in a solution, indicated as the negative log of that concentration. A pH of 7 is neutral, lower numbers are more acidic, and higher numbers are more basic.

What Did You Learn?

Multiple choice questions: choose the best answer.

1. The basic unit of an element is one:
   a. Electron
   b. Molecule
   c. Smidgeon
   d. Atom
   e. Proton

2. The nucleus of an atom contains:
   a. Protons
   b. Neutrons
   c. Both of the above
   d. Neither of the above

3. Electrons orbit atomic nuclei:
   a. Randomly
   b. In organized energy levels
   c. No they don't; they are in the nucleus
   d. In one orbit only

4. The second energy shell can contain up to _____ electrons.
   a. 0
   b. 2
   c. 8
   d. 16
   e. None of the above

5. For electrons to enter the third energy level, there must already be _____ in orbit around the nucleus.
   a. 4
   b. 8
   c. 12
   d. 26
   e. None of the above is correct.

6. A positively charged ion is _____.
   a. An anion
   b. A cation
   c. Both of the above
   d. Neither of the above

7. The number of electrons that the outer energy level needs to either gain or lose is that atoms _____.
   a. Valence
   b. Combining capacity
   c. Both of the above
   d. Neither of the above

8. Sodium chloride is held together by a/an _____ bond.
   a. Hydrogen
   b. Polar covalent
   c. Nonpolar covalent
   d. Ionic
   e. Savings

9. Which of the following is attracted to an anion?
   a. Another anion
   b. A cation
   c. Both of the above
   d. Neither of the above

10. A water molecule is held together by a _____ bond.
    a. Hydrogen
    b. Polar covalent
    c. Nonpolar covalent
    d. Ionic
    e. Savings

11. _____ bonds contribute greatly to the shape of proteins.
    a. Hydrogen
    b. Polar covalent
    c. Nonpolar covalent
    d. Ionic
    e. Savings

12. The valence of carbon is _____.
    a. Two
    b. Four
    c. Six
    d. Eight
    e. None of the above

13. The ratio of _____ in a carbohydrate is 2:1.
    a. Oxygen to carbon
    b. Oxygen to hydrogen
    c. Hydrogen to helium
    d. Hydrogen to oxygen
    e. None of the above. All of these ratios may be variable in carbohydrates.

14. Hexose is a _____.
    a. Monosaccharide
    b. Disaccharide
    c. Polysaccharide
    d. Polypeptide
    e. None of the above

What Did You Learn? (continued)

15. Hexose contains _____ carbons.
    a. Three
    b. Four
    c. Five
    d. Six
    e. Seven

16. Glucose is a _____.
    a. Monosaccharide
    b. Disaccharide
    c. Polysaccharide
    d. Polypeptide

17. Glucose is bound together to form glycogen by _____ synthesis reactions.
    a. Hydrolytic
    b. Decarboxylic
    c. Dehydration
    d. Magical

18. A triglyceride is _____.
    a. A carbohydrate
    b. A lipid
    c. A protein
    d. A nucleic acid
    e. None of the above

19. A triglyceride contains:
    a. One fatty acid and two glycerols
    b. One fatty acid and three glycerols
    c. Three fatty acids and one glycerol
    d. Three fatty acids and two glycerols
    e. None of the above

20. A saturated fatty acid contains all of the _____ it can hold.
    a. Carbon
    b. Oxygen
    c. Hydrogen
    d. Double bond

21. A monounsaturated fatty acid has one _____.
    a. Carbon
    b. Oxygen
    c. Hydrogen
    d. Double bond

22. A chain of amino acids is a _____.
    a. Carbohydrate
    b. Lipid

c. Protein
d. Nucleic acid

23. The identity of an amino acid is determined by its _____.
    a. Central carbon
    b. Carboxyl group
    c. Amino group
    d. Side chain
    e. Hydrogen

24. An enzyme is a:
    a. Carbohydrate
    b. Lipid
    c. Protein
    d. Nucleic acid

25. Which of the following is not found in DNA?
    a. Adenine nucleotides
    b. Thymine nucleotides
    c. Cytosine nucleotides
    d. Guanine nucleotides
    e. Uracil nucleotides

26. Water is a _____ solvent.
    a. Polar
    b. Nonpolar
    c. Either of the above
    d. Neither of the above

27. NaCl is _____.
    a. An acid
    b. A base
    c. A salt
    d. None of the above

28. H_2CO_3 is _____.
    a. An acid
    b. A base
    c. A salt
    d. None of the above

29. The pH scale is:
    a. Based on the molarity of hydroxyl ions
    b. Logarithmic
    c. Both of the above
    d. Neither of the above

30. A solution with a pH of 10 is:
    a. Acidic
    b. Basic
    c. Neutral
    d. None of the above

3 Understanding Your Cells

What You Will Learn

- What your smallest living components are.
- The names and functions of your cells' organelles and what the substances stored in your cells are called.
- How your cell membranes control the passage of substances into and out of your cells.
- Passive and active transport mechanisms that move substances into and out of your cells.
- How your cell generates ATP and how it uses it as a fuel.
- The structure and composition of the skeleton of your cells.
- How your cells reproduce.
- How your cells gain specialized functions and forms.

3.1 Introducing: Your Cells!

Wow, we're about to learn about the cell. Big deal, you say? It is a big deal. Your cells are your smallest living units. Yes, I did say living. You began as only one cell, and now your cells number in the many trillions. You originally were only one type of cell, but now you have many individual types of cells, all working together as a large community of individuals to form the complete you. Here we will examine the cell in some detail. This will help you to understand how cells work together to complete the many complex processes that go into keeping you alive.

■ Who Studies Cells?

Cell biologists are scientists who study cells and develop the knowledge you are about to gain. By studying the cell, they have provided insight into some of the fundamental questions regarding life, disease, and the continuation of our species. Many cell biologists specialize in some particular aspect of this discipline. They may study the biochemistry of the cell or use electron microscopes to further elucidate the fine structure of cells. Some cell biologists specialize in the function of one organelle or activity of the cell. Cell biology is a fascinating field, perhaps one that you will choose to follow.

What Did You Learn? (continued)

Short answer questions: answer briefly and in your own words.

1. Describe the structure of an atom, including where each of its components is to be found.

2. Distinguish between ionic, polar covalent, nonpolar covalent, and hydrogen bonds.

3. Which carbohydrate is a major source of energy in our bodies, in what form is it stored in our cells, and what type of reaction allows us to store it and release it from storage?

4. How are our organic molecules related to each other? What does this tell you about our ability to use the various organic molecules that are included in our diet?

5. What do enzymes do, and what type of molecules are they?

6. Explain what characteristic of proteins allows them to fill their many roles in our bodies. What is responsible for this characteristic? What could happen if one amino acid is substituted for another in a protein? (Think. There are a number of possible effects.)

7. What is the role of ATP and how does it fulfill that role? Why is ATP necessary?

8. Describe why water is important in our bodies. What abilities of water and features of the water molecule enable it to provide for our needs?

9. Two related reactions are frequently used to join or take apart molecules in our bodies. Identify these reactions, describe how they work, and explain why this system works well for us.

10. Define the terms *salt, acid,* and *base.*

11. Briefly explain the pH scale. Why do we need this scale?

12. Why is some basic knowledge of chemistry necessary for someone who wants to understand the human body? How might this knowledge benefit you <u>personally</u>?

Cytology is a related field. Cytologists examine the structure or anatomy of cells and are part of the medical team that diagnoses disease. They use microscopes to examine cell samples collected by physicians and other medical practitioners. Special dyes and stains are used to highlight features of the cell. Now they also use computers with image analysis software to aid in their work. This field also may appeal to you.

A Naming Dilemma

You may notice that some of the things we will learn about in this and subsequent chapters will have two or more names. That was not done specifically to confuse students; that is merely a side benefit of this practice. Often structures are studied by people working in different disciplines at the same time. Each discipline applies its own terminology to the object of study, and only at some later date does some other researcher figure out that they have all been looking at the same thing. By then it is difficult to consolidate the terminology, so we end up with multiple names. Also, names may be given at different times in history, and old names are often not completely dropped. In this text, I will try to keep this repetition to a minimum.

Many of the concepts we learned in the chemistry chapter (Chapter 2) will be applied here. You will begin to see how the information you are learning builds and why these foundation materials are necessary. Proceed and enjoy the time you will now spend learning about the cell.

3.2 The Organelles: Organs for Your Cells

You have many organs in your body. Even before completing your current study, I am sure you could name many of them and give some of their functions. Can't we all picture a kidney, a heart, or a brain? Don't we all have some idea about what these organs do? Your cells have small structures within them (or surrounding them, in the case of your cells' membranes) that perform specific functions for them, just as your organs perform functions for you. These subcellular structures act as little organs and are called organelles. The organelles can be seen in **FIGURE 3.1**. Please refer back to this figure as you read about the organelles. Don't confuse them with substances stored within the cell. Stored substances are collectively called inclusions, and we will consider these separately.

Note that the area of your cells between the membrane and the nucleus (two organelles that we will

soon consider) is called the cytoplasm. Most of our organelles are found in the cytoplasm. Also found here is a liquid called cytosol. Our discussion of organelles will start with the first one encountered as we examine a cell: the cell membrane.

Your Cells' Membranes

The cell membrane, plasmalemma, or plasma membrane is to your cell what your skin is to your body. It limits the cell, separating what is inside of the cell from the outside environment. It is selectively permeable. This means that it allows certain substances, but not other substances, to pass through it. It is flexible and self-repairing if punctured. What gives this membrane these special characteristics? The material of which it is made: phospholipids.

Those Amazing Phospholipids

The main material of the plasma membrane is a phospholipid bilayer. So, what is a phospholipid bilayer? The term *bilayer* implies two layers; the term *phospholipid* implies lipids bound to phosphates. Each molecule of phospholipid has a phosphate head and two lipid tails (**FIGURE 3.2**). The phosphate head is polar, just as water is polar. Polar molecules tend to be attracted to water. We refer to this characteristic as being *hydrophilic*. The polar phosphate head is hydrophilic. The lipid (fatty acid) tails, like other lipids, are nonpolar. Water and nonpolar molecules are not attracted to each other; in fact, they repel each other. This characteristic is called *hydrophobic*. Many lipids, including the fatty acid tails of the phospholipid molecule, are hydrophobic. Think about how greasy cooking pans do not come clean when rinsed with water. Water simply causes the fats to congeal. This is because many lipids are hydrophobic. Phospholipids contain hydrophilic and hydrophobic moieties and are, therefore, *amphipathic*.

So, if we had a small amount of phospholipid and we dropped it into water (Figure 3.2), how would the molecules orient themselves? Their heads would be attracted to the water and would point outward. Their tails would point inward, shielded from the water by their phosphate heads. In this way, they would form a small sphere. If we had a larger amount of phospholipid and exposed it to water, it would self-assemble into a double sheet. The hydrophilic phosphate heads would again point toward the water, while the hydrophobic fatty acid tails would point toward each other in the middle of the membrane. This could form a larger sphere, with water on the inside and the outside of the sphere. This is exactly the arrangement we have in our plasmalemma, except that it is not exactly water, but an aqueous solution that is on either side of

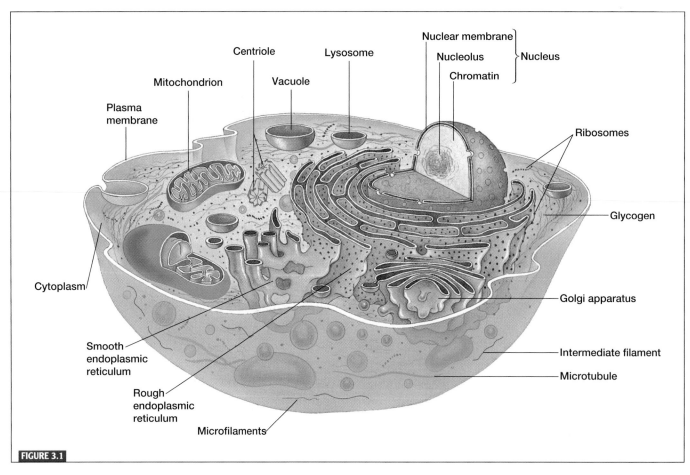

FIGURE 3.1

The cell.

the membrane. Outside of the cell, we have our extracellular fluids, which we will learn about in our next two chapters. Inside of the cell, we have a gel-like substance called *cytosol*. The cytosol surrounds and supports the organelles and inclusions within the cytoplasm. The plasmalemma separates the cytoplasm of the cell's internal environment from the cell's external environment.

Membrane Proteins: Like Floating Toys

But wait; there's more to the cell membrane than that. There are numerous proteins that have specific functions associated with the plasma membrane (**FIGURE 3.3a**). Some of these proteins extend through both layers of the membranes. These are called integral membrane proteins. These are often channels (tunnel-like molecules) through which specific substances, such as ions, may pass. They may also be enzymes that act as molecular pumps to move substances through the membrane. More on that in a few minutes.

Other proteins do not span the entire thickness of the membrane, but are associated with either the internal or external surface, and may extend partway into the

membrane. These are called peripheral proteins. These may be enzymes that speed up specific reactions that the cell needs to conduct near the membranes. They may also serve as anchors for specific carbohydrates that the cell uses to identify itself to other cells or to communicate with other cells. When proteins and carbohydrates are associated in this way, we refer to them as glycoproteins. Note that carbohydrates may also be anchored to the membrane by attachment to certain lipids. Carbohydrates exist as a sort of "fuzz" on the cell surface, called the *glycocalyx*.

Let's picture the membrane in the following way. Imagine a swimming pool filled with water. Onto the water, let's float hundreds of tennis balls, enough to form a complete layer over the entire surface (Figure 3.3b). The water in the swimming pool is the inside of the cell, the air above the swimming pool is the outside of the cell, and the layer of tennis balls is the phospholipid bilayer of the plasmalemma. Now, place a few floating air mattresses on the tennis balls. They are light enough to sit on the tennis balls without pushing them aside and making contact with the air and water at the same time.

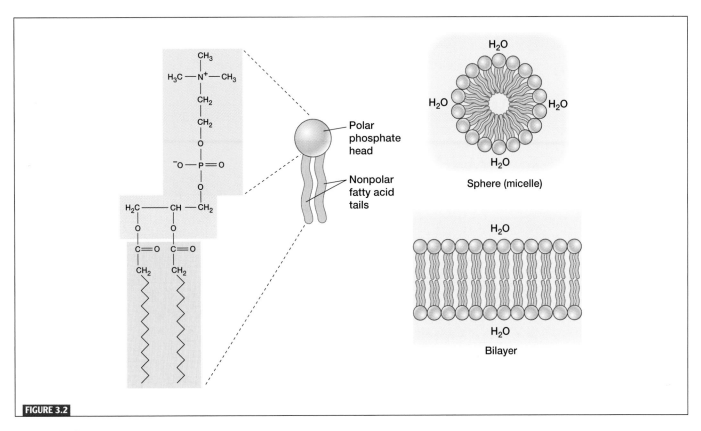

Phospholipids.

These are the peripheral proteins. Finally, let's put in a few of those floating toys, the large blow-up kind in the form of sea serpents and things like that. You know the kind; they have weighted bottoms that allow them to float upright and bob along in the water. These would extend through the tennis ball layer with their bottoms in the water and their heads in the air. These are our integral proteins.

What would happen if a strong wind began to blow? Our floating objects other than the tennis balls would be pushed to one end of the pool (Figure 3.3c). The layer of tennis balls would remain intact and merely be pushed aside slightly to allow our sea serpent toys to pass through. When the wind stopped, the toys would again drift around and become dispersed throughout the pool. A similar phenomenon exists in the cell membrane. In laboratory experiments, we can cause the peripheral and integral proteins to move to one area of the membrane without making holes in the continuous layer of phospholipid (without interrupting membrane integrity).

Now, what would happen if you were to do a "cannonball" into the pool? The tennis balls would allow you to pass through, but would seal over again after you went through. Our cell membrane is similarly self-sealing after a puncture. (Too bad it is not strong enough to use to make tires!) This whole block of information about the cell membrane—how it contains proteins within it or on either of its surfaces, how these proteins can move around, and how it can seal after a puncture—is all part of a system for describing the cell membrane called the Fluid-Mosaic Model.

Selective Permeability: Movement Across the Membrane

To consider how the membrane is selectively permeable, we need to think about how molecules move and specifically how they pass through membranes. Let's think about that in general and then return to the cell.

Diffusion: A Skunk's Defense

Look around the room you are now in. If a skunk came into this room and "let loose" in the farthest corner from you (**FIGURE 3.4**), would you ultimately smell the skunk odor? Yes, you say? Why? How do the molecules of "skunk juice" reach you? They reach you through a process called diffusion. Diffusion is the means by which molecules move from a region of their higher concentration to a region of their lower concentration. If you have two regions that differ in their concentration of some

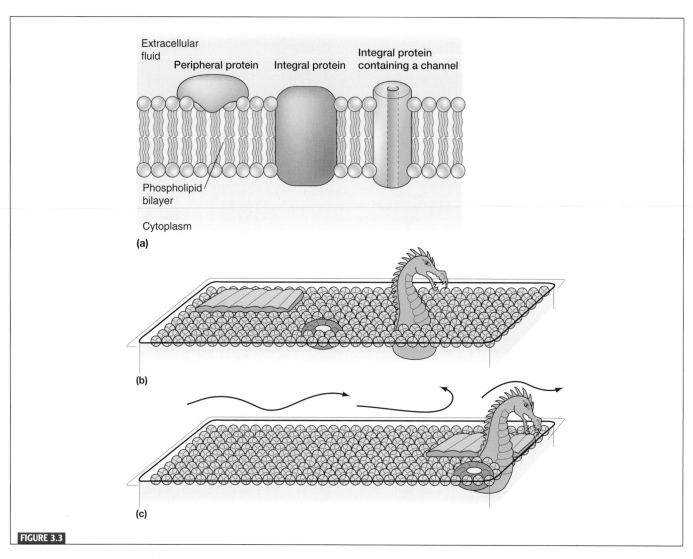

FIGURE 3.3

Membrane associated proteins (a). Note how pool toys among tennis balls are similar to membrane proteins in the phospholipid bilayer (b and c).

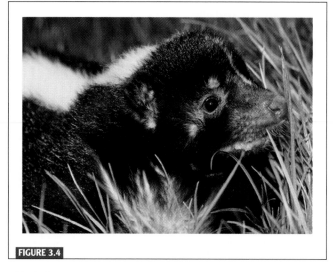

FIGURE 3.4

Think about how the skunk's odor would spread by diffusion.

substance, you have a concentration gradient. Diffusion occurs down a concentration gradient. Simply, the molecules that the skunk releases will diffuse throughout the room until their concentration is the same throughout the room. We would then say that we have reached equilibrium: there no longer is a concentration gradient. The same thing happens to molecules released into water. Picture a swimming pool again, this time with the filter pump turned off so the water is not circulating. Dump a case of green Kool Aid powder in one corner of the pool (**FIGURE 3.5a**). The whole pool will eventually turn green as the Kool Aid diffuses throughout the pool. (Don't try this at home!)

Osmosis: Kool Aid in the Pool

Now, let's picture that swimming pool again. We could suspend a special membrane across the pool and seal it

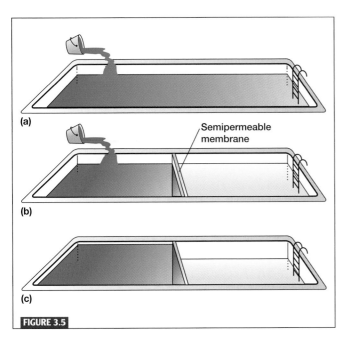

FIGURE 3.5

Diffusion (a) and osmosis (b and c) in a swimming pool. Notice the change in water levels between panels b and c.

to the sides and bottom of the pool (Figure 3.5b). This membrane has holes in it that allow water to pass through, but are so small that the molecules of green Kool Aid cannot pass through. What happens if we now dump a case of Kool Aid powder in one corner of the pool? First, wouldn't the water on that side of the membrane all turn green? Absolutely, but the water on the other side of the membrane would have to stay clear. Remember that the Kool Aid powder cannot pass through the membrane, but that the water can pass through. The concept of diffusion tells us that molecules move from a region of their higher concentration to a region of their lower concentration (down a concentration gradient), and as Scotty would have told Captain Kirk (original *Star Trek*), "You canna change the laws of physics, Captain." In other words, neither our semipermeable membrane nor the fact that we're dealing with water negates the law of diffusion. That's a long way around to the question "What's the water going to do?" On which side of the membrane is our water the most concentrated? Remember, the water is our solvent, the Kool Aid is our solute, and we have an aqueous solution of Kool Aid. We have a higher concentration of Kool Aid on the side where we dumped it, as we have no Kool Aid on the other side. We must have a higher concentration of water where we have a lower concentration of Kool Aid, so that our water will move through the membrane from the side where we have only water to the side where we dumped the Kool Aid (Figure 3.5c).

What we have just depicted is called osmosis. Osmosis is the movement of water across a semipermeable membrane from a region of its higher concentration to a region of its lower concentration. Essentially, it is diffusion of water across a semipermeable membrane. At some point, as the level of water rises on the Kool Aid side of the pool, the pressure of that water will block the flow of more water through the membrane. That pressure is called the osmotic pressure. As we will learn, osmotic pressure is important to cells.

So, where were we? We were learning about the ways in which substances move across the cell's plasma membrane. One way must be osmosis if the plasma membrane is semipermeable, permeable to water, and in an aqueous environment. (It is all of these things.) What determines which substances can cross the membrane? One factor is size. If a molecule is small enough, it can pass through small pores within the membrane. Water is one such molecule. Solubility in lipids is another factor. Picture a ghost in the cartoons that can pass right through a wall. If a molecule is lipid soluble and the membrane is mainly lipid (phospholipid), that molecule can pass through the membrane (**FIGURE 3.6**). Steroid hormones, oxygen, carbon dioxide, and alcohol are examples of lipid soluble substances that can pass through the cell membrane. The presence of a specific channel or carrier molecule is another factor that determines whether a molecule can pass through the cell membrane. We already learned that some of the integral proteins are channels. These channels allow specific substances to pass through the membrane. In many cases, these channels allow specific ions such as sodium

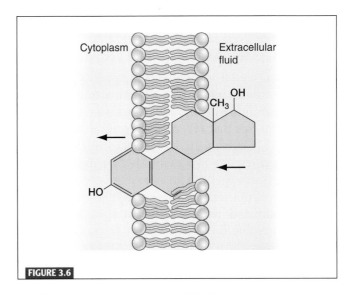

FIGURE 3.6

Lipids can pass through the phospholipid bilayer.

(Na^+), potassium (K^+), or calcium (Ca^{++}) to pass. These channels generally have gates within them that allow these ions to pass only under specific conditions. We will learn more about this later on.

Facilitated Diffusion: Back to Our Pool Toys

Other molecules have a different form of carrier. Let's think back to our swimming pool with the tennis balls, air mattresses, and sea serpent toys for a minute. Could a bird pass through the tennis balls into the water? Probably not; a bird is not big enough or powerful enough to move the tennis balls aside and enter the water. What would happen if the bird landed on the head of the floating sea serpent toy? That might upset the balance of the toy and cause it to tip over, dunking its head and the bird through the tennis balls into the water (**FIGURE 3.7**). If the bird then let go of the serpent's head, the bird might be left in the water as the head bobbed back up. If a bird that was in the water grabbed onto the head as it was bobbing up, it might be carried through the tennis balls in the opposite direction out into the air. Can't you see how a similar molecular mechanism might carry molecules through the membrane that otherwise might not be able to pass through? That is called facilitated diffusion. Facilitated diffusion is still diffusion, the movement of molecules from a region of their higher concentration to a region of their lower concentration, but it involves the use of a carrier molecule. Glucose, a monosaccharide that we learned about in the last chapter (remember, it is a fuel used by the cell for energy), is carried through the cell membrane by facilitated diffusion. For facilitated diffusion to work, the cell must have a carrier for the specific molecule that needs to be carried across the cell membrane. These carriers are highly specific, each carrying only one molecule or a few closely related molecules.

Active Processes: And Now with Energy!

Each system we have discussed thus far involves the movement of substances across the cell membrane without the expenditure of any energy by the cell. These are passive processes that rely on a concentration gradient to achieve a net movement of substances. By that, I mean that in these passive processes, the net movement of substances is always from an area of greater concentration to an area of lesser concentration. Passive processes move substances down a concentration gradient. Active processes involve the use of energy to transport substances across the cell membrane. Unlike diffusion, which is always down a concentration gradient, these active processes can move substances in either direction and can, in fact, even generate a concentration gradient,

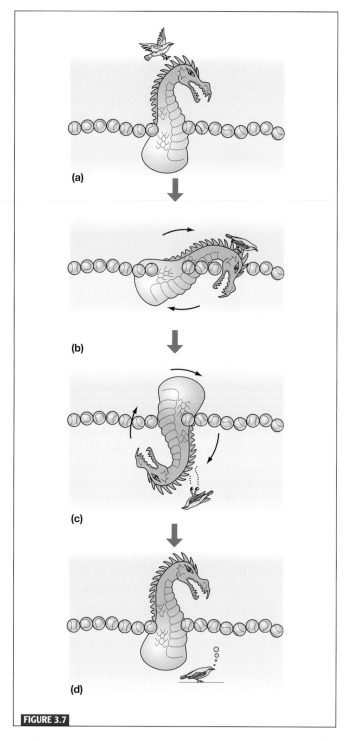

(a)

(b)

(c)

(d)

FIGURE 3.7

A demonstration of facilitated diffusion. The bird (molecule) can't pass through the phospholipid bilayer without a carrier (the floating toy). No energy is used in this transport mechanism.

causing a substance to become more concentrated on one side of the cell membrane. Have you ever been in a house that had a wet basement or in a leaky boat? In either case, water can enter the building or boat passively. It floods in because there is much water outside and much less (hopefully) inside. You must run a pump to remove the water, and the pump requires the use of energy, generally electricity.

Active Transport: Molecular Pumps

One active process is called active transport. Active transport involves the use of molecular pumps to move substances across the cell membrane. Let's think about those molecular pumps for a moment. To what chemical class do you think those pumps would belong? Did we learn about a class of molecules that often serve as molecular machines? Proteins often serve as molecular machines, specifically the proteins we call enzymes. Enzymes speed up some chemical reaction. They take a chemical reaction that can occur without the use of enzymes and greatly increase the rate of that reaction. They act as catalysts of that reaction. In this case, the reaction they speed up is the breakdown of ATP to ADP. What does this reaction liberate? If you answered "a phosphate group," you are correct, but what is the goal of that reaction? The goal is to liberate energy that can be used for some other purpose. The purpose in these molecular pumps is to move some atom across the cell membrane. These atoms are often ions. For instance, a calcium ATPase (Ca++ATPase) would break down ATP (hence, the term *ATPase,* the *-ase* indicating that it breaks down or cleaves ATP) and use that energy to pump calcium across a membrane.

Sometimes active transport involves molecular pumps that move two ions at the same time. This is referred to as co-transport if both are moving in the same direction, and counter-transport if they are moving in opposite directions. One such system is the sodium-potassium ATPase (Na+K+ATPase). This enzyme pumps sodium out of the cell and potassium into the cell, and is, therefore, an example of counter-transport (**FIGURE 3.8**).

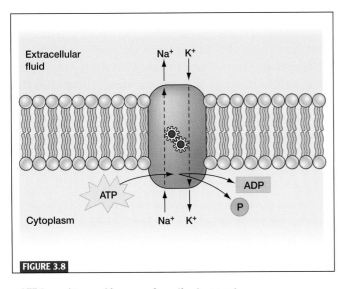

FIGURE 3.8

ATP is used to provide energy for active transport.

Endocytosis: Several Neat Processes

Another active process is endocytosis. Endocytosis is a mechanism, or actually a group of mechanisms, that cells use to move large molecules or even droplets or particles into the cell. A few forms of endocytosis exist. If very large particles need to be engulfed by the cell, phagocytosis is used. Let's break down that term. *Phago-* indicates eating and *-cytosis* indicates the cell; *phagocytosis* means cell eating. In phagocytosis, the cell detects some object in its environment that it needs to engulf. It moves toward this object using chemotaxis. Think of this as cell smelling. Just as you might smell good food cooking on a barbeque and move toward the source of the aroma, the cell detects the object and moves toward it. The cell moves sort of like the "Blob That Ate Toledo" from the horror movies. As it moves, the cell sends out pseudopodia (*pseudo-* = false, *-podia* = feet; *pseudopodia* = false feet) that it ultimately wraps around the particle. Because the plasmalemma is self-sealing, the membranes fuse when the pseudopodia touch each other on the opposite side of the particle, and the particle is encased in a membrane sack, or phagocytotic vesicle, within the cell's cytoplasm. Notice how this is depicted in **FIGURE 3.9**. Only certain cell types can perform phagocytosis. The prime example is the macrophage (*macro-* = big, *-phage* = eat; this cell is the "big eater"). Macrophages are involved in keeping our tissues free from debris, such as would form at a site of injury.

Another form of endocytosis is pinocytosis. This can be thought of as cell drinking. Pinocytosis is similar to phagocytosis, except that pseudopodia are not involved, and usually only small droplets or very small particles, such as individual large molecules, are engulfed. Most cells are capable of pinocytosis. One more form of endocytosis requires a specific receptor on the cell surface for the molecule being engulfed. This is called receptor-mediated endocytosis and is used to carry substances such as certain amino acids and vitamins into cells. This process is otherwise similar to pinocytosis and is common among most cell types.

It is important to note that just as endocytosis is used to bring substances into cells, a related process called exocytosis is used to remove substances from cells. Exocytosis is very similar to pinocytosis, but works in the opposite direction.

■ The Nucleus: Your Cell's Most Prominent Organelle

The nucleus is the next organelle we will consider (Figure 3.1). The nucleus is the largest and most prominent organelle within the cell. If you have ever examined cells

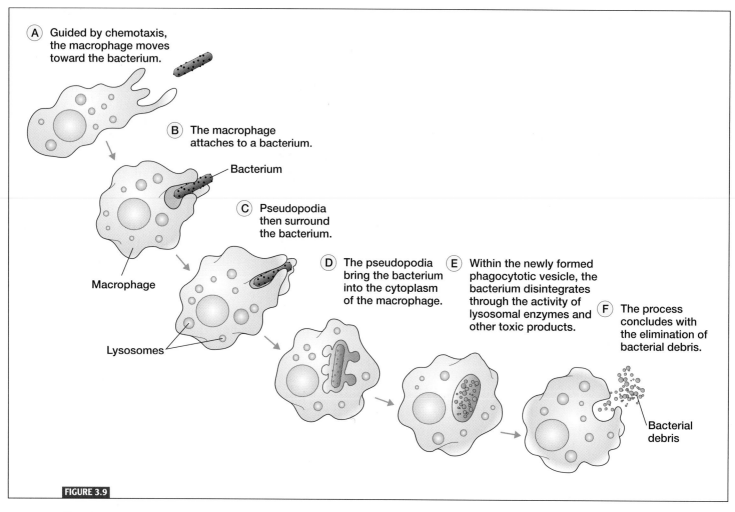

A Guided by chemotaxis, the macrophage moves toward the bacterium.

B The macrophage attaches to a bacterium.

Bacterium

C Pseudopodia then surround the bacterium.

Macrophage

D The pseudopodia bring the bacterium into the cytoplasm of the macrophage.

E Within the newly formed phagocytotic vesicle, the bacterium disintegrates through the activity of lysosomal enzymes and other toxic products.

F The process concludes with the elimination of bacterial debris.

Lysosomes

Bacterial debris

FIGURE 3.9

Phagocytosis.

under the microscope, you undoubtedly noticed their nuclei. Most cells have one nucleus, although certain cell types, such as skeletal muscle and osteoclasts, have multiple nuclei. Cells with many nuclei are sometimes called giant cells or syncytia. Red blood cells are the only mature, living human cells that lack nuclei.

The nucleus is surrounded by the nuclear membrane, a double layer of the same phospholipid bilayer we have already considered. A small space, the perinuclear cisterna, exists between the two layers, and pores extend through the nuclear membrane periodically. This membrane surrounds a substance similar to cytosol called nucleoplasm or karyolymph. Within this gel-like substance we find the nucleolus, which we will discuss shortly, and the genetic material of the cell. The genetic material of the cell is composed of DNA. Recall that DNA was described in the previous chapter as a nucleic acid composed of a double chain of nucleotides. Four different nucleotides are used to construct this chain, and the order in which they occur has specific meaning. The

DNA acts as a blueprint for our proteins; the order of nucleotides in our DNA specifies the order of the amino acids in our proteins. We will discuss protein synthesis in detail in Chapter 14. As we consider how proteins are synthesized, the role of our DNA will become clear. For now, remember that the order of the nucleotides in our DNA specifies the order of the amino acids in our proteins, and in this way our genetic material contains the plan by which we are constructed.

Most of the time, our DNA is spread out in the form of fine threads called chromatin. Some of this chromatin is packed more densely than the rest of our chromatin. The densely packed chromatin is called heterochromatin and, under the microscope, is seen as darkly staining regions of the nucleus. The less densely packed chromatin is called euchromatin and stains less darkly. Euchromatin is actively involved in protein synthesis, whereas heterochromatin is not currently in use. A number of relatively small proteins called histones are responsible for organizing the DNA.

During cellular reproduction, as the nucleus prepares to divide, the DNA must be replicated and packaged into a condensed form so that each daughter nucleus ends up with the proper genetic content. Each unit of this packaged form of DNA is called a chromosome. Note that nuclei that are not undergoing division do not contain chromosomes, but contain chromatin fibers instead. People are often confused about this, thinking that chromosomes are always present in the nuclei. If that were the case, our cells would be unable to produce proteins and would die. We will learn more about cell division later in this chapter and in Chapter 14.

■ The Nucleolus: A Potential Source of Confusion

The nucleus also contains a structure called the nucleolus. Notice how similar the words nucleus and nucleolus look. As similar as they look to you as you relax, reading this text, they might look even more similar during a classroom examination. Always read these words carefully during an exam to see that you do not confuse them and answer a question incorrectly because of that confusion.

As I was saying, the nucleus contains the nucleolus (Figure 3.1). Nucleoli are largely made of RNA, the other nucleic acid we learned about in Chapter 2, although some DNA and proteins are also present. They are the site of ribosome production; ribosomes are the next organelle that we will discuss.

■ Ribosomes: Two Subunits, One Organelle

Ribosomes are organelles that are distributed throughout the cytoplasm (Figure 3.1). Cells generally have a great number of ribosomes. Ribosomes are composed of a specific form of RNA called ribosomal RNA (rRNA). The rRNA is organized into two subunits that must come together for the ribosome to function. This organelle is the site of protein synthesis; it provides the actual location where amino acids are bound together to form the protein chain. This fascinating process will be covered in Chapter 14.

Ribosomes exist in two forms. Some ribosomes are scattered throughout the cytoplasm. These are called free ribosomes and are the site of production of proteins for use within the cell's cytoplasm. The proteins of the cytoskeleton are examples of proteins for use within the cytoplasm. The other form of ribosomes is called bound ribosomes. These are attached to another organelle, the endoplasmic reticulum. Bound ribosomes are the site of production of proteins for export from the cell or insertion into the cell membrane. The protein hormone insulin is an example of an exported protein, and the $Na^+K^+ATPase$ is an example of a protein for insertion into the cell membrane.

■ Endoplasmic Reticulum: Seeded or Plain?

The endoplasmic reticulum is a series of large channels that extend throughout the cytoplasm (Figure 3.1). They are each surrounded by a phospholipid bilayer that is continuous with the outer layer of the nuclear membrane. This is an amazing organelle. The membrane of the endoplasmic reticulum can be thought of as the bench top of the cell. Cells obviously have a lot of synthetic processes occurring within them; in other words, they make a lot of things. If you were to make something, you would need a place to work, a place to assemble that thing. This is also true of your cells. The endoplasmic reticulum provides that surface.

Two types of endoplasmic reticulum exist. One form has ribosomes bound to its surface; the other does not. To picture the two forms, think about bread or rolls you might eat. You could have a seeded roll with sesame seeds on its surface, or you could have a nonseeded roll. Both are basically the same thing, except for that one difference. The same is true of the endoplasmic reticulum.

Granular or rough endoplasmic reticulum (RER) has ribosomes bound to its surface. This is the site of synthesis of proteins for export from the cell or for insertion into the cell membrane. As amino acids are added to the newly formed protein, this chain extends into the central open area of the RER. This open area is called the lumen or the cistern. Here, the newly synthesized protein may be modified in a variety of ways, or it may be packaged for modification elsewhere in the cell, or for export from the cell.

Agranular or smooth endoplasmic reticulum (SER) has no ribosomes on its surface. This is the site where many lipids and carbohydrates are produced. It is also the site of other chemical reactions. When we study the liver, we will learn that the cells of the liver, the hepatocytes, have the amazing ability to break down and inactivate many of the toxins we encounter. This detoxification occurs in the hepatocytes' SER. Frequent exposure to certain toxins (barbiturates, for example) will result in the production of more SER within hepatocytes to increase their ability to detoxify (inactivate) these sleep-inducing drugs. This is why habitual barbiturate users must repeatedly increase their intake of these drugs to induce the same effect.

The lumen (an open area within any round or tubular structure is its lumen) of either type of endoplasmic reticulum is also used for storage and transport. Because the endoplasmic reticulum extends throughout the cell, this also makes perfect sense.

■ Golgi Apparatus: Like a Stack of Pita

This interesting organelle was, until the advent of electron microscopy, thought by some to be merely an artifact of how we examined cells, not an actual organelle. It is, in fact, an organelle that is similar to, and functionally related to, the endoplasmic reticulum. To picture a Golgi apparatus, imagine a stack of pita bread. You know what pita bread is; it is that flat bread that is hollow in the center. You open it up and put good things inside for a nice light sandwich. Imagine a stack of those, say six or eight high, sitting near the nucleus. Instead of being made out of dough, they are made out of phospholipid bilayer. Each layer has a hollow lumen or cistern, and that is where the functions of this organelle take place.

The function of the Golgi is to modify and package secretory proteins. Proteins for secretion are produced where? Right: in the RER. Once the chain of amino acids is synthesized, the protein may not be completely finished. It may need to have pieces clipped off and/or have other molecular moieties (a fancy word for pieces) added to it. For instance, many proteins are not complete until a carbohydrate moiety is added, making a glycoprotein. Here is where that modification would be completed. To carry the protein from the RER to the Golgi, a small bleb of membrane containing the protein pinches off from the RER and travels to the Golgi, where it fuses with the membrane of the Golgi. Remember that this is possible because the phospholipid bilayer is self-sealing. It arrives at the first layer of Golgi, nearest the nucleus, where some modifications are performed. Then, a bleb from that layer carries the protein to the next layer of Golgi to complete other modifications. When all modifications are complete, a bleb of Golgi membrane, called a secretory vesicle, carries the protein to the cell surface, where it fuses with the cell membrane, releasing the finished protein to the outside of the cell. This is an example of exocytosis, mentioned previously. See **FIGURE 3.10** for clarification.

■ Lysosomes: They Really Are Organelles

A little while back, we learned that cells can move substances and particles across their cell membranes and into vesicles within their cytoplasm through processes such as phagocytosis and pinocytosis. Once there, what happens to them? Well, the cell must have some way to break down these things once they are within those vesicles. They use lysosomes to do this. Lysosomes were once thought to be inclusions, vesicles of stored substances. Now that we understand their functions, we realize that they actually are organelles. Lysosomes are vesicles of phospholipid membrane surrounding hydrolytic en-

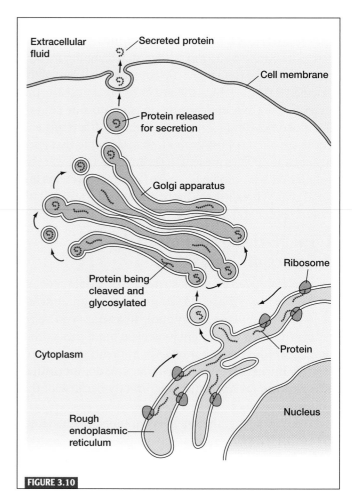

FIGURE 3.10

Protein synthesis, processing, and secretion.

zymes. Let's think about that for a minute; in Chapter 1, we learned that hydrolysis meant to break (cleave) a bond using water and that enzymes were protein "machines" that speed up chemical reactions. A hydrolytic enzyme, therefore, must be one that causes hydrolysis to occur. These enzymes and other substances within the lysosomes allow the cell to digest whatever is in phagocytotic or pinocytotic vesicles. Since both possess a membrane of phospholipid bilayer, they are able to fuse together, combining their contents within one lumen.

A similar role for the lysosomes comes into play as other organelles wear out. Many organelles do not last for the entire life of the cell. Injurious events experienced by the cell may hasten the wear and tear on specific organelles. When organelles wear out, they are removed from service and replaced. This process, called autophagy (*auto-* = self, *-phagy* = to eat; *autophagy* = self eating), is similar to phagocytosis, although it occurs within the cell. The organelle is surrounded by a vesicle of membrane. This autophagocytotic vesicle fuses with a lysosome, and the organelle is broken down for recycling.

Lysosomes are produced in the same way that proteins are prepared for export. The hydrolytic enzymes are synthesized in the RER and modified by the Golgi apparatus. They are then packaged in vesicles by the Golgi and released into the cytoplasm, but not secreted from the cell. They remain within the cytoplasm to perform their vital function.

Mitochondria: Let's Get Energized

Now here is an amazing organelle. People often refer to the mitochondria as the "powerhouse" of the cell. Mitochondria are the main site of ATP production, and you remember that ATP is the fuel on which molecular processes run. ATP is cleaved to ADP, releasing one phosphate group and energy. That energy is used to power many vital processes. More on this after we think about the structure and general features of mitochondria.

Mitochondria are composed of one sack of phospholipid bilayer inside of another sack of phospholipid bilayer, with a space between them and a space in the center (**FIGURE 3.11**). You can imagine this by picturing one small balloon held within another larger balloon. The only problem in picturing it that way is that the inner membrane of the mitochondria is thrown into folds to increase its surface area, while the inner balloon has no folds. These folds are called cristae. The great surface area provided by the cristae gives lots of surface area on which the many chemical reactions of the mitochondria can occur. The area in the center of the mitochondria is filled with a gel-like substance called matrix. DNA is present in the matrix. This DNA, called mitochondrial DNA, is composed of circular fragments similar to that found in bacteria. It encodes some, but not all, of the enzymes needed for mitochondrial function. The remaining enzymes are encoded by the DNA within the nucleus.

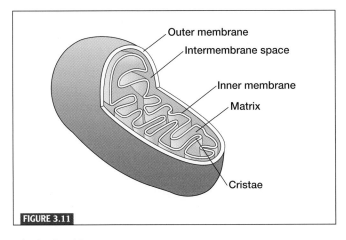

Outer membrane
Intermembrane space
Inner membrane
Matrix
Cristae

FIGURE 3.11

A mitochondrion.

Since mitochondria are the main site of ATP production within the cell, it makes sense that cells that are more active and need more energy would have more mitochondria. That is the case. In fact, if a cell increases its level of activity and needs more energy, its mitochondria will divide to become more numerous and also become larger to meet this new demand. This is one of the changes that occur in muscle cells as you increase your level of daily exercise (and you know what a good idea that is).

Why Do We Generate ATP?

So, what actually goes on in the mitochondria, where does that ATP come from, and why is this necessary? Human beings and other animals are examples of heterotrophs. Heterotrophs are organisms that must take in preformed foods as they cannot harvest energy from the sun, or from other sources, for the production of organic molecules. Autotrophs, such as plants, can gather energy in that way, and we take advantage of their ability to do so by consuming them or other animals who have consumed them. So, we use these preformed organic molecules (food) to provide us with the raw materials and energy we need to process those materials and perform other functions.

Glucose is the main organic molecule we use as fuel to produce our ultimate fuel, the fuel on which our molecular machinery runs, ATP. Remember that our molecular machinery, the enzymes that pump our ions, contract our muscles, and enable us to grow, think, and do all of the things we do, runs on ATP. We must use another source of energy to produce that ATP. Glucose is the main source of energy we use to produce that ATP. This is not as complicated as it sounds. Perhaps you have seen the small electrical generators that some people take camping or use when there is a power outage. These little generators use gasoline, an energy source these people have available, to produce electricity, the energy source these people need. That is exactly what our cells do; they use glucose, an available energy source, to produce ATP, the needed energy source. Molecules other than glucose can be used for this purpose, but glucose is the main energy source. Glucose is available in our diets. Nonglucose monosaccharides in our diet can be converted into glucose; even fatty acids and amino acids from the fats and proteins we eat can be used to produce glucose, or can be used directly by our mitochondria.

How Do We Generate ATP?

ATP generation is a multistep chemical process that, to be honest, many students find difficult to understand. Some of this difficulty lies in the fact that it is easy to become frustrated and decide, "I just can't do this." Well, you can do this! I will go through this process slowly and in a stepwise fashion. Read carefully, look at the diagram, and think. If you don't understand one of the steps, spend a little more time on it. I'm sure you can do this.

We will first consider aerobic cellular respiration, the process that operates when oxygen is available (because it usually is). After you understand this, we will move on to what happens when oxygen is not available: anaerobic cellular respiration.

Aerobic Cellular Respiration

Aerobic cellular respiration is a multistep process used to harvest the energy present in the food we eat and store that energy as ATP, the fuel that runs the machinery of our cells (**FIGURE 3.12**). Aerobic cellular respiration uses glucose as the "input" fuel and requires the presence of oxygen. The final products are ATP, carbon dioxide, and water. The whole process, which yields 38 ATP, is summed up in the following formula (note that $C_6H_{12}O_6$ is, in this case, glucose):

$$C_6H_{12}O_6 + 6O_2 \rightarrow 6H_2O + 6CO_2$$

Now, how can we go about this? Let's break it down into its individual steps, and then I will explain it one step at a time. The first step is called glycolysis. Glycolysis is the initial breakdown of glucose and produces very little ATP, but is a necessary step because we have to prepare the glucose molecule for the steps that follow. Glycolysis occurs in the cytoplasm and breaks one molecule of glucose (a six-carbon molecule) into two molecules of pyruvic acid (three carbons each). Each of the later steps occurs in the mitochondria. The next step is such a small one that some people treat it as part of our third step. For completeness, we will count it as a separate step. It is called the transition reaction, and in it each molecule of pyruvic acid is converted into a molecule of acetic acid, which is then bound to a carrier. More on that in a moment.

Next, we have the third step (some would say the second step), the citric acid cycle. The citric acid cycle is also called Krebs cycle, or the tricarboxylic acid (TCA) cycle. We will stick to the citric acid cycle. In this step, the acetic acid from our transition reaction is used to produce citric acid. The citric acid is then broken down, producing another molecule of ATP.

In our final step, electron transport, we rely on a phenomenon that I have not yet mentioned. Each of the previous steps has included oxidation-reduction reactions. Oxidation reactions involve the loss of electrons from

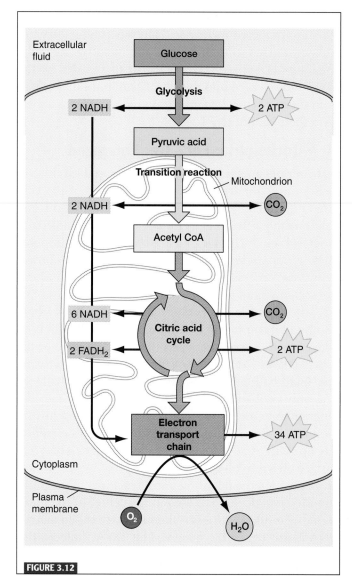

FIGURE 3.12

ATP production by aerobic cellular respiration: glycolysis, the transition reaction, the citric acid cycle and the electron transport chain. For further details, see Appendix D.

molecules. In organic molecules, oxidation generally involves the loss of hydrogen ions. Reduction reactions involve the gaining of electrons (or hydrogens in the case of organic molecules) by a molecule. Oxidation-reduction reactions involve the transfer of electrons (hydrogens) from one molecule to another in a coordinated fashion. Each hydrogen transferred represents energy taken from the oxidized molecule and given to the reduced molecule.

In each of our first three steps (glycolysis, transition reaction, and the citric acid cycle), electrons (hydrogens) are released (by oxidation) from our glucose or glucose breakdown products (pyruvic acid and citric acid) and transferred (by reduction) to carrier molecules called coenzymes. The coenzymes used have included

NAD, which becomes NADH when it is reduced (picks up electrons and hydrogens by reduction), and FAD, which becomes FADH$_2$ when it is reduced. Our final step, electron transport, involves the use of these high-energy (reduced) electron carriers and a chain of cytochromes (coenzymes) to produce lots of ATP. In a way, the real goal of the earlier steps was the reduction of NAD and FAD for use in electron transport.

Now let's look at each of these steps in a little more detail. Ready? Here we go!

Glycolysis

Glycolysis begins as glucose enters the cell. Glucose is transported across the cell membrane by facilitated diffusion. Since facilitated diffusion, like all diffusion, is bidirectional, we need a way to keep the glucose in the cell and keep more glucose entering the cell. The first step in glycolysis takes care of that for us. In the first step, we use an ATP to phosphorylate glucose. That means we convert ATP to ADP and stick the liberated phosphate on the glucose. This renders the glucose unable to move back through the membrane (we've trapped it) and also helps maintain the gradient necessary for glucose to diffuse into the cell (once phosphorylated, it is no longer "glucose"). That works so well that we do it again. Now our glucose really is no longer glucose; it has two phosphate groups on it, and additionally, it has been converted to a fructose.

Now wait right there, you say! We have used up two ATP molecules when we are supposed to be making ATP! You are right, but the old adage is true: you have to spend money (ATP) to make money (ATP). Don't worry; we'll make lots more.

So, now our glucose has been converted to another monosaccharide (fructose) and had two phosphates added to it. It's time to split it in two. We split this one diphosphorylated six-carbon monosaccharide into two phosphorylated three-carbon monosaccharides. We will continue altering these two three-carbon molecules through several steps until we end up with two pyruvic acid molecules. Our $C_6H_{12}O_6$ glucose becomes two $C_3H_4O_3$ pyruvic acids. That means that we have some energy available (we've been splitting bonds) and some hydrogens available. What happened to this stuff?

With the energy we liberated, we produced a total of four ATP molecules (two per pyruvic acid). Since we used two ATP molecules early in this step, we have a net gain (profit) of two ATPs. This is not really that much, but it is better than a loss. We used the hydrogens liberated to reduce two NAD molecules to two NADH molecules that we can use in the electron transfer step. We also ended up with two pyruvic acid molecules that are still loaded with energy. We're ready for our next step: the transition reaction.

The Transition Reaction

This is the easiest step of all. There's nothing to worry about here.

Our two pyruvic acid molecules enter a mitochondrion (not necessarily together, but we'll assume they are sticking together). The problem is that mitochondria need acetic acid, not pyruvic acid. That's O.K., though; that's the reason for the transition reaction.

In the transition reaction, our three-carbon pyruvic acids are changed into two-carbon acetic acids. This involves oxidation (loss of hydrogen) and decarboxylation (loss of a carbon). So, what can we do with the carbon we cleave off? Since oxygen, from the pyruvic acid, stays with the carbon, we make carbon dioxide (CO_2) in this step. For each pyruvic acid that enters this step, we make one CO_2; since there are two pyruvic acids per glucose (in our previous step), we make two CO_2 molecules per glucose.

Now, since we oxidized the pyruvic acid, what do you suppose we do with the hydrogens? We stick them onto NADs. For each molecule of pyruvic acid, we produce one NADH; since we have two pyruvic acids per glucose (in our previous step), we make two NADH molecules per glucose. Again, we will use these reduced coenzymes when we get to the electron transfer step.

There is one more thing to think about, however. Our acetic acid is not actually ready for our next step. To enter the citric acid cycle, it needs to be bound to a vitamin B$_5$ derivative called coenzyme A (CoA). That too is part of this step. Acetic acid is bound to CoA, producing an active acetate known by its friends as acetyl CoA. We can now take our acetyl CoA into the citric acid cycle.

The Citric Acid Cycle

O.K., this is a little bigger step, but you can handle it. It's a cycle, which means once you've been through it, you can go around again and again until you really figure it out. Let's start with what we need to make it work. We need to bring our two-carbon acetyl CoA into this cycle (remember, we have two of these for every one glucose with which we started). Our acetyl CoA binds to the already present four-carbon oxaloacetic acid (part of the machinery of this cycle), making the six-carbon citric acid (the name told you that it had to be in here somewhere). The citric acid is what we will "work on" in this cycle.

In the next step, we decarboxylate the six-carbon citric acid, making a five-carbon molecule. The carbon that was released kept two oxygens, resulting in CO_2. We also carry out an oxidation and bind the hydrogen to an NAD, making an NADH molecule. This works so well that we do it again, going from our five-carbon molecule to a four-carbon molecule, again producing one CO_2 and reducing one NAD to NADH.

Now that we are back to a four-carbon molecule, we need to convert it into oxaloacetic acid so that we can continue the cycle with the next acetyl CoA that comes along. We do this through a series of oxidation-reduction reactions. In the process, we produce one molecule of ATP and reduce yet another NAD, and an FAD, which becomes $FADH_2$.

So, we get back to our starting point. What did we end up with? From one acetyl CoA, we produced two carbon dioxides, three NADH, one $FADH_2$, and one ATP. Since we have two acetyl CoA molecules for every glucose molecule with which we started, double these numbers when tallying up our score. As already stated, we will take these reduced coenzymes (NADH and $FADH_2$) into our final step, electron transport.

The Electron Transport Chain

Have you ever watched a group of grandparents sitting on a park bench? One, all the way at the end, will take out a stack of pictures of his (or her) grandchildren and pass them along one at a time. As each grandparent looks at each picture, it energizes him or her to display a big smile before passing it along (although undoubtedly they are thinking that this kid is not half as cute as his or her grandchild). This is how the electron transport chain works, although we're not dealing with grandparents and pictures.

The electron transport chain is a group of respiratory enzyme complexes composed of cytochrome coenzymes and other protein and protein-metal molecules. These complexes are located on the inner membrane of the two-membrane mitochondrial structure. The first enzyme complex in the chain receives hydrogens directly from the reduced NAD or FAD of our previous steps. They separate the hydrogen atoms into a proton and an electron, and pass electrons along, one to the next by oxidation reduction reactions, like our grandparents and their pictures. The protons (which we will call "hydrogens" for the sake of our discussion) are ejected from the respiratory enzyme complex. It is interesting to note that many toxins—cyanide, rotenone, and certain mercury compounds as examples—cause their toxic effect by interfering with this electron transport chain.

The ultimate fate of these electrons is that a molecule of oxygen (O_2) will be split into two oxygen ions ($2O^-$) by the delivery of these electrons. This results in the release of lots of energy. The cell needs to capture this energy. Just as each grandparent was energized to smile by each picture he or she was passing along, each respiratory enzyme complex is energized to pump hydrogen ions (protons) across the inner mitochondrial membrane by the electron it is passing along. In this way, we end up with lots of hydrogen outside of that inner membrane (in the space between the two mitochondrial membranes), and not much inside the mitochondrion.

So, what would the protons do if they could pass through the inner mitochondrial membrane? That's right; they would diffuse back into the center of the mitochondrion. The only way they can do this is by passing through channels that are present in the integral membrane protein complexes called ATP synthases. ATP synthase uses this flow of hydrogen to run its machinery, just like the old mills used a water wheel to capture the energy in flowing water to do work. ATP synthase uses the flowing hydrogens to phosphorylate (add a phosphate to) ADP, producing ATP. There is our oxidative phosphorylation, or production of ATP. That's what all this discussion has been about.

For each NADH, this step can generate three molecules of ATP. For each molecule of $FADH_2$, this step can produce two ATP molecules. We started with one molecule of glucose, so let's keep score. We had two reduced NADs from glycolysis, two more reduced NADs from the transition reaction, and six reduced NADs from the citric acid cycle. The citric acid cycle also gave us two reduced FADs. If we add them up, we have 10 NADH, which will produce a total of 30 molecules of ATP. Our two $FADH_2$ will give us four more ATPs, so that's a total of 34 ATPs. Since we already produced two ATP molecules in the first step (glycolysis), and two more in the citric acid cycle (one per each acetylCoA), we have produced a total of 38 molecules of ATP from the breakdown of our one molecule of glucose. Therefore, at peak efficiency, for each molecule of glucose consumed, we have gained 38 molecules of ATP.

Oh, by the way, the two oxygen ions that were formed as the electrons from this chain split an O_2 molecule each bind to hydrogen ions and produce a molecule of water.

I hope you followed all of that. It really is not that hard, but it is somewhat complicated. Go through it a few times, and write it down in an outline as you do. Look over Figure 3.12 carefully; then move on to our brief discussion on anaerobic cellular respiration.

Anaerobic Cellular Respiration

If you made it through our previous section, this will be easy. In fact, you already know most of it.

What happens when you run? Right. You eventually get out of breath and slow down. Why does that happen? Because you use up your supply of ATP in your muscles, and you can't deliver enough oxygen to those muscles to produce enough ATP to keep you going (a more accurate description of this is coming in Chapter 9, but this will do for now). So, your muscle cells have to switch to anaerobic cellular respiration. Let's think about how that works.

It starts the same way the aerobic system did, with glycolysis. But, since oxygen isn't present, NADH can't get rid of its hydrogens; they have no place to go. You see, if there is no oxygen present, there is nothing with which to make water (so the "grandparents won't pass along the pictures"); hydrogen is backing up. This makes the tissues acidic, and bad things begin to happen.

In your muscles, the NADH gives the hydrogens back to the pyruvic acid, converting the pyruvic acid into lactic acid. There's really nothing for these cells to do with lactic acid at this point, so that is the end of the story until more oxygen comes along. Some of the lactic acid will make its way to the liver, which can convert it back to glucose for storage as glycogen or use it in its own mitochondria. The rest of it acidifies your tissues and contributes to your need to breathe heavily at the end of the race.

Back to Our Mitochondria

So, here you see why mitochondria are considered the powerhouses of the cell. Muscle cells, neurons, and other highly active cells use lots of energy. They need lots of mitochondria to fulfill these needs. We must eat lots of energy-rich foods to supply them with the glucose and other molecules needed to convert ADP into ATP.

If you have found this topic fascinating, good news; we will revisit carbohydrate metabolism repeatedly throughout this book. If, on the other hand, you found this material difficult and confusing; don't despair. This is the most difficult section on this topic. Review it; look carefully at the diagrams. Write down what you have learned and what you actually understand about this topic. Don't be negative and say you understand nothing. Think. I am sure you know more than you are admitting to yourself. After writing down what you know, look over the "What You Should Know" section at the back of this chapter. Then look back into the chapter to fill in your knowledge. Go over it slowly, allowing each step to sink in. If you continue to have trouble, see your instructor. I am sure that he or she will be glad to help you.

A Slight Detour

We now have only one more organelle to consider. That is the centriole. The best time to think about that organelle is as we discuss the cytoskeleton. Therefore, let's move on to the cytoskeleton and include the centrioles there.

3.3 The Cytoskeleton: A Skeleton for Your Cells

The cytoskeleton is a special group of organelles. Just as you have a skeleton that is important in supporting your body, aiding in movement, and organizing the structure of your body; your cells have their own skeletal structure to do those things for them. This is the cytoskeleton.

Three Major Cytoskeletal Components

There are three major components to the cytoskeleton: microfilaments, microtubules, and intermediate filaments (Figure 3.1). They are described in **TABLE 3.1**. Microfilaments are approximately 6 nM in diameter. For information on these measurements, see Appendix A for details of the metric system. For comparison, 6 nM are equal to less than one one-thousandth the diameter of a red blood cell. Microfilaments are the smallest diameter component of the cytoskeleton, and are composed of the protein actin. Individual actin molecules bind to each other to form filaments. This is a common feature among structural proteins, so let's consider some terminology here. When we have individual molecules that have the ability to bind together, we call them monomers. Once they have bound to each other, we call them polymers. The process is called polymerization. Actin monomers polymerize into polymers in

Table 3.1   The Cytoskeleton

Cytoskeletal Component	Diameter*	Protein
Microfilaments	6 nM	Actin
Intermediate Filaments	12 nM	Keratin
		Vimentin
		Desmin
		Neurofilaments
		GFAP
Microtubules	24 nM	Tubulin

*These diameters are meant to show relative size and are somewhat variable depending on the preparation techniques used before measurement.

the form of filaments. It is these filaments that make up the microfilaments. We will learn about actin's role in muscle contraction elsewhere in this book (Chapter 9); however, actin and a group of actin binding proteins are found in many cell types.

Microtubules are made of the protein tubulin. As its name implies, tubulin polymers are tubular in structure. This is the component of the cytoskeleton with the largest diameter, approximately 24 nM. Their tubular design allows them to function in transport within the cell and in the movement of other structures within the cytoplasm. The centrioles are organelles made out of tubulin. In the centrioles the tubulin tubules are arranged as nine sets of three tubules each. This organelle is shown in Figure 3.1. The mitotic spindle is made up of microtubules and centrioles, and plays an important role in cell division (considered later in this chapter and in Chapter 14).

The intermediate filaments are intermediate in diameter, between the microfilaments and the microtubules. They were the third component of the cytoskeleton to be discovered and have survived a bit of controversy regarding their existence early on and their composition later on. We now know that they exist in almost all cell types, but their composition varies among cell types. Five different classes of proteins make up the intermediate filaments, varying with individual cell types. We will consider this fascinating topic further in our next chapter. You will then learn which cells express (produce) which intermediate filament protein and why that concept helps us to understand the many cell types in the body. Intermediate filaments give support to the cell, contributing to its shape and the location of organelles relative to each other and to the membrane within the cell.

FIGURE 3.13 shows a micrograph of the intermediate filaments in human cell grows in culture. This figure presents an accurate depiction of the cytoskeleton. Note how it is arranged as a fine network throughout the cell. See also that the net is most dense around the nucleus and in areas associated with the cell membrane. It is easy to understand from this picture that the cytoskeleton plays a major role in cell shape, movement, and the organization of the cytoplasmic space.

3.4 Cytoplasmic Inclusions

Before we get too far away from organelles, we need to think about the fact that not everything found within a cell is an organelle or a component of the cytoskeleton. It's sort of like your kitchen. Is everything in your kitchen an appliance? Sure, the stove is an appliance, and so is

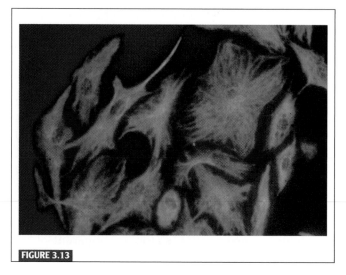

FIGURE 3.13

Photomicrograph of intermediate filaments in cells grown *in vitro* (cultured cells).

the refrigerator. They are appliances because they perform active functions just the way your organelles perform active functions in your cells. But the jar of peanut butter is not an appliance. Neither is the loaf of bread. They are simply stored goods.

Just like your kitchen can contain stored goods, so can your cells. We call these stored goods cytoplasmic inclusions. Cytoplasmic inclusions may be stored lipids, like the lipid droplet seen in adipose cells. They may be granules of glycogen, stored glucose (Figure 3.1). They may even be composed of debris left over after all the good materials from autophagy have been recycled. The cell can't find anything to do with that leftover junk. Rather than discard it, some cells are "pack rats" and store it away. This material is called lipofuscin, or wear-and-tear pigment. It, too, is a cytoplasmic inclusion. Chronic injury to cells that store lipofuscin will result in increased lipofuscin storage. In this way, pathologists examining heart tissue (cardiac muscle stores lipofuscin) can get some idea of its history. High amounts of lipofuscin would indicate ongoing disease (i.e., blocked arteries over a period of time).

3.5 Cell Division: Reproducing Your Cells

All right, we have thought about the components of individual cells and the fact that you were once only one cell, but now are composed of very many cells. How do these concepts relate to one another? There must be some way of getting from one cell to many cells, and it must somehow involve the organelles we have learned about. There is, and it does. We are now going to learn about cell division.

■ Mitosis and Cytokinesis: Two Big Events

Cell division, as I am presenting it here, actually involves two distinct processes: mitosis and cytokinesis. The term *mitosis* is used synonymously with cell division by some people. It is, in fact, only one part of cell division. The term *mitosis* indicates one form of division of the nucleus. We will learn about the other form of nuclear division in Chapter 14.

For cell division to be complete, we must have division of the cytoplasm as well as division of the nucleus. Division of the cytoplasm is called *cytokinesis*. Mitosis plus cytokinesis equals cell division. Mitosis can occur without cytokinesis. Think about that for a minute. What would happen if mitosis occurred and cytokinesis did not occur? You would end up with one cell with two nuclei. If that process was repeated, you could end up with one cell containing many nuclei. That does sometimes happen. *Syncytia* are cells with many nuclei. We will learn about these cells later on. Mitosis is actually only one of two processes that can result in syncytia.

■ The Cell Cycle: Taking a Larger View

Meanwhile, back to cell division. Let's start with a larger view of life. Think about the life of a human. Don't we have some form of a life cycle? We are born. We grow and develop through a number of stages. We may or may not reproduce, and may even reproduce many times. We may cease reproducing at some point. The cell too goes through a cycle called the cell cycle. This cycle is depicted in **FIGURE 3.14**. Notice that it consists of two circles, almost a figure eight. One circle has several phases, labeled mitosis, G_1, S, and G_2. This circle depicts the life of a cell that is actively dividing. Each time the cell completes one revolution of this cycle, it has divided into two cells. G_1 represents the time just after cell division in which the daughter cells are growing to their mature size. This is sometimes referred to as the resting phase, but the cell is not actually resting during G_1; it is carrying out the many functions a living cell must perform. It is essentially doing its "job." S phase represents the time that is spent replicating DNA in preparation for the next cell division. During the G_2 phase, the cell manufactures many of the substances needed for division. These three phases (G_1, S, and G_2) are grouped together into a time period called interphase. More on interphase in a moment.

The next phase of the cell cycle is labeled mitosis, and you already know what that means. You will note that the mitosis phase is subdivided into smaller units. We will consider those as the phases of mitosis in a moment. First, however, let's think about the other circle in our diagram of the cell cycle. This circle is labeled G_0. The G_0 phase is where we find cells that are

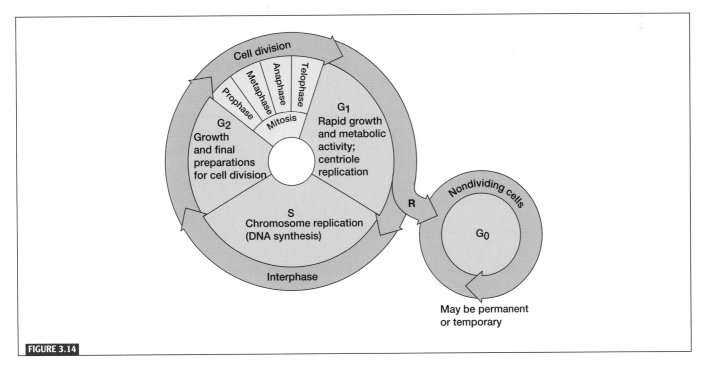

FIGURE 3.14

The cell cycle.

not actively dividing. Some cells, neurons for example, may cease division permanently. Some cells, those of the liver for example, may actually cease division for years, but resume division if the need for more of their type arises. These nondividing cells are in the G_0 phase, which is also a part of interphase. They may be very active from the standpoint of other functions, but they are not dividing. The point in their cycle where they make that decision to divide or not divide is labeled R and is called the restriction point.

■ The Phases of Mitosis: I Prefer My Anatomy Teacher

Now back to mitosis. Scientists look at complicated activities, systems, or whatever else they might be studying and break them down into understandable units. Different scientists might break down the same system into different units, based on their own need for understanding. The cycle of cell division has been broken down differently by different scientists. The scheme we will use is shown in Figure 3.16. Here we find five stages, a description of what occurs in each, and a diagram of cells in each stage. It is important that you learn the names of these stages and what happens in each stage. We will need this information in Chapter 14 as we examine the other form of nuclear division, called meiosis. It is often helpful to use a mnemonic device to assist us in this type of learning. To do this, take the first letter of each term and make up a sentence of words beginning with the same letters. interphase, prophase, metaphase, anaphase, and telophase can be transformed into I prefer my anatomy teacher.

There are a few additional facts you will need to understand mitosis as presented in this diagram. You will recall that the centrioles are organelles composed of tubulin, similar to the microtubules. It is during mitosis that the centrioles perform their function. During prophase, chromatin fibers condense, or pack, into chromosomes. Chromosomes are tightly packed DNA that are prepared for division. Four types of chromosomes are shown in **FIGURE 3.15**. Note that chromosomes are each made up of two identical units called chromatids, and these are joined in a constricted area called the centromere. Also during prophase, the centrioles (two per cell) move to the opposite ends, or poles, of the cell. From the centrioles, microtubules extend from pole to pole and from pole to chromosome. These microtubules make up the mitotic spindle. The action of the mitotic spindle and the centrioles is responsible for splitting the chromosomes and moving the chromatids away from one another as the nucleus divides. Note these features in

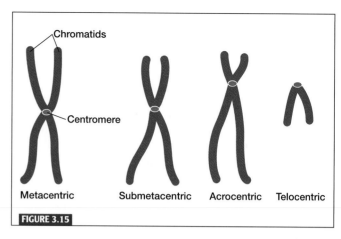

FIGURE 3.15

Chromosomes.

FIGURE 3.16. Note also that if cytokinesis is to accompany mitosis, it begins late in anaphase and is completed in telophase. This completes the cycle and results in two daughter cells.

Well, now that we see how cells divide, we can understand how we each began as one cell, but are now many cells. But here is a question to ponder: what type of cell were you when you began? You now have liver cells, neurons, muscle cells, and many other cell types. How did the one cell you were when you began become these many different cell types? This occurred through a process called differentiation, the topic we will next consider.

3.6 Differentiation: How Your Cells Become All That They Can Be

The many people you know have a lot of different vocations. Perhaps you know a scientist, a physician, a policeman, a farmer, and a pianist (**FIGURE 3.17**). Do they all perform the same tasks? Sure, they must all do some things like eating, sleeping, and paying taxes. But what about the things that the policeman does as part of his or her profession? Does the pianist do those things too? Probably not. Very few pianists examine crime scenes and arrest criminals. Could the pianist become a policeman tomorrow, if he or she chose to change jobs? Again, probably not. That career shift would require some major reeducation. Also consider when they became part of their profession. No matter how great a child prodigy the pianist might have been, she was not born a pianist. At birth she did not belong to any of those professions. No infant does. The infant grows, learns, gains specialized skills and abilities, and at some point becomes proficient

Stage	Description	Diagram

Interphase:
– Resting stage between divisions.
  This does not mean that the cell is resting; it may be quite active metabolically. It is simply resting from division.
– DNA replication occurs late in interphase.

Prophase:
– Chromatin fibers condense into chromosomes.
– Centrioles separate and move toward opposite poles.
– Mitotic spindle forms: this is composed of two sets of microtubules
   Continuous microtubules extend pole to pole (centriole to centriole)
   Chromosomal microtubules extend from centromeres (constricted region on the chromosome) to the centrioles at the poles
– Nuclear membrane disassembles and nucleoli become less distinct.

Metaphase:
– Centromeres line up along equatorial plane.

Anaphase:
– Division of centromeres: chromosomes split and chromatids move to opposite poles.

Telophase:
– Return to interphase conditions.
– Chromatids uncoil into chromatin fibers.
– Nuclear membrane reassembles.
– Nucleoli becomes more distinct.
– Centrioles replicate.

If cell division is to be complete, cytokinesis begins in late anaphase with the formation of a cleavage furrow around the cell. Cytokinesis is completed during telophase.

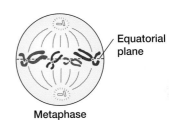

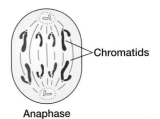

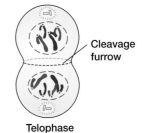

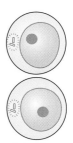

FIGURE 3.16

Mitosis and cell division.

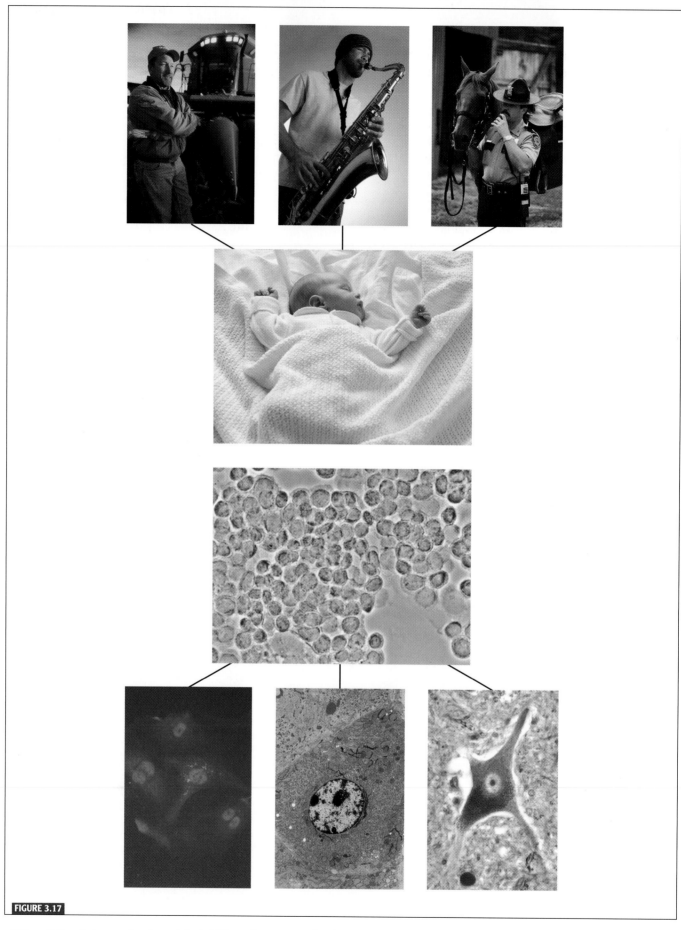

FIGURE 3.17

Differentiation. Just as people gain specialized abilities as they mature, cells gain specialized structures and functions through differentiation.

at performing the tasks necessary to join the workforce and be a professional. Now let's look at what cells do.

Your "original" cell was like the infant just described. It could not inactivate toxins the way your hepatocytes (liver cells) can or transmit impulses the way your neurons can or store energy the way your adipose cells can. It had no specialized functions. Other than the processes common to all living cells, its only function was a highly nonspecialized one: it could divide. As it became many cells, some of these gained special features. They activated specific genes that encoded certain proteins that caused them to alter their form and their organelle content until they had abilities their predecessors lacked (Figure 3.17). In a word, they differentiated.

Differentiation is defined as the process whereby cells gain specialized structures and functions. They also may give up non-specialized functions in the process. As a cell becomes completely differentiated, it may lack the ability to divide. This completely differentiated cell is said to be terminally differentiated. It is completely specialized to perform its particular function. A differentiated neuron can transmit electrical impulses; a differentiated skin cell can protect the surface of the body. In many tissues, a non-terminally differentiated population of cells remains present throughout life. These cells are present to act as a reservoir of dividing cells to replenish the terminally differentiated cells with their daughter cells. These cells are the stem cells of that tissue. Stem cells are the cells present in a tissue that have retained their ability to divide. It is the daughter cells of these stem cells that will differentiate and become the mature cells of that tissue, if more of those cells are needed.

This completes our discussion on the cell. Make sure you have learned the concepts listed in the "What You Should Know" section. If there is something about which you are not clear, go back to it before considering the next chapter. Test yourself with the questions contained in the "What Did You Learn?" section. Remember, these features are here to help you master this material. Use them to honestly assess your skills and make any adjustments necessary before it's too late.

Breaching Homeostasis . . . When Things Go Wrong

Disease and Injury at the Cellular Level

Although the focus of this text is the normal anatomy and physiology of the human body, some information regarding diseases or injuries to the body may help us understand normal functioning. Think about your car: don't you learn the most about how it works when something goes wrong with it? Well, at the end of certain chapters in this text we will have brief discussions about diseased or injured states that relate to the normal conditions we have been discussing. These sections are titled "Breaching Homeostasis: When Things Go Wrong . . ." for reasons that will become apparent when you read Chapter 5. For now, let's think about injured cells.

Injured cells? Sure. Although you may normally think of a person as having an injury or a disease, these phenomena actually occur at the cellular and molecular level. The signs and symptoms of injury or disease we observe in individuals are actually manifestations of chemical and cellular events.

Cells experience injury in a number of ways: they may lack some substance they need to function, they may encounter some toxin that keeps them from functioning properly, or they may experience some trauma, a physical injury that disrupts them in some manner.

So, let's think of some examples of these types of cellular injury. First let's think about what happens when a cell lacks some substance that it needs. This type of injury is called a deficiency. Many types of deficiencies exist. Stroke (blockage of an artery supplying the brain), drowning, strangulation, dietary malnutrition, and genetic abnormalities that limit the absorption of specific substances from the digestive tract may all lead to a deficiency. During a stroke or cerebrovascular accident, an artery that supplies blood to the brain becomes blocked. The cells that normally receive their nutrients from that artery suddenly have lost their supply. Although cells die through several types of injury during stroke (see the "Breaching Homeostasis" section of Chapter 12), one form of injury experienced in that area is due to a deficiency of oxygen (needed for aerobic cellular respiration) and glucose (needed also for energy). The lack of oxygen and glucose leads to a lack of ATP and an inability to maintain the activity of molecular pumps (ATPases) in the cell membrane. This disrupts membrane integrity and leads to cell death.

What about toxins? Toxins, sometimes called poisons, are molecules that interrupt normal cell functions. Cyanide, a toxin you have probably heard of, binds to the cytochromes involved in electron transport inhibiting the ability of cells to produce ATP. (You will note that many forms of injury result ultimately in inhibition of ATP synthesis.) You may have heard about toxins present in poisonous mushrooms. One such toxin, muscarine, is a parasympatheticomimetic, meaning that it binds to receptors on cell membranes and mimics the activity of a neurotransmitter in the parasympathetic nervous system (Chapter 12); in doing so, it may reduce cardiac and respiratory levels below those needed to sustain life. One final example is that of tetrodotoxin, the poison found in puffer fish. The species of puffer fish used in the Japanese delicacy Fugu carries tetrodotoxin in their internal organs. If that dish is not properly prepared and tetrodotoxin is consumed, it binds to the sodium channels of integral membrane proteins in neurons and inhibits neuronal function. This too is an example of an injury at the cellular level (blockage of the sodium channels) leading to morbidity (disease or injury).

Trauma covers a wide array of potential injuries. The term *trauma* implies injury from a physical event rather than a chemical event. Mechanical pressure, radiation injury, hyperthermia (excessive heat), and hypothermia (excessive cold) are all examples of trauma. Traumatic injuries affect cells by disrupting cell membranes, altering the shape of proteins within cells thereby inhibiting their activity, and in some cases by causing the production of toxins within the affected cell.

Cells adapt to injurious events in an attempt to survive, just as people do. They may increase in size (hypertrophy) by adding organelles to overcome the injurious agent. They may instead become smaller (atrophy). They may also increase their rate of proliferation (undergo hyperplasia). When the injury is too severe, or persists for a long period, cells may undergo necrosis (die).

What You Should Know

1. Your cells are your smallest living units.
2. Organelles are subcellular structures that perform specific functions within your cells.
3. Substances are stored within your cells as structures termed inclusions.
4. Your cell membranes or plasmalemma are constructed of a phospholipid bilayer with hydrophilic phosphate heads sandwiching the hydrophobic fatty acid tails.
5. Contained within the plasmalemma are the organelles and inclusions, in a gel called the cytosol.
6. Integral proteins span your cells' plasmalemma, while peripheral proteins are associated with the inner or outer surface of the membrane.
7. The plasmalemma is selectively permeable, allowing some substances to cross, but excluding others.
8. Diffusion, facilitated diffusion, and osmosis are passive transport mechanisms.
9. Active transport requires energy, usually in the form of ATP.
10. Endocytosis is a form of active transport that includes phagocytosis and pinocytosis.
11. Your cells' most prominent organelle is the nucleus.
12. DNA in the nucleus is usually in the form of chromatin fibers.
13. The nucleolus, also found in the nucleus, is the site of ribosome production and is largely made of RNA.
14. Ribosomes are the site of protein synthesis and may be bound to the endoplasmic reticulum or free in the cytoplasm.
15. The endoplasmic reticulum may be granular (with ribosomes) or agranular (without ribosomes).
16. Granular (rough) endoplasmic reticulum is the site where proteins are synthesized for export from the cell, or inclusion in the cell membrane.
17. Agranular (smooth) endoplasmic reticulum is the site of many chemical reactions, including the production of lipids and carbohydrates, and the breakdown of toxins.
18. The Golgi apparatus is located near the nucleus and is the site for the production of lysosomes and the modification of proteins produced by the rough endoplasmic reticulum.
19. Lysosomes, membrane-bound vesicles containing hydrolytic enzymes, are important for autophagy and following endocytosis.
20. Mitochondria are important organelles in the production of ATP.
21. Aerobic cellular respiration requires oxygen and yields 38 molecules of ATP per molecule of glucose, and involves the following steps: glycolysis, the transition reaction, the citric acid cycle, and electron transport.
22. During glycolysis, which occurs in the cytoplasm, one molecule of glucose is converted into two molecules of pyruvic acid; although we produce four ATP molecules, we use two in the process.
23. During the transition reaction (which occurs in the mitochondria), pyruvic acid is converted into acetic acid, which will be bound to coenzyme A, forming acetyl CoA. We also produce NADH for use in electron transfer. Carbon dioxide is a byproduct of this step.
24. In the citric acid cycle, our two-carbon acetic acid is bound to the four-carbon oxaloacetic acid, making the six-carbon citric acid. The citric acid is then converted back to the four-carbon molecule by the stepwise removal of two carbons. In doing this, we produce two carbon dioxides, three NADH, one ATP, and one $FADH_2$ per citric acid, and have again prepared our oxaloacetic acid to receive acetyl CoA.
25. The electron transport chain uses a group of respiratory enzyme complexes on the inner mitochondrion membrane to take hydrogens from NADH and $FADH_2$, which are then separated into protons and electrons. The electrons are passed from one enzyme complex to the next.
26. Energy released by the passing of these electrons is used to pump the hydrogen nuclei (the protons) from the center of the mitochondrion into the space between the two mitochondrial membranes.
27. The hydrogen nuclei diffuse back into the center of the mitochondrion through channels in the enzyme ATP synthase.
28. This movement of protons is used by the ATP synthase to phosphorylate ADP, producing ATP.
29. Anaerobic cellular respiration occurs when oxygen is not available. It is not nearly as efficient as aerobic respiration and it acidifies your tissues.
30. Microfilaments of actin, microtubules of tubulin, and intermediate filaments containing keratin, vimentin, desmin, neurofilaments, or GFAP make up the cytoskeleton.

What You Should Know (continued)

31. The cell cycle encompasses all phases of your cell's life; nuclear division, or mitosis, makes up one part of that cycle.
32. Mitosis plus cytokinesis equals cell division.
33. Specific activities of mitosis are arranged into five phases: interphase, prophase, metaphase, anaphase, and telophase
34. Differentiation is the process whereby cells gain specialized structures and functions.

What Did You Learn?

Multiple choice questions: choose the best answer.

1. _____ is another term for your cells' membranes.
   a. Cytoplasm
   b. Plasma
   c. Plasmalemma
   d. None of the above

2. Cell membranes are composed primarily of:
   a. Protein
   b. Polysaccharides
   c. Glycogen
   d. Phospholipids
   e. PVC

3. In a phospholipid bilayer, the hydrophobic fatty acid tails face:
   a. The internal and external environment of the cell
   b. Other fatty acid tails within the membrane
   c. They are randomly arranged.
   d. Fatty acid tails do not exist.

4. Channels through a membrane are likely to be in:
   a. Integral membrane proteins
   b. Peripheral membrane proteins
   c. Either of the above
   d. Neither of the above

5. The plasmalemma is:
   a. Fluid
   b. Self-repairing
   c. Semipermeable
   d. All of the above
   e. None of the above

6. Which of the following is an active process (requires energy)?
   a. Diffusion
   b. Osmosis
   c. Both of the above
   d. Neither or the above

7. What form of energy is used during facilitated diffusion?
   a. ATP
   b. ADP
   c. Glucose
   d. Triglycerides
   e. None of the above

8. Pseudopodia are used in:
   a. Phagocytosis
   b. Pinocytosis
   c. Both of the above
   d. Neither of the above

9. The nucleolus is predominantly made of:
   a. DNA
   b. RNA
   c. Both of the above
   d. Neither of the above

10. Insulin, a protein exported from the cells that produce it, is synthesized by:
    a. Free ribosomes
    b. Ribosomes on the rough endoplasmic reticulum
    c. Smooth endoplasmic reticulum
    d. None of the above

11. Toxins encountered by your cells are likely to be detoxified in the:
    a. Rough endoplasmic reticulum
    b. Smooth endoplasmic reticulum
    c. Golgi apparatus
    d. Nucleus
    e. Nucleolus

12. The Golgi:
    a. Modify and package secretory proteins
    b. Produce lysosomes
    c. Both of the above
    d. Neither of the above

What Did You Learn? (continued)

13. Which of the following does not occur in the mitochondria?

    a. Glycolysis

    b. The citric acid cycle

    c. Electron transport

    d. None of the above occurs in the mitochondria.

    e. All of the above occurs in the mitochondria.

14. Which of the following produces the most ATP?

    a. Glycolysis

    b. The citric acid cycle

    c. Electron transport

    d. None of these produce ATP

    e. Each of these steps produce a similar amount of ATP

15. Which of the following has the largest diameter?

    a. Microtubules

    b. Microfilaments

    c. Intermediate filaments

    d. Their diameters are all the same

16. Which of the following is composed of actin?

    a. Microtubules

    b. Microfilaments

    c. Intermediate filaments

    d. They are all composed of actin

    e. None of these are composed of actin

17. During which phase of mitosis do centrioles replicate?

    a. Metaphase

    b. Telophase

    c. Interphase

    d. Prophase

    e. Anaphase

18. During which phase of mitosis do chromosomes line up along the equatorial plane?

    a. Metaphase

    b. Telophase

    c. Interphase

    d. Prophase

    e. Anaphase

19. Put the following in their proper order:

    1. Metaphase

    2. Telophase

    3. Interphase

    4. Prophase

    5. Anaphase

    a. 3,4,1,2,5

    b. 3,4,1,5,2

    c. 1,5,4,2,3

    d. 2,4,3,5,1

    e. 2,1,3,4,5

20. Cells gain specialized structures and functions through:

    a. Mitosis

    b. Meiosis

    c. Diversion

    d. Graduation

    e. None of the above

Short answer questions: answer briefly and in your own words.

1. Please draw a diagram of a cell, showing the organelles. Label these organelles and list their functions.

2. Please draw a diagram of the plasmalemma showing orientation of the molecules of which it is composed. Include peripheral and integral proteins, and list some functions of these molecules.

3. Imagine that you are a scientist working on a new drug that will repair damage to the DNA that results in cancer. Where, within the cell, would that new drug have to be able to reach? What might keep that drug from reaching that part of the cell? What steps might you take to ensure that it reaches its target?

4. How do your cells generate the fuel they use to power their molecular machinery?

5. Think about the functions of the mitochondria. What would happen to the cell if the mitochondria stopped functioning? What other changes would that lead to?

6. Imagine that you have fallen down, scraped your knee, and driven bacteria and particles of dirt into the wound. Describe the manner in which your cells will remove that debris from the wound. What will they do with that debris once they have internalized it?

7. Describe the way in which your cells reproduce; include the terms for reproduction of the nucleus and the cytoplasm, and the stages of nuclear division.

8. Imagine that you work at a job that exposes you to low levels of an industrial chemical every day. Your hepatocytes, in trying to rid you of this mild toxin, actually turn it into a much more toxic substance. You have worked at this job for decades, and a new employee has just been hired to assist

What Did You Learn? (continued)

you. He has never been exposed to this chemical. During his first day on the job, there is a major spill of this substance and you are both badly exposed. Which of you is more likely to die from this large exposure? Please explain your answer in terms of the organelles involved.

9. Your liver cells differ from your bone cells in a number of ways. How do these cells differ from the early embryonic cells that were present at the beginning of your life? How are these differences generated?

10. Early embryonic stem cells can differentiate into any cell type in the body. If you could generate stem cells in adults and control their differentiation, what medical conditions do you think you could cure? What would be some potential uses for that technology?

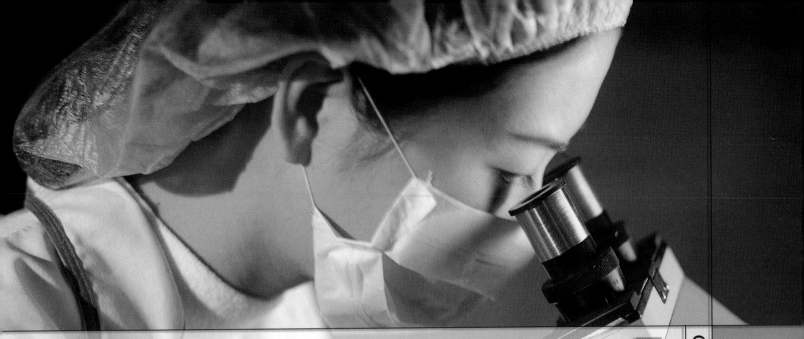

Construction Materials of Your Body: The Tissues

CHAPTER 4

What You Will Learn

- What tissues are and how they are used to construct our bodies.
- The names, characteristics, and examples of each of our five classes of tissue.
- The types of epithelial cells and the uses for each type.
- How the surfaces of epithelial cells may be modified to meet specific needs.
- The types of connective tissue and how they differ in composition and characteristics.
- The terms *parenchyma* and *stroma,* and how these concepts help us understand physiology.

4.1 Why Are We Interested in Tissues?

If you wanted to learn to be a builder or an architect, would it be enough to study fully constructed buildings? Wouldn't you also have to learn about the materials that are used to construct them? For a moment, think about the home in which you live (**FIGURE 4.1**). What was used to construct the outside walls? Perhaps they are brick or cement. They may be wood or wood covered with a modern plastic material. In any case, you can be sure that those materials were chosen because they met the need for strength, weatherproofing, and durability in the elements that walls require. Underneath this covering, you might find materials chosen for their ability to sup-

port the weight of the roof or upper floors, for their insulating properties, or for meeting other structural requirements. Additionally, you would find an electrical system made from materials with specific characteristics, such as the ability to conduct an electrical current or the ability to insulate against such a transfer of charge. Flexibility and longevity of these materials might also be considerations.

Now, what about the human body? Is it not also true that we are constructed of a variety of materials with specific characteristics that fill specific needs? Just as someone who wants to understand buildings must know the materials from which they are constructed, someone who is trying to understand the human body (such as you) must understand the materials from which the body is constructed. We learned about cells

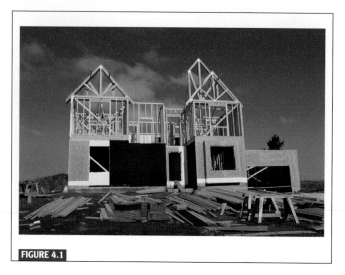

FIGURE 4.1

Like the construction materials used in buildings, tissues are the construction materials of the body.

in Chapter 3. Among the things we learned were the facts that they are the basic living units of our bodies and that there are many types of cells. Cells are organized into tissues; groups of similar cells working together to perform specific functions. These tissues are the construction materials of the body. In this chapter, we will learn about the tissues.

4.2 How to Learn This Information

It is important that you spend some time on the material presented in this chapter. Many students are anxious to move as quickly as possible into the chapters dealing with the systems of the body. Their desire for that information is understandable; it certainly is interesting subject matter! However, a little more time spent on the information contained in this chapter will be of benefit in the long run. It will save you a great deal of time when studying later chapters and will deepen your understanding of the information contained in those chapters. As you move through this book, you will need to know which tissues are present in specific locations throughout the body. If you know the abilities and characteristics of the various tissues, you will not have to memorize any of that material. Based on your knowledge of tissues, you will be able to reason out, on your own, which tissue belongs in a particular location. What could be a lot of memorization instead will become a sort of game in which you think about what tissue you would use in a specific location if you were designing the body. In no time you will find that you can choose the right tissue for each purpose. You will

also retain this ability much better than you would retain a memorized list of locations and tissues.

4.3 The Five Classes of Tissue

How Did We Settle on Five Classes?

As the study of anatomy progressed through the ages, people began to study the microscopic anatomy of the body (**FIGURE 4.2**). This science, called histology, greatly deepened our understanding of how the body works. Histology involves the examination of very thin sections of tissue through the microscope.

Histologists (microscopic anatomists) began to notice that some tissues had certain characteristics in common. To make sense of this information, they tried to group tissues together into categories. Some considered only three categories, while others chose four or five categories. Valid arguments could be made for each of these schemes. What was needed was a way to distinguish between the categories of tissues independent of their microscopic anatomy. Perhaps a biochemical marker could be found that would separate tissues into unique classes. During the 1970s and 1980s, such markers were found. In the years that followed, highly useful tools were developed from this knowledge. Read on and imagine how diagnostic pathologists use this information daily to determine the specific diagnosis of various cancers and how researchers use this information as they study differentiation of stem cells and how various cell types travel throughout the body and interact with each other.

So That's Why We Learned about Intermediate Filaments!

In Chapter 3, we learned about the cytoskeleton. We learned of three major components of the cytoskeleton: microtubules composed of tubulin, microfilaments composed of actin, and intermediate filaments composed of five classes of related proteins. At that time, you read that we would return to intermediate filaments later in this book. Now it's time to learn about the role of the intermediate filaments in our understanding of the tissues.

The five classes of intermediate filaments are expressed (produced by cells) in a tissue-specific manner. That means that each type of tissue expresses one specific type of intermediate filament. Notice, in **TABLE 4.1**, that there are five classes of tissue. Special features characterize each class of tissue, and each class expresses a specific intermediate filament protein. In the paragraphs that follow, and in later chapters, we will explore these classes of tissue in more detail.

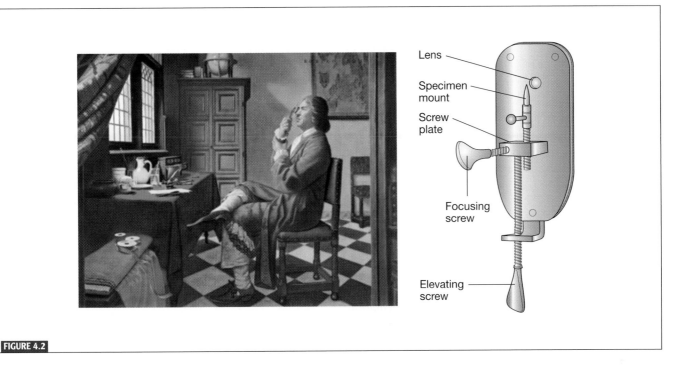

FIGURE 4.2

Seventeenth-century scientist Anton van Leeuwenhoek and his microscope.

Epithelial Tissues: Linings

Think of any surface in your body: perhaps the outer surface, or the surface of a body cavity, or even the surface of a duct within an organ. All of these surfaces are lined with cells. The cells that line these surfaces are all epithelial cells, components of the tissues we call epithelium. As such, they share a number of features in common. These features are listed in **TABLE 4.2**.

Characteristics of Epithelial Cells

We have already learned that epithelial cells all express keratin as their intermediate filament proteins, but what about their morphological characteristics, those observed by the histologists who first defined this category. Well, the first and most obvious characteristic is that epithelia are always lining something. In some cases it may be more difficult to see what they are lining than in other cases, but this is a basic underlying feature of epithelia. Another characteristic is that they sit on a basement membrane. A basement membrane is a thin membrane made of protein, glycoprotein, and proteoglycan, which anchor the epithelial cells in place.

The next characteristic is that they have intercellular junctions (**FIGURE 4.3**). These are special features of the plasmalemma where the cells are in contact with each other. One type, the tight junction, locks cells together, making them difficult to dislodge and creating a tight seal between them. Another type, the gap junction, contains minute channels that allow ions to move between cells. This serves as a form of communication

Table 4.1 The Five Classes of Tissue

Tissue Type	Major Characteristics	Intermediate Filament
Epithelium	Lining	Keratin
Mesenchymal derivatives	Connective tissues, "packing," support	Vimentin
Muscle	Contractility	Desmin
Nervous	Electrical activity, receive and respond to stimuli	Neurofilaments
Glia	Support for the central nervous system	GFAP

Table 4.2 Common Characteristics of Epithelial Cells

Line some surface
Express keratin intermediate filament proteins
Sit on a basement membrane
Have intercellular junctions
Are avascular

among adjacent cells. Note that for cells to have intercellular junctions, they must be situated in direct contact with each other and, therefore, must not have a lot of intercellular space.

The final characteristic is that they are avascular. Please note that the prefix "a" before a word indicates the absence of that item. Since vascular refers to blood vessels, the term *avascular* indicates that no blood vessels are present. Epithelial tissues lack blood vessels. The nutrients needed by epithelial tissues are supplied by vasculature present in tissues deep to the epithelial basement membrane.

Functions of Epithelia

What are epithelia there for anyway? Cells have jobs to perform, just like people. This is as true of epithelia as it is of other cells. The types of jobs performed by epithelia are many and highly varied. We will learn about them in great detail throughout this textbook. For now, a simple list will suffice. Epithelia are involved in the following functions: protection, secretion, excretion, absorption, and in certain cases, sensory reception, and contraction.

There are a number of different types of epithelia that are specialized for performing specific functions. They can be distinguished from one another in several ways. First, the shape of individual cells present within the epithelium determines the type of epithelium. Second, the organizational arrangement of one layer or multiple layers determines another characteristic of the epithelial type. Finally, the presence of specialized features on the superficial (apical) surface gives further detail to their type and function.

Epithelial Cell Shapes

TABLE 4.3 and **FIGURE 4.3** demonstrate the various shapes of epithelial cells. They also indicate the activities for which each shape best equips these cells, and presents analogies you can use to think about the relationship between shape and function.

As you can see, like the shingles on your roof, squamous cells present little surface area on their sides to catch against passing fluids or other forces, making them resistant to loss by abrasion. Further, if substances are to diffuse through the epithelium (remember, those substances must be able to pass through the phospholipid bilayer of the plasmalemma), a squamous cell is thin enough to allow rapid diffusion. Other cell shapes would present a larger distance for the molecules to cross, thus slowing the rate of diffusion.

Cuboidal cells have a greater volume of cytoplasm. More time would be required for substances to diffuse

Table 4.3   Epithelial Cell Shape

Epithelial Cell Type	Shape	Characteristic	Analogy
Squamous	Flat	Allows easy diffusion	Window screens are thin to allow breezes to easily pass through.
		Resists loss by lifting	Roofing shingles are flat to resist lifting by the wind.
Cuboidal	Cube shaped	More cytoplasmic space for organelles	A small workshop needs space for tools and supplies.
		Short enough to allow easy transport through the cell	
Columnar	Column shaped	Ample cytoplasmic space for synthetic organelles and for storage of products	A large factory needs room for machinery and storage of goods before shipping.

through these cells, making them a poor choice for a location where that is a prime activity. However, what would be required if active transport from one surface of the cell to the other surface (through the cell) were to be a major activity? For one thing, an ample source of energy would be required. That means lots of mitochondria. Think about the shape of a squamous cell. Does that cell have enough room within it to hold all those mitochondria? Won't this cell also need lots of rough endoplasmic reticulum to produce the integral membrane proteins that serve as molecular pumps? These organelles require space, more space than is present in a squamous cell.

Another use for the cuboidal cell is synthetic activity, where relatively small amounts of a substance need to be produced at one time. Hormones are an example of this type of product. A certain volume of cytoplasm is required to house the synthetic organelles, but not an excessively large cytoplasmic volume.

Columnar cells, on the other hand, have a very high cytoplasmic volume. Think of a cell that will be called upon to produce large quantities of some substance. It may also be required to store that substance in bulk for release at some specific time. Mucus is produced in this way. Columnar cells are just the cells for this purpose.

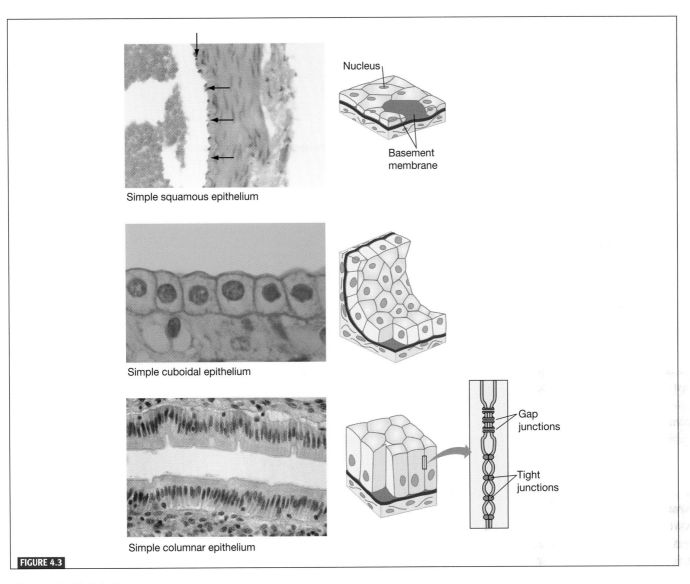

Simple squamous epithelium

Simple cuboidal epithelium

Simple columnar epithelium

Nucleus

Basement membrane

Gap junctions

Tight junctions

FIGURE 4.3

Shapes of epithelial cells.

Epithelial Organizational Arrangements

Epithelial cells can be present in one layer (*simple epithelia*), multiple layers (*stratified epithelia*), or an arrangement that looks like multiple layers when, in fact, only one layer is present (*pseudostratified epithelia*). **FIGURE 4.4** demonstrates each type. Where would you expect to find simple epithelia? Would it be present in locations exposed to abrasion? No, you would not find simple epithelia in those locations. Simple epithelia are restricted to locations that do not experience physical abrasion. How about locations where the epithelia are involved in absorption or secretion? Those would be good locations for simple epithelia. Epithelial cells arranged in that way would have access to a vascular supply located below their basement membranes (remember, epithelia are avascular) for the materials needed to synthesize their product or to carry away the substances they absorb. They would also have direct access to the lumen of the structure that they line.

Stratified epithelia are found in places where abrasion is likely to occur. As you move about during the day, doesn't the surface of your body come into contact with other surfaces, some of which are abrasive? You might brush against the wall as you pass down the crowded corridor of your school. You might scrape against the basketball court after you block an opponent's shot. Even the clothes you wear abrade the surface of your body as you move about. Surfaces exposed to such abrasion need protection. Stratified epithelia offer protection; if the cells of the very top layer are scraped off, there are other cells located below them to maintain the body's protective barrier. Much of the dust we encounter every day is actually abraded epithelial cells!

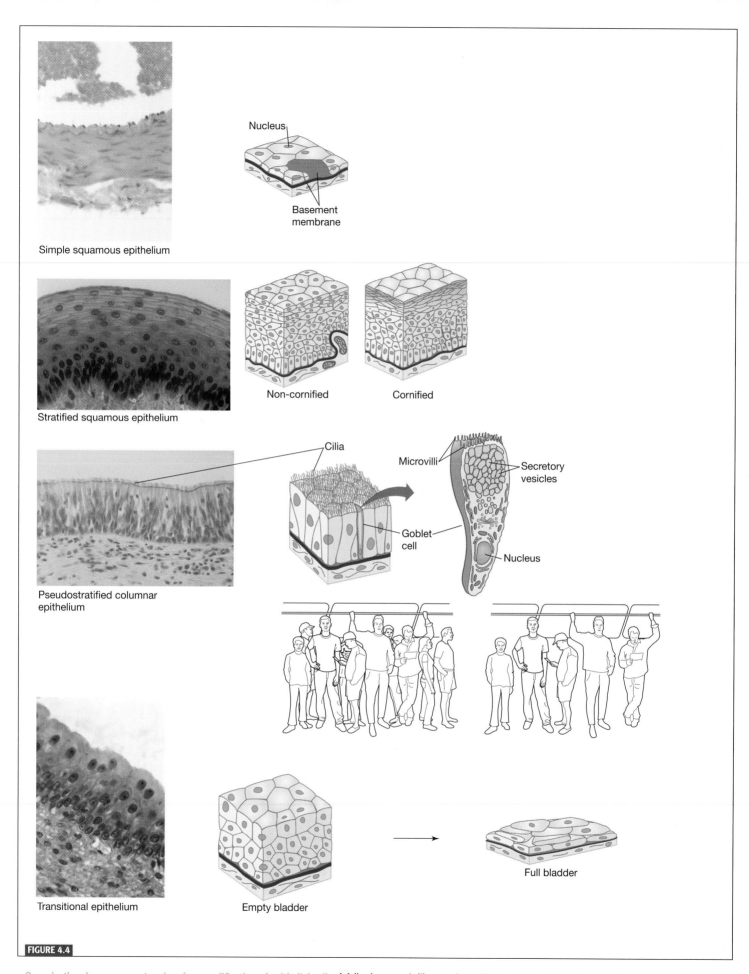

Nucleus

Basement membrane

Simple squamous epithelium

Stratified squamous epithelium

Non-cornified

Cornified

Cilia

Pseudostratified columnar epithelium

Microvilli

Secretory vesicles

Goblet cell

Nucleus

Transitional epithelium

Empty bladder

Full bladder

FIGURE 4.4

Organizational arrangement and surface modification of epithelial cells. A full subway car is like pseudostratified epithelium. Even after several people leave, the car still appears full.

When examining a stratified epithelium under the microscope, remember to look at the cells of the most superficial layers to determine which type of stratified epithelium you are examining. The shape of the cells in the deep layers does not indicate the epithelial type. The cells of the deep layers (the basal layers) are the stem cells of the stratified epithelium, dividing to provide new cells. As the daughter cells move from the basal layer toward the superficial layers, they differentiate, taking on the characteristics of the mature epithelium. These changes include a change in shape of the individual cells to that of their specific type, such as squamous or cuboidal.

Pseudostratified epithelia look stratified on quick examination, but when you look more closely, you see that every cell is in contact with the basement membrane, whether it reaches the luminal surface or not. This is an important distinction to make between stratified epithelia and pseudostratified epithelia. There is no true layering in pseudostratified epithelium. Why would cells be arranged in this manner?

Imagine a subway train in a very busy city at rush hour (Figure 4.4). As the train pulls into the station, the platform is crowded with tired, hungry people in a hurry to get home. The doors open and the train fills with passengers. So many people get on the train that they are all pressed together. Their arms are pressed to their sides; no one has even an inch in which to move. As the train reaches the first station outside the city, several passengers get off. The same thing happens at the next few stations. If you would look into the train, however, it would still look completely full. Passengers were initially so crammed together that, as some of them leave, the rest simply relax and expand a little. Every inch of floor space is still occupied.

That is how it is with cells in a pseudostratified epithelium. The cells are so tightly packed together that if some were to die, the rest would still completely cover the basement membrane. In this way, they would continue to serve as a protective barrier over the basement membrane, protecting the underlying tissues from exposure. The cells that line airways, such as the trachea, are composed of pseudostratified epithelium. If exposure to cold dry air, dust, fumes, or respiratory viruses were to cause the death of some of these cells, there would still be enough cells present to maintain a protective barrier.

One more epithelial type should be considered at this time. Think about the activities of your urinary bladder. Perhaps you use the restroom before you enter the classroom. Lectures can be very long, however, and by the time the lecture ends, your bladder may feel as if it is about to burst! What has happened to the size and shape of your bladder? As your bladder fills with urine,

its walls get stretched. As it empties, the walls regain their smaller dimension. The epithelium that lines the bladder has to be able to stretch and recoil, yet maintain a protective barrier over the basement membrane at all times. To accomplish this, the bladder is lined with an epithelium composed of multiple layers of irregularly shaped cells. These cells alter their shape as they are stretched. In an empty bladder, the cells are round to pear shaped. As the bladder wall is stretched, they flatten out. Due to their ability to change shape, these cells are called transitional epithelium.

Epithelial Cell Surface Modifications

We have discussed the types of epithelial cells based on shape and organizational arrangement. There are several potential modifications of the these cell types to be considered (see Figure 4.4). The surfaces of individual epithelial cells can be described as follows. The *basal surface* is the one that is against the basement membrane, the "bottom" of the cell. The *lateral surfaces* of the cell are the "sides" of the cell, facing adjacent cells. The *apical surface* is the "top" of the cell, the exposed surface.

How could we increase the exposed surface area of a cell? We could form the plasmalemma of the apical surface into a great number of fingerlike projections. There are many instances in which this is a desirable feature, such as when the surface of the cell is used for absorption. An example of this is the cells that line the small intestine. Much absorption of digested substances from food must occur here. By folding the apical surface of these cells, we have much more surface area available through which absorption can occur. These fingerlike projections are called microvilli. Epithelial cells that possess microvilli are said to have a brush border because of the brushlike appearance it gives these cells.

There are also epithelia that need to be able to move a substance (mucus, for example) along their surface. How can that be accomplished? When you are cooking a soup, don't you place a spoon in the soup and move it about to stir it up, to move the contents of the pot around? Just as you can place a spoon in the soup and stir, epithelial cells may have projections on their apical surface called cilia that they can move to propel substances such as mucus. They move their cilia in a beating motion, which causes the mucus to move in one direction. Epithelia that possess cilia are referred to as ciliated epithelia. One example would be the pseudostratified ciliated columnar epithelium of the trachea.

A special modification is present in the apical layers of some stratified squamous epithelia. The stratified squamous epithelium that lines the outer surface of your body (the epithelium of your skin) must be highly resistant to abrasion. This resistance is accomplished by covering this epithelium with a layer of dead cells. This layer acts as a sort of armor over your body (see Chapter 20). It is especially thick in areas exposed to heavy abrasion, such as your palms and your heels. This feature is called *cornification*, and these epithelia are called cornified stratified squamous epithelia. Perhaps you have noticed that if you perform hard work for a period of time, such as preparing and planting your garden in the spring, you will develop calluses on your hands. Calluses are thickenings of this cornified layer. Cornification is sometimes referred to as *keratinization;* however, as we know that all epithelia contain keratin, this term is somewhat misleading.

Cornification is not found in locations that are kept moist, even if abrasion occurs at that site. The presence of a cornified layer is not compatible with moisture, which is present in these locations as a lubricant. Think about how the skin of your fingers wrinkles when you keep your hands in water too long. This wrinkling is caused by the absorption of water by your fingers' cornified layer. *Noncornified* stratified squamous epithelium is found in locations that are exposed to abrasion but need to be kept lubricated. Two such locations are the vagina and the oral cavity. Imagine trying to eat crackers if your oral cavity was not lubricated!

One additional modification that we need to consider involves nearly the entire cell, as opposed to just the surface. Imagine a cell that makes a large quantity of some substance and needs to be able to accumulate this product for release all at once. A very large cytoplasmic inclusion would be present in this cell just for this purpose. In fact, this inclusion might fill the majority of the volume of this cell. Wouldn't columnar cells be the best type to house this inclusion? The cells that I am referring to are called goblet cells. Notice in Figure 4.4, the gobletshape of the mucus-filled inclusion in these cells. Goblet cells are a special type of columnar cell that serves as a unicellular (single-cell) gland. Goblet cells are abundant in places that need much mucus, such as the trachea and large intestine.

We are now ready to begin thinking about which epithelia we will find in specific locations. **TABLE 4.4** presents several examples. We will continue to expand this list as we explore the body in later chapters.

■ *Mesenchymal Derivatives:* A Fancy Term for Some Simple Tissues

The next class of tissue we will consider is the mesenchymal derivatives. This class is often referred to as connective tissues; however, *mesenchymal derivatives* is a more precise term. All tissues in this class are derived from the embryonic tissue known as mesenchyme. Some are typical connective tissues; others have characteristics similar to the typical connective tissues but are specialized in one or more ways.

Characteristics of Mesenchymal Derivatives

So, what are the characteristics of mesenchymal derivatives? Unlike epithelia, the cells in the mesenchymal derivatives are not closely packed. In fact, there is usually a great deal of space between the cells in these tissues. This space is filled with extracellular matrix. In typical connective tissues, the extracellular matrix is composed of protein fibers and a gel-like substance called amorphous ground substance.

Table 4.4	Examples of Epithelia in Selected Locations
Epithelium	**Location and Function**
Simple squamous	Lining the alveoli in the lungs, allowing rapid exchange of gases between the blood and the external environment. Also lining capillaries to allow rapid exchange between the blood and the surrounding tissues.
Simple cuboidal	Lining tubules in the kidney, adding substances to the developing urine (tubular secretion) and removing needed substances from the developing urine (tubular resorption).
Simple columnar	Lining the intestinal tract, producing mucus, and absorbing nutrients. Often includes goblet cells.
Pseudostratified ciliated columnar	Lining the trachea and major bronchi, producing and moving mucus to trap and remove dust. Includes goblet cells.
Noncornified stratified squamous	Lining the mouth and regions of the pharynx through which food travels, providing protection from abrasion in a moist environment.
Cornified stratified squamous	Covering the surface of the body (the skin), providing protection from abrasion, becoming thicker and more resilient with increased exposure to abrasion.
Transitional	Lining the urinary bladder, stretching and recoiling to provide protection as the bladder fills and empties.

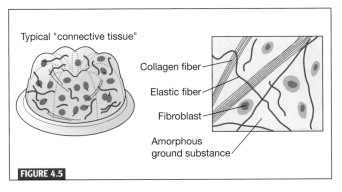

Typical "connective tissue"

Collagen fiber

Elastic fiber

Fibroblast

Amorphous
ground substance

FIGURE 4.5

Mesenchymal derivatives (connective tissues) are composed of cells and extracellular matrix. Extracellular matrix consists of fibers and amorphous ground substance.

Types of Mesenchymal Derivatives: A Recipe for Jell-O Salad

To understand the differences between the various mesenchymal derivatives, we need to be able to picture the cells and matrix in our minds. Let's think about something that is put together in a similar manner (**FIGURE 4.5**). Have you ever eaten a salad of Jell-O containing pieces of fruit? Let's now think about a hypothetical Jell-O salad. In this salad, we will use three ingredients: Jell-O, grapes, and pasta. If we use green grapes and linguini in one salad, and purple grapes and angel hair (very thin) pasta in another salad, wouldn't we have two different salads? We could continue to make these variations, using regular spaghetti and concord grapes in yet a third salad. Incidentally, I do not recommend eating Jell-O salad made with my recipe; it is for instructive purposes only! The variations in this recipe are very similar to the variations used to produce the different types of connective tissue.

The fibers of mesenchymal derivatives compare to the pasta in our salad. There are three different types of fiber used in our connective tissues. Collagenous fibers are the largest diameter fibers (like the linguini pasta in our illustration). They are made of the protein collagen and are very strong. Elastic fibers, composed of the protein elastin, are highly elastic (stretchy). They are thinner than collagenous fibers (like the regular spaghetti in our illustration). Finally, the reticular fibers are the thinnest fibers used in connective tissue (just as the angel hair pasta is the thinnest pasta in our illustration). These fibers are also composed of collagen.

The cells of mesenchymal derivatives are analogous to the grapes in our salad. The presence of different types of cells would result in different connective tissues. Alterations to the amorphous ground substance would be similar to using different flavors or consistencies of Jell-O. Amorphous ground substance is made up of a variety of proteins, glycoproteins, and proteoglycans.

Typical Connective Tissues

The typical connective tissues are presented in **TABLE 4.5**. The first connective tissue we will discuss is loose connective tissue (**FIGURE 4.6**). It is called *loose* connective tissue because of the loose arrangement of fibers and cells in the amorphous ground substance. The major cell type present is the fibroblast. As a mesenchymal derivative, this cell expresses vimentin as its intermediate filament protein. Fibroblasts are generally spindle shaped and are widely scattered throughout the extracellular matrix. These cells produce and maintain the fibers and ground substance of this matrix.

The main fiber type of loose connective tissue is the collagenous fiber. Here they are not abundant enough to add strength, but are loosely arranged to add bulk or dimension. It is in this and one other type that we truly see connective tissue as a "packing," a tissue that takes up space, much as styrofoam pellets or crumpled newspaper take up space around objects packed in a box.

Table 4.5   The Typical Connective Tissues

Connective Tissue	Location and Function
Loose connective tissue	Beneath the skin, around muscles, and in other locations where "packing" is required. This tissue changes shape, cushioning the structures it surrounds, as the body moves.
Dense irregular connective tissue	In organ capsules, it provides strength where forces are applied in many directions.
Dense regular connective tissue	In tendons and ligaments, acting as cables connecting together muscles and bones.
Elastic connective tissue	Provides elasticity to the walls of the great arteries, the vocal cords, the anterior abdominal wall, and other locations.
Adipose tissue	Typical locations include the breast, buttocks, and other subcutaneous sites. Also found in the mesentary and other internal locations. Serves as a reservoir for energy, a thermal insulator, and a cushion.
Reticular connective tissue	Provides a fine scaffolding within our hematopoietic organs, giving support and three-dimensional structure.

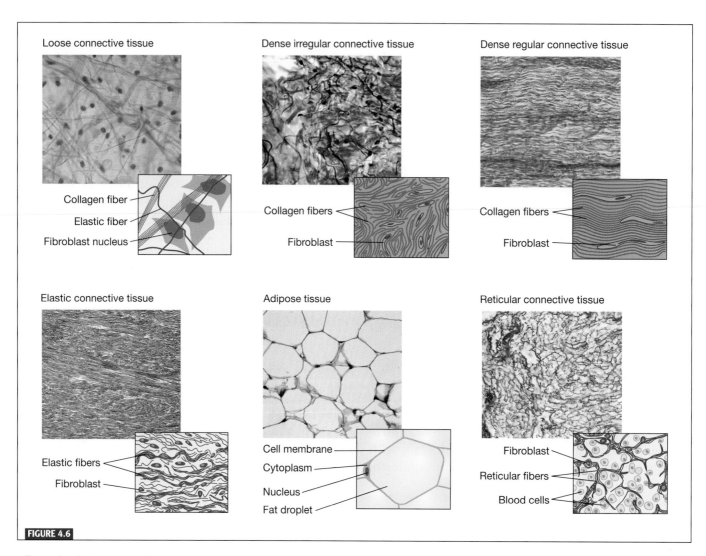

FIGURE 4.6

Types of typical connective tissues.

Dense connective tissue has the same cells, ground substance, and fibers as loose connective tissue, but here the fibers are abundant and densely arranged. So densely-packed are these fibers that there is little space left for cells and blood vessels. This tough tissue is, therefore, very slow in healing after injury (think, for example, of a torn tendon). To use our Jell-O salad analogy, the difference between loose connective tissue and dense connective tissue is the amount of linguini in the salad. Dense connective tissue has much more collagenous fiber (linguini) than loose connective tissue. Dense connective tissue is used where strength is needed; the dense arrangement of collagenous fibers provides much strength. There are two types of dense connective tissue, based on how the fibers are organized.

In dense irregular connective tissue (Figure 4.6), the fibers run in all directions. This form is used where tension will be applied to the connective tissue in multiple directions. Picture a basketball. Fibers are used in con-

struction of a basketball so it will retain its shape as it is filled with air and exposed to the extreme forces applied as it is dribbled, passed, and bounced. The forces applied to organs, such as the kidney and testes, are similar. As these organs produce their respective products (urine and sperm), these products must be pushed out of the organ and down a tube. There is, of course, resistance to flow in this tube. We will learn about this resistance in Chapter 19. To picture this resistance, think of exhaling through your garden hose. Even with both ends open, you will feel resistance as you blow through the hose. In the case of these organs, such resistance could result in retained product and swelling of the organ if some mechanism were not in place to counteract that force. A capsule of dense irregular connective tissue fills that need. Fibers run in all directions because the forces that would swell the organ are applied in all directions.

Dense regular connective tissue is found in locations where strength is needed, but force is applied in one direction only. Here, all of the collagenous fibers are arranged parallel to one another (Figure 4.6). In our Jell-O salad analogy, picture making this salad with raw linguini and not stirring the Jell-O as we put in the linguini. Tendons and ligaments are made of dense regular connective tissue. Tendons attach muscle to bone; ligaments attach one bone to another bone. The forces being overcome in both cases are in one direction only. The tendons and ligaments, therefore, work much like the cables that hold up a suspension bridge.

Elasticity is the ability to return to shape after stretching. In locations where elasticity is required, we find elastic connective tissue (Figure 4.6). Again we find fibroblasts as the main cell type and a ground substance similar to that in loose and dense connective tissues. Here, however, the main fibers are not collagenous, but elastic fibers made of elastin. These are very stretchy fibers and have a wavy appearance when not stretched. Elastic connective tissue is found in the walls of the great arteries that must stretch as the heart forces blood into them. They must then recoil as the heart stops ejecting blood between contractions. We will learn more about this interesting phenomenon in Chapter 16.

Adipose tissue is similar to loose connective tissue except that an additional cell type has been added in very large quantities (Figure 4.6). That cell is the adipocyte or fat cell. Adipocytes are adapted for the storage of large quantities of fat. This allows adipose tissue to act as a reservoir of energy, to serve as thermal insulation (built-in long underwear), and to provide a cushion underneath our skin. We learned about the storage of energy as lipids in Chapters 2 and 3.

The last typical connective tissue we must consider is reticular connective tissue (Figure 4.6). The term *reticular* indicates the concept of a network. Reticular fibers (the finest fibers, like angel hair pasta) are found in reticular connective tissue.

Our blood-forming (hematopoietic) organs have a complex three-dimensional structure. To produce and maintain this structure, some framework or scaffolding must be in place. Strength is not a major requirement of this framework, but it must not occupy too great a space or these organs would have to be excessively large. Reticular connective tissue meets those requirements. We will see evidence of reticular connective tissue in the structure of organs such as the spleen and lymph nodes.

Cartilage

Cartilage is another form of mesenchymal derivative. Again our Jell-O salad analogy applies. Think of Jell-O Jigglers, the extra-thick form of jello, made so kids can carry it around and eat it out of their hands. Well, if we make our Jell-O salad with Jell-O Jigglers rather than conventional Jell-O, we will have something similar to cartilage.

In cartilage, changes have been made to the amorphous ground substance so that it has a firm, almost plastic texture. You have probably seen cartilage when eating chicken. The white covering seen on the ends of bones, in joints, is cartilage.

Another difference between typical connective tissues and cartilage is the cell type present. The fibroblasts of typical connective tissues have been replaced with chondrocytes. The word root *chondro-* implies cartilage, so chondrocytes are "cartilage cells." Chondrocytes are loosely scattered throughout the extracellular matrix, but each chondrocyte is found in a small cavity in the matrix called a lacunae. The term *lacuna* means "little lake." Chondrocytes produce and maintain the amorphous ground substance and fibers of cartilage.

Three types of cartilage exist, their differences mainly being which fibers are present within each type (**FIGURE 4.7**). Hyaline cartilage is the white material found on the articular surfaces of bones, that is, where bones meet within joints. Hyaline means glassy, as it looks similar to white glass. The name hyaline was given before the invention of plastic; however, to the touch, hyaline cartilage seems much more like plastic than glass. Hyaline cartilage contains relatively few fibers (Figure 4.7). This tissue provides a smooth surface for movement and a cushion to absorb shock where bones meet.

Fibrocartilage is found where additional strength is required, such as in the intervertebral disks between the vertebrae in your spinal column. These disks serve as a cushion between vertebrae and aid in movement. The addition of collagenous fibers to the same ground substance and cells as are found in hyaline cartilage results in fibrocartilage (Figure 4.7).

Elastic cartilage results from adding elastic fibers to the cartilage extracellular matrix. Just as collagenous fibers contributed strength to fibrocartilage, elastic fibers contribute elasticity (flexibility) to elastic cartilage (Figure 4.7). The pinna of your outer ear contains a core of elastic cartilage. Notice how you are able to fold your pinna and it returns to its original shape. Elastic cartilage provides this flexibility.

Other Mesenchymal Derivatives

Bone is a mesenchymal derivative, but will be discussed only briefly here. Chapter 6 deals extensively with bone as a tissue. Although not a typical connective tissue, it does have the characteristic features we have been discussing (**FIGURE 4.8**). There are several cell types present, and almost a third of the extracellular matrix is composed of fibers. The amorphous ground substance of

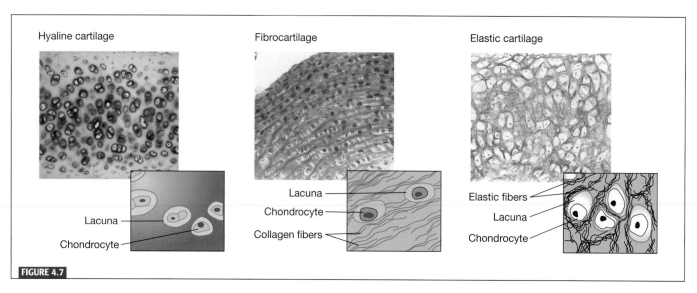

FIGURE 4.7

Types of cartilage.

bone contains calcium salts that have precipitated, making the extracellular matrix hard. This would be similar to adding cement to our Jell-O salad recipe! We will discuss this in greater detail in Chapter 6.

Blood is another atypical connective tissue. Blood certainly has cells present within it (Figure 4.8). It also has amorphous ground substance, but in this case it is liquid, not gel or solid. It is as if the Jell-O in our salad did not set, but stayed liquid. This ground substance is called plasma. Are fibers present in this connective tissue? Yes, but in an unconventional form. While the blood is flowing within your blood vessels, the protein fibrinogen, of which these fibers are composed, is in solution as individual molecules, referred to as monomers.

When a blood vessel is damaged and bleeding begins, a complex series of enzymatic reactions take place that ultimately cleave a piece off of fibrinogen, converting it into fibrin. Fibrin molecules bind to each other forming polymers in the form of fibers. These are the fibers of this connective tissue and are one component of a blood clot. Blood and blood clotting will be considered in detail in Chapter 16.

■ Other Tissues: Beyond Lining and Packing

We began our discussion of tissues with the thought that there are five classes of tissue. Thus far we have discussed two of the five classes. We will now consider the

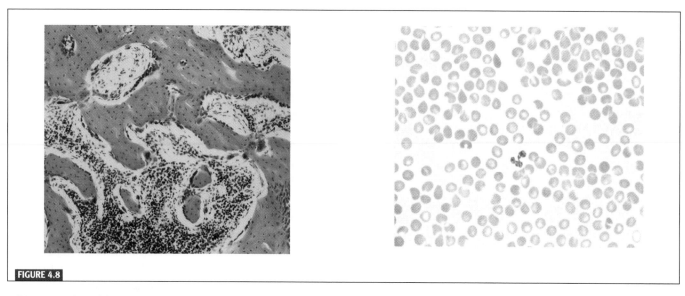

FIGURE 4.8

Other mesenchymal derivatives include bone (left) and blood (right).

other three. You will notice that we are spending relatively little time on these remaining classes of tissue. That is because each of them will be covered in detail in later chapters.

Muscle Tissue: Three Types

Muscle is composed of cells specialized in their ability to generate a force by contraction. Desmin is their intermediate filament, although it has little to do with this ability to contract. There are three different types of muscle. They will be introduced briefly here, but more details on muscle will be presented in Chapter 9.

Skeletal muscle is the tissue we typically think of as muscle. It is the muscle over which we have voluntary control. It is attached to our bones by tendons and is responsible for the motion of our bodies, our posture, and the production of heat.

Smooth muscle is the muscle responsible for movement within our internal organs. Your ability to move food and waste through your digestive tract, control the flow of blood through your arteries, and have the hair stand up on the back of your neck when you are scared is the responsibility of smooth muscle. Structurally, smooth muscle cells differ greatly from those of skeletal muscle. We do not have voluntary control over the contractions of our smooth muscle; therefore, they are said to be involuntary.

Cardiac muscle is the muscle of the heart. The contractions of cardiac muscle are also involuntary. They are forceful and rhythmic, with a rhythm generated within the muscle itself. It is structurally different from either of the muscle types described previously.

Nervous Tissue

Nervous tissue . . . tissue about to have an exam! No, not really! Nervous tissue is composed of cells called neurons and is found throughout the nervous system. These cells have the ability to generate an electrical charge across their membrane and to release that charge as a wave of depolarization along the length of the cell. This allows for quick communication within the nervous system and throughout the body. This rapid communication system is necessary for the maintenance of homeostasis. We will learn about your body's electrical activities in Chapter 8 and about the details of these cells in Chapter 11. Recall that the intermediate filaments found within nervous tissue are neurofilaments.

Glial Tissue

The term *glia* means "glue." This tissue serves the same functions in the central nervous system that connective tissue serves in the rest of the body. For that reason, some anatomists classify this tissue as part of nervous tissue. We know, however, that glia expresses its own intermediate filament, GFAP. We, therefore, consider it a separate class of tissue. We will learn the details of this tissue in Chapter 11.

4.4 Parenchyma and Stroma: Useful Concepts

Let's think about your school for a minute. What is the actual function of your school? Educating students would be a pretty good answer, although it may also have other functions. Who among the people at your school actually educates students? The instructors (teachers, professors, or other educators) teach the students. They can be said to be doing the actual "work" of your school, but what about the other people who work there? Aren't there also lots of support people (administrators, secretarial staff, custodial and maintenance personnel) without whom the instructors could not function? This same situation exists in your organs.

In learning about the five classes of tissue, you may have figured out that each organ actually has a mixture of different tissues within it. These tissues are arranged in ways that allow the organ to carry out its functions. Some of the tissues actually do the work of that organ, while others are there to support those tissues doing that work. For example, one function of the kidney is the production of urine. This fluid is produced through a three-step process involving filtration, adding substances to the filtrate (tubular secretion) and removing other substances from the filtrate (tubular absorption). The epithelial cells of the kidney are responsible for those processes. We would say that the epithelial cells are doing the work of that organ. We call the cells that do the work of an organ the parenchyma of that organ. Those epithelial cells are the parenchyma of the kidney.

The parenchyma of an organ must be organized and supported. Recall how we learned earlier in this chapter that the cells of an organ must have a structure or scaffolding on which they are arranged to have the proper three-dimensional structure. The tissues that support the parenchyma are called the stroma. The stroma of the kidney includes various mesenchymal derivatives and blood vessels.

The concepts of parenchyma and stroma will be referred to repeatedly throughout this text. While not always the case, the parenchyma will often be epithelial, and the stroma often will be composed of mesenchymal derivatives. In the nervous system, we will find a parenchyma of nervous tissue and a stroma of glial tissue and mesenchymal derivatives.

Breaching Homeostasis . . . When Things Go Wrong

This "Breaching Homeostasis" section does not deal with a disease; rather, it presents information on a technique used to study tissues, learn about normal and abnormal activities in the body, and diagnose diseases.

Histotechnology: How Microscope Slides Are Prepared

In hospitals, whenever tissues are removed from the body, they are examined by pathologists. Pathologists diagnose diseases based on the microscopic examination of tissues. For a Pathologist to examine tissues under the microscope, very thin sections of the tissue must be prepared. This process is also used in research laboratories and to prepare the slides used to teach microscopic anatomy. At various places in this book, you will find photographs taken by a camera attached to a microscope (photomicrographs) or drawings of such photographs. You may also have the opportunity to examine tissue sections through a microscope if the course you are now taking (or subsequent courses) offers laboratory sessions. An understanding of how the specimens were prepared will help you to develop a three-dimensional concept of the tissue or organ you are studying, based on the two-dimensional image you are viewing. The flowchart presented in **FIGURE 4.9** follows a piece of tissue from an organ through histologic examination (examination through the microscope). As you examine this figure, think about the chemical concepts discussed in Chapter 2 and how we use these concepts in the biological laboratory.

Histotechnologists, the people who prepare tissues for histologic examination, are highly trained professionals. Every day in hospital, research, and educational laboratories, histotechnologists, in a real blend of art and science, use the concepts you have recently learned to prepare tissues for examination. Perhaps you would like to consider this exciting and rewarding career!

In recent decades, technology has been developed to allow us to identify the locations of specific molecules within tissues. One such technology, called immunohistochemistry, uses antibodies, products of the immune system, to locate specific molecules (antigens). After reading Chapter 21, you will understand how this works. This technology has been instrumental in many of the recent breakthroughs in our understanding of the body. It is also used extensively in the diagnosis of disease. Another technology, called *in situ* hybridization, allows us to identify individual cells that are ex-

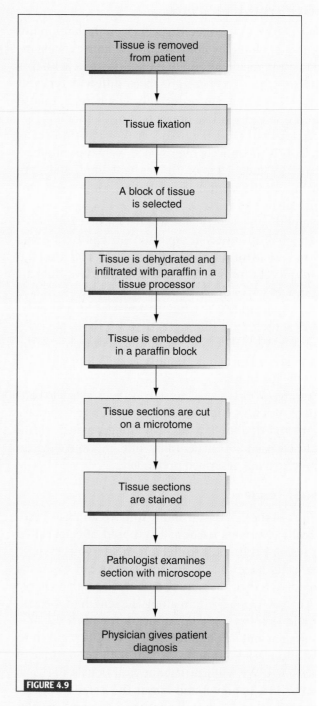

FIGURE 4.9

Preparation of tissues for histologic examination.

pressing specific genes. The specificity of such techniques allows scientists to answer questions that could not even be dreamt of less than a generation ago.

What You Should Know

1. Tissues are groups of similar cells working together to perform specific functions.
2. Tissues are the "construction materials" of our bodies.
3. Although they can be divided in a variety of ways, when defined by intermediate filaments, there are five classes of tissue.
4. Epithelial cells line surfaces, sit on a basement membrane, have intercellular junctions, are avascular, and express keratin as their intermediate filament protein.
5. Epithelial cells range from the flat squamous type to tall columnar cells, and may be simple (one layered), pseudostratified, or stratified (multilayered).
6. Stratified squamous epithelia may be cornified or noncornified.
7. Some types of epithelial cells may possess microvilli or cilia.
8. Goblet cells are unicellular glands that produce mucus and accumulate it for later secretion.
9. All forms of connective tissue are derivatives of the embryonic tissue mesenchyme.
10. Cells of the mesenchymal derivatives have much space between them, which is filled with extracellular matrix.
11. Extracellular matrix is composed of amorphous ground substance and fibers, their composition varying among the types of connective tissues.
12. Three types of muscle tissue exist: skeletal muscle, which is found in the muscles we control voluntarily; smooth muscle, which is the muscle of our internal organs and is involuntary; and cardiac muscle, which is the muscle of our heart and is also involunary.
13. Nervous tissue and glial tissue are found in your nervous system.
14. The term *parenchyma* indicates the cells that perform the actual work of an organ.
15. The term *stroma* indicates the cells that support the parenchyma of an organ.

What Did You Learn?

Multiple choice questions: choose the best answer.

1. A group of similar cells working together to perform a specific function is:
   a. An organ
   b. A piano
   c. A tissue
   d. An organelle
   e. None of the above

2. There are _____ types of intermediate filament proteins.
   a. Two
   b. Three
   c. Four
   d. Five
   e. Six

3. Which of the following is not true of epithelial tissues?
   a. They are avascular.
   b. They line some surface.
   c. Keratin is their intermediate filament type.
   d. They sit on a basement membrane.
   e. All of the above are true.

4. The epithelial cell type shown here is:
   a. Simple cuboidal
   b. Stratified squamous
   c. Pseudostratified columnar
   d. Transitional
   e. Simple squamous

5. The epithelial cell type shown here is:
   a. Simple cuboidal
   b. Stratified squamous
   c. Pseudostratified columnar
   d. Transitional
   e. Simple squamous

6. The epithelial cell type shown here is:
   a. Simple cuboidal
   b. Stratified squamous
   c. Pseudostratified columnar

What Did You Learn? (continued)

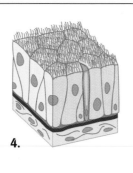

4.

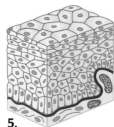

5.

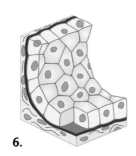

6.

d. Transitional

e. Simple squamous

7. When considering a stratified epithelium, which layer do we examine to determine which type of stratified epithelium it is?

a. The most superficial layer

b. The most basal layer

c. The intermediate layers

d. None of the above is correct.

8. Which type of epithelium would be best in a location where you need to produce mucus and protect a basement membrane despite losing cells to environmental contaminants and infectious agents periodically?

a. Simple columnar

b. Stratified squamous

c. Pseudostratified columnar

d. Transitional

e. Simple squamous

9. You would use _____ epithelium in a location exposed to much abrasion.

a. Simple columnar

b. Stratified squamous

c. Pseudostratified columnar

d. Transitional

e. Simple squamous

10. Epithelial cells that need to carry out much absorption would possess _____ on their apical surfaces.

a. Cilia

b. Microvilli

c. Either of the above

d. Neither of the above

11. Which of the following is not a mesenchymal derivative?

a. Bone

b. Typical connective tissues

c. Cartilage

d. Blood

e. All of the above are mesenchymal derivatives.

12. The main difference between loose and dense connective tissues is that dense connective tissue has more _____.

a. Amorphous ground substance

b. Elastic fibers

c. Fibroblasts

d. Collagenous fibers

e. None of the above

13. _____ connective tissue is found in the walls of our great arteries.

a. Dense regular

b. Dense irregular

c. Elastic

d. Loose

e. Reticular

14. Which of the following is not true of adipose tissue?

a. It is a mesenchymal derivative.

b. It serves as a reservoir for energy.

c. It serves as a thermal insulator.

d. It serves as a cushion.

e. All of the above are true of adipose tissue.

15. What type of cartilage is found on the articular surfaces of bones?

a. Hyaline

b. Elastic

What Did You Learn? (continued)

    c. Fibrocartilage

    d. None of the above

16. Which of the following contains more collagenous fibers?

    a. Fibrocartilage

    b. Hyaline cartilage

    c. They contain equal amounts of collagenous fibers; it is in elastic fibers that they differ.

    d. Neither contains any collagenous fibers at all.

17. Chondrocytes are found in _____.

    a. Typical connective tissue

    b. Cartilage

    c. Blood

    d. All of the above

    e. None of the above

18. The intermediate filament of muscle is _____.

    a. Keratin

    b. Desmin

    c. GFAP

    d. Vimentin

    e. Neurofilaments

19. Contractions of which of the following are voluntary?

    a. Cardiac muscle

    b. Smooth muscle

    c. Both of the above

    d. Neither of the above

20. The cells that perform the actual function of an organ are its:

    a. Parenchyma

    b. Stroma

    c. Pachyderma

    d. Strumming

Short answer questions: answer briefly and in your own words.

1. Briefly list the characteristics of each of the tissue types.

2. Why is the body constructed of tissues of a variety of types? What benefits does this variety provide?

3. List five types of epithelium and give a place where you would expect to find each type.

4. What type of connective tissue would you expect to find in the capsule of the kidney (be specific)? How about in a tendon? If you have given two different answers for these questions, how do these connective tissues differ and what determines where you find them?

5. Describe the three components that are found in all connective tissues. Are any of these different in blood than in a typical connective tissue (loose connective tissue, for example)? Please explain your answer: why is this so?

6. Define the terms *parenchyma* and *stroma* and give two examples of each. Why must our organs contain both?

7. An organ is injured in a way that enables the stroma to regenerate, but not the parenchyma. What impact will that have on the subsequent functioning of that organ?

5 Viewing the Body As a Whole

What You Will Learn

- How your organs are organized to carry out their tasks.
- The names and functions of each of your organ systems.
- The concept of homeostasis.
- How homeostasis is regulated and maintained.
- The role of precise terminology in anatomy and physiology.
- The anatomical position.
- The terminology used to identify locations on and in the human body.
- The location, name, and contents of each of your body cavities.

Let's think big! We are finally ready to begin thinking about the body on a larger scale. We must cover some of the basics regarding how we arrange the organs of the body into groups based on their functions. We must then think about how these units work together, with one goal in mind: that of keeping the body alive. We will also consider some terminology that will allow us to communicate effectively regarding the locations of the anatomy we will study. Then our foundation will be complete, and we can begin to build upon it.

5.1 Organ Systems: A System for Organizing Your Organs

Let us think for a moment about your house. Do you have a sink with a faucet in your house? How about some water pipes? Is there a toilet present somewhere? You most likely said yes to all of these questions. If so, can you give us a term that unites all of these things? Of course, they are part of your house's plumbing system. We can carry out a similar exercise for other components of your house. You know that the lighting fixtures, the electrical outlets, the wiring, and a number of other components are all part of the electrical system. This knowledge requires some understanding of the functions of these items. If you did not know what these things did, you might not know that these household features could be grouped in this way.

A similar situation exists in your body. Some of your organs have interrelated functions. Sometimes, organs performing related functions are directly connected to each other. An example of this would be the relationship of your stomach to that of your small intestine. Even if we did not know what these two organs did, we would bet that their functions were related, based on how they are connected together. But how about your pituitary gland, located in your head, and your adrenal glands, located near your kidneys? Without some knowledge of their functions, would we group them together? Probably not. We are about to list groups of organs together based on their functions. We call these groups our "organ systems." This allows us to explore the functions of the organs in a context that makes sense. **TABLE 5.1** lists our organ systems, gives representative organs, and gives functions for each.

You will notice that the remainder of your textbook is arranged according to your organ systems. By grouping the organs we study into their respective systems, we can gain a more integrated understanding of their functions. Ultimately, we will be able to look back and understand how these systems work together to keep us alive.

5.2 Homeostasis: What a Concept!

What are our organs actually attempting to achieve? In other words, what is their common goal? Simply put, their goal is to keep us alive. Is that so difficult? Perhaps it would not be if we lived in a laboratory environment with a constant setting of light, heat, humidity, nutrients, etc. However, that is not how we live. In the span of a few moments, we may experience the searing heat of the beach in the sun and the cold wetness of a dip in the ocean. Humans live in environmental conditions ranging from desert heat to arctic cold (**FIGURE 5.1**); while living in those varied environments, we carry out a wide range of activities. One moment we may be resting comfortably, expending little energy; the next moment, we may be sprinting along expending great energy, generating lots of heat and metabolic waste. Through these varied environments and activities, our body's internal environment must remain relatively constant. That is the goal of our organ systems: to keep the internal environment of our body constant, despite where we are and what we are doing. The concept of this internal constancy has a name:

Table 5.1 The Organ Systems		
System	**Representative Organs/Structures**	**Representative Functions**
1. Skeletal system	Bones, joints, marrow	Support, protection, leverage for movement, hematopoiesis (blood formation)
2. Muscular system	Skeletal muscles, tendons	Movement, posture, heat production
3. Nervous system	Brain, spinal cord, nerves, sense organs	Regulation of body activities
4. Endocrine system	All hormone producing glands, i.e., pituitary, adrenal, pancreas	Regulation of body activities
5. Reproductive system	Ovaries, testes, vagina, penis, associated ducts and structures	Reproduction
6. Cardiovascular system	Heart, blood vessels	Transportation of gases, nutrients, and wastes
7. Respiratory system	Lungs and associated airways	Exchange of gases between the internal and external environment
8. Digestive system	Esophagus, stomach, intestines, associated glands	Ingestion, digestion, and absorption of nutrients, elimination of wastes
9. Urinary system	Kidneys, urinary bladder, ureters, urethra	Elimination of wastes, regulation of blood composition
10. Integumentary system	Skin, sweat glands, hair follicles	Protection, temperature regulation
11. Immune system	White blood cells, bone marrow, lymph nodes, thymus	Protection

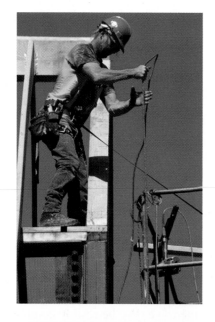
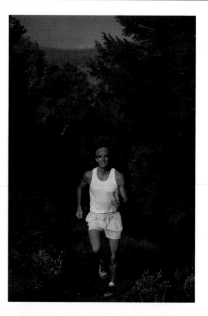
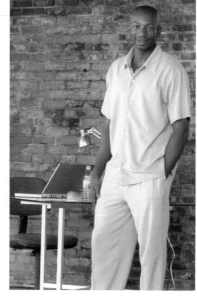
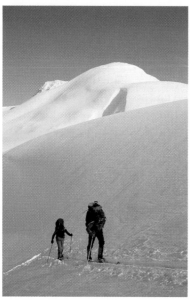
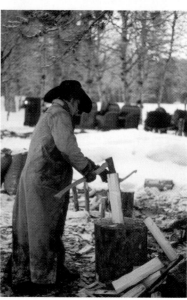

FIGURE 5.1

Our organ systems enable us to maintain homeostasis despite changes in our environment or level of activity.

homeostasis. The *homeo-* portion of this word indicates sameness; the *-stasis* portion indicates standing. It is like "standing" in that there is a steady state of conditions within, despite influences that would cause those conditions to change. We also have a term for those influences that would cause those conditions to change: *stress*. Stress is anything that happens to the body that challenges homeostasis. Stress can be external, such as exposure to the heat of the sun or a cold driving wind. Stress can also be internal, such as the effects of high blood pressure or recurring unpleasant thoughts.

■ Stress and Its Consequences

Despite our body's attempts to maintain homeostasis, stress can have its consequences. A short-term or mild deviation from homeostasis results in injury or disease. A longer-term or more severe deviation from homeostasis can result in death. The reason for this has to do with some of the first things we learned in this text. We learned that our bodies are large sacks of chemicals. Reactions among these chemicals, collectively called metabolism, are necessary for life to exist. These chemical reactions, many of which require the activity of enzymes, occur properly only within a very narrow range of environmental conditions (pH, temperature, pressure, etc.). So, how does our body maintain homeostasis?

■ Regulation of Homeostasis

First, as a way of regulating homeostasis, we have two systems that monitor the internal and external environments. These two main regulators of homeostasis are the nervous system and the endocrine system (**FIGURE 5.2**). The nervous system uses electrical impulses to monitor these environments and to signal necessary reactions to effectors throughout the body. Electrical impulses allow rapid monitoring and response, making the nervous system our fast-acting regulator of homeostasis. The endocrine system uses chemical messengers to convey this type of information. Chemical messengers work more slowly than electrical impulses; hence, the endocrine system is our slow-acting regulator of homeostasis.

■ Mechanisms in the Maintenance of Homeostasis

It is, of course, one thing to be able to sense the conditions of the internal environment, and yet another to be able to do something to alter those conditions. What tools does the body use to make changes as needed? One major tool that the body uses is moving fluids. The body uses a variety of moving fluids to even things out, to transport nutrients and wastes to the proper locations, to balance temperatures and pH, and to impact all the other aspects of homeostasis.

Many of these fluids are extracellular or outside of our cells. These include our blood, which is usually the first moving fluid to come to mind; our lymphatic fluid; our cerebrospinal fluid; and our interstitial fluid (**FIGURE 5.3**). Interstitial fluid is the fluid that bathes the

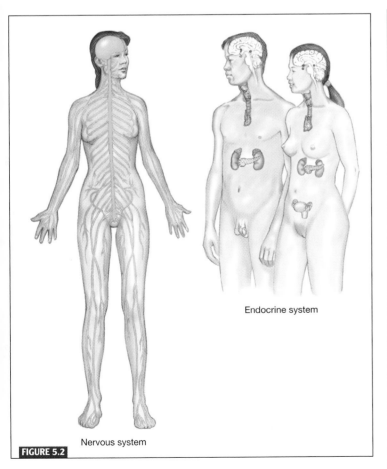

Endocrine system

Nervous system

FIGURE 5.2

Regulators of homeostasis. The nervous system is the fast-acting regulator of homeostasis and works through electrical impulses. The endocrine system is the slow-acting regulator of homeostasis and works through chemical messengers called hormones.

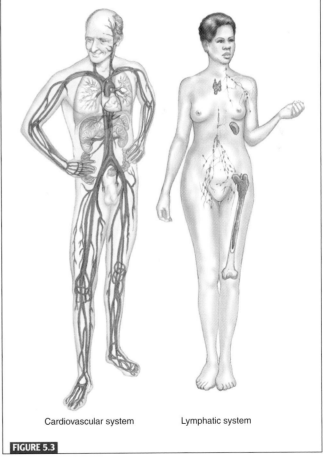

Cardiovascular system   Lymphatic system

FIGURE 5.3

A main mechanism in the maintenance of homeostasis is that of moving fluids. Blood and lymphatic fluids are two examples.

cells in our tissues. The term *interstitial* means lying between. The interstitial fluid lies between our cells. We will learn the details of these fluids in Chapters 12 and 16.

Homeostasis also involves intracellular fluid, the fluid within our cells. Cytoplasm, that gel-like substance surrounding our organelles, is one of the fluids used in the maintenance of homeostasis. Its composition varies from that of our extracellular fluids, but is also dependent on those fluids. The interstitial fluid is the reservoir from which our cells draw their intracellular fluid and the receptacle for the wastes they must eliminate. The blood and lymphatic fluid carry nutrients into the tissues and wastes away from the tissues. These moving fluids work together as one single unit, just as the water

of our planet; whether in streams, lakes, bays, oceans, or the clouds, all comprise one unit.

■ The Role of Negative Feedback

When homeostasis is challenged, our organ systems respond by altering conditions to counteract that challenge. Let's start by thinking about your home. Assume that you have heating and air conditioning in your home, and that they both are controlled by a thermostat (**FIGURE 5.4**). What happens if the air in your home gets too hot? The air conditioner comes on, lowering the temperature back to a preset range. If the air becomes too cold, the air conditioner will not come on; the heater will come on, moving the temperature in the opposite direction. The systems in your home react when

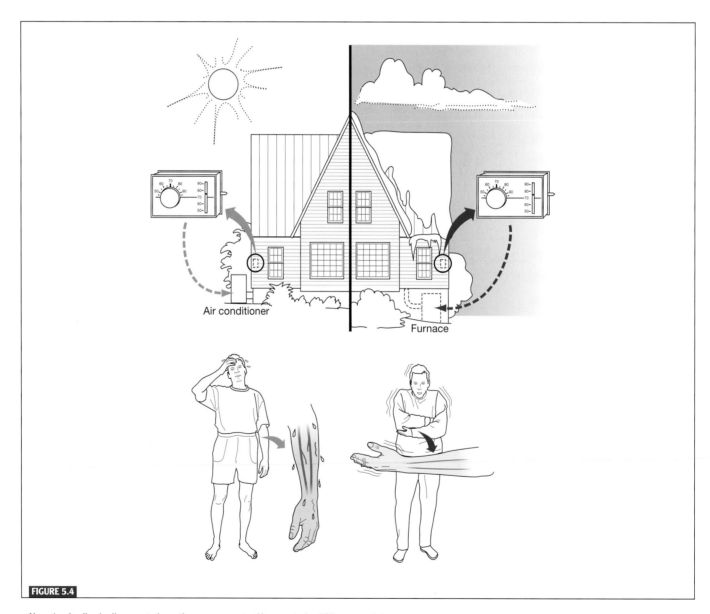

FIGURE 5.4

Negative feedback allows us to keep the many aspects of homeostasis within appropriate ranges.

the temperature exceeds a preset range by moving the temperature in the opposite direction, returning it to within the desired range. This is exactly what happens in your body.

If you were to work out in the sun on a hot day, your body would heat up. As your body temperature rises, your nervous system detects this movement away from homeostasis, the preset temperature range, and takes steps to counteract this change (Figure 5.4). It would cause you to sweat. Sweating wets the surface of the body. The value of this is that when water evaporates, it absorbs a large quantity of heat. Remember that we learned this as one of the reasons why water is important for our bodies. Water absorbs lots of heat as it changes from liquid to vapor.

This cools the surface of the body. We must, however, cool the core of the body. To do this, your nervous system will also signal blood vessels just beneath your skin to dilate. This increases blood flow to the surface of your body. The blood flowing just beneath your skin will be cooled by the evaporation of the sweat; as it recirculates through your tissues, it will distribute that coolness and absorb the heat of those tissues, then lose that heat at the body's surface. Once your body has returned to homeostasis, these cooling systems will be shut off; your body will not be cooled below homeostasis.

What would happen, on the other hand, if you were waiting for a bus on a cold blustery day? As your body cooled, you would again be leaving the normal temperature range (homeostasis), but in the opposite direction. Now your body must conserve heat and perhaps generate more heat. To conserve heat, blood flow to your skin would be reduced. Diverting that moving fluid away from the surface of the body keeps the blood from being cooled and then carrying that coolness into the core of the body. Instead, heat is held in the core of the body. Also, to generate heat, you would begin to shiver. Shivering involves rapid cycles of contraction and relaxation of the skeletal muscles. This muscle activity generates heat. Blood flow is increased within the skeletal muscles and the muscle activity heats the blood. The blood then carries this heat to organs in the core of the body.

There are a couple of important points we just learned. First, you see that a movement in one direction triggered a movement in the opposite direction. When your body became too hot, steps were taken to cool it. If your body became too cool, steps were taken to warm it. This is called negative feedback. Negative feedback is used to maintain homeostasis. In the entire body, under the conditions of homeostasis, we have very few examples of positive feedback, and these are limited to systems that are self-limiting. Positive feedback is a system in which a change in one direction triggers a further change in the same direction. Return to the example of your house; positive feedback would dictate that if your house became too hot, the heat would come on. See why this would only work in self-limiting processes? We will cover these rare cases as we come to them. For now be aware that negative feedback is the standard for maintaining homeostasis.

The second important point is that moving fluids were used to maintain your body temperature. Do you see that the moving fluid in your blood picked up heat at one location and released heat at another location? It then returned to the hot location and cooled it off by picking up more heat. Moving fluids can as easily distribute gasses, such as carbon dioxide and oxygen, wastes, nutrients, and buffers that will stabilize pH. Moving fluids are very important in the maintenance of homeostasis.

Everything we will learn in this text regarding the physiology of our bodies will assume that the body is in homeostasis. Homeostasis is the underlying theme of physiology. Pathology, the study of disease processes, involves the functions of the body outside of homeostasis. After you complete your current study of anatomy and physiology, perhaps you will go on to study pathology. It is a very exciting discipline and will help you to more fully comprehend anatomy and physiology.

5.3 The Language of the Anatomist: Why It Is Important

Why do we care about the precise use of terminology in our study of anatomy and physiology? Isn't any terminology good enough if it gets across the general idea? No. We must use the precise language of anatomy for several important reasons. If we do not use precise language, we might not communicate the thought that we intended to communicate. For example, if I tell you that the adrenals are above the kidneys and I am picturing the body in an upright position while you are picturing the body lying down, we might come up with very different locations for the adrenals. Also, as you move out of the classroom and try to communicate your knowledge with others, your proper use of the language of anatomy and physiology will indicate to others that you have learned your subject properly. Our correct use of language is one way we demonstrate our knowledge to those around us. This can be very important in both the academic and employment arenas. Also, you might need to communicate these things with people whose primary language is not English. If they have been trained in this discipline, they will know this terminology and be able to understand you, even if their English and your use of their native language are not strong. So, what language do we need? What terminology must we master? New terminology will be distributed throughout this text. We merely need to lay a foundation here that we can build upon.

■ Locational Terminology

First, let's consider a few facts about the body. Our body has a tube-in-a-tube body plan. That means we are basically tube shaped and have a tube, the digestive tract, running through us. Second, we need to know that we are bilaterally symmetrical. This simply means that there is a central line running through us by which we can be divided into two approximately equal halves. You have a right half that is essentially equal to your left half. If you took a big saw and cut me in half right down the middle, each half would have one eye, one ear, one nostril, one kidney, one arm, and one leg. If you were slightly to one side of that line or cut on a different angle, you would not end up with two equal halves. That is what it means to be bilaterally symmetrical.

Notice in **FIGURE 5.5a** that the body is shown in a particular position. This position is one where the subject is standing erect facing the observer. The arms are at the subject's sides with the palms facing forward (not the natural position for the palms to face). The feet are flat on the floor. This is the anatomical position. Any time we are referring to locations within the body, we must use the anatomical position as our reference position. In other words, always refer to the location of one structure

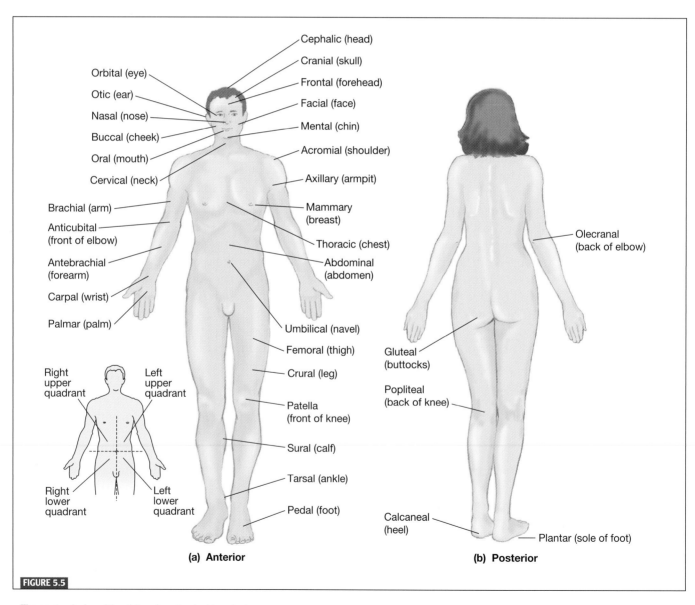

Cephalic (head)
Cranial (skull)
Orbital (eye)
Frontal (forehead)
Otic (ear)
Facial (face)
Nasal (nose)
Mental (chin)
Buccal (cheek)
Acromial (shoulder)
Oral (mouth)
Cervical (neck)
Axillary (armpit)
Brachial (arm)
Mammary (breast)
Anticubital (front of elbow)
Thoracic (chest)
Antebrachial (forearm)
Abdominal (abdomen)
Carpal (wrist)
Palmar (palm)
Umbilical (navel)
Femoral (thigh)
Crural (leg)
Patella (front of knee)
Sural (calf)
Tarsal (ankle)
Pedal (foot)

Right upper quadrant
Left upper quadrant
Right lower quadrant
Left lower quadrant

Olecranal (back of elbow)
Gluteal (buttocks)
Popliteal (back of knee)
Calcaneal (heel)
Plantar (sole of foot)

(a) **Anterior**   (b) **Posterior**

FIGURE 5.5

The anatomical position (a) and anatomical terminology.

versus another as if the body is in the anatomical position, even if at that very moment the body is in another position. Figure 5.5 identifies a number of structures by their common and medical names. I am sure you already know their common names, so learning their medical names will not be difficult.

TABLE 5.2 lists a number of terms that are used to indicate the location of structures with respect to other structures. These terms are used for locations on the body in the same way that you would describe locations in your neighborhood. For example, you might say, "My home is east of Main Street" or "My school is just past the movie theatre." We use similar language in locating structures in the body. You might say, "My mouth is inferior to my nose." This indicates that in the anatomical position your mouth is located below your nose. It is very important that you learn this table, as we will use these terms extensively in upcoming chapters and you will not want to have to look them up each time. Notice that many of these terms are grouped to-

Table 5.2   Locational Terminology

Term	Definition	Example
Medial	Toward the midline of the body	Your nose is medial to your eye. (Your nose is nearer to the midline than your eye.)
Lateral	Away from the midline of the body	Your ear is lateral to your eye. (Your ear is further away from your midline than your eye.)
Intermediate	Between two structures	Your eye is intermediate to your nose and your ear. (It is between your nose and ear.)
Anterior	Toward the front surface of your body	Your nose is an anterior structure. (It is on your front surface.)
Posterior	Toward the rear surface of your body	Your kidneys are posterior to your intestines. (They are behind your intestines.)
Ventral	Toward the front surface of your body	Your navel is a ventral structure. (It is located on your front surface.)
Dorsal	Toward the rear surface of your body	Your spinal cord is a dorsal structure. (It is toward your back surface.)
Superior	Above or higher than	Your head is superior to your neck. (Your head is above your neck.)
Inferior	Below or lower than	Your chest is inferior to your neck. (Your chest is below your neck.)
Superficial	Toward the surface of your body	Your skin is superficial to your muscles. (Your skin is closer to the surface than your muscles are.)
Deep	Away from the surface	Your brain is deep to your skull. (Your brain is further from the surface than your skull is.)
Ipsilateral	Same side	Your right ear is ipsilateral to your right eye.
Contralateral	Opposite side	Your left ear is contralateral to your right eye.
Proximal*	Closer to the beginning or site of attachment	Your elbow is proximal to your wrist. (Your elbow is closer to the attachment of your arm to your trunk than your wrist is.)
Distal*	Further from the beginning or site of attachment	Your colon is distal to your small intestines. (The digestive tract is a tubular structure; the colon is further from the beginning of the tube than the small intestine is.)
Parietal	See the discussion on body cavities later in this chapter.	
Visceral	See the discussion on body cavities later in this chapter.	

* Terms used in tubular structures or in the limbs.

gether in pairs. These pairs are opposites of each other. Notice also that in two instances (*posterior* and *dorsal*; *anterior* and *ventral*), two terms are interchangeable in humans. This is not true when these terms are applied to species that walk on four legs.

The best way to learn these terms is to practice them in your daily conversation. Use them in describing the location of objects you encounter, not just anatomical structures. Think up examples of them on your body. Practice them as you go through your day. This has a

number of advantages. If you use public transportation and practice aloud, you might find that you have an empty seat next to you more often!

■ Planes of Section

No, we are not talking about the rolling grasslands of a place called Section. The term *plane* refers to a flat surface. The term *section* refers to cutting the body or some portion of the body. Look at **FIGURE 5.6**. It shows a body cut through at different angles. Each of these cuts has a

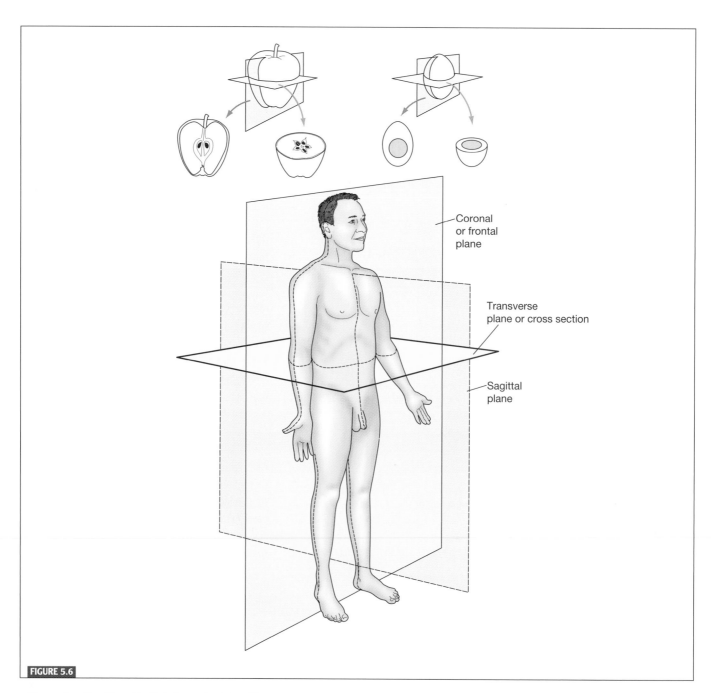

FIGURE 5.6

Planes of section. The subject is in the anatomical position.

name. These are referred to as the planes of section. It is important to know the planes of section for our discussions on the internal structure of organs. To understand how organs work, we must understand their structure or design. We study this structure by looking at diagrams of cut surfaces of organs. The plane of the sections shown in these diagrams determines the orientation of your view. Think about an apple. If we cut an apple in half in one plane, the core resembles a vase. If we cut in the opposite plane, we see a wheel with five spokes (Figure 5.6). A similar effect can be seen by cutting a hard-boiled egg. Notice how in one plane the yolk is central, in the other plane it is toward one end. In some planes we do not see any yolk at all. These effects must be taken into account when viewing the cut surface of an organ, or for that matter cut sections of tissues under the microscope. By learning these planes of section now, you will save considerable confusion in the future.

The frontal or coronal plane divides the body or organ into anterior and posterior parts (Figure 5.6). The transverse plane or cross section divides the body or organ into superior and inferior parts. The sagittal plane divides the body or organ into right and left parts. If it is in the midline of the body, the parts are equal and it is called a midsagittal section. If it is to one side of the midline, the parts are not equal and it is called a parasagittal section.

■ Body Cavities

Within your body, there are spaces that contain your organs (**FIGURE 5.7**). This makes perfect sense, doesn't it? If you opened your body and removed your organs, a cavity must be present where your organs were located. These are called the body cavities. There are two major cavities, the dorsal cavity and the ventral cavity. These are subdivided as follows. The dorsal cavity consists of the cranial cavity, which contains the brain, and the vertebral canal, which contains the spinal cord. The ventral body cavity consists of the thoracic cavity, which is superior to the diaphragm, and the abdominopelvic cavity, which is inferior to the diaphragm. The diaphragm is a sheet of muscle that is important in breathing.

The thoracic cavity is divided into two pleural cavities (right and left), which contain the lungs. The mediastinum is a mass of tissue that separates the two pleural

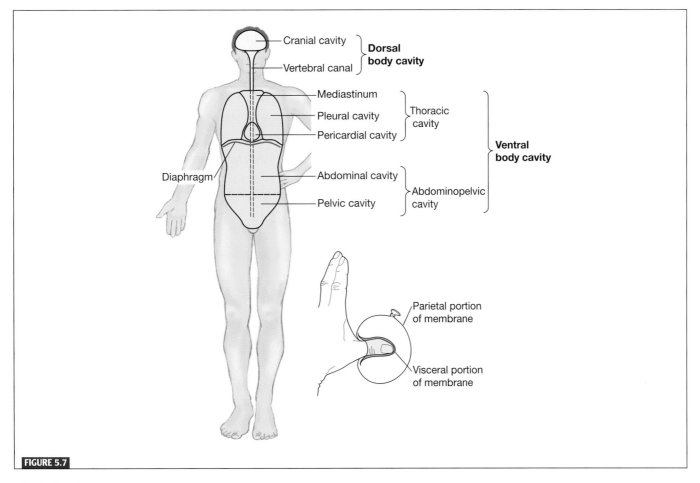

FIGURE 5.7

The body cavities.

cavities from each other. It also contains a third subdivision of the thoracic cavity, the pericardial cavity. The pericardial cavity contains the heart.

The abdominopelvic cavity can be divided along an imaginary line into the abdominal cavity and the pelvic cavity. The abdominal cavity contains organs such as your stomach, intestines, liver, and pancreas. The pelvic cavity, which is the inferior portion of the abdominopelvic cavity, contains the internal organs of reproduction and the urinary bladder.

Each cavity and each organ within each cavity is lined by a thin membrane called a serous membrane. It is not called this because it cannot take a joke (serous, not serious); serous indicates a thin, watery fluid. A serous membrane secretes a small amount of a thin, watery fluid. This fluid lubricates your organs and the walls of your cavities so they don't wear out as you move around. This membrane is actually one continuous membrane stretched around the cavity and each organ.

Picture a partially filled balloon. Now, press your thumb into the balloon. Your thumb is within the cavity that is inside the balloon, but is surrounded by the membrane of the balloon so it is not in contact with the portion of the balloon that is lining the cavity (Figure 5.7). Your organs and cavities are surrounded with a serous membrane in the same way. Picture your thumb as your

heart, the space within the balloon as the pericardial cavity, and the balloon as the serous membrane. Do you see that the serous membrane is continuous, but one portion is in contact with the organ and another portion is in contact with the walls of the cavity? The portion that surrounds the organ is the visceral portion; in this example, it is the visceral pericardium. The portion that surrounds the cavity is the parietal portion; in this example, it is the parietal pericardium. The membrane of each cavity has its own name. The pleural cavities contain the pleura; the abdominopelvic cavity contains the peritoneum. There is a visceral and a parietal component of each. Collectively, the epithelial component of these membranes is called mesothelium. There will be more on these cavities and membranes as we come across them.

We have now completed our foundation materials on the body as a whole. Please take the time now to memorize the terminology covered. I cannot stress enough how much that information will help you to succeed in later chapters. Also, go through the facts listed that follow and consider your understanding of them. Any that you do not understand, please review. Again, I am sure your instructor will be glad to go over any of these topics with you as long as you have spent time trying to understand them first. Next, why not try the questions in the "What Did You Learn?" section?

What You Should Know

1. Your organs are grouped into organ systems based on their functions.
2. Eleven organ systems exist and you must know the names and representative organs and functions of each.
3. Homeostasis is the normal state of our body's internal environment relative to physical and chemical parameters. These conditions must be kept relatively constant despite changes in our external environment and activity level.
4. Things that challenge homeostasis are referred to as stress.
5. A short-term or minor deviation from homeostasis results in injury or disease.
6. A severe or long-term deviation from homeostasis may result in death.
7. Homeostasis is regulated by the nervous and endocrine systems.
8. Moving fluids, including blood, lymphatic fluid, cerebrospinal fluid, and interstitial fluid play a major role in the maintenance of homeostasis.
9. Negative feedback is the response most often used in maintaining homeostasis.
10. The use of proper terminology allows us to communicate precise information about the body to others. It is important for us to know and use proper terminology.
11. The anatomical position is one in which the subject is standing erect, facing the observer with his or her arms at their sides, palms facing forward, and feet flat on the floor.
12. Our bodies have two major cavities that are further subdivided into other cavities.
13. The dorsal body cavity is composed of the cranial cavity and the vertebral canal.
14. The ventral body cavity is composed of the thoracic cavity and the abdominopelvic cavity.
15. The thoracic cavity may be subdivided into the pleural cavities, the pericardial cavity, and the mediastinum.
16. Serous membranes line each of our body cavities and the organs that reside within them.

What Did You Learn?

Multiple choice questions: choose the best answer.

1. The kidneys belong in which organ system?
   a. Muscular
   b. Endocrine
   c. Respiratory
   d. Digestive
   e. Urinary

2. The pituitary belongs to which organ system?
   a. Muscular
   b. Endocrine
   c. Respiratory
   d. Digestive
   e. Urinary

3. Which of the following is correct regarding the organs in an organ system?
   a. To be in the same organ system, two organs must be directly connected to each other.
   b. To be in the same organ system, two organs must have interrelated functions.
   c. Both of the above are correct.
   d. Neither of the above is correct.

4. Gasses are exchanged between the internal and external environments in the _____ system.
   a. Muscular
   b. Endocrine
   c. Respiratory
   d. Digestive
   e. Urinary

5. The concept of homeostasis involves which of the following?
   a. Maintenance of optimum concentrations of gasses, ions, and water
   b. Maintenance of optimum pressures
   c. Maintenance of optimum temperature
   d. All of the above
   e. None of the above

6. Feedback systems are used in the maintenance of homeostasis. _____ feedback is seen almost exclusively in the normal functioning of the human body.
   a. Positive
   b. Neutral
   c. Negative
   d. Feedback. What's that?

7. Anything that happens to the body that challenges homeostasis is considered _____.
   a. Regulation
   b. Negative feedback
   c. Sagittal
   d. Stress
   e. None of the above

8. Of the following organ systems, which is involved in regulation of homeostasis?
   a. Nervous system
   b. Endocrine system
   c. Both of the above
   d. Neither of the above

9. Which fluid bathes the cells in our tissues?
   a. Intracellular fluid
   b. Interstitial fluid
   c. Blood
   d. None of the above

10. The human body is said to have bilateral symmetry because it:
    a. Is a tube-in-a-tube
    b. Has a dorsal and ventral body cavity
    c. Can be separated into two approximately equal halves
    d. Has a head at one end and feet at the other
    e. None of the above is correct

11. The term *plantar* refers to the:
    a. Hip
    b. Shoulder
    c. Posterior portion of the knee
    d. Anterior surface of the hand
    e. None of the above

12. If a patient came to you complaining of pain in his left antecubital area, you would request that he remove his:
    a. Hat
    b. Shirt
    c. Pants
    d. Dentures
    e. Insurance card

13. The subject faces _____ when in the anatomical position?
    a. To the left
    b. Forward (toward the observer)
    c. Backward (away from the observer)
    d. To the right
    e. Any direction; it's random

14. Your nose is _____ to your mouth.
    a. Superior
    b. Inferior
    c. Lateral
    d. Medial

What Did You Learn? (continued)

15. Your wrist is _____ to your elbow.
    a. Proximal
    b. Distal
    c. Ipsilateral
    d. Contralateral

16. Please identify the plane of section indicated.
    a. Midsagitttal
    b. Parasagittal
    c. Coronal
    d. Transverse

17. Please identify the plane of section indicated.
    a. Midsagitttal
    b. Parasagittal
    c. Coronal
    d. Transverse

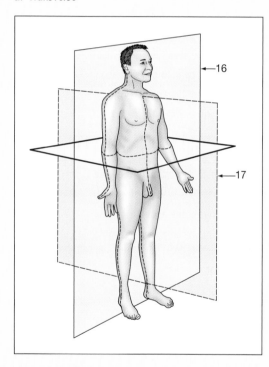

18. The body cavity that contains the internal organs of reproduction is the:
    a. Thoracic cavity
    b. Dorsal cavity
    c. Pelvic cavity
    d. Abdominal cavity
    e. Pericardial cavity

19. The mediastinum is found in the:
    a. Thoracic cavity
    b. Dorsal cavity
    c. Pelvic cavity

    d. Abdominal cavity
    e. Pericardial cavity

20. The _____ portion of a serous membrane directly surrounds the organs within a body cavity.
    a. Visceral
    b. Parietal

Short answer questions: answer briefly and in your own words.

1. Define the term *organ system* and explain what we must know to place an organ in its appropriate system.

2. List five organ systems, give their functions, and indicate the organs that belong within these systems.

3. Describe negative feedback and positive feedback, and indicate which is most important in the maintenance of homeostasis. Why is this form of feedback important?

4. Imagine that instead of negative feedback, positive feedback was being used to regulate blood pressure. You are now experiencing a slight elevation in blood pressure. What will happen next? Why will this happen? To what further changes will this lead?

5. How are moving fluids used in the maintenance of homeostasis? List these fluids and explain how they contribute to the maintenance of homeostasis.

6. Thinking of the environment in which you live, can you think of any manmade devices that imitate our bodies in the use of moving fluids for the regulation of that device's "homeostasis?" Please describe that device and the use for that moving fluid.

7. Use each of the following terms correctly in a sentence, demonstrating your understanding of the term:
   Lateral
   Intermediate
   Posterior
   Inferior
   Contralateral
   Distal
   Parietal

8. List the proper medical term for each of the following:
   Forehead
   Eye
   Head
   Cheek
   Thigh
   Calf
   Shoulder
   Armpit

Our Journey Continues

Congratulations, you now have laid a solid foundation on which to build your understanding of the human body. This does not mean that your study of the human body has not yet begun. On the contrary, just as a foundation is an integral part of a house, so this foundation is an integral part of your understanding of the human body. Without this knowledge, organs are merely "black boxes" in which magic occurs. With this knowledge, the inner workings of the human body become fascinating processes that you can understand and explain to others.

So, now we resume our study of the body, one organ system at a time. We will begin with the systems that provide support and motion to the body. Read on and learn the many fascinating attributes of your skeletal and muscle systems.

6 Your Living Bones

What You Will Learn

- The functions of your skeletal system.
- The components of the extracellular matrix of bone.
- What cells types are present in bone.
- The structures of dense and spongy bone.
- The names of the parts of a typical long bone.
- The membranes associated with bone, their composition, and their function.
- How your bones are formed, how they grow, and how they are maintained.

6.1 The Many Functions of Your Bones

It is easy to imagine the role our skeletal systems play in supporting our bodies. There are, however, a great many other functions provided by our skeletal systems. We will learn about those functions in the section that follows.

If we had no bones, we would not be able to stand, sit, or move. Our bones provide us with the support necessary to do these things and with attachments for muscles, allowing them to affect our position and movement. Without the bones to pull against, in their current arrangement, our muscles would be totally ineffective. Think also of the protection that our bones give to our

soft tissues. Your brain is a relatively soft organ. It would not withstand the many bumps you gave it as you rough-housed as a child, and perhaps still give it through the activities you enjoy, were it not protected by that tough internal helmet, your skull. How about the organs of your thoracic cavity? Proper functioning of your heart and lungs is critical for your moment-to-moment survival. Your thoracic organs are well protected by your flexible but durable rib cage. The ribs provide a shield against a hostile world, protecting our internal organs. You may think of other locations in your body in which your organs are protected by the bones that encase them.

Our bones are living things. Perhaps when you examined a skeleton, you had the impression that the bones were somewhat cementlike. Although they share some characteristics with that building material, they are, in fact, active, living organs. Because minerals make up a large part of bone and because bones are living things, we are able to move certain minerals into and out of bone as needed. Homeostasis dictates that we must have a specific level of calcium in our circulating fluids at all times. Calcium is necessary for activities like muscle contraction and nervous system functioning. Without the proper level of calcium in our blood, we would die. However, we do not walk around eating yogurt all day (not a bad idea, though; how about with strawberry preserves in it, yum!). We must have a system for increasing blood calcium when we are not taking any in, and for storing calcium for future use when we are consuming it. Our skeletal systems provide us with a reservoir for this purpose.

But what about other forms of storage? Can we use our bones to store anything else? Sure we can. Have you ever had a nice piece of meat that had a bone in it (**FIGURE 6.1**)? Perhaps the vegetarians among us have not had this experience but have seen this bone anyway. I'm talking about the cut of meat that has a section of a leg long bone in it so it looks like a ring of bone. Did you notice what was within the core of that ring of bone? In adult humans (and obviously other animals, too), the marrow cavity in our long bones contains yellow marrow. Yellow marrow is composed of adipose tissue. What did we learn about adipose tissue in Chapter 4? We learned that adipose tissue is similar to loose connective tissue with a large number of adipocytes added. Adipocytes are mesenchymal

derivatives that have differentiated with the specialized ability to store fats. Fats are stored energy (think about that the next time you put on a few pounds). Our bones, therefore, are a site of fat (energy) storage.

One last function before we move on. Where do the cells of your blood originate? Obviously, they are produced within your body. The process by which we produce blood cells is called *hematopoiesis*. Hematopoiesis (big word for blood-cell production) occurs in, among other places, red bone marrow. When you were very young (maybe you still are?), you had red bone marrow even in the shafts of your long bones. Now, red bone marrow is found in the middle of your flat bones, such as your ribs, your sternum, your pelvis, and in the ends of your long bones. Perhaps you or someone you know has donated bone marrow to aid an ill person. Most likely, the bone marrow was removed from one of these locations.

So, there we have the functions of your bones: support and aid in movement, protection, storage of minerals and fat, and hematopoiesis (see **FIGURE 6.2**).

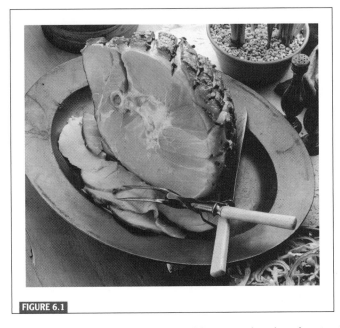

FIGURE 6.1

You may have noticed a ring of bone containing marrow in a piece of meat. Your long bones are similarly constructed.

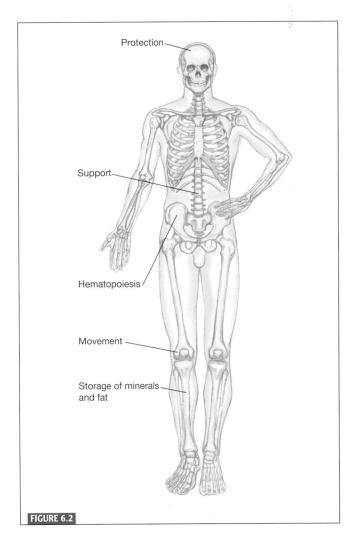

FIGURE 6.2

The functions of your skeletal system.

6.2 Bone As a Connective Tissue

The cells of your bones are mesenchymal derivatives; therefore, your bones are connective tissues. What were the three components of connective tissues (think: Jell-O, spaghetti, and grapes)? Ah, yes; amorphous ground substance, fibers, and cells. Let's start with the amorphous ground substance. In most connective tissues, the amorphous ground substance is composed of proteins, glycoproteins (a molecule of mostly protein and a little carbohydrate), and proteoglycans (a molecule of a little protein and lots of carbohydrate). In bone, however, that amorphous ground substance becomes mineralized. This means that mineral salts become deposited within it. In fact, if we were to dry out bone (remove all the water) and weigh what remains, we would discover that these mineral salts make up about two-thirds of the dry weight of bone. This is why a cleaned, dried skeleton is so durable. The two most abundant mineral salts of bone are calcium phosphate $[Ca_3(PO_4)_2(OH)_2]$ and calcium carbonate $(CaCO_3)$. This accounts for the use of bone as a reservoir for calcium and phosphate. Smaller amounts of other minerals, such as magnesium hydroxide, fluoride, and sulfate, are also present.

As for the fiber component of this connective tissue, many collagen fibers are present. Again in that dried bone sample I mentioned, the remaining one-third of the dry weight is mostly protein, collagen fibers. Histologists often have to prepare histologic sections of bone for examination under the microscope. If only the structure of the extracellular matrix needs to be examined, bone can be ground down to very fine sections with abrasives for examination; it is like using sandpaper to sand away until a transparent piece is left (**FIGURE 6.3a**). If the cells of bone must be examined, we need to section the bone on a microtome, as discussed in Chapter 4 (Figure 6.3b). How could we cut that hard substance? Simply remove the mineral salts and all we would have left would be the collagen fibers, some other matrix molecules, and the cells. That is done by placing the bone in an acid (usually formic acid) until the salts dissolve. There is enough strength and flexibility in the collagen fibers that remain to allow us to bend the bone into a knot without breaking it (Figure 6.3c). Now, onto the cells of bone.

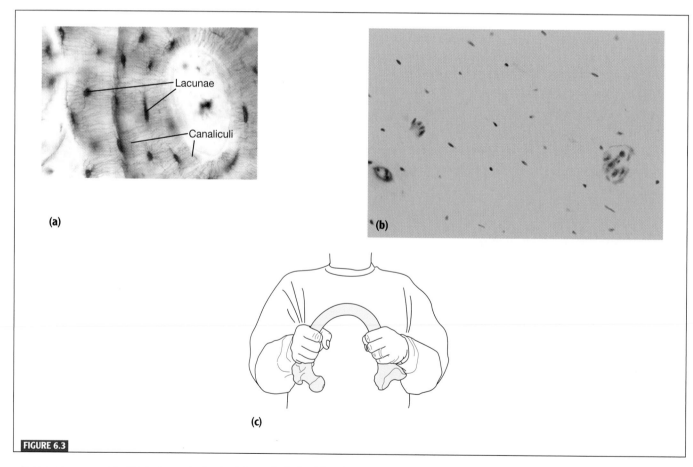

(a)

(b)

(c)

FIGURE 6.3

Bone can be prepared for histologic examination by drying and grinding (a) or decalcification and sectioning (b). Ground preparations allow us to examine the extracellular matrix, while decalcified sections enable examination of the cells of bone. Once the minerals are dissolved from its matrix, bone becomes flexible (c).

The Cells of Bone

In bone, we have four cell types to consider (**FIGURE 6.4**). All of these cells are mesenchymal derivatives; however, three are directly related to each other, and one is less related. Let's start with the three-cell lineage that includes the cells that make bone. The least differentiated cells of this lineage are the stem cells of bone. These stem cells are called osteoprogenitor cells. Osteoprogenitor cells divide to produce additional cells of this lineage. Some of these daughter cells differentiate into osteoblasts, the cells that produce bone matrix. Osteoblasts produce bone by laying down the extracellular matrix of bone. As they produce bone matrix around themselves, they find that they are enclosed in a small cavity, completely surrounded by matrix. This is sort of like painting yourself into a corner in three dimensions (hope they are not claustrophobic!). This cavity is called a lacuna, meaning little lake. These lacunae are connected to each other by little canals called canaliculi. Sounds quite nice, actually; little lakes connected by little canals. With a little rowboat, we'd be all set. At this point, osteoblasts can produce no more bone matrix. If they did, where would they put it? They differentiate into cells that do not produce bone matrix, but simply maintain bone matrix. These cells are called osteocytes. So, osteoprogenitor cells become osteoblasts, which produce bone. Osteoblasts become osteocytes, which maintain bone.

Now for the fourth cell type. Just as we have the ability to make bone matrix, we also have the ability to degrade, or teardown, bone matrix. We must have that ability if we are to repair bone over time and if we are to be able to release the minerals we have stored in the bone as we need those minerals. The cell that degrades bone

matrix is the osteoclast. Osteoclasts are in the monocyte-macrophage lineage. Macrophages, you recall, are cells that can perform phagocytosis. Monocytes are white blood cells that can differentiate into macrophages. Cells of the monocyte-macrophage lineage are found in tissues throughout the body. They have a specific name in many organs because they either take on a different form in that organ or simply because they were named before there was knowledge of how they related to the lineage. In bone, the resident macrophage population has become syncytia, or giant cells with many nuclei. They become syncytia by fusing together many individual cells into one large cell. Remember that the plasmalemma is a self-sealing phospholipid bilayer. This allows individual monocyte-derived cells to fuse into one osteoclast. Osteoclasts resorb bone matrix and reside in a hole called a pit of resorption, or Howship's lacunae. Think of this as being like a rock quarry, a pit from which marble or granite is being removed (see Figure 6.9). The large wall of stone is being chipped away from one side, leaving a pit. Osteoclasts resorb bone by releasing acid and proteolytic enzymes into the pit of resorption. The acids dissolve the mineral salts of bone matrix, releasing them into the interstitial fluid, where they diffuse into the blood and are carried away (again, our moving fluids). The proteolytic (protein-cutting) enzymes break down the collagen fibers so that the smaller peptides and amino acids of which they are composed are also carried away.

Osteoclast activity is controlled by hormones, among other influences. Parathyroid hormone increases osteoclast activity, increasing the amount of bone being resorbed and, therefore, the amount of calcium released into the blood. This elevates blood calcium levels. The hormone calcitonin decreases osteoclast activity, reducing the amount of bone being resorbed, and increases calcium deposition into bone matrix, decreasing the level of calcium in the blood. We will consider the details of this control in Chapter 13. We will learn more on why osteoclast activity is necessary as we consider bone remodeling.

The Structure of Bone

There are structurally two types of bone: dense bone and spongy bone (**FIGURE 6.5**). We will consider each separately.

Dense bone, also known as compact bone, is the form of bone we might typically think of as bone. The example of the bone in the meat that I used a little while ago is dense bone. The shafts of our long bones, such as the bones in our arms and legs, are composed of dense bone. Dense bone has a fascinating internal microscopic architecture, despite its uniform appearance. If we cut a transverse section (think; you learned what that means in the previous chapter) of the shaft of a long bone and examine

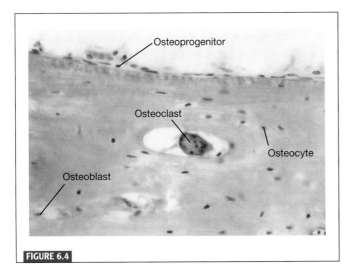

FIGURE 6.4

The cells of bone. Osteoprogenitor cells, osteoblasts, and osteocytes are related cell types, while osteoclasts are related to monocytes and macrophages.

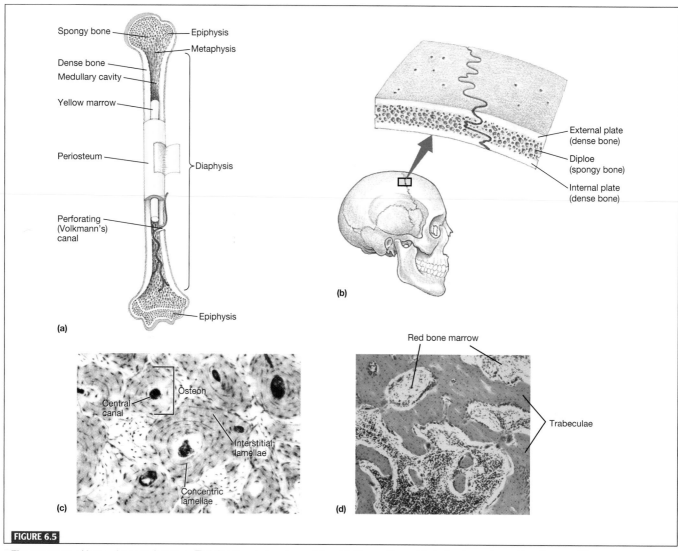

FIGURE 6.5

The two types of bone, dense and spongy. Their locations in long bones (a) and flat bones (b), and their structures: dense (c) and spongy (d).

it under the microscope, we will see that the bone tissue is made up of smaller units called osteons or haversian units. Examine Figures 6.5c and 6.3a as you read this description. Each osteon has, at its core, a central canal. Central canals, also called haversian canals, contain small blood vessels and nerves. Layers of calcified bone matrix surround the central canals. To imagine this, picture an onion cut in cross section, such that the rings of onion tissue are shown. Now, picture that onion as tubeshaped like a leek, not globeshaped. The layers of onion tissue correspond to the layers of bone tissue or concentric lamellae. The lacunae, containing osteocytes, are between the concentric lamellae and are interconnected by canaliculi. The canaliculi contain fine extensions from the osteocytes as if they are holding hands from one lacuna to the next through the canaliculi. The canaliculi and lacunae also contain interstitial fluid, which bathes the osteocytes, just as it bathes cells throughout our bodies. This arrangement allows nutrients, gasses, and wastes to diffuse to and from the osteocytes. Volkmann's canal, or perforating canal, conveys blood vessels from the exterior of the bone to the central canals and the cavity in the center of the shaft (the medullary or marrow cavity).

Interstitial lamellae lie between the osteons and look like incomplete osteons. This is because they are incomplete osteons, left over during the remodeling process. We will learn about that process later in this chapter.

Spongy bone, also called cancellous bone, has a very different architecture (Figure 6.5d). We find spongy bone at the ends of our long bones and within our flat bones, for example, the bones of the skull and the pelvis. Spongy bone gets its name from the minute spaces it contains. It is composed of small interconnecting plates of bone tissue called trabeculae or spicules. Trabeculae are surrounded by red bone marrow, the tissue responsible for hematopoeisis.

6.3 A Typical Bone: Naming the Parts of a Long Bone

As long as we're learning the structure of bones, let's learn the parts of a couple of typical bones. Although, based on their shape, bones exist in several forms, we will concentrate on long bones, such as the bones of your arms and legs, and flat bones, such as the bones of your skull. The other forms of bone are variations on these major types.

Let's start with long bones. To imagine a typical long bone, imagine what a cartoon caveman would use for a club (a femur, perhaps), or think of the bone you end up with after you eat a turkey drumstick (yum). This is also shown in Figure 6.5. The shaft of the long bone is called the diaphysis. Each end of the long bone is called the epiphysis. There is a proximal epiphysis and a distal epiphysis (quick, which is which?). The place where the epiphysis and diaphysis meet is called the metaphysis. A cavity is present in the middle of the shaft of a typical long bone. This cavity, called the medullary or marrow cavity, contains red bone marrow for hematopoeisis when we are young and yellow marrow for energy storage as we grow older.

Flat bones, such as your skull, are relatively thin and, as the name implies, flat. The core of a flat bone is composed of spongy bone. The spaces within the spongy bone contain red bone marrow throughout life. Superficial and deep to this core, we find thin plates of dense bone. The central spongy bone core is called the diploe; the layers of dense bone located superficial and deep to the diploe are called the internal and external plates or tables.

■ The Membranes of Bone

Bones are covered with connective tissue membranes (**FIGURE 6.6**). The surface of bones, whether long or flat, are covered with a membrane called periosteum. Periosteum has two layers. The deep layer, directly adjacent to the bone tissue, is mainly composed of osteoprogenitor cells. These stem cells provide the bone with replacement osteoblasts as needed. The superficial layer, a glistening, silvery-white layer, is of dense, irregular connective tissue. This allows the attachment of tendons and ligaments to the bone. Tendons attach muscles to bones, allowing the muscles to apply force to the bones. Ligaments attach bones to other bones at our joints so we don't go to pieces.

Cavities within our bones, such as our medullary cavity, central canals, perforating canals, and the surfaces of our trabeculae, are covered with another mem-

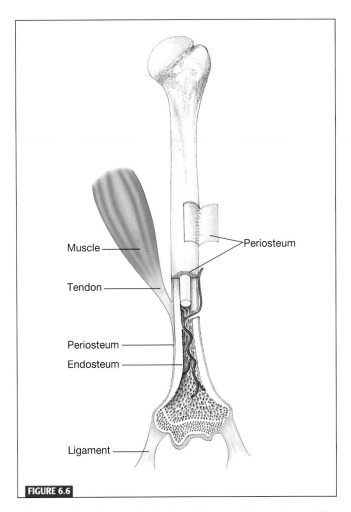

FIGURE 6.6

Periosteum lines the superficial surface of bones and is continuous with tendons and ligaments. Endosteum lines the medullary cavity.

brane, the endosteum. Endosteum is composed mainly of osteoprogenitor cells and does not have the dense irregular connective tissue layer of the periosteum.

The arrangement of these membranes makes perfect sense. Where we need to attach connective tissue structures to our bones, we have a two-layer covering that allows us to do so. Where we do not have to attach connective tissue structures, we do not have the dense connective tissue membrane. In either location, we have abundant osteoprogenitor cells, the stem cells of our bones.

6.4 Life As a Bone: Osteogenesis, Growth, and Remodeling

O.K., time to think about the life of a bone. It's pretty interesting stuff, really. Think about it. Originally, you had no bones. So, where did they come from? How did they develop their shapes? Later on they had to get larger: not just longer or wider, but larger in all dimensions. They also had to repair the wear-and-tear damage we do to them daily, not to mention any fractures we might have developed. So, let's take it in that order: life as a bone, part 1, osteogenesis.

■ Osteogenesis: Formation of Your Bones

Osteogenesis: big word, easy concept. *Osteo-* refers to "bone";*-genesis* refers to "formation of." Formation of bone is our current topic (**FIGURE 6.7**). If you were going to make a complex three-dimensional structure out of a material that is tough to work with, wouldn't you start with a material that is easier to work with and convert it to the difficult material later on, if you could? Don't some sculptors work that way, first producing their creations in a malleable material, such as wax, and then using that object to cast the actual metal sculpture? A similar process occurs with the formation of our bones. Long bones have thickness and other complex dimensions to them. In the developing embryo, they are first formed of hyaline cartilage. As the embryo develops, the cartilage is replaced by bony tissue that is ultimately remodeled into compact bone. This occurs in a stepwise manner, beginning with the diaphysis and ending with the epiphyses. The process of bone formation involving cartilage in this way is called endochondrial ossification. Endochondrial indicates that it occurs within cartilage.

The formation of our flat bones does not require a cartilage model. Since they are to be flat in shape (picture the bones of your cranium, those that surround your brain), they are easily modeled by a membrane of connective tissue. This connective tissue is then replaced by bony tissue that is remodeled into spongy bone and later gains its internal and external plates of compact bone. It is interesting to note that, at birth, some of these connective tissue membranes have yet to become ossified; they exist as soft areas in the infant's skull. These soft areas, called fontanels, give the brain room to grow and allow some distension of the skull, easing delivery of the infant. The process of forming bone using a connective tissue model is called intramembranous ossification.

■ Growth: Enlarging Your Bones

Naturally, your bones have to be able to grow. Let's think about how our long bones grow. That will allow

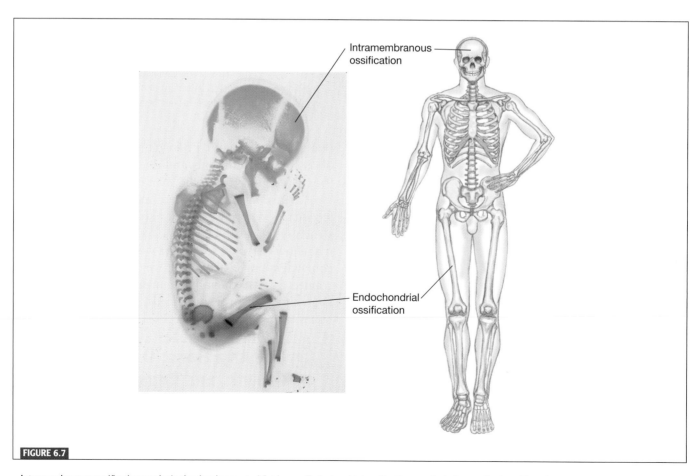

Intramembranous ossification
Endochondrial ossification

FIGURE 6.7

Intramembranous ossification results in the development of flat bones. Endochondrial ossification results in the production of long bones.

us to consider how we gain height and how our bones gain girth. You know that our long bones have the ability to get longer when we are young and lose that ability as we age. In fact, right before they lose that ability, we have a growth spurt and gain a lot of height all at once.

When we are young and our bones are still growing, we have a structure called the epiphyseal plate, where our diaphyses meet our epiphyses. The epiphyseal plate is composed of four layers of cartilage, each of which has its own name and function. See **FIGURE 6.8a** for the details of this structure. The layer nearest the epiphyses is called the zone of reserve cartilage. It is made of hyaline cartilage and does not directly participate in the lengthwise growth of long bone. It merely anchors the epiphysis to the epiphyseal plate. The next layer is the zone of proliferating cartilage or hyperplastic cartilage. Hyperplastic implies hyperplasia. *Hyper-* means increased, and *-plasia* means growth by cell division. This is an area in which

the cartilage cells, chondrocytes, are rapidly dividing. The chondrocytes lie in rows looking like stacks of coins. The next layer is the zone of hypertrophic cartilage. Hypertrophic implies *hypertrophy*, which means rapidly increased growth through increased cell size, not increased cell number. Here the chondrocytes are not dividing; each cell is getting larger and is making extracellular matrix. Although the cells are still in rows, the individual cells are further apart, due to this increase in matrix. The fourth layer is called the zone of calcified matrix. In this zone, the chondrocytes have died. They release substances when they die that cause calcium salts to precipitate from the interstitial fluid. This causes the matrix to become hardened. The death of these chondrocytes involves apoptosis or cell suicide. The hardened matrix perpetuates this process. Osteoclasts are resorbing the calcified matrix at the diaphyseal edge of this zone, and osteoblasts are replacing that calcified matrix with newly formed bone through the process of re-

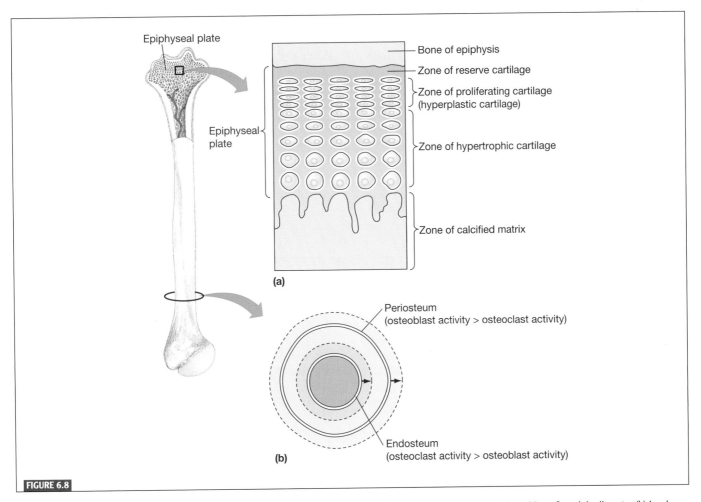

FIGURE 6.8

Lengthwise growth (a) occurs in the epiphyseal plate until puberty when the epiphyseal plate closes, becoming the epiphyseal line. Growth in diameter (b) involves altered rates of osteoclast and osteoblast activity at the periosteum and endosteum.

modeling. Be sure to study Figure 6.8a to fully understand how this process increases the length of your bones.

The lengthwise growth of long bones is dependent on good nutrition and the presence of several hormones. Human growth hormone (hGH) is necessary for this process. Thyroid hormone increases the rate of growth. The sex hormones estrogen and testosterone greatly increase the rate of growth. This is why around puberty and at the start of sex hormone production, adolescents have such a rapid spurt of growth. It is as if the gas pedal of the epiphyseal plate has been pushed to the floor. However, just as in your car, pushing the pedal to the floor has its costs. If you hold your car's gas pedal to the floor constantly, your car may go very fast; but you will quickly ruin your engine. The sex hormones cause rapid growth at the epiphyseal plate but quickly "burn out" the plate. The plate becomes replaced with a bony line (epiphyseal line) in a process called "closure of the epiphyseal plate." After closure of the plate, we are no longer capable of lengthwise growth of long bone and, therefore, stop becoming taller.

As you grow taller, you are growing in other ways too. Your bones need to become larger in diameter to support your increased weight and the increased power of your muscles. This is done by balancing the activity of osteoblasts with that of osteoclasts. If, just deep to the periosteum (superficial surface of your long bones), we have more osteoblast activity than osteoclast activity, what would happen to the outer diameter of the bones? Think about it. At that surface, we are making more bone than we are removing. Wouldn't that cause the bones to increase in diameter? Sure it would. Now, don't we have to increase the diameter of the medullary cavity at the same time? If we did not increase the diameter of the

medullary cavity as our bones grew, we would have great big bones with massively thick walls and tiny medullary cavities. Our bones would weigh so much that we would have trouble moving. So, how can we make the medullary cavity larger using the same two tools (osteoblasts and osteoclasts) we used to make the overall bone diameter greater? We can do this by having more osteoclast activity than osteoblast activity at the endosteum. Think about it; we are removing more bone than we are laying-down. See Figure 6.8b to clarify this concept.

■ Remodeling: Keeping Your Bones New

Remodeling, kind of like kitchens and bathrooms, right? Actually it is very much like what we do to buildings. Just as you may remodel rooms in your home to upgrade them and keep them functional, you need to replace bone matrix to keep your bones strong. The manner in which this is done may already be apparent to you. You already know the cell types and their functions; think about how you would remodel bone using those cells as "workers."

To replace old bone matrix, you must first remove it. What cell type would remove the matrix? Osteoclasts could, of course, perform that function (**FIGURE 6.9**). Their use of acids to dissolve mineral salts and proteolytic enzymes to break down the collagen fibers of bone has already been mentioned. Think about the lysosomes that contain these catalytic chemicals. Can't you picture how these lysosomes can fuse with the cell membrane and release their contents onto the bone matrix? This would then dissolve away matrix, forming a pit of resorption, which the cell moves into as it continues its work. In

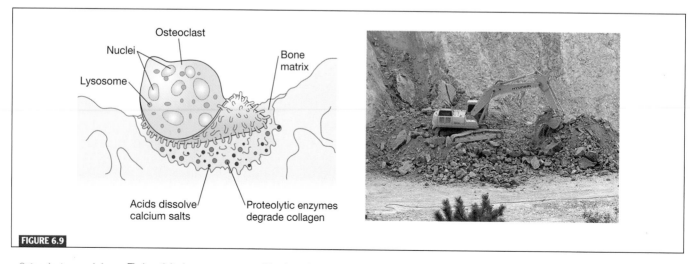

FIGURE 6.9

Osteoclasts resorb bone. Their activity in some ways resembles that which occurs in a quarry. Refer to Figure 6.4 for a photomicrograph of an osteoclast.

dense bone, this resorption begins in the central canal of osteons and works through the layers of concentric lamellae toward the outside of the osteon. Regions of the osteon that are not resorbed will become interstitial lamellae, lying between the newly formed concentric lamellae.

What cell type will build new bone matrix? Right again, osteoblasts. Where do the osteoblasts originate? They come from osteoprogenitor cells. Osteoprogenitor cells proliferate and produce new daughter cells. Some of the daughter cells differentiate into osteoblasts and make new bone matrix at the remodeling site. As they build new concentric lamellae, they find themselves encased in lacunae. When they become encased in this way, they can no longer produce new matrix (they have nowhere to put it), so they differentiate into osteocytes. Layer by layer, a new osteon is produced. Remaining pieces of the old concentric lamellae become interstitial lamellae, lying between the new osteons. This is similar to the way in which parts of old buildings may become incorporated into of newer, larger buildings, as each successive generation adds onto the buildings. Large medical centers in big cities are places where you might have seen this method of building, adding new structures onto older existing ones. See **FIGURE 6.10** for clarity.

What determines the rate of resorption in our bones? Also, what determines how thick the walls of our bones become? These two phenomena are related. Do you travel over any large bridges? Some large bridges carry a great amount of traffic. The safety of these passing vehicles must be assured. Bridge inspectors must frequently examine the bridges for signs of wear. Worn structural members must be replaced. If the amount of wear becomes too great, the bridge must be made stronger. The same type of inspection and reconstruction goes on in your bone.

As you stress your bones, such as when you walk, run, or exercise, the bone matrix flexes. This causes the minerals in the bones to move slightly and creates very slight electrical currents in the bone. The more the bones flex, the more current is generated. The electrical current stimulates the cells of the bone to increase the rate of remodeling and the amount of bone matrix produced. This increases the strength of the bone; this strength reduces the amount that the bones flex as you exercise. This, in turn, reduces the amount of current that is generated, keeping remodeling and bone thickness from becoming too great. There it is again, negative feedback in action.

If you were to become a couch potato and stop exercising all together, your rate of remodeling would decrease and the walls of your bones would become thinner. If you were to increase the amount of exercise you receive, you would cause more stress to your bones (like the bridge carrying more traffic and bigger trucks). The rate of remodeling would have to increase to repair the damage that the increased exercise would cause. The walls of your bones would become thicker to provide more support, so you would not cause damage that would lead to bone failure, a fracture. Providing the stress needed to maintain bone has been a problem in the development of strategies for extended space travel. When people spend time in space with reduced gravity, the stress on their bones is greatly diminished. This leads to reduced bone mass, which, in turn, causes problems when they return to the earth.

One last topic related to remodeling: What happens when we actually break a bone? When we fracture a bone, we activate a multi-stepped process that culminates in replacing the damaged bone matrix (**FIGURE 6.11**). The blood and debris left by the injury must be removed, and ultimately the damaged matrix must be replaced. Fortunately, our mesenchymal cells are very good at this process. Both endochondrial and intramembranous ossification resume in the site of injury, just as they occurred during embryonic development. This process replaces the lost tissue. Successive rounds of remodeling replace all of that matrix until, with proper nutritional homeostasis and immobilization of the wound, none of the damaged matrix remains. With the proper conditions, several years after a fracture, the only evidence of its existence may be thickened periosteum and endosteum. One type of fracture that may have added

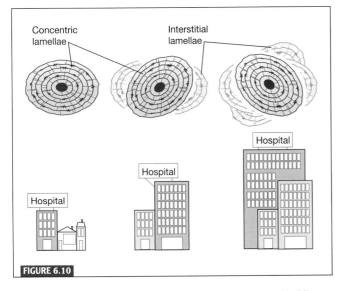

FIGURE 6.10

Remodeling of haversian units (osteons) resembles remodeling of buildings. Some portions of older osteons remain as interstitial lamellae when new concentric lamellae are laid down.

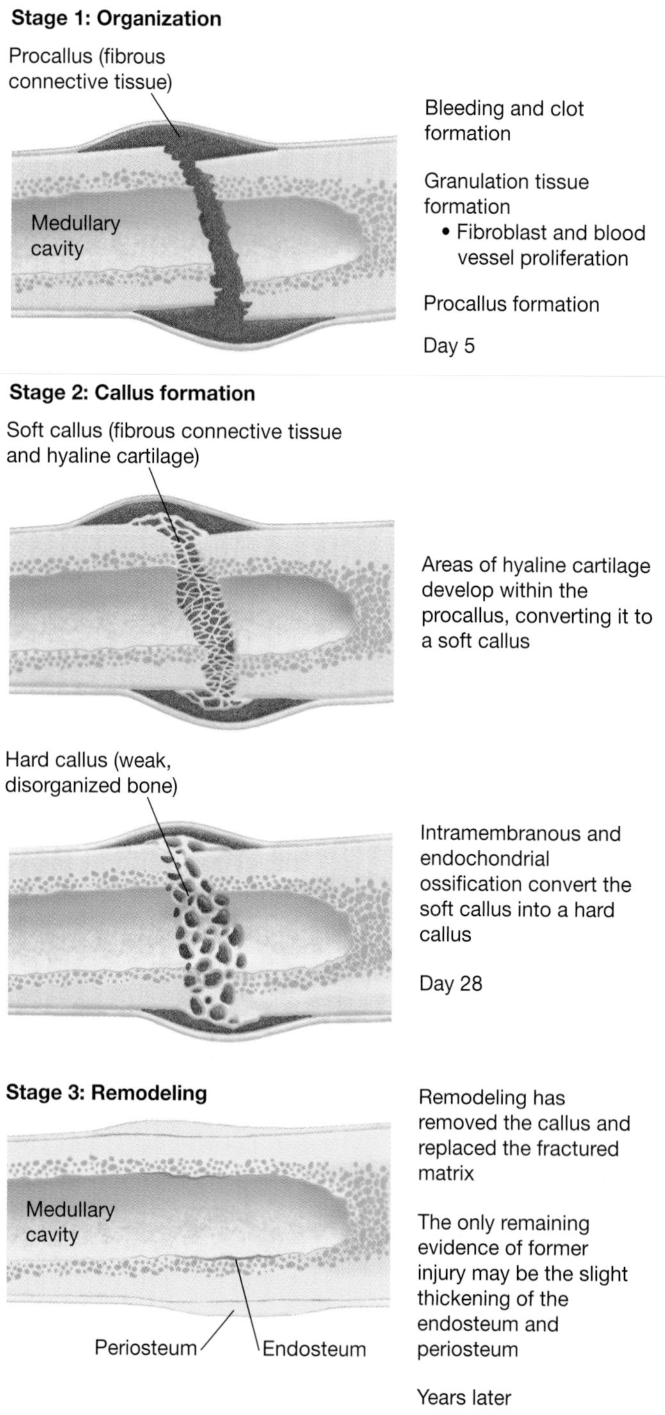

Stage 1: Organization

Procallus (fibrous
connective tissue)

Medullary
cavity

Bleeding and clot
formation

Granulation tissue
formation
• Fibroblast and blood
vessel proliferation

Procallus formation

Day 5

Stage 2: Callus formation

Soft callus (fibrous connective tissue
and hyaline cartilage)

Areas of hyaline cartilage
develop within the
procallus, converting it to
a soft callus

Hard callus (weak,
disorganized bone)

Intramembranous and
endochondrial
ossification convert the
soft callus into a hard
callus

Day 28

Stage 3: Remodeling

Medullary
cavity

Periosteum   Endosteum

Remodeling has
removed the callus and
replaced the fractured
matrix

The only remaining
evidence of former
injury may be the slight
thickening of the
endosteum and
periosteum

Years later

FIGURE 6.11

Bone healing following a fracture.

complications is a fracture involving the epiphyseal plate in a young person (before closure of the plate). This can cause premature closure of the plate and a reduced potential for future growth in that region. So, if you are young and intend to break a long bone, avoid breaking it near the epiphyses, or else!

We have now completed our discussion on the general physiology of bones. The next chapter will cover the specifics of the anatomy of your skeleton. Please make sure you are clear on all of the concepts presented in this chapter by using the "What You Should Know" and "What Did You Learn?" features before proceeding.

Breaching Homeostasis . . . When Things Go Wrong

Osteoporosis

The maintenance of homeostasis often depends on a delicate balance between competing, opposing activities. The maintenance of our bones is no exception. If you think for a moment about remodeling, you will realize that the balance between the resorptive activity of osteoclasts and the productive activity of osteoblasts must be balanced or homeostasis will be breached. Before the age of about 28, osteoblast activity predominates over osteoclast activity to varying degrees for our bones to grow. Ideally, in later years, the resorption and deposition of bone matrix are equal. This, however, is not always the case. In this section, we will briefly discuss a disorder that occurs when this balance is upset.

Osteoporosis, a name we have all heard, actually means "porous bones." It is a disease that exists in a few different forms, all of which are characterized by a measurable loss of bone mass. The bone loss is the effect of an imbalance between bone resorption and bone deposition: resorption outpaces production. This is an extremely prevalent disease, more common in women than men, affecting approximately 25% of women in their 60s and costing U.S. society an estimated $10 billion annually.

Based on etiology (cause), we observe two forms: primary and secondary. Primary osteoporosis is the most common form and we will discuss it momentarily. Secondary osteoporosis can occur at any age and is caused by some identifiable pathologic process. Etiologies for secondary osteoporosis include endocrine conditions, such as increased activity of the adrenal cortex or thyroid gland, and reduced activity of the ovaries or testes; nutritional imbalances, such as insufficient calcium or vitamin C in the diet, and the inability to absorb nutrients in the digestive tract; immobilization for an extended period, such as could occur after traumatic injury or from a chronic disorder. Interestingly, chronic alcoholism contributes to risk of secondary osteoporosis, but it is not known whether this is due to a toxic effect of alcohol, liver disease induced by alcohol, the malnutrition often associated with excessive alcohol consumption, or some combination of these effects.

Now, back to primary osteoporosis: we identify two forms based on the pathology observed. Type I (postmenopausal) osteoporosis occurs in women, with fractures beginning about 10 years after menopause. Loss of spongy bone exceeds the loss of compact bone. Crush fractures of vertebrae and the distal end of the radius are the most common manifestations.

Type II (senile) osteoporosis has an equal prevalence in men and women, and is seen in those over 70 years of age. The loss of spongy and compact bone is comparable to the proportion of these two types of bone, and much of this loss is in long bones. Fractures are common in the proximal femur, mainly in its neck. Multiple wedge-shaped microfractures of the vertebral bodies are common, mostly anteriorly, and result in a loss of stature and a stooped posture. Approximately 50 percent of 80-year-olds show evidence of these fractures.

So, how can we avoid these disorders? The time to initiate your strategy is while you are still young. Eating a diet rich in calcium, with sufficient levels of vitamin D (necessary for calcium absorption in your digestive tract), is a good start. Talk to your health-care provider about whether dietary supplements are right for you. Also important is sufficient exercise: remember the link between exercise and bone size. Keep in mind, however, that when taken to an extreme, exercise can cause harm. In young women, extreme exercise (most commonly seen in runners) can result in amenorrhea (cessation of menstruation). This amenorrhea can lead to osteoporosis.

How can older people reduce their risk? Proper diet and moderate exercise are still important. Supplementary estrogen may be useful in postmenopausal women, but there are risks that need to be considered. Discuss this issue with your health-care provider to get the advice that's right for you. There are even drugs currently on the market (biophosphonates) that bind to bone and inhibit osteoclast activity. For those experiencing excessive bone loss, these might be the right solution. Discuss this, too, with your health-care provider.

What You Should Know

1. Your skeletal system, composed mainly of bone, provides you with support, aid for motion, protection of vital organs, storage of minerals and fat (energy), and is the site of hematopoeisis.

2. Bone is a connective tissue and, as such, is composed of cells and an extracellular matrix of amorphous ground substance and fibers.

3. The amorphous ground substance of bone, unlike that of other connective tissues, is mineralized with calcium salts: the main calcium salts of bone are calcium carbonate and calcium phosphate.

4. The fibers of bone are mainly made of collagen and account for one-third of the dry weight of bone.

5. The calcium salts of bone matrix provide rigidity and hardness; the collagen fibers provide strength.

6. The four main cell types of bone are osteoprogenitor cells, osteoblasts, osteocytes, and osteoclasts. The first three of these are directly related to each other. The fourth is in the monocyte-macrophage lineage.

7. Osteocytes reside in lacunae interconnected by canaliculi.

8. Osteoclasts reside in Howship's lacunae or pits of resorption, and resorb bone during remodeling.

9. Dense bone (compact bone) is composed of haversian units.

10. Spongy bone (cancellous bone) is composed of trabeculae (spicules).

11. A long bone consists of a diaphysis (shaft) and two epiphyses (ends); the diaphysis meets the epiphysis at the metaphysis.

12. In adults, the medullary cavity of long bones contains yellow marrow.

13. Flat bones contain a core of spongy bone sandwiched between plates of dense bone.

14. Red marrow is found in flat bones and in epiphyses, even in adults.

15. Periosteum is the membrane of dense connective tissue and osteoprogenitor cells that surrounds our bones; endosteum is the membrane mainly composed of osteoprogenitor cells that lines the medullary cavity of our bones.

16. Osteogenesis, the formation of bones during embryonic development, can occur in a preformed cartilage model (endochondrial ossification) or a connective tissue membrane (intramembranous ossification).

17. Lengthwise growth of long bones occurs at epiphyseal plates. Closure of these plates after adolescence eliminates the ability of these bones to increase in length.

18. Our bones are remodeled throughout life, replacing potentially damaged matrix with new matrix.

19. The rate of bone remodeling is directly related to the amount of stress to which we expose our bones: within reason, exercise results in stronger, healthier bones.

What Did You Learn?

Multiple choice questions: choose the best answer.

1. Which of the following is not a function of the skeletal system?

   a. Support

   b. Protection

   c. Hematopoeisis

   d. Storage

   e. Each of the above is a function of the skeletal system.

2. Which of the following cell types is not directly related to the others?

   a. Osteocytes

   b. Osteoprogenitors

   c. Osteoclasts

   d. Osteoblasts

   e. All of the above are directly related to each other.

3. Which of the following is not a major mineral salt of bone?

   a. Calcium chloride

   b. Calcium carbonate

   c. Calcium phosphate

   d. All of the above are major mineral salts of bone.

   e. None of the above is a major mineral salt of bone.

4. What percentage (by weight) of the extracellular matrix of bone is protein (i.e., collagen)?

   a. 5

   b. 10

   c. 25

What Did You Learn? (continued)

d. 33

e. 66

5. The extracellular matrix fibers of bone are largely composed of:

   a. Keratin

   b. Vimentin

   c. Tubulin

   d. Collagen

   e. Laminin

6. Which of the following cell types is found in Howship's lacunae?

   a. Osteocytes

   b. Osteoprogenitors

   c. Osteoclasts

   d. Osteoblasts

   e. All of the above

7. Which of the following contains haversian units?

   a. Compact bone

   b. Spongy bone

   c. Both of the above

   d. Neither of the above

8. Which of the following contains lacunae?

   a. Compact bone

   b. Spongy bone

   c. Both of the above

   d. Neither of the above

9. Which of the following contains canaliculi?

   a. Compact bone

   b. Spongy bone

   c. Both of the above

   d. Neither of the above

10. Which of the following contains trabeculae?

    a. Compact bone

    b. Spongy bone

    c. Both of the above

    d. Neither of the above

11. Identify the parts of the long bone indicated:

    a. Epiphysis

    b. Diaphysis

    c. Metaphysis

    d. None of the above

12. Identify the parts of the long bone indicated:

    a. Epiphysis

    b. Diaphysis

    c. Metaphysis

    d. None of the above

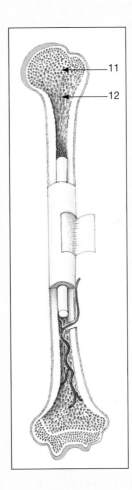

13. In adults, red marrow is found in:

    a. The medullary cavity of long bones

    b. The spaces between trabeculae in flat bones

    c. Both of the above

    d. Neither of the above

14. In adults, hematopoeisis occurs in:

    a. The medullary cavity of long bones

    b. The spaces between trabeculae in flat bones

    c. Both of the above

    d. Neither of the above

What Did You Learn? (continued)

15. Which of the following is attached to the superficial surface of bones?

    a. Periosteum

    b. Endosteum

    c. Both of the above

    d. Neither of the above

16. Which of the following has a layer that is composed of dense connective tissue?

    a. Periosteum

    b. Endosteum

    c. Both of the above

    d. Neither of the above

17. In mature adults, the lengthwise growth of long bone occurs at:

    a. The epiphyseal plate

    b. The epiphyseal line

    c. The articular surface

    d. All of the above

    e. None of the above

18. Which of the following cells resorb bone?

    a. Osteocytes

    b. Osteoprogenitors

    c. Osteoclasts

    d. Osteoblasts

    e. All of the above

19. Which of the cells produce bone?

    a. Osteocytes

    b. Osteoprogenitors

    c. Osteoclasts

    d. Osteoblasts

    e. All of the above

20. Of the following, who has heavier long bones?

    a. A marathon runner

    b. A couch potato

    c. Could be either; it's random

Short answer questions: answer briefly and in your own words.

1. List the functions of your skeletal system and briefly discuss how each is accomplished.

2. Bone is a mesenchymal derivative (connective tissue). Describe the components of bone that make it a connective tissue. Include in your description a discussion of the cell types found in bone.

3. How are bones formed during embryonic development? Please describe the two processes involved.

4. Think about the process of bone formation during fracture repair. How does this process resemble that which occurs during embryonic osteogenesis? What does this tell us about the genes that are active during embryogenesis? What could be the potential implications of this for the regeneration of other organs?

5. Draw and label an epiphyseal plate. List the function of each of the layers. What happens to this structure after adolescence?

6. Describe the process of remodeling in bone and include the role of each cell type in this process.

7. What changes could you make personally to develop and maintain good skeletal health as you age? Be specific in the lifestyle changes that you could make to achieve this goal. Include the physiologic basis for each of the changes you list. Why not implement these changes in your life?

8. Draw and label a diagram of the structure of spongy bone and compact bone. Indicate where we could find each of these types of bone.

CHAPTER 7

The Ankle Bone's Connected to the . . .: The Anatomy of Your Skeleton

What You Will Learn

- Tips to improve your ability to memorize the gross anatomy of the body.
- The skeleton is divided into axial and appendicular components.
- The names and locations of the bones of the axial skeleton.
- The names and locations of the bones of the appendicular skeleton.
- The generic names and descriptions of the features of bones.
- A functional classification scheme for the articulations (joints).
- A structural classification scheme for the articulations.
- The movements of synovial joints.

7.1 How to Know the Bones: A Strategy for Learning

We are about to embark on the first real gross anatomy exercise in this textbook. The skeletal system is a great place to begin our practice of learning the gross anatomy for several reasons. First, it is a system of easily visualized structures. Since the skeleton supports our bodies, it has a shape similar to that of our bodies. It is very easy to imagine the bones that lie deep to our soft tissues. In many instances, we can even palpate (feel) them through the soft tissues. This makes learning the bones easier than some of the other anatomy we will learn later on.

Second, by learning the bones before learning the anatomy of other systems, we have a built-in series of landmarks we can use to describe other locations in the body. By using our directional terms (I am sure you spent the time necessary to be able to now use those terms without looking them up) and our skeletal landmarks, all of our later gross anatomy will be much easier.

Third, the gross anatomy of the skeletal system is easy enough that it will not overburden you, yet complex enough that you can use it to hone your memorization skills and develop strategies for learning that will benefit you throughout your study of the human body. You may also find these strategies useful in other subjects or in other aspects of your life. So, let's begin by thinking about these strategies.

You know that you have to learn the names and locations of a lot of bones. How do you go about such a task? Like so many things in life, the overall task looks large, but if you break it down into smaller components, it's really not so bad. In this case, it is simple to divide the learning into smaller units. Follow the sections and diagrams as they occur in this text. Learn the bones of one skeletal structure completely before moving onto the next structure. Then, when you do move on, continue to review the bones you have already learned each time you sit down to study new ones. This keeps those you have already learned fresh in your memory. This also puts you in the proper frame of mind to learn the new material and reinforces the fact that you absolutely can learn this material. You may even want to review what you have learned during any free moment you have as you go about your busy day. Simply point to the location of a bone and name that bone. You might want to do this mentally as opposed to physically, or only when you are alone or with those who understand what you are doing. Nothing will clear an elevator as fast as someone pointing to parts of their body and naming bones. Then again, that might be a good thing.

Now, let's say you are studying the bones of the upper limb. There are still a lot of bones to learn, even in that one structure. How do you do it? I recommend you break that structure down further. Again, this has been done in the diagrams; follow the diagrams, learning one at a time. Be careful, however, to learn the bones, not the diagrams. Take, for instance, the bones of the wrist, the carpal bones. If you learn the diagram rather than the bones, you might run into problems when confronted with the opposite limb (right versus left), or with the opposite view (posterior versus anterior) of the same limb. How can we overcome this difficulty? Very easily; always start at a landmark and work through the bones in the same order, naming each one in turn. In the case of the carpal (wrist) bones, it is simple. You will note that they are arranged essentially in two rows of four bones each. The proximal row articulates (has joints) with the radius and ulna bones of the arm, while the distal row articulates with the metacarpals. Now, also notice that the thumb makes a great landmark, both because of how it extends from the hand at an angle different from that of the fingers and because it has only two phalanges, as opposed to three in the fingers. So, always start in the proximal row of carpals at the one nearest the thumb. Work through that row and then go back to the beginning of the distal row (thumb side again) and work through those four bones. Think about the names of the bones and how they relate to one

another. Try to make up a story based on the meanings of the names of the bones (scafoid = skiff or boat, lunate = moon, triquetrum = three sided, pisiform = pea shaped; "We went out in a boat under the moon to a three-sided island and ate peas"). If that technique doesn't work for you, use the first letter of each name in the group to make up a sentence of words beginning with the same letters: scafoid, lunate, triquetrum, pisiform, trapezium, trapezoid, capitate, hamate; "Some lazy teachers pretend to teach chimpanzees hopscotch." This is called a mnemonic device and is a very handy tool for use during memorization. Remember, we already used a mnemonic device while learning the stages of mitosis. One additional hint you might want to use involves what to do when two names that begin with the same letter occur together. From our carpal example, note trapezium and trapezoid. Don't you think that it would be easy to get confused during an exam as to which of these two similar terms comes first? Simply make a mental note each time you see this situation as to whether the terms are in alphabetical order or not. In this case, they are. It is easier to remember that than it is to arbitrarily remember which comes first.

That's about it for tips on memorization. One additional point about this chapter you will notice is that, for most bones, only the name of the bone is given in the diagrams. Often when people begin studying the body, they try to learn everything at once. In the case of the skeletal system, they try to learn the names of all of the bones and the names of the features on these bones at the same time. The names of individual bone features are beyond the scope of this text. The names of a few specific bone features are given because these are features that will be useful to you later on in your reading. In some cases, these features are useful landmarks that can be observed from the surface of the body. Table 7.3 appears later in the chapter and presents the generic names of bone features. By reviewing that information, you will be able to identify, in most cases, the feature being referred to on any given bone.

Once you begin learning the bone names, you will find it is not that difficult. You will also be surprised how useful this knowledge can be, even in your daily life. Think of the fun you can have the next time you are at a Halloween party and someone is there dressed as a skeleton. Anyway, let's begin.

7.2 The Skeleton: Subdivisions

As previously suggested, we can divide the bones of the skeleton in a variety of ways that make them easier to learn. The skeleton can be divided into two general components: the axial skeleton and the appendicular

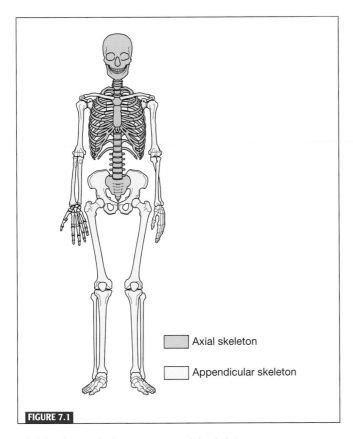

FIGURE 7.1

Axial and appendicular components of the skeleton.

Axial skeleton

Appendicular skeleton

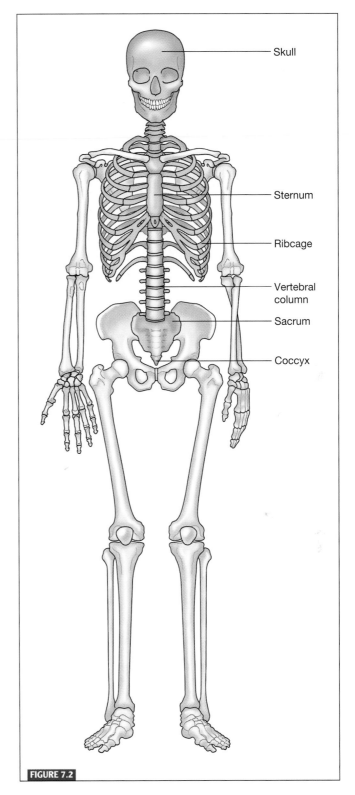

Skull

Sternum

Ribcage

Vertebral column

Sacrum

Coccyx

FIGURE 7.2

Major bones of the axial skeleton.

skeleton (**FIGURE 7.1**). This is the plan we will follow in learning the bones. The axial skeleton includes the bones of the head, neck, and trunk. The appendicular skeleton includes the bones of the limbs and the bones that attach the limbs to the trunk. We will begin with the axial skeleton.

■ The Axial Skeleton

The axial skeleton includes the bones of the axis or midline of the body. This includes the bones of the head, the neck, and the trunk. **FIGURE 7.2** demonstrates which bones are included in the axial skeleton. We will begin with the bones of the head, the skull.

The Skull

FIGURE 7.3 shows the bones of the skull. These bones are listed in **TABLE 7.1**. Again, begin at one location and work your way through the bones in the same order each time. I suggest beginning with the forehead (frontal bone) and moving up over the top of the skull, then around the side of the skull, and finally down the face to the hyoid bone, which is actually in the upper throat region. You will notice that the bones are listed in this order in the table.

We need to consider a few points about the bones of the skull before we move on. The nasal chonchae are plates of bone that extend into the nasal cavity. On each

side, two are part of the ethmoid bone and an additional one is a separate bone. These plates swirl the air inhaled through the nose. This is important in conditioning the air so it will not damage delicate tissues lower in the airways. We will discuss that in detail in Chapter 17.

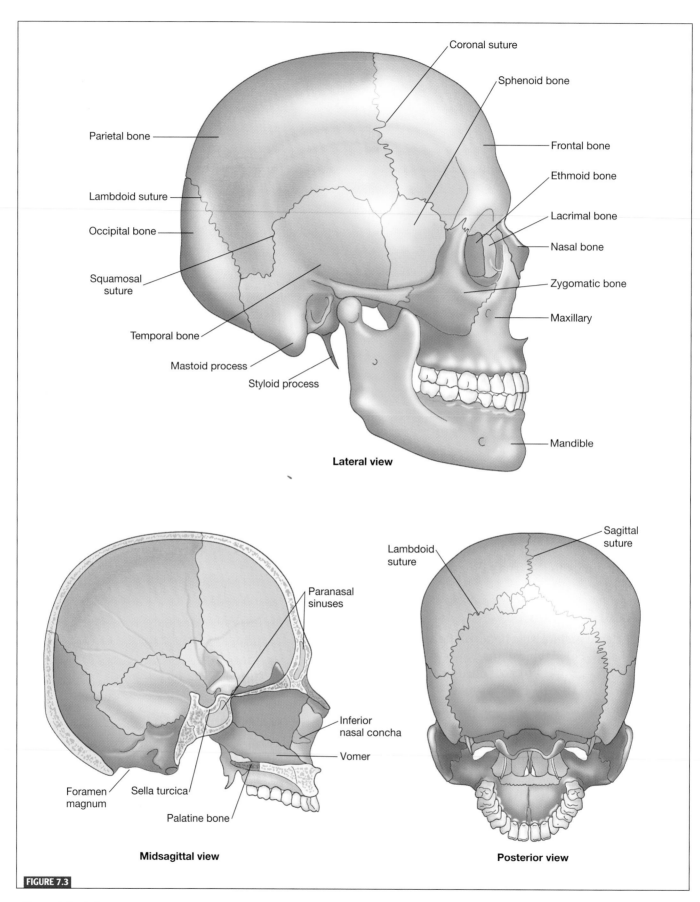

Lateral view

Midsagittal view

Posterior view

FIGURE 7.3

Bones of the skull.

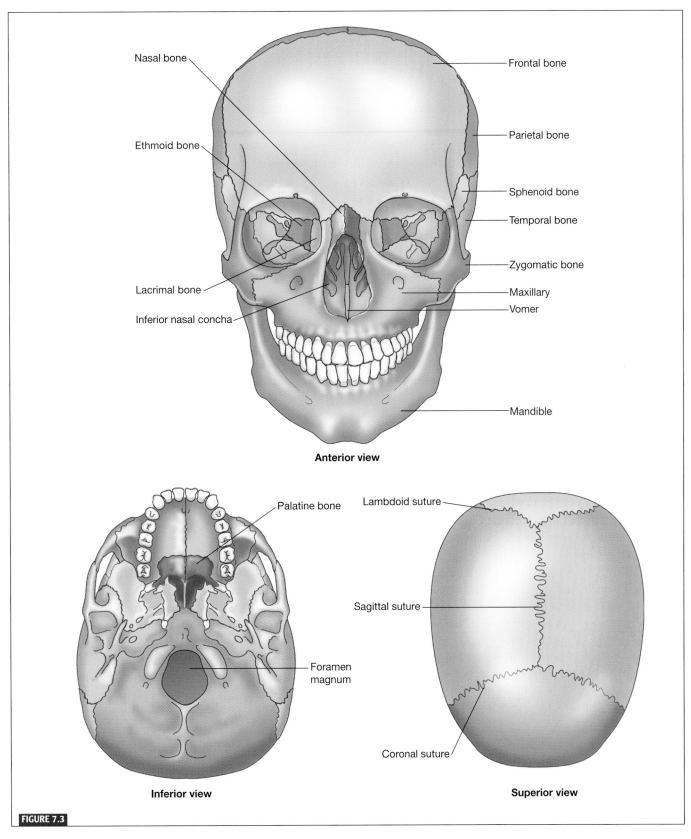

Nasal bone

Ethmoid bone

Lacrimal bone

Inferior nasal concha

Frontal bone

Parietal bone

Sphenoid bone

Temporal bone

Zygomatic bone

Maxillary

Vomer

Mandible

Anterior view

Palatine bone

Foramen magnum

Inferior view

Lambdoid suture

Sagittal suture

Coronal suture

Superior view

FIGURE 7.3

(*Continued*)

Table 7.1	The Bones of the Skull	

Bone	Number Present	Special Features/Memory Aids
Frontal*	1	Forehead, in the front
Parietal	2	Just posterior to the frontal
Occipital	1	Most posterior bone in the skull, contains the foramen magnum
Temporal	2	In the temple region
Sphenoid*	1	Extends across skull, includes the sella turcica
Zygomatic	2	Cheekbones
Maxillary*	2	Includes anterior portion of the hard palate (hard portion of roof of mouth), articulates with upper teeth
Nasal	2	Bridge of the nose
Lacrimal	2	Think lacrimation (production of tears from lacrimal glands)
Ethmoid*	1	Bone of complex shape, includes medial portion of eye socket and portions of the nasal cavity; also includes superior and middle nasal conchae (turbinates)
Inferior nasal concha	2	The largest nasal concha (turbinates)
Vomer	1	Nasal septum
Palatine	1 (fused)	Posterior part of hard palate
Mandible	1	Lower jaw, articulates with lower teeth
Hyoid	1	Not actually part of the skull, but this is a convenient place to mention it; anchors base of the tongue, does not directly articulate with other bones

*Includes paranasal sinuses.

Paranasal sinuses are small air spaces within the bones of the skull. Bones that contain paranasal sinuses include the frontal, sphenoid, maxillary, and ethmoid bones. These sinuses are important for several reasons. They play a role in conditioning the air we breathe. They act as small resonance chambers, altering the sounds of our voices and allowing us to be heard clearly. You have probably noticed that when your sinuses are inflamed and filled with mucus, due to a cold or allergy, your voice does not project clearly. That is because the ability of the paranasal sinuses to resonate sound has been impaired. They also help to somewhat lighten the bones of the skull.

One feature mentioned previously is the sella turcica of the sphenoid bone. The sella turcica is a pit on the superior surface of this bone. It faces the inferior surface of the brain. This structure surrounds the pituitary gland, which we will learn much more about in Chapter 13.

An additional feature you will want to know is the foramen magnum. The foramen magnum (meaning big hole) is the opening through which your brain and your spinal cord connect to each other. This is an opening through the occipital bone.

Figure 7.3 also demonstrates features called sutures. Sutures are a form of articulation or joint between bones.

We will learn more about articulations later in this chapter. For now, it is important that you learn the names of these sutures, the joints between the bones of your skull.

The Vertebrae

The vertebrae are the bones that make up our vertebral column, commonly called our necks and our backbones. We will need to know a number of features of these bones, as well as the various regions of the vertebral column, how many vertebrae are present in each, and what curves the vertebral column follows. These curves provide flexibility to the column when bearing a load or experiencing an impact. If the vertebral column was straight and you landed hard on your feet, this structure would experience a hard impact. The curves allow it to flex under this load, reducing the probability of damage. We will specifically name two of the vertebrae. **TABLE 7.2** and **FIGURE 7.4** contain much of this information.

Now, some additional information about the vertebrae. Let's start with the typical vertebra shown in Figure 7.4. While a thoracic vertebra is shown here, other vertebra, except C1 (the atlas) and C2 (the axis), are similar. By knowing the features of these vertebrae, you will know the basics of other vertebrae. The atlas and axis will be considered separately. Notice that vertebrae

Table 7.2	The Vertebrae			
Region	**Number of Vertebrae**	**Curvature**	**Special Features/Memory Aids**	
Cervical	7	Concave	Vertebra C1 is the atlas; vertebra C2 is the axis	
Thoracic	12	Convex	The ribs articulate with these vertebrae	
Lumbar	5	Concave	These are the heaviest vertebrae	
Sacral	5	Convex	These are fused into one structure (the sacrum)	
Coccygeal	3–5	Convex	These are variable in number and may fuse together as we age; these are our "internal tail"	

have a structure called a body. This is the anterior portion of the vertebral column and carries the weight of the body. Intervertebral disks composed of a fibrocartilage body (the annulus fibrosus) with a gel-like fluid center (the nucleus pulposus) provide a cushion between the bodies of the vertebrae and allow flexibility to our vertebral columns. It is these disks that can compress or rupture, causing considerable back pain and mobility problems to the affected individuals.

You will also notice that the vertebra have a vertebral arch that surrounds the vertebral foramen or canal. The vertebral arch is made up of the pedicle (means feet), or sides, of the arch and the lamina, or top, of the arch. The vertebral foramen is the canal where we find the spinal cord. Notice also that there are several other features associated with the arch. The transverse processes and the spinous process are spinelike projections that extend off the arch. These provide sites of attachment for muscles that allow us to bend our vertebral columns in various directions. Feel your vertebral column with your fingers and you will be able to identify your spinous process. The superior and inferior articular facets are the points of articulation between vertebrae. The term *articular* refers to a joint between bones, and the term *facet* refers to a flat, smooth place on a bone where it articulates with another bone. Thoracic vertebrae also have costal articular facets for joints with individual ribs (costal indicates rib). Some thoracic vertebrae share such a facet with the adjacent vertebra. In these cases, the rib actually splits its articulation between two vertebrae. These vertebrae then each have a demifacet (*demi* = half) for a rib articulation.

Where do nerves from the spinal cord enter and exit the vertebral foramen? Nerves must extend from the spinal cord to structures throughout the body, so how do they get there? Notice that there are no lateral holes or foramen through vertebrae for this purpose. Instead, there is a notch on each side of the inferior aspect of the vertebral arch for this purpose. Since this creates a fora-men (hole) between vertebrae, we call this the intervertebral foramen. You can see how a compressed intervertebral disk could crush a spinal nerve (ouch!), since spinal nerves exit and enter between, not through, vertebrae.

We now need to consider the atlas and the axis. What was Atlas' role in mythology? Didn't he hold up the world? So, doesn't it make sense that the atlas (the first cervical vertebra) holds up your head? Facets on the atlas articulate with facets on the occipital bone of your skull, allowing you to nod your head in the "yes" manner. Your second cervical vertebra is called the axis. In the anterior midline, you will notice a feature called the dens, or odontoid process. The term *odontoid* means "toothlike." This process has a toothlike appearance. The odontoid process articulates with a facet on the atlas. This articulation allows you to shake your head in the "no" manner. When someone has a fatal whiplash injury in an automobile accident, what has most often occurred is that the odontoid process has penetrated the soft tissue of the brain stem through the foramen magnum, where the brain joins the spinal cord.

The Ribs and the Sternum

The ribs form a strong, yet flexible shield around the vital organs of our thoracic cavity. These organs must be protected, as our life depends on their unimpaired functioning. However, for these organs to function, we must be able to alter the volume of our thoracic cavity. This is why the ribcage must be flexible. The term *costal* refers to the ribs. For example, the intercostal muscles are the muscles that are associated with our ribs. Please look at **FIGURE 7.5** for the configuration of our ribs. Note that the ribs articulate with our thoracic vertebrae. Also note that in the anterior midline, most of our ribs articulate with the sternum. Ribs that articulate directly with the sternum are called true ribs. Ribs 1 (most superior) through 7 are true ribs. False ribs are those that do not directly articulate with the sternum. Ribs 8

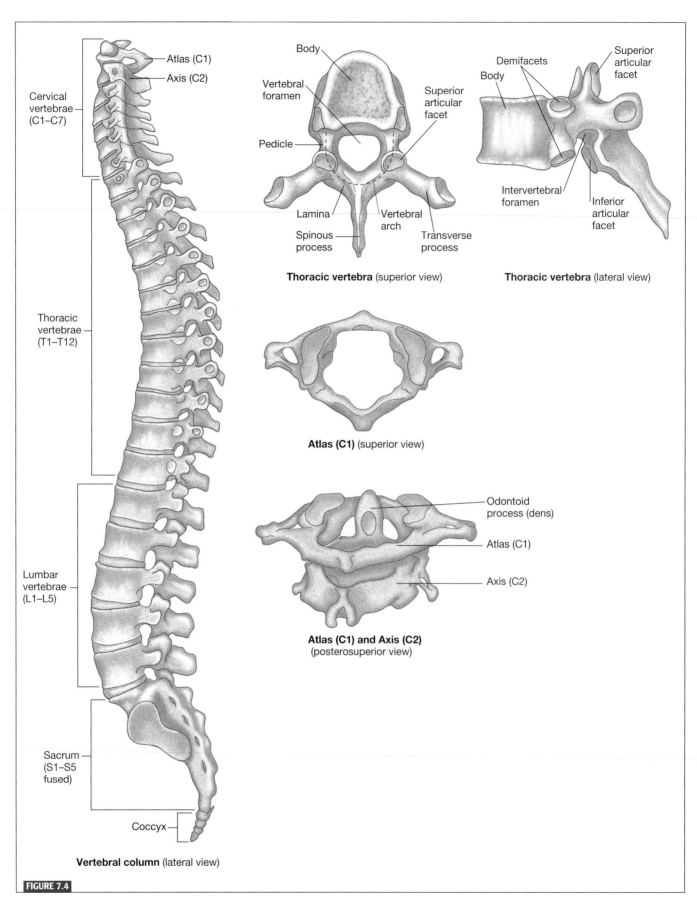

Thoracic vertebra (superior view)

Thoracic vertebra (lateral view)

Atlas (C1) (superior view)

Atlas (C1) and Axis (C2)
(posterosuperior view)

Vertebral column (lateral view)

FIGURE 7.4

The vertebral column and features of selected vertebrae.

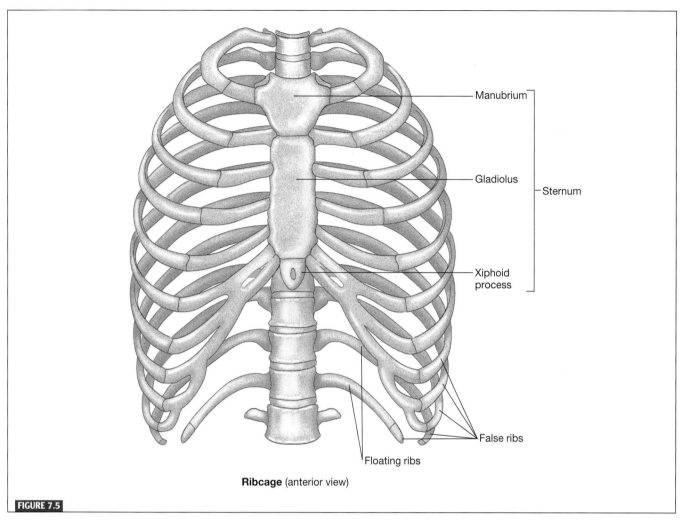

Ribcage (anterior view)

FIGURE 7.5

The ribcage including the sternum.

through 12 (most inferior) are false ribs. Ribs 8 through 10 articulate only indirectly with the sternum. The cartilage that links them to the sternum actually joins together with the cartilage of rib 7, indirectly linking them to the sternum. Ribs 11 and 12 do not articulate with the sternum at all. You can feel this on your own ribs by gently pressing in the inferior region of your rib cage. You will find the free anterior ends of these two ribs with your fingers. For this reason, in addition to being false ribs, ribs 11 and 12 are also called floating ribs.

Now that I have mentioned the sternum (breast bone) several times, perhaps we should consider it. The sternum is made up of three separate, or not so separate, structures in the anterior midline of your thoracic cavity. Figure 7.5 also illustrates the sternum. The most superior bone of the sternum is the manubrium. The first rib articulates with the manubrium, while the second rib articulates with the joint between the manubrium and the next bone of the sternum. This next bone of the sternum is the largest of the three bones. It is called the body, or gladiolus, of the sternum. The term *gladiolus* is Latin for "little sword." It may help you to remember this term if you think, not of a little sword, but instead of the word "gladiator." Gladiators carried shields, didn't they? Since the gladiolus is the largest bone in the sternum, it serves us as a shield (a fact that might help you to remember the term *gladiolus*). Ribs 2 through 10 articulate either directly or indirectly with the gladiolus.

The third bone of the sternum is, for much of our life, not a bone at all. Extending from the inferior aspect of the gladiolus, there is a small pointed structure called the xiphoid, or xiphoid process. The term *xiphoid* comes from the Greek word meaning "sword"; the anatomist who coined the terms for the sternum must have been really stuck on the idea of its resembling a sword. Early in life, the xiphoid is made of hyaline cartilage. By about age 40, it is converted to bone. It may or may not completely fuse with the gladiolus. Overzealous CPR sometimes can fracture the xiphoid and drive it into the underlying organs, causing them injury.

■ The Appendicular Skeleton

The appendicular skeleton includes the bones of the limbs and the bones that connect the limbs to the trunk (**FIGURE 7.6**). The bones that connect the arms to the trunk are called the pectoral girdle. The bones that connect the legs to the trunk are called the pelvic girdle. We will begin with the arms and pectoral girdle.

The Pectoral Girdle and Arms

The bones of the upper limbs (arms) and the pectoral girdle are shown in **FIGURE 7.7**. The pectoral girdle attaches

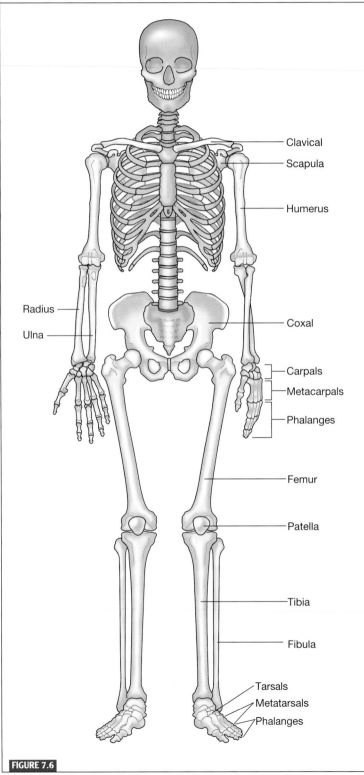

FIGURE 7.6

Major bones of the appendicular skeleton.

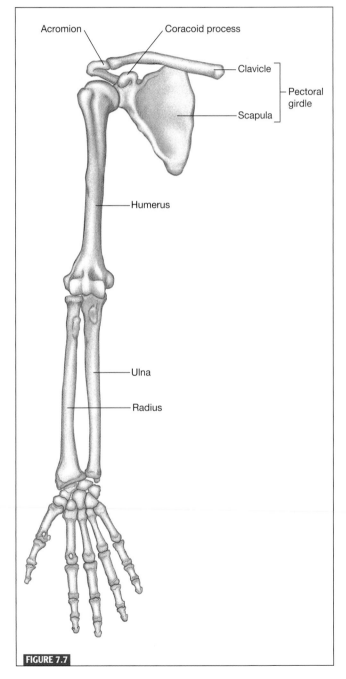

FIGURE 7.7

Bones of the pectoral girdle and arm.

the upper limbs or arms to the trunk. The pectoral girdle consists of two bones on each side of the body. The clavicle is the anterior bone of the pectoral girdle (**FIGURE 7.8**). This relatively fine bone has an elongated s-shape and extends from the sternum to the scapula. After viewing the area shown in the diagram, feel your clavicle with your fingers. The clavicle is one of the most frequently broken bones in the human body. This is due to the amount of strain placed on this bone when someone falls onto an extended arm.

The scapula (shoulder blade) makes up the posterior portion of this girdle (Figure 7.8). By following your clavicle laterally with your fingers, you will find the location where it meets the scapula. The scapula has a flattened, triangular shape with prominent ridges. By rotating your shoulder anteriorly, you may reach back with your opposite arm and feel the shape of your scapula. This bone provides a site of attachment for muscles affecting move-ment of your shoulder. It articulates with the humerus, the proximal bone of your forelimb.

You know that your arm consists of an upper region and a lower region. The upper or proximal region of your arm has the humerus as its support (**FIGURE 7.9**). The humerus extends from your scapula to your elbow. At your elbow, your lower arm (the distal portion) begins. Two bones make up the supporting structure of your lower arm. With your body in the anatomical position, the ulna is the medial bone and the radius is lateral. This sometimes confuses students during an exam (again,

Pectoral girdle (anterior view)

Acromion
Corocoid process
Clavicle
Glenoid fossa
Scapular notch
Body

Pectoral girdle (posterior view)

Clavicle
Acromion
Glenoid fossa
Spine

FIGURE 7.8

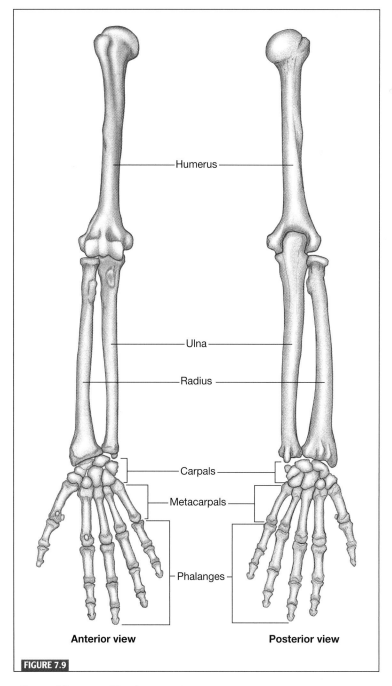

Humerus
Ulna
Radius
Carpals
Metacarpals
Phalanges

Anterior view **Posterior view**

FIGURE 7.9

The pectoral girdle including features of the scapula.

Bones of the arm and hand.

you knew it the night before, but . . .). As you are trying to remember which bone is which, wouldn't you be likely to scratch your head and make the sound "Um"? That's the clue, "Um" tells you that the ulna is medial. (O.K., so some of these hints are a little hokey. As long as they work, who cares?)

The ulna and the radius extend from the elbow to the wrist. At the wrist, we encounter the carpals, the bones given as an example in the beginning of this chapter. Students also sometimes confuse whether it is the carpals or the tarsals that are in the wrist (the tarsals are in the ankle). To remember this, simply recall that carpal tunnel syndrome involves the wrist; hence, the carpals are in the wrist. (Or, if you were to grab a carp [fish], you would use your hand, not your foot.)

Meanwhile, back at the carpals. The carpals are composed of eight small bones. These bones are arranged into two rows, as shown in **FIGURE 7.10**. Learn the bones in the manner described in the beginning of this chapter. You are likely to encounter a different view of the wrist at some point, so simply memorizing this diagram won't do.

Moving distally, we next encounter the metacarpals, or bones of the hand. Note the presence of sesamoid bones associated with the metacarpals in Figure 7.10. Sesamoid bones are located within tendons and may vary among individuals. They articulate with the distal row of the carpals and with the phalanges. The phalanges are the bones of the thumb and fingers. The same term applies to the bones of the toes (later). Although the fact that the thumb has two phalanges, while the fingers have three each, seems to be a good way to identify the thumb as a landmark in a diagram or radiograph, use caution. It is not that uncommon for people to lose the distal phalanx (singular for phalanges) from one or more of their fingers. This can lead to confusion. It is best to identify the thumb based on how it attaches to the carpals, and after that, determine that the little finger does, in fact, have all of its phalanges.

The Pelvic Girdle and Legs

The pelvic girdle consists of a bone on each side of the body (the coxal bones) that articulates with the sacrum in your posterior midline and with each other in your anterior midline (**FIGURE 7.11**). Each coxal bone is actually made up of three bones each, which fused as you developed (**FIGURE 7.12**). The three bones that make up the coxal bones are the ilium, the ischium, and the

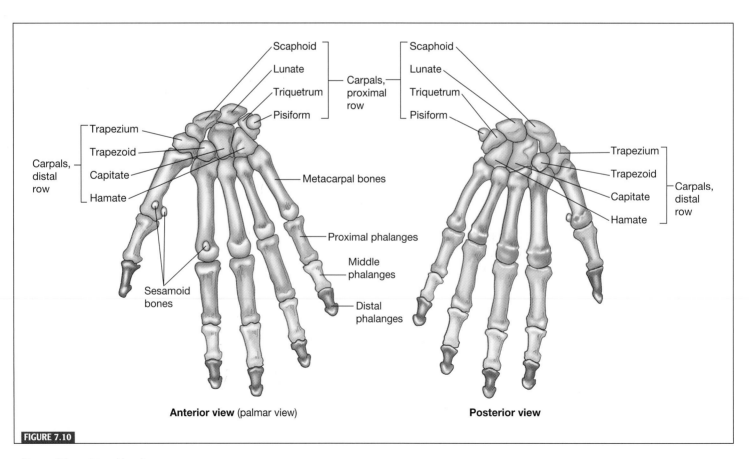

Anterior view (palmar view)   **Posterior view**

FIGURE 7.10

Bones of the wrist and hand.

pubis. The term *coxal* comes from the root *coax*, meaning hip. The ilium (meaning groin or flank) makes up the largest portion of the coxals. It comprises the posterior and superior region of the coxals and you can palpate the superior border of this bone (the iliac crest) laterally in your lower back. This region of the ilium is called the iliac crest and is the site of attachment for several muscles controlling movement of the hips. The ischium lies between the ilium and the pubis. It makes up the posterior and inferior region of the coxals. The pubis includes the anterior portion of this bone. The two pubis bones meet at a joint called the symphysis pubis. We will learn more about this joint shortly. The pelvic brim outlines an open region through the coxal bones. During delivery, the infant must pass through the opening through the pelvis. This fact, together with the greater weight and more powerful musculature of the male (in general), dictates that the coxals are shaped differently between the two sexes. Figure 7.12 demonstrates these differences.

The femur, which is the bone of the thigh, articulates with the coxal bones at a special ball and socket joint. We will discuss joints (articulations) later on in this chapter, but for now, let's consider this interesting joint. A ball and socket joint allows us to rotate our legs in any direction. When you consider all that we do with our legs, this is a good thing. Consider the shape of the socket, however. The socket is called the acetabulum. It has a concave shape to accept the ball with which it articulates. This is a complex shape for the body to form. Do you think the acetabulum is part of the ilium, ishium, or pubis bone? If you answered "all three," you are right. Note in Figure 7.12 that the three bones join together through the acetabulum.

The bone of the proximal region of the leg is the femur (**FIGURE 7.13**). The head of the femur is the ball that articulates with the acetabulum. This head is mounted on a neck, a projection from the femur. Two ridges extend from the proximal region of the femur for the attachment of muscles. The lateral ridge is the greater trochanter, and the medial ridge is the lesser trochanter. The powerful muscles that control the movements of the upper leg make these ridges necessary.

Two bones articulate with the distal end of the femur. The tibia is one of two bones that extend through the distal portion of the leg (the calf). It directly articulates with the femur. The patella, or kneecap, is a sesamoid bone that articulates with the femur. The kneecap adds to the strength of contraction of one of the muscles used to bend the leg at the knee by extending the leverage of this muscle. It also stabilizes the knee when it is in the bent position.

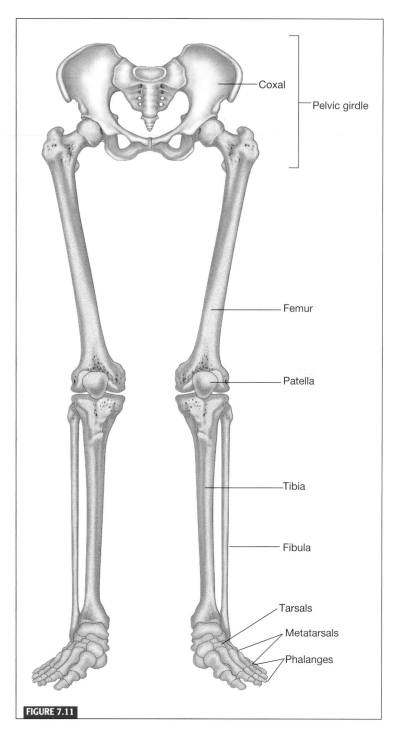

FIGURE 7.11

Bones of the pelvic girdle and legs.

The calf, or distal region of the leg, is supported by two bones, the tibia and the fibula. The tibia is the larger of these two; it articulates with the femur proximally and with the talus of the tarsals, or ankle bones, distally. The fibula articulates with the tibia, not the femur, at its proximal end. It articulates with the tibia and the talus distally. See Figure 7.13 for a diagram of this arrangement. From

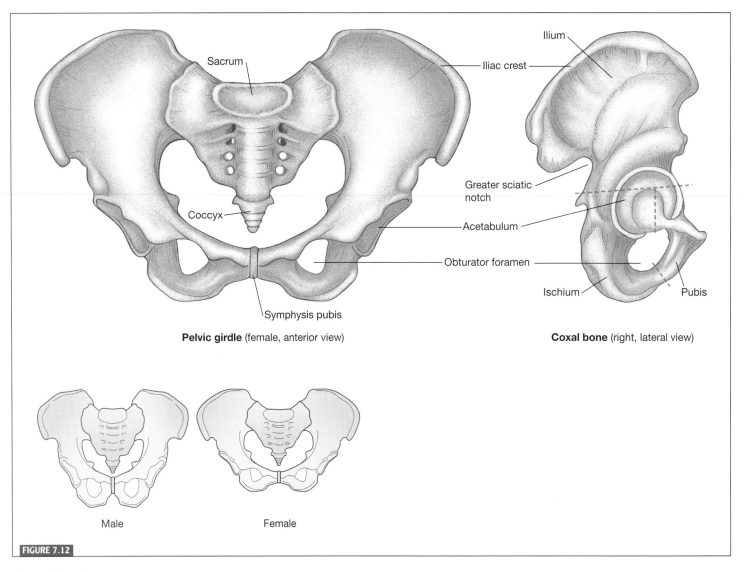

Pelvic girdle (female, anterior view)

Coxal bone (right, lateral view)

Male   Female

FIGURE 7.12

The pelvic girdle.

this arrangement, can you determine which of these two bones is actually bearing the weight of the body?

We are now at the ankle, and here we find the tarsal bones. In the wrist, numerous carpal bones were present; similarly, we find several tarsal bones in the ankle. Again, be sure to remember that the carpals are in the wrist, and that the tarsals are in the ankle. The tibia and fibula directly articulate with the most superior tarsal bone, the talus (talus means ankle). The talus, in turn, articulates with the calcaneus (means heel) and the navicular (boat shaped). The calcaneus is the largest of the tarsals and makes up the heel of your foot. The navicular bone articulates with the first, second, and third cuneiform (cone-shaped) bones and with the cuboid bone. The cuboid also articulates with the calcaneus. The three

cuneiform bones and the cuboid bone each articulate with the metatarsals. So, that was a lot of explanation for something that can easily be seen in Figure 7.13.

How can you remember all this? You have seven tarsal bones. The most superior of these is the one with the name that means ankle (talus). The largest of these is the one with the name that means heel (calcaneus). Just anterior to these you have two bones, the navicular and the cuboid. The navicular is medial (n is closer to m alphabetically). Anterior to the navicular, you have the three cuneiforms. Instead of numbering them, you can refer to them as the medial (first), intermediate (second), and lateral (third) cuneiform. There you have the ankle.

Next, we have the bones that extend the length of the foot. These are the metatarsals (analogous to the

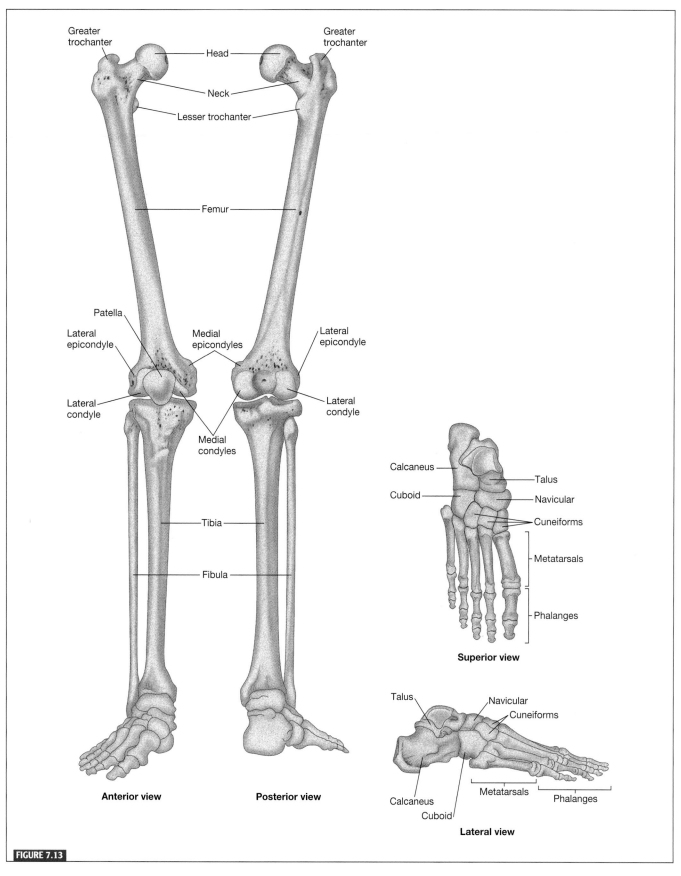

FIGURE 7.13

Bones of the leg and ankle.

metacarpals in the hand). The toes contain the pha-langes, just as the fingers did, and they are in the same arrangement. We have three phalanges in each toe, ex-cept in our big (great) toe, which has only two.

7.3 The Generic Features of Bones

We have now examined all of the bones. **TABLE 7.3** lists the generic terms for the features of the bones. By features, I mean things like holes, grooves, and ridges. Every fea-ture of each bone has a specific name. This amount of detail is beyond the scope of this text, as previously mentioned. If you are interested, there are many texts available with which you can expand your knowledge. You are now developing a solid base on which you can expand. By knowing the generic terms for the features, you will be in an excellent position to discuss the skele-tal system and understand what others tell you about it. Please spend some time familiarizing yourself with the information contained in that table.

We need now to consider how the bones join to-gether. That brings us to our next topic, the articulations.

7.4 The Articulations: What Kind of a Joint Is This Anyway?

O.K., here we are at a joint; what kind of a joint is it? That is what we are about to learn. Joints (articulations) are the places where two bones meet, or in some cases where bones meet cartilage or teeth. There are a num-ber of different types of joints in our skeletal systems and several different ways of categorizing them. We will use two systems of categorization. One system will be based on how they function; the second will be based on their structure. Much of this information will be pre-sented in the form of tables, as it is very straightforward and easy to learn. Synovial joints comprise one type; we will spend the majority of our time on this type, as it is the most interesting and complex.

■ Functional Classification of the Articulations

Functionally, there are three classes of articulations. Those joints in which the opposing bones are unable to move are called synarthroses (synarthrosis is singular). Next, we have joints in which limited movement is pos-sible; these are called amphiarthroses. Finally, we have the diarthroses, or freely movable joints. We will see ex-amples of each of these in our next section. To remem-ber these, recall that we are going from immovable to freely movable, and the first letter of each category spells the word <u>sad</u>.

■ Structural Classification of the Articulations

The structural classification of our joints is determined by which tissue is present within the joint. We learned about the types of connective tissues in Chapter 4. Now we will see those connective tissues in various joints in the body. We have four categories of joints: bony joints, fibrous joints, cartilaginous joints, and synovial joints. Each of these categories has several subcategories in-cluded within them. This information is presented in **TABLE 7.4**. Although Table 7.4 contains the information we need on the bony, fibrous, and cartilaginous joints, more time must be spent on synovial joints.

Synovial Joints

Synovial joints have a fascinating structure that allows us to move smoothly and easily. This amazing capac-ity for motion is due to the fact that each synovial joint has a space within it; this space separates the articu-

---

Table 7.3   The Features of Bones

Category	Feature	Description
Openings extending through bones	Foramen	A round hole through a bone
	Meatus	A tubelike canal through a bone
	Fissure	A narrow, cracklike opening through a bone, or between adjacent bones
Features on bone surfaces	Sulcus	A groove or trenchlike depression on the surface of a bone
	Fossa	A rounded depression on the surface of a bone
	Facet	A flat, smooth surface used for articulation
	Process	Any structure protruding from the surface of a bone

Table 7.5   Terminology Describing Movements of the Human Body

Name of Movement	Description
Flexion	Decrease the angle of a joint to move bones closer together (bend your elbow).
Extension	Increase the angle of a joint to move bones apart (straighten your elbow).
Hyperextension	Extend a joint past the straight position (bend backwards).
Abduction	Move a limb away from the midline (lift your leg laterally from the anatomical position).
Adduction	Move a limb toward the midline (return your leg to the anatomical position).
Circumduction	A complex movement in which a limb describes a cone in the air (with your arm or leg stiff, move that limb so your hand or foot completes a circle).
Lateral rotation	Turn a structure away from the midline (from the anatomical position, turn your head to one side).
Medial rotation	Turn a structure toward the midline (return your head to the anatomical position).
Elevation	Move a structure superiorly (shrug your shoulders).
Depression	Move a structure inferiorly (pull your shoulders down).
Protraction	Move a structure anteriorly (jut out your jaw).
Retraction	Move a structure posteriorly (pull your jaw in).
Dorsiflexion	Specific for the ankle and foot, move superiorly (arch your foot up).
Plantar flexion	Specific for the ankle and foot, move inferiorly (arch your foot down).
Inversion	Specific for the ankle and foot, rotate soles medially (face soles toward each other).
Eversion	Specific for the ankle and foot, rotate soles laterally (make soles face outward).
Supination	Specific for forearm, rotate palms anteriorly or superiorly (flex elbow, then rotate forearm as if to collect money in your hand).
Pronation	Specific for forearm, rotate palms posteriorly or inferiorly (flex elbow, as if to dump dust from your hand).
Opposition	Move one digit across the hand (place your thumb across your palm, as if to hold onto a rope).

What You Should Know

1. By developing and using a strategy, your memorization skill can be improved, thereby aiding your progress in anatomy and physiology.

2. The axial skeleton includes the bones of the head, neck, and trunk.

3. The appendicular skeleton includes the bones of the limbs and the bones that attach the limbs to the trunk.

4. You must be able to identify the name and location of each bone in the axial and appendicular skeletons.

5. Paranasal sinuses are found in the frontal, sphenoid, maxillary, and ethmoid bones.

6. There are seven cervical vertebrae, and together they have a concave curvature.

7. Cervical vertebra number one is the atlas and number two is the axis.

8. The 12 thoracic vertebrae together have a convex curvature.

9. The five lumbar vertebrae together have a concave curvature.

10. The five sacral vertebrae are fused into a convex structure.

11. The coccygeal vertebrae are variable in number and may fuse as we age.

12. Vertebral features you must know include the body; vertebral foramen; arch, including pedicle and lamina; transverse and spinous process; articular facets and demifacets; and intervertebral foramen.

13. Ribs 1 through 7 are true ribs, 8 through 12 are false ribs, and 11 and 12 are also floating ribs.

14. The sternum includes the manubrium, the gladiolus, and the xiphoid.

What You Should Know (continued)

15. The pectoral girdle and pelvic girdle are components of the appendicular skeleton.

16. The pectoral girdle attaches the arms to the trunk.

17. The pelvic girdle attaches the legs to the trunk.

18. You must know all of the bones of the appendicular girdles and limbs.

19. The carpal bones are found in the wrist and include the scaphoid, lunate, triquetrum, pisiform, trapezium, trapezoid, capitate, and hamate bones.

20. The tarsal bones are found in the ankle and include the talus, calcaneus, navicular, cuboid, and the first, second, and third cuneiforms.

21. While each bone feature has a specific name, many of these names include the generic term for that type of feature. You must know these generic terms.

22. Synarthroses are immovable articulations, amphiarthroses are slightly movable articulations, and diarthroses are freely movable articulations.

23. A synostosis is a bony articulation.

24. Categories of fibrous joints include suture, syndesmosis, and gomphosis.

25. Categories of cartilaginous joints include synchondrosis and symphesis.

26. Synovial joints are freely movable and contain a synovial space.

27. Each type of movement in a synovial joint has a name. You must know these names.

What Did You Learn?

Multiple choice questions: choose the best answer.

1. _____ is the bone of your cheek.
   a. Zygomatic
   b. Maxillary
   c. Lacrimal
   d. Temporal
   e. Ethmoid

2. _____ include the anterior portion of the hard palate.
   a. Zygomatic
   b. Maxillary
   c. Lacrimal
   d. Temporal
   e. Ethmoid

3. Of the following, which does not contain a paranasal sinus?
   a. Sphenoid
   b. Ethmoid
   c. Frontal

   d. Mandible
   e. Maxillary

4. The sagittal suture is found between which bones?
   a. The two parietals
   b. The parietals and the frontal
   c. The occipital and the sphenoid
   d. The temporal and the occipital

5. The sella turcica is a feature of which bone?
   a. Maxillary
   b. Zygomatic
   c. Sphenoid
   e. Ethmoid

6. Which of the following contribute to the acetabulum?
   1. Ilium
   2. Ischium
   3. Pubis
      a. 1,2,3
      b. 1,2

What Did You Learn? (continued)

  c. 2,3

  d. 1,3

  e. 1 only

7. Which of these features is on the lateral aspect of the proximal end of the femur?

  a. Greater trochanter

  b. Lesser trochanter

  c. Both of the above

  d. Neither of the above

8. The hyoid bone directly articulates with the:

  a. Vertebrae

  b. Ribs

  c. Manubrium

  d. Clavicle

  e. None of the above

9. Identify this location or structure:

  a. Fibrous capsule

  b. Synovial membrane

  c. Synovial space

  d. Articular cartilage

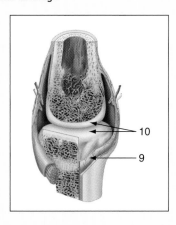

10. Identify this location or structure:

  a. Fibrous capsule

  b. Synovial membrane

  c. Synovial space

  d. Articular cartilage

11. A round hole through a bone is a _____.

  a. Fissure

  b. Foramen

  c. Meatus

  d. Fossa

  e. Process

12. A symphesis is a:

  a. Synarthrosis

  b. Amphiarthrosis

  c. Diarthrosis

13. Identify the bone indicated:

  a. Hamate

  b. Capitate

  c. Triquetrum

  d. Trapezoid

  e. Trapezium

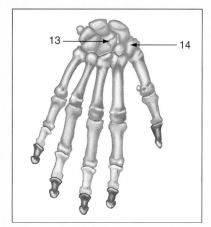

14. Identify the bone indicated:

  a. Hamate

  b. Capitate

  c. Triquetrum

  d. Trapezoid

  e. Trapezium

What Did You Learn? (continued)

15. Identify the bone indicated:
    a. Humerous
    b. Radius
    c. Ulna
    d. Tibia
    e. Fibula

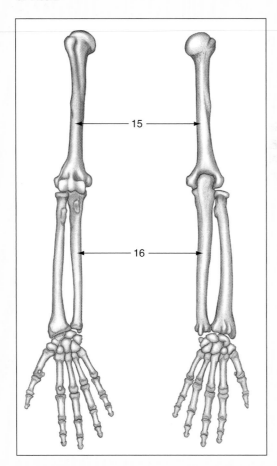

16. Identify the bone indicated:
    a. Humerous
    b. Radius
    c. Ulna
    d. Tibia
    e. Fibula

17. Identify the feature indicated:
    a. Transverse process
    b. Body
    c. Spinous process
    d. Superior articular facet
    e. Demifacet

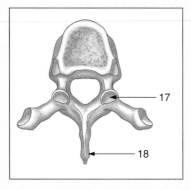

18. Identify the feature indicated:
    a. Transverse process
    b. Body
    c. Spinous process
    d. Superior articular facet
    e. Demifacet

What Did You Learn? (continued)

19. Identify the bone indicated:

   a. Coxal

   b. Sacrum

   c. Radius

   d. Clavicle

   e. Fibula

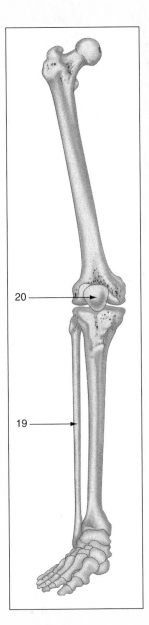

20. Identify the bone indicated:

   a. Tibia

   b. Patella

   c. Radius

   d. Clavicle

   e. Fibula

Short answer questions: answer briefly and in your own words.

1. What is meant by the terms *axial skeleton* and *appendicular skeleton?*

2. Draw a simple diagram of a lateral view of the vertebral column. Label the regions of this structure, indicate how many vertebrae are present in each region, and show the proper curve for each region.

3. Why does the vertebral column have curves? What would happen if these curves were not present?

4. Draw a superior view of one vertebra and label its parts.

5. Define the following terms:

   Foramen

   Fissure

   Fossa

   Facet

   Sulcus

6. Describe the following movements:

   Abduction

   Circumduction

   Protraction

   Eversion

   Pronation

8 The Body Electric: Electrical Activities in Your Body

What You Will Learn

- How ion gradients can be generated across a cell membrane.
- How ion gradients across a cell membrane can result in an electrical potential.
- What molecular pump is responsible for generating this electrical potential.
- How membrane potential can be depolarized and repolarized.
- What molecular event can trigger this depolarization and repolarization.
- How chemically and electrically gated channels participate in this process.
- That a wave of depolarization and repolarization spreading along the cell membrane is an action potential.
- The basic structure of synapses and neuroeffector junctions.
- How the all-or-none principle applies to action potentials.

8.1 What . . . Electricity in My Body?!!!

Absolutely, electrical activity does play a major role in your body. In Chapter 4, we learned that the nervous system is the fast-acting regulator of homeostasis. We also learned that the muscle system provides the force needed for movement and posture. To function, both of these systems require electrical activity. In this chapter, we will learn exactly what is meant by electricity in your body and how that electrical activity is generated. Although a number of cell types have this ability, it is most well developed in neurons and muscle cells. Please keep these cells in mind as you read this material. This is a very interesting aspect of our metabolism and crucial for understanding some concepts that we will learn in upcoming chapters, so read on.

8.2 Ions and Gradients: Membrane Polarization

Think back to Chapter 2 for a minute (chemistry, remember?). What did we learn about ions? Ions are charged atoms or groups of atoms. We can call them charged particles. Did they all have the same charge? No, some were positively charged and some were negatively charged. We have a name for each; positively charged ions are called cations, and ions with a negative charge are anions.

Now, how was a gradient defined? A gradient is the condition where we have more of a substance (a higher concentration) at one location than at another location (a lower concentration exists at the second location). Usually this concentration gradient exists across a membrane.

■ It's All about Cats and Dogs

Have we thought enough on the molecular level yet? O.K., let's move on to bigger things. You are sitting in your classroom. No other people are with you, but the room is full of animals, dogs and cats to be specific (**FIGURE 8.1a**). You look into the hallway and see the same thing: lots of dogs and cats. There are about the same number of dogs and cats per unit area in the room as there are outside the room. That means that the animals are in about the same concentration in either place. That means there is no concentration gradient.

Next, you decide that there are too many animals in the room. You begin to shoo animals out the door into the hallway. After a few minutes, there are far fewer animals in the room than there are out in the hallway. You have developed an animal gradient (Figure 8.1b). What would happen if you now left the doorway and did not close the door behind you? The cats and dogs would redistribute themselves so that there was no longer a concentration gradient. More cats and dogs would enter the room than would leave the room until their concentrations were again balanced.

What would happen, instead, if you were to stand in the doorway and toss dogs out of the room and cats into the room? Every time you tossed one dog out, you tossed one cat in. Would you develop an animal gradient? Think now: one dog out, one cat in. No, you would not develop an animal gradient. How about a cat gradient? Yes, there would ultimately be more cats in the room than outside the room. A dog gradient would also be established with more dogs out than in. You would have developed two independent gradients (Figure 8.1c).

If you still wanted to bring cats into the room and toss dogs out (cats are better than dogs, after all), but you also wanted to develop an animal gradient (overall, a higher concentration of animals outside the room than inside the room), how would you accomplish that? Again, paws (pun intended) to think about your dilemma; you want to move cats in and dogs out, but you want not just a cat gradient and a dog gradient, you want an animal gradient

too. How would you do that? O.K., you could move unequal numbers of cats and dogs. Let's say for every two cats you move into the room, you toss three dogs out of the room (Figure 8.1d). You would ultimately have a cat gradient (more cats in than out), a dog gradient (more dogs out than in), and an animal gradient (more animals out than in). Great, we have it all figured out. Be sure to look at the cartoons of Figure 8.1 to clarify this point.

■ Meanwhile, Back at the Ions

Do you have the feeling that we're not just talking about cats and dogs, but about ions? That's right, so let's make the switch to ions. The dogs are sodium ions, which carry a positive charge and are, therefore, cations (Na^+). The cats are potassium ions and also carry a positive charge: cations again (K^+). Instead of you standing in the doorway of your classroom, we have a molecular pump sitting in a cell membrane (**FIGURE 8.2a**). Review time again; the cell membrane is made of what? The molecular pump is a what? Think about it, don't just read on. Thinking about it is the only way you will actually learn it. So, what did you answer? The cell membrane is phospholipid bilayer that is impermeable to these ions. The molecular pump is an integral membrane protein, an enzyme. If this pump were to move only sodium ions out of the cell, a sodium gradient would be established (Figure 8.2b). Since sodium has a positive charge, an electrical gradient would also be established with more positive charges outside the cell than inside the cell.

What would happen if this pump were to transport sodium ions out of the cell and potassium ions into the cell? If it pumped equal amounts of these two ions in opposite directions, a sodium gradient would be established (more Na^+ out than in) and a potassium gradient would be established (more K^+ in than out), but no electrical gradient would be established (Figure 8.2c). Equal amounts of ions of the same charge would have been moved in opposite directions; hence, no electrical gradient. But what would happen if this pump were to move unequal amounts of sodium and potassium in opposite directions, pumping three sodium ions out of the cell for every two potassium ions into the cell, for instance. A sodium gradient would be established and a potassium gradient would be established, as already described. An electrical gradient would also be established, with the outside of the cell becoming more positive when compared to the inside of the cell (Figure 8.2d). We have established an electrical gradient, or a charge, across the cell membranes. The cell membrane is now polarized in that it has a positive side and a negative side. We have been discussing membrane polarization. Note how this

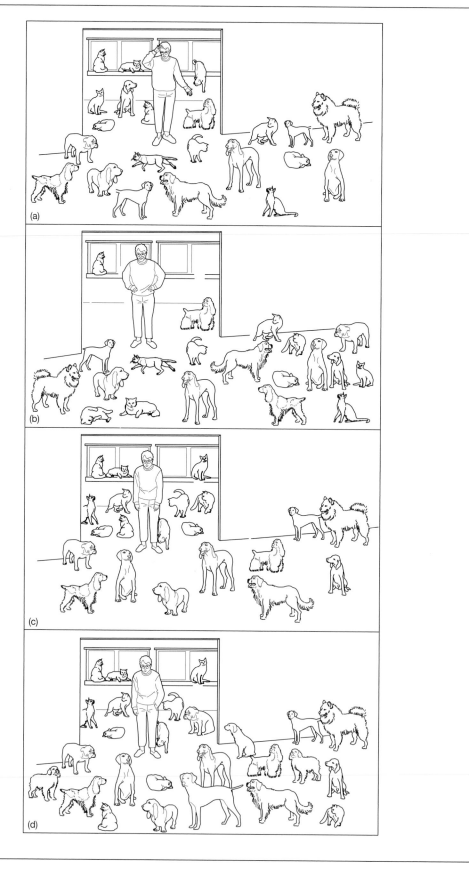

FIGURE 8.1

Like ions, we can establish gradients of animals. In (a), no gradients exist. The distribution of animals in the classroom is similar to that in the hallway. In (b) the student has established a gradient between the classroom and the hallway. He has moved most of the animals out of the room. In (c) the student has established a dog gradient (most of the dogs are in the hallway) and a cat gradient (most of the cats are in the classroom) but no overall animal gradient (similar numbers of animals are present in the room and in the hallway). In (d) the student has again established a dog gradient (most of the dogs are in the hallway) and a cat gradient (most of the cats are in the room), but because he has moved more dogs out of the room than cats into the room (i.e., 2 cats in for every 3 dogs out), he has also established an animal gradient. There are more animals (total) in the hallway than there are in the room. Notice that the student has expended energy moving the animals.

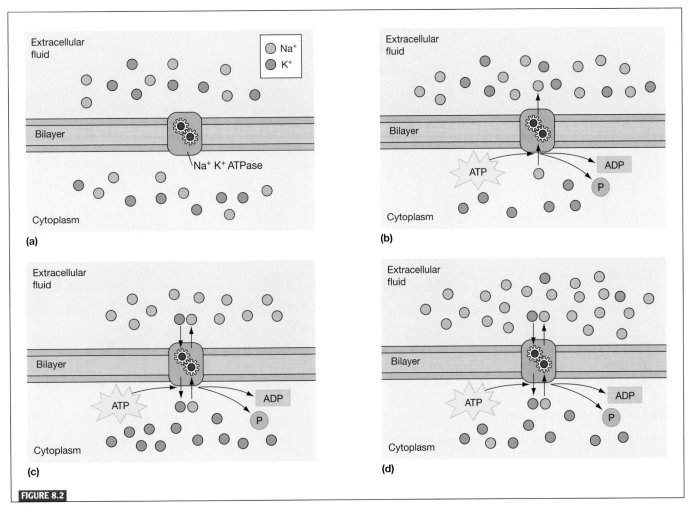

FIGURE 8.2

Like the animals shown in Figure 8.1, here we are establishing gradients of ions. In (a) no gradient exists across the cell membrane. In (b), a sodium ATPase has pumped Na$^+$ ions out of the cell, establishing a Na$^+$ gradient across the cell membrane. In (c), a Na$^+$K$^+$ ATPase has pumped Na$^+$ ions out of the cell and K$^+$ ions into the cell. It has established a sodium gradient and a potassium gradient, but no total ion gradient exists across the cell membrane. In (d), the Na$^+$K$^+$ ATPase has pumped three Na$^+$ out of the cell for every two K$^+$ it pumped into the cell. This has established three gradients across the membrane: a Na$^+$ gradient, a K$^+$ gradient, and a cation gradient (more cations out of the cell than in the cell). In this way, the membrane has become polarized. Note that the pump has used energy in the form of ATP to generate these gradients. Na$^+$K$^+$ ATPases are distributed throughout the membranes.

makes the cell membrane like a battery (see **FIGURE 8.3**). Isn't that great? Just by moving some ions, we have turned our cell into a small battery.

8.3 Molecular Pumps: That's Some Fancy Enzyme

Before we go on, let's get a few things straight about that molecular pump. We have already decided that it is an enzyme and an integral membrane protein (you, of course, remember what it means to be an integral membrane protein). Since it is an enzyme, it must catalyze, or speed up, some chemical reaction. Does it need energy to perform this pumping? Sure it does. After all, it can't use diffusion to establish a gradient; it must use an active transport mechanism (Chapter 3). What would it use for

energy? Right again, ATP; it must cleave ATP into ADP and a phosphate group to release energy to perform this pumping activity. There is the reaction it catalyzes; hence, it is an ATPase. We call it the sodium-potassium ATPase, or Na$^+$K$^+$ATPase. Since it is pumping two things in opposite directions, it is involved in countertransport (cotransport would be pumping two things in the same direction). Also, since it generates an electrical charge, we refer to it as an electrogenic pump. To put it all together, the Na$^+$K$^+$ATPase is an electrogenic molecular pump that transports three Na$^+$ out of the cell for every two K$^+$ it moves into the cell.

Do you have any batteries? Maybe you even have some of the small rechargeable type (ecologically and economically more sound than the disposable type; why not get those next time?). Do those batteries do you any

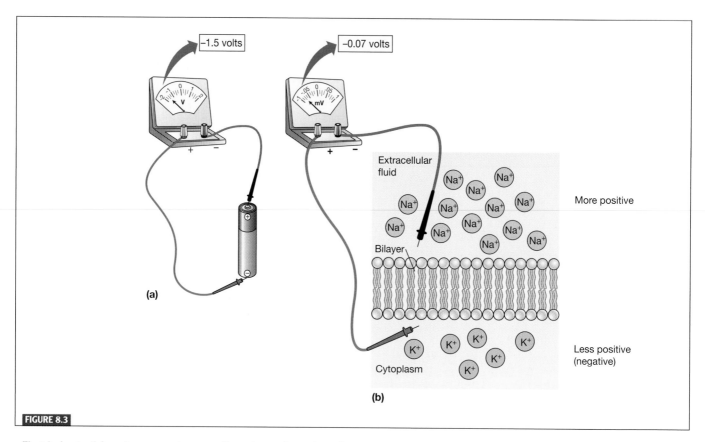

FIGURE 8.3

Electrical potential can be measured across cell membranes just as it can be measured in a battery. A typical electrically active cell such as a neuron, measures approximately −70 mV.

good at all unless you discharge them? Obviously, at some point those batteries are fully charged; lots of positivity at one end, lots of negativity at the other end. But if you use them, let's say in a small tape recorder to record your anatomy and physiology instructor's excellent lectures for your repeated listening pleasure (only with permission, of course), they become discharged. In using the energy stored in these batteries, you must destroy the charge gradient. They are only of use when you are discharging them. See an analogy coming?

How about your cells? So, we have established that some cell membranes become polarized, or "charged up" by the electrogenic Na⁺K⁺ATPase. Once the electrical gradient is established, we must have some way to use this gradient, just as you use a battery. We use a battery by depleting the energy gradient stored within it. We use the membrane polarization in the same way. Let's now see how that works.

8.4 Membrane Depolarization and Repolarization

We can use a voltmeter to measure how much energy (electrical potential) is stored in a battery, perhaps to

test our battery and see if it is still "good." For instance, a little AA battery that you would use in a small tape recorder would be fully charged at 1.5 volts. What would happen if you switched the electrodes on your voltmeter to the opposite poles of the battery (Figure 8.3a)? It would read −1.5 volts at a full charge. The negative or positive reading is simply a matter of perspective. Now, let's consider the polarized cell. If you used a tiny voltmeter to measure the potential across the cell membrane (see Figure 8.3b), it would give you a very small but measurable reading. Although this reading will vary somewhat between different types of polarized cells, 70 mV (that is 70 millivolts or thousandths of a volt, 0.07 volts) is a good average for our consideration. Since we are looking from the perspective of inside the cell, which is more negative than the outside, we will have the electrodes of our small voltmeter positioned to read −70 mV. For the sake of our discussion, the charge of a fully polarized cell is −70 mV. We call this the cell's resting membrane potential.

Now, if you use the AA battery for a while (to listen to an anatomy and physiology lecture a few times) and test it again, the charge would be reduced. As the battery "goes dead," the reading in volts you will measure will be reduced. To use the charge in our cell membrane, we must also discharge it somewhat. This is called membrane depolarization because the membrane is becoming less polarized. How could we depolarize a cell membrane? We could allow ions to flow across the membrane. Specifically, sodium channels that open when we need to depolarize the membrane, allowing sodium ions to rush in (down their concentration gradient), would make the inside of the cell less negative (more positive) with respect to the outside of the cell (**FIGURE 8.4**). This would depolarize the membrane, wouldn't it? Consider that point for a minute; at rest, the outside is more positive

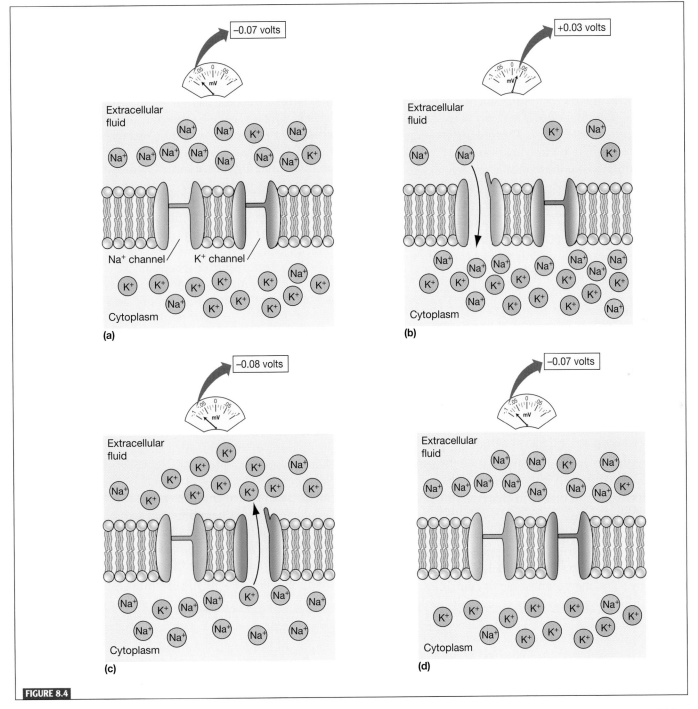

FIGURE 8.4

Opening ion channels can alter membrane potential. In panel (a), Na⁺ and K⁺ channels are closed, and the membrane is polarized to resting membrane potential. In panel (b), an open Na⁺ channel causes membrane depolarization. In panel (c), the Na⁺ channel has closed and the K⁺ channel has opened, causing membrane repolarization. Panel (d) shows that our membrane has returned to resting membrane potential because only a small amount of ions move during the depolarization and repolarization event. To aid your understanding, the voltage-gated sodium channel depicted has been simplified. It is shown with only one gate while it actually has two gates.

than the inside. When the positive ions that are outside the cell enter the cell, the outside becomes less positive and the inside becomes more positive. That is how the membrane depolarizes. Integral membrane proteins distributed throughout the cell membrane contain sodium channels that, when conditions are right, open very briefly to allow sodium to rush in. As the membrane depolarizes, these channels close again. In effect, they contain molecular gates that allow this to happen.

Now, here is a small glitch. When our AA battery is completely discharged (depolarized), our voltmeter reads zero volts. We would assume that the same would be true of our polarized cell, as we currently understand it. Not so, however. Our cell, starting with a resting membrane potential of −70 mV, actually "depolarizes" to approximately +30 mV. The polarity reverses from negative to positive by moving past the zero point. We started with more sodium outside the cell and an excess of potassium inside the cell. Both of those ions have positive charges. When sodium ions become balanced across the cell membrane, the potassium ions are still in excess within the cell. This accounts for the somewhat confusing reversal of polarity. This process is still, however, called membrane depolarization.

The cells that have the capacity for electrical activity must be able to return quickly to the polarized state, to resting membrane potential. How can we return them to resting membrane potential most quickly? It would be easy at this point to be confused into thinking that since the $Na^+K^+ATPase$ (sodium-potassium pump) develops the initial polarization, it should also repolarize the cell after depolarization. That's not how it works, however. Although the sodium-potassium pumps are running all the time to keep the membrane fully charged, they work like very slow battery chargers. They keep the cell membrane polarized by working continually, but do not have enough power to charge it quickly when it becomes depolarized.

To quickly repolarize the cell membrane, potassium channels open briefly, allowing potassium ions to flow through them. Potassium channels, like sodium channels, are integral membrane proteins containing an opening controlled by a gatelike portion of the molecule. As potassium ions move down their concentration gradient (from inside the cell to outside the cell), the inside of the cell becomes more negative again, and resting membrane potential is restored. This process is called repolarization. Excessive movement of the potassium ions results in a slight, temporary hyperpolarization of the membrane. All of this is depicted in Figure 8.4. Look it over and consider what is happening carefully before moving on.

Lightning Strikes: Initiating the Electrical Event

So, what triggers this depolarization and repolarization anyway? Let's call this deplorization and repolarization event an action potential. We will define the term *action potential* more fully later. It begins at one point on the cell's surface and spreads across the membrane like a wave across a pond or a fire through a brush field. We will return to how it spreads in a moment; first, let's think about the point where it begins. The most common way in which the depolarization and repolarization event begins is through the binding of a receptor and a ligand. Think of a lock and a key. The receptor is like a lock. Every receptor has some molecule that binds to it. That is why it is called a receptor; it receives some molecule. The molecule that binds to a receptor is called its ligand. The ligand is like the key in our lock and key analogy. The ligand fits into some part of the receptor. In doing so, it causes some change in the three-dimensional structure of the receptor. The ligands that are released from neurons to initiate an action potential in another neuron or in a muscle cell are called neurotransmitters. The receptors we have been discussing are called neurotransmitter receptors.

Acetylcholine is the neurotransmitter that causes action potentials in skeletal muscle cells. Numerous neurotransmitter receptors play a role in the initiation of action potentials in neurons. We will learn about them in Chapter 11. We will learn about the structures that release and receive neurotransmitters later in this chapter and in more detail in Chapters 9 and 11.

When molecules of acetylcholine (neurotransmitter) bind to the receptors located at some point on the cell's surface, the change that occurs in the receptor involves the opening of a chemically gated sodium channel. The channels are "chemically gated" because it is a chemical event (the binding of ligand to the receptor) that causes the channels to open (**FIGURE 8.5**). Once they open, depolarization has begun in that area of the membrane. Now, a second type of ion channel is brought into play.

Distributed throughout the cell membrane, we find voltage-gated sodium channels and voltage-gated potassium channels (as shown in Figure 8.4). These channels do not rely on the binding of ligand to a receptor to open them. Instead, they are activated by specific electrical conditions. When the membrane is at resting membrane potential, the channels are closed. When the membrane depolarizes slightly, the gates in the channels are triggered and the channels open. The point at which this occurs is called threshold. Threshold may be in the range of 10–15 mV above resting membrane potential. For our discussion, we will consider it as 10 mV. If the membrane depolarizes up to −60 mV, the cell has reached threshold. When it reaches threshold, the sodium channels open rapidly and then reclose. This causes the affected area of membrane to completely depolarize. The same event (reaching threshold) causes the potassium channels to open slowly. At about the same time that the sodium channels close, the potassium channels are fully open, allowing repolarization. The potassium channels then close and the whole system is reset.

If the chemically gated sodium channels in one specific location are activated to the point of threshold, this event will begin. That area of membrane will be sufficiently depolarized to activate the voltage-gated sodium and potassium channels. When that area has completely depolarized, the surrounding area reaches threshold and completely depolarizes. Then the area surrounding it reaches threshold, so it too completely depolarizes. In each case, depolarization is followed by repolarization. It is similar to the way in which a brushfire spreads. Lightening strikes one point in a field, starting it on fire. The area immediately around that fire gets so hot that it starts to burn, then the area surrounding that burning area gets hot enough that it starts to burn, and so on. As the fire spreads, the area behind it stops burning, since it has consumed all of the fuel. We, therefore, get a wave of fire spreading from one point, with an extinguished area following after the wave of fire. That is exactly how the wave of depolarization and repolarization spreads across the cell surface (**FIGURE 8.6**). We call this moving wave of depolarization and repolarization an action potential. The action potential is the mechanism that carries information along a neuron, and by which a muscle contraction is stimulated throughout a muscle cell. The action potential begins in a location where chemically gated sodium channels are present. They are present in locations called postsynaptic membranes in neurons and motor endplates in muscle cells. These are parts of structures called synapses or neuroeffector junctions. We will briefly discuss these structures in our next section.

First, however, one small point is needed here for clarity. Only a minute amount of ions actually moves with each action potential. Even if we were to stop the action of the sodium-potassium ATPase completely, the cell would be capable of many action potentials. Just as a battery can power many flashes in a flashlight, the fully charged neuron or muscle cell is capable of many action potentials without "recharging."

8.5 Synapses and Neuroeffector Junctions

Neurons interact with each other in structures called synapses. Neurons interact with muscle cells and other

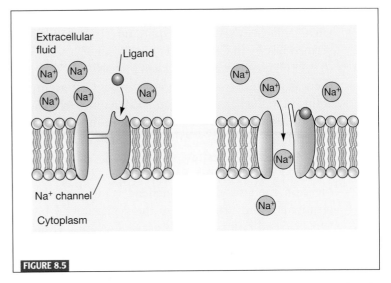

FIGURE 8.5

A chemically gated sodium channel in a neurotransmitter receptor. The binding of neurotransmitter (its ligand) to the receptor opens the channel.

cell types (collectively called effector cells) in structures called neuroeffector junctions. Sometimes, people use the term *synapse* for either of these structures because they are very similar. Some neurophysiologists take offense to that, though, so be careful with your use of these terms. For the purposes of our discussion, I will use the term *synapse* to mean either a true synapse or a neuroeffector junction. Also, here I am only describing one

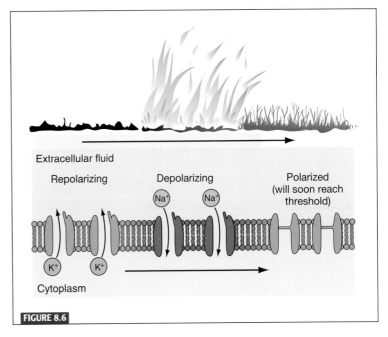

FIGURE 8.6

An action potential (a wave of depolarization and repolarization) moves along the cell surface like a grass fire spreads across a field.

type of synapse: a chemical synapse. Another type, electrical synapse, exists but is quite rare, and will be described briefly in Chapter 11.

A chemical synapse is shown in **FIGURE 8.7**. Note that there is a gap between the two neurons that are interacting in this synapse. This gap, the synaptic cleft, makes the movement of an electrical impulse unidirectional between these two neurons: it moves in one direction only. When an action potential moves down the neuron shown at the top of the diagram, it progresses through the axon, then through the telodendria (also called axon terminals), and ultimately to the synaptic end bulbs. Synaptic end bulbs contain vesicles (synaptic vesicles) of neurotransmitter. When the action potential reaches the synaptic end bulb, voltage-gated calcium channels in the membrane of the end bulb open, and calcium diffuses in. (Calcium is not present in the synaptic end bulb at rest; it is removed by a calcium ATPase.) The presence of calcium causes the synaptic vesicles to fuse with the plasmalemma and release their contents (neurotransmitter) into the synaptic cleft. This release is an example of exocytosis, as described in Chapter 3.

Neurotransmitter molecules then diffuse across the synaptic cleft and bind to the neurotransmitter receptors on the membrane on the opposite side of the cleft. This is what triggers the action potential in the second neuron or effector cell, as described previously. Ultimately, neurotransmitter molecules are broken down by enzymes present in the synaptic cleft, enabling their rapid removal from the cleft and their receptors. Examine the synapse shown in Figure 8.7 and familiarize yourself with the names of the parts of the synapse. We will revisit synapses in Chapters 9 and 11.

8.6   How Your Electrical Cells Are Like Toilets: The All-or-None Principle

What happens when you push the little lever on your toilet? Obviously, it flushes. Next, consider what would happen if you merely rested your finger on the little lever. Would it flush? No, of course not; you must push hard enough to get a flush. How about if you pushed really hard; would you get a bigger flush? Heck, no. Your toilet is capable of one size flush and one size flush only. This is just like the electrical activity in the cells we've been discussing. If your stimulus is too small (a sub-threshold stimulus), you get no action potential. If you have a threshold stimulus, you get an action potential. If you have a larger-than-threshold stimulus, you still get the same-sized action potential. See, just like your toilet. This phenomenon is called the all-or-none principle.

Now, what happens if you flush and then immediately push the lever again? Do you get a second flush? No, the toilet is still busy with the first flush. The same thing happens in these cells. There is a brief period of time, after a stimulus, in which an additional stimulus will not produce an additional action potential. This is called the absolute refractory period.

Have you ever flushed a toilet and then, as it was filling back up, tried to flush it a second time. You may have found that the usual stimulus didn't work, but if you held the lever down a bit longer than usual (used a larger stimulus), you could get a second flush. Again, the same thing happens in these cells. There is a certain time period, after a stimulus, during which a second stimulus will produce a second action potential, but only if it is a larger stimulus than usual. This is called the relative refractory period, and it roughly corresponds to the period in which the membrane is hyperpolarized by the excess movement of potassium ions. See **FIGURE 8.8**

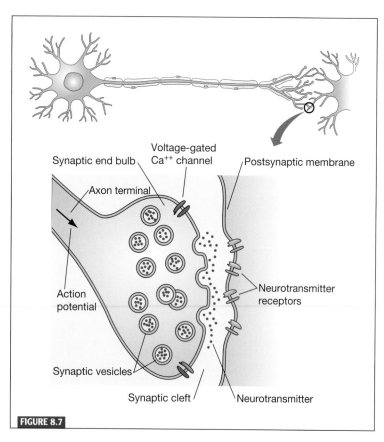

Synaptic end bulb

Voltage-gated Ca++ channel

Postsynaptic membrane

Axon terminal

Neurotransmitter receptors

Action potential

Synaptic vesicles

Synaptic cleft

Neurotransmitter

FIGURE 8.7

A chemical synapse.

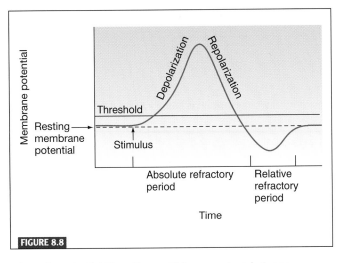

FIGURE 8.8

An action potential. The entire event takes approximately 4 msec.

for these time periods, as well as the overall timing of an action potential.

We have just completed a block of highly conceptual information. Be sure that you are clear on the topics considered here before moving on. Please sit for a few moments and make sure that you understand the points listed in "What You Should Know" before continuing on. You should try to picture an action potential in a "cartoon" fashion in your head. Try to envision neurotransmitter binding to receptors and opening chemically gated sodium channels, starting the process. Then picture voltage-gated sodium channels carrying the wave of depolarization across the cell membrane, and voltage-gated potassium channels carrying the wave of repolarization behind it. If you can do this, you are ready to move on. Next, we consider the exciting world of muscle cells.

What You Should Know

1. Electrical activity is important for many of the functions that regulate and maintain homeostasis.
2. Gradients of atoms can be established across the cell membrane by the action of molecular pumps.
3. If the atoms used to establish a gradient across a membrane are ions, an electrical potential will be generated.
4. An electrical potential can be generated by pumping two ions with the same charge in opposite directions across the cell membrane, if different amounts of the two ions are moved.
5. The molecular pumps that establish these gradients are ATP-splitting enzymes.
6. The $Na^+K^+ATPase$ is an electrogenic molecular pump that transports three sodium ions out of the cell for every two potassium ions it pumps into the cell.
7. Depolarization of the membrane is necessary to use this electrical charge.
8. A wave of depolarization followed by repolarization that moves along the cell membrane is called an action potential.
9. Chemically gated sodium channels can initiate action potentials.
10. Voltage-gated sodium channels carry the wave of depolarization along the membrane.
11. Voltage-gated potassium channels carry the wave of repolarization along the membrane.
12. Chemically gated sodium channels are found in some neurotransmitter receptors in synapses and neuroeffector junctions.
13. If the membrane depolarizes to a point called "threshold," an action potential will be initiated.
14. A larger-than-threshold stimulus will not generate a larger action potential; a subthreshold stimulus will not initiate any action potential. This is the basis of the all-or-none principle.
15. An absolute refractory period follows an action potential. During this period, no new action potential can be generated.
16. A relative refractory period also follows an action potential. During this period, a larger than normal stimulus is required to generate an action potential.

What Did You Learn?

Multiple choice questions: choose the best answer.

1. A positively charged atom or group of atoms is called:
   a. An anion
   b. A cation
   c. A dogion
   d. None of the above

2. We have a _____ when we have more of one substance on one side of a membrane than we have of that substance on the other side of the membrane.
   a. Potential
   b. Graduation
   c. Polarization
   d. Gradient
   e. Solution

3. Can two independent gradients exist across a membrane at the same time?
   a. Yes
   b. No
   c. Maybe (don't pick this one)
   d. Maybe not (don't pick this one either)

4. The molecular pumps that move ions across membranes are _____.
   a. Enzymes
   b. Integral membrane proteins
   c. Both of the above
   d. Neither of the above

5. Why is the Na⁺K⁺ATPase electrogenic?
   a. It pumps sodium against a concentration gradient.
   b. It requires energy in the form of ATP.
   c. It transports sodium and potassium in opposite directions.
   d. It transports unequal amounts of sodium and potassium in opposite directions.
   e. It transports sodium and potassium in the same direction.

6. At resting membrane potential (when the membrane is polarized), there is _____ sodium outside the cell than inside the cell.
   a. More
   b. Less
   c. The same amount in both locations
   d. It varies

7. At resting membrane potential (when the membrane is polarized) there is _____ potassium outside the cell than inside the cell.
   a. More
   b. Less
   c. The same amount in both locations
   d. It varies

8. Potassium is _____.
   a. An anion
   b. A cation
   c. A dogion
   d. None of the above

9. Sodium is _____.
   a. An anion
   b. A cation
   c. A dogion
   d. None of the above

10. A wave of depolarization and repolarization spreading along a cell membrane is called _____.
    a. A gradient
    b. A threshold
    c. An action potential
    d. A contraction

11. A stimulus that is smaller than threshold will produce:
    a. No action potential
    b. A smaller than usual action potential
    c. An action potential of the usual magnitude (size)
    d. A larger than usual action potential

12. A stimulus that is larger than threshold will produce:
    a. No action potential
    b. A smaller than usual action potential
    c. An action potential of the usual magnitude (size)
    d. A larger than usual action potential

13. A molecule that binds to a receptor is referred to as that receptor's _____.
    a. Ion
    b. Channel
    c. Legume
    d. Ligand
    e. None of the above

14. The action potential's wave of depolarization spreads across the cell as _____ rushes in through voltage-gated channels.
    a. Sodium
    b. Calcium
    c. Chloride

What Did You Learn? (continued)

d. Potassium

e. None of the above

15. The action potential's wave of repolarization spreads across the cell as _____ rushes out through voltage-gated channels.

    a. Sodium

    b. Calcium

    c. Chloride

    d. Potassium

    e. None of the above

16. The initial event that begins the action potential involves the binding of a ligand to a receptor that contains a _____ potassium channel.

    a. Voltage-gated

    b. Chemically gated

    c. Both of the above are correct.

    d. Neither of the above are correct.

17. Identify the structure indicated.

    a. Telodendrion

    b. Synaptic end bulb

    c. Synaptic vesicle

    d. Synaptic cleft

    e. Neurotransmitter receptor

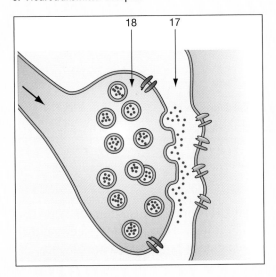

18. Identify the structure indicated.

    a. Telodendrion

    b. Synaptic end bulb

    c. Synaptic vesicle

    d. Synaptic cleft

    e. Neurotransmitter receptor

19. _____ is contained within synaptic vesicles.

    a. Calcium

    b. Neurotransmitter

    c. Sodium

    d. Potassium

    e. None of the above

20. An action potential in an axon results in neurotransmitter being released into the _____.

    a. Synaptic end bulb

    b. Synaptic cleft

    c. Synaptic vesicle

    d. Great rift valley

Short answer questions: answer briefly and in your own words.

1. What is an ion gradient? How is an ion gradient established across a membrane? How does an ion gradient across a cell membrane result in an electrical potential?

2. What is the role of the sodium potassium ATPase in establishing an electrical potential? Describe how the sodium potassium ATPase works.

3. Describe an action potential. How does it spread along the cell membrane? What initiates it?

4. In what ways does your body rely on these cellular electrical activities? What would happen if you were not able to generate an electrical potential across your cell membranes, or you were unable to generate an action potential?

5. Explain the all-or-none principle. What is the result of a subthreshold stimulus? How about a larger than threshold stimulus?

6. Draw and label a synapse. What do synapses do?

7. Why are neurotransmitters necessary? After their release, how are they removed from the synaptic cleft? What would happen if they could not be removed from the synaptic cleft?

8. What is the difference between voltage-gated ion channels and chemically gated ion channels? What are the differences between the roles that these two different channels play?

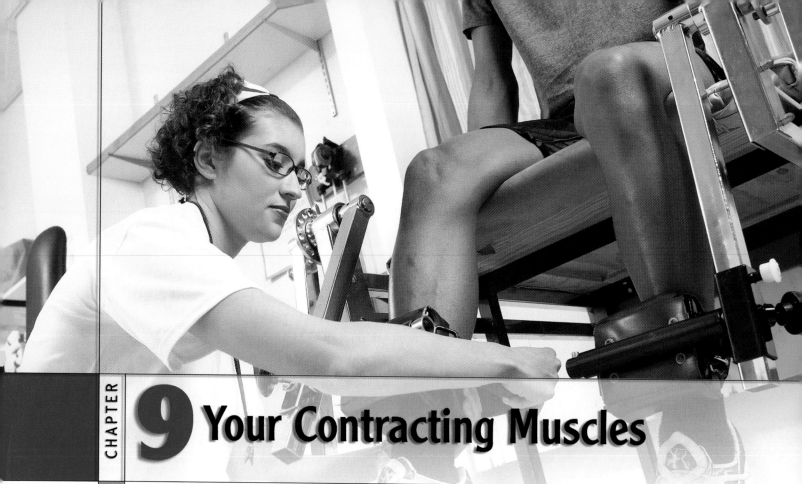

9 Your Contracting Muscles

What You Will Learn

- The functions of your muscle system.
- Details of the three types of muscle.
- The structure of an individual skeletal muscle fiber.
- The structure of the protein contractile machinery of muscle cells.
- The steps involved in muscle contraction.
- The types of contractions of individual fibers.
- How multiple fibers work together to produce a sustained contraction of the desired force.
- Different types of skeletal muscle fibers have different contraction and fatigue characteristics.
- Where the energy comes from for contraction and relaxation.

9.1 Functions of the Muscle System

Whenever we think of the muscle system, its contractile ability is the first thing that comes to mind, as well it should; that is a truly amazing ability. Think about it. These cells have the ability to forcefully shorten. They also have the ability to be stretched, return to their original shape, and shorten again. How do we make use of these remarkable abilities? We use this capacity for generating force to lift objects, move about, and alter our immediate environment in many ways. Haven't you gotten up and moved from a sunny area to the shade on a

hot day? Haven't you also done the opposite on a cool day? These uses of our muscle system and their role in the maintenance of homeostasis are obvious.

How about less obvious uses? Are you breathing right now? I sure hope you are. If you are not, you will not make it to the end of this chapter and you will miss a lot of useful information. How do you breathe? What moves the air into and out of your lungs? The action of the muscle system does. As we will learn in Chapter 17, air is pulled into the lungs by changes in the volume of your thoracic cavity. These changes are the result of the contraction of muscles, such as your external intercostals (think now, what would the term *intercostals* mean?) and your diaphragm. Obviously, breathing is included in the functions of the muscle system.

What position are you in as you read this book? Are you sitting up, standing, or perhaps lying down (don't go to sleep, this is good stuff)? Our ability to hold a posture involves partial contraction of our muscles. This partial contraction must be maintained for long periods of time; think about how long you hold your head up on any given day. The amount of contraction used must not be too great or fatigue would set in and we would be uncomfortable from the rigidity. It must also not be too little, as we would slump down and not maintain the position desired. Posture is a role of the muscle system.

Finally, heat production is a role of the muscle system. As much as 85 percent of the heat generated by our bodies is generated by our muscle system. When you are cold, you begin to shiver. Shivering is the repeated cycle of contraction and relaxation of your muscles. This contraction and relaxation generates heat. This heat is carried through your body by the moving fluids with which you are now familiar, warming the body so that shivering is no longer required (hopefully).

9.2 The Three Types of Muscle

How can we recognize muscle tissue? What characteristic would distinguish muscle cells from other cell types? If you answered "the ability to contract," I'm sorry to tell you that some other cells also have that ability. Think back to what you have learned about the five tissue types. What distinguished muscle tissue? Right, the presence of intermediate filaments composed of desmin. If we look for desmin in the body, we will find it in muscle cells in a wide variety of places, however, not just in the muscles that are connected to our bones. There are actually three types of muscle, and only one of the three makes up the muscle system. **TABLE 9.1** and **FIGURE 9.1** present the three types and help you to distinguish among them. I would learn this table if I were you; it looks like the kind of thing your instructor might ask on the next exam.

Smooth muscle is not the muscle of the muscle system. Smooth muscle is the muscle of our internal organs, such as our digestive tract and our muscular arteries. We cannot voluntarily contract our smooth muscle cells. Smooth muscle cells are relatively small and are torpedo-shaped, or pointed on both ends. We refer to this shape as fusiform. Smooth muscle cells generally contract either as individual cells or as small groups of cells. As their contractions are slow, this arrangement allows the development of waves of contraction, such as the peristalsis seen in the digestive tract. We will learn more about the functions and distribution of smooth muscle in later chapters.

Skeletal muscle is the muscle of the muscle system. These are the cells that make up your skeletal muscles. They are sometimes referred to as *striated muscles*; however, this term is somewhat misleading. Striations are microscopic lines that appear when we use certain staining techniques and run across each cell. They are caused by the alignment of the contractile machinery of the cell, and are present in skeletal and cardiac muscle. Because both of those cell types have striations, skeletal muscle should not be referred to simply as striated muscle. Skeletal muscle cells are also called muscle fibers due to their long, narrow shape. One individual cell may exceed 30 centimeters in length. Thirty centimeters is approximately 1 foot. Imagine a cell of that length! It is easy to see why a cell of that length would need multiple nuclei. These cells may have hundreds of nuclei. We refer to cells with many nuclei as syncytia, or giant cells. The nuclei of skeletal muscle fibers are not in the center of the fiber, as in other muscle types. The nuclei are pushed to the border of the cell, just deep to the cell membrane. Sometimes, in fact, in cross section it may appear as if the nuclei are outside the cell. This is because the nuclei are actually bulging out the membrane as they are pushed to the periphery by the contractile machinery of the cell. The contractions of skeletal muscle fibers are generally under voluntary control, but involuntary or reflex contractions also occur. Think, for instance, of how you breathe without thinking about it, or how you turn quickly toward the sound of a loud crash without thinking about it.

Table 9.1 The Three Types of Muscle

Type	Striation	Shape/Size	C.S.Size (µm)	Nuclei	Organization	Contractions
Smooth	No	Fusiform 30–200 µm	5–10	Single central	Single cells	Involuntary, slow
Skeletal	Yes	Cylindrical up to 30 cm	10–100	Multiple peripheral	Syncytia	Voluntary, quick, forceful
Cardiac	Yes	Irregular, branching 150 µm	10–20	One or two central	Functional syncytia	Involuntary, rhythmic

C.S. indicates cross sections.

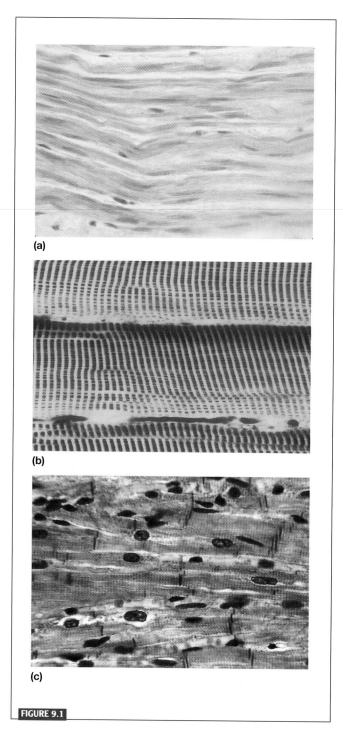

FIGURE 9.1

The three types of muscle fibers: (a) smooth, (b) skeletal, and (c) cardiac.

The contractions of cardiac muscle cells, the muscle cells of the heart, are certainly not under voluntary control. The heart develops its rhythm of contraction within specialized cardiac muscle cells. The entire mass of cardiac muscle cells acts as if they are one giant cell, even though they are many individual cells. For this reason, we refer to their organizational arrangement as a functional syncytium; they function like one large

multinucleated cell. The membranes between cardiac muscle cells, where individual cells join each other, are modified to allow this to happen. Here we find structures called intercalated disks. Intercalated disks are areas of membrane containing small pores called gap junctions, which allow ions to pass from one cell to the next. It is this passage of ions that allows these cells to contract in unison. We will learn a great deal more about these cells in Chapter 16.

The rest of this chapter will focus on the cellular physiology of skeletal muscle cells (fancy way of saying "how skeletal muscle cells work"). The other types of muscle function similarly, but with various subtle alterations. If you understand the activities of skeletal muscle cells, it is easy to understand the activities of other types of muscle. As already stated, cardiac muscle cells will be presented in greater detail in Chapter 16.

9.3 A Skeletal Muscle Cell

Muscle cells, also called muscle fibers or myofibers, have many interesting features. Some of these features allow them to have their special ability to contract. We will also see, however, that some of their features are very similar to those of other cells, but muscle physiologists have given them special names in muscle cells (every discipline has its quirks). We will start by identifying a few characteristics and parts of muscle cells. See **FIGURE 9.2** for further details.

■ Special Features of Muscle Cells

Some of the special features of muscle cells are obvious the minute you begin to examine them. First of all, let's consider their great size. Imagine a cell that can be more than a foot long. That is one extremely large cell! Its prodigious number of nuclei is also an amazing feature. The plasma membrane of a muscle cell is a polarized membrane, as we have just learned in Chapter 8. This membrane has a special name in muscle fibers; it is called sarcolemma. The cytoplasm also has a special name, sarcoplasm. The root *sarco* comes from the Greek term for "flesh," so we will see this term applied repeatedly to features of muscle.

Smooth endoplasmic reticulum in muscle is called sarcoplasmic reticulum (**FIGURE 9.3**). This organelle is different in muscle cells than in other cell types, however. It has been modified for the storage of calcium. Certain portions of the sarcoplasmic reticulum have been dilated into sacks called terminal cisterns. The membrane of the sarcoplasmic reticulum contains integral proteins that act as calcium ion pumps. This pump, a Ca^{++}ATPase, removes calcium from the sarcoplasm and stores it in

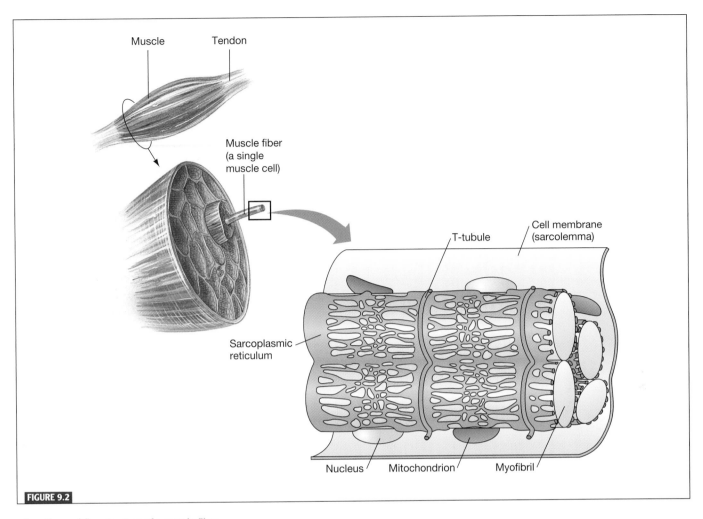

FIGURE 9.2

Location and fine structure of a muscle fiber.

the terminal cisterns of the sarcoplasmic reticulum. This membrane also contains voltage-gated calcium channels that will open, releasing calcium into the sarcoplasm under appropriate electrical conditions. This release, triggered by an action potential, allows the calcium concentration to increase as much as 1,000-fold within the sarcoplasm. The calcium will again be removed from the sarcoplasm by the calcium ATPase after the action potential has passed. If action potentials are repeated at a high frequency, the sarcoplasmic calcium level will remain elevated. We will discover the role of calcium in muscle cell activity shortly.

An additional interesting feature of the myofiber is the T-tubule, or transverse tubule. Transverse tubules are tubelike extensions of the sarcolemma that extend into the sarcoplasm. Imagine a bowl full of Jell-O covered with plastic wrap. Now, push your fingers into the Jell-O. The plastic wrap would surround your fingers like tubes, extending into the Jell-O. That is what these T-tubules are like. The plastic wrap is analogous to the

sarcolemma; the Jell-O is the sarcoplasm. The portion of the plastic wrap that surrounds your fingers and extends into the Jell-O is the T-tubules. These are located directly along the sides of terminal cisterns. In fact, for every one T-tubule, we find two terminal cisterns. This combination is called a triad (Figure 9.3).

Finally, we need to recall the synapse or neuroeffector junction mentioned in Chapter 8 (**FIGURE 9.4**). We learned that a neuroeffector junction exists where neurons meet other cell types, such as muscle cells. Again, we will use the terms *synapse* and *neuroeffector junction* interchangeably. The synapse includes the synaptic end bulb of the neuron, the synaptic cleft that separates the two cells, and the motor endplate of the muscle cell. This motor endplate is a special feature of the muscle cell and contains neurotransmitter receptors. The neurotransmitter used in these neuroeffector junctions is acetylcholine so these are acetylcholine receptors. The motor endplate also contains the enzyme acetylcholinesterase for removing neurotransmitters from the

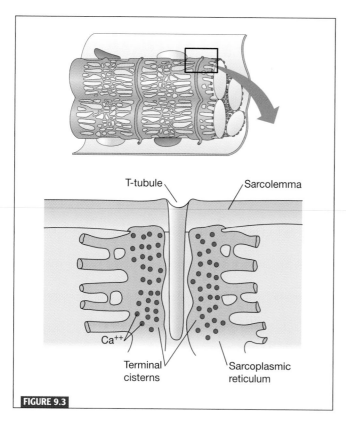

FIGURE 9.3

A triad: two terminal cisterns and one T-tubule.

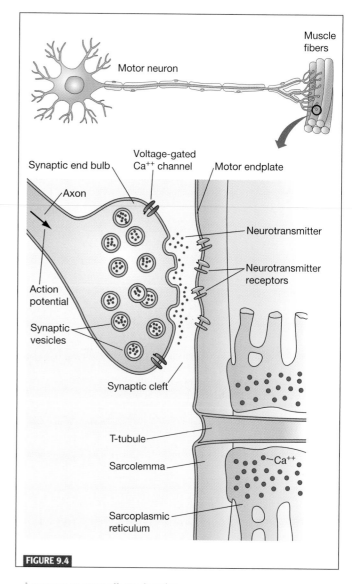

FIGURE 9.4

A synapse or neuroeffector junction.

synaptic cleft. Without these enzymes, once activated, a muscle cell would remain contracted for life. This would make life very short indeed!

■ The Contractile Machinery

The cytoskeleton in a myofiber is very different from that of other cells. Sure, we have intermediate filaments and microtubules, as we do elsewhere. As you know, the intermediate filaments of muscle cells are made of the protein desmin. But the arrangement of certain other components of the cytoskeleton is very different from what we see elsewhere. There are large structures, 1–2 micrometers in diameter, running the entire length of the myofiber (**FIGURE 9.5**). These are called myofibrils and are made up of myofilaments. There are two types of myofilaments: thick myofilaments and thin myofilaments.

Thick myofilaments are composed of myosin. Myosin is a protein shaped like a hockey stick (Figure 9.5). The shafts of the hockey sticks bind together into bundles, making a long fiber. The blades of these hockey sticks extend out of the bundle, making it look like a frayed piece of yarn. The part of the myosin molecules that sticks out of the fiber (the hockey stick blade) is referred to as the myosin cross bridge or side arm.

Under appropriate conditions, the side arm will bind to actin. It is also an ATPase: it cleaves ATP to ADP + P, releasing energy. The myosin side arm has two forms: (1) a high-energy state, after it has cleaved ATP and gained the energy from that reaction; and (2) a low-energy state, after it has used that energy and changed its shape.

The thin myofilament is somewhat different in that it is made up of several proteins (Figure 9.5). The backbone of the thin myofilament is composed of the protein tropomyosin. The tropomyosin backbone is decorated along its length with two other proteins. The more numerous of these two is actin. Actin is a myosin-binding molecule. Specifically, actin has a binding site that, when available, attaches to the myosin side arm. Also decorating the tropomyosin backbone is the protein tropo-

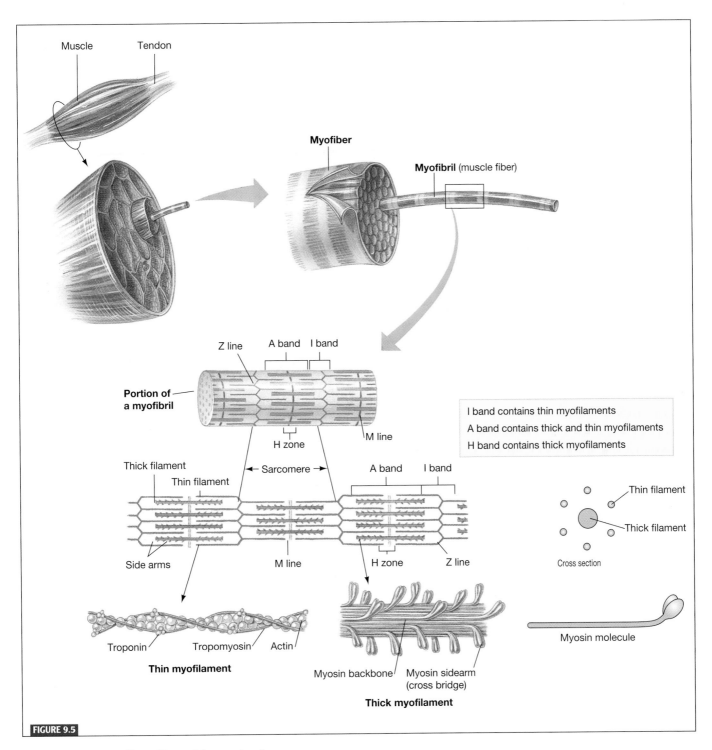

Muscle Tendon

Myofiber

Myofibril (muscle fiber)

Z line A band I band

**Portion of
a myofibril**

H zone M line

I band contains thin myofilaments

A band contains thick and thin myofilaments

H band contains thick myofilaments

Thick filament

Thin filament

Sarcomere

A band I band

Thin filament

Thick filament

Side arms

M line

H zone Z line

Cross section

Troponin Tropomyosin Actin

Thin myofilament

Myosin backbone Myosin sidearm
(cross bridge)

Myosin molecule

Thick myofilament

FIGURE 9.5

Details of the contractile machinery of the muscle cell.

nin. Troponin has several interesting functions: it is a calcium-binding molecule, and it influences tropomyosin to "cover" actin, rendering it unable to bind the myosin side arm. Let's think about that for a moment. Tropomyosin has two possible confirmations (shapes) that are influenced by troponin. When calcium is not bound to troponin, troponin pushes tropomyosin into a form that covers actin, making it unavailable to bind myosin. When troponin binds calcium, it changes the shape of tropomyosin, causing it to uncover actin, allowing it to bind myosin.

Look at Figure 9.5 for the arrangement of the thick and thin myofilaments. This will show you several things, most notably, that there are six thin myofilaments for every one thick myofilament. The myosin side arms of the thick myofilaments extend outward, toward the thin myofilaments. The muscle fiber or myofiber is the cell; the myofibrils are the smaller structures within the myofiber that run the length of the myofiber (each myofiber has many of these). The myofibril is made up of many thick and thin myofilaments, and for each thick myofilament there are six thin myofilaments.

Now, let's think about where striations come into all of this. We have already learned that skeletal muscle cells are striated, that is to say, they have striations or fine lines running across them. These striations appear because the arrangement of thick and thin myofilaments in each myofibril results in their lining up across the myofiber. That sounds more complicated than it is. Look at Figure 9.5. Notice that the myofibril has regions that contain both thick and thin myofilaments (called the A bands). Other regions contain only thin myofilaments (I bands) or only thick myofilaments (H zones). By lining up these regions in a repeating pattern across

all of the myofibrils, we develop stripes across the cell. These regions are diagrammed in Figure 9.5. Note that one complete unit of these repeating structures is called a sarcomere. We will consider these sarcomeres as we discuss the manner in which muscle cells contract. We can view the entire process from the standpoint of one sarcomere. As the myofiber contracts, each individual sarcomere shortens.

■ The Sliding-Filament Theory: It's Just Like Rowing a Boat

As we have been examining the inner structure of the myofibril, what we have actually been examining is the contractile machinery of the cell. These proteins work like small machines, pulling the ends of the cell closer together. The theory that explains how these proteins work together to cause a forceful shortening of muscle cells is called the sliding-filament theory. That theory is outlined below as a multistep process. Read over that process now, and examine **FIGURE 9.6** as you do.

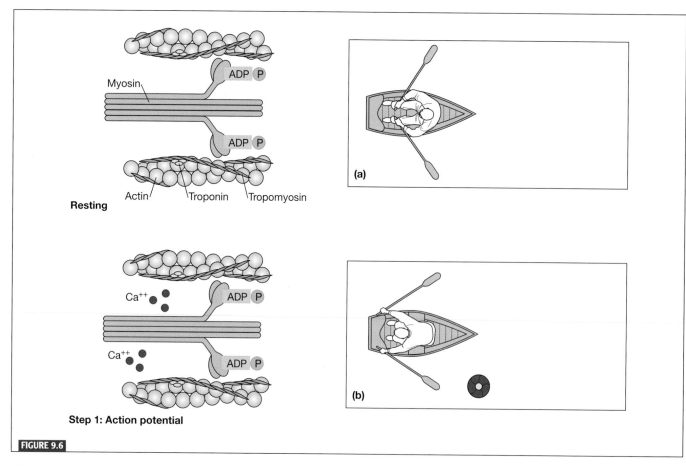

FIGURE 9.6

The sliding-filament theory: how muscle fibers contract. Note how the rowing motion mimics the sliding filaments. See text for details.

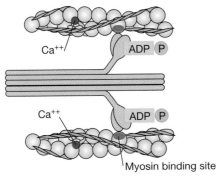

Ca++

ADP P

Ca++

ADP P

Myosin binding site

Step 2: Myosin-actin binding

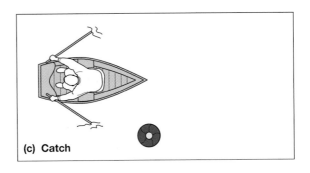

(c) Catch

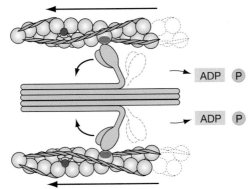

ADP P

ADP P

Step 3: Power stroke

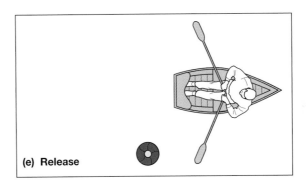

(d) Drive

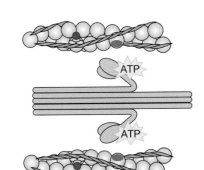

ATP

ATP

Step 4: ATP binding and actin-myosin release

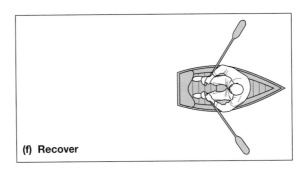

(e) Release

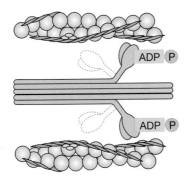

ADP P

ADP P

Step 5: ATP cleavage

(f) Recover

FIGURE 9.6

(Continued)

The Resting State (Conditions Preceding Step One)

This is what we would find before the muscle begins to contract. ATP has already bound to the myosin side arm and been cleaved to ADP + P. This has converted the side arm to its high-energy state. Calcium is not present in the sarcoplasm at this time, having been stored away in the terminal cisterns. Nothing more can happen until calcium is present.

Step One: The Action Potential

An action potential must be triggered in the muscle cell for a contraction to begin. To accomplish this, neurotransmitter molecules must be released from the motor neuron that innervates this muscle cell. They diffuse across the synaptic cleft and bind to the neurotransmitter receptors in the motor endplate. This opens the chemically gated sodium channels in the receptors and begins the action potential. As the action potential spreads along the sarcolemma, it also travels down the T-tubules. Here, the action potential causes voltage-gated calcium channels in the terminal cisterns to open. This causes release of calcium into the sarcoplasm, making it available to bind to troponin. The presence of calcium allows the contractile machinery to become active.

Step Two: Myosin-Actin Binding

The binding of calcium to troponin causes a conformational change (change in shape) in the troponin. This, in turn, pulls tropomyosin away from actin, uncovering the myosin-binding site on actin. Actin and the myosin side arm now bind to each other. The energy liberated when ATP was cleaved is used to create their bond.

Step Three: The Power Stroke

The binding of actin to the myosin side arm causes a conformational change in the side arm called the power stroke. In the power stroke, the side arm pivots in such a way that the thick and thin filaments slide past each other. This is the step that actually shortens the sarcomere. At the same time, the ADP and P that have been bound to the endplate are released. The side arm has now changed to its low-energy state.

Step Four: Actin and Myosin Release

The empty ATP binding site on the myosin side arm is again filled with another ATP molecule. This causes another change in confirmation in the side arm. This results in release of the actin by the side arm.

Step Five: ATP Cleavage

ATP is cleaved by the myosin side arm, converting the side arm from its low-energy state to its high-energy state. This pivots the side arm back to its starting position. If calcium is still present, actin will still be available for binding, allowing the cycle to repeat. If calcium has been returned to the terminal cisterns, the cycle will not repeat and the muscle fiber can relax. ATP must be present for the muscle fiber to relax because the myosin side arm needs to bind ATP to be able to release actin and to cleave the ATP to return to its high-energy state. Also, ATP must be present to enable the calcium ATPase to remove calcium from the sarcoplasm. Think about this the next time you get muscle cramps after vigorous exercise (see the following for further discussion on this topic).

This is a very complex process, so don't be frustrated if at first you don't get it. Let's use a larger example to help you understand this. Have you ever rowed a boat? Rowing is great fun and can be vigorous exercise. It is a quiet, healthful, nonpolluting way to explore the aquatic and marine environments. Let's have a rowing lesson.

In Figure 9.6, panel a shows a rower (me) preceding the first step in this rowing exercise. Note that my oars are not in contact with the water, yet are in the "high-energy" position, the position from which I could exert power. The boat is the thick myofilament, the oar is the myosin side arm, and the water is the thin myofilament. In the next step (panel b), I get the notion that it is time to row. This is analogous to step one, the action potential, in the muscle cell. If I were a muscle cell, calcium would now be available. The life-ring in the water represents calcium. Panel c shows contact between the oars and the water (called *catch* in rowing terms). This is similar to step two, binding of the actin to the myosin side arm. Next, I undergo a change in confirmation (panel d). This alters the angle of the oars to the boat and propels the boat forward (called *drive* in rowing terms). This is the same as the power stroke (step three) in our muscle cell. Note that this propels the boat through the water just as it causes the thick and thin myofilaments to slide past each other. Next (panel e), I lift the oars from the water (*release* in rowing terms) just as the actin and myosin side arms release each other in step four of muscle contraction. In step five of muscle contraction, the side arms pivot back to their high-energy position, ready to make another cycle, if conditions allow. This is shown in panel f and is called *recover* in rowing terms. Note that in rowing, one cycle does not move the boat very far. I must perform several cycles to cover any distance. So too in muscle contraction; a "twitch," or single contraction of a muscle fiber caused by a single stimulus, involves many cycles.

Twitches and Tetany: The Types of Contractions

A single action potential in a single, isolated muscle fiber will cause a single, short contraction. This contraction, lasting only about 0.1 seconds, is called a twitch. If we plot that twitch on a graph (a myogram), it would look like that shown in **FIGURE 9.7a**. Note that we first have a latent period of about 0.01 seconds (10 milliseconds), corresponding to the time necessary for the spread on the action potential across the cell and the release of calcium into the sarcoplasm. Next, we have a contraction period of approximately 40 milliseconds, followed by a 50 millisecond relaxation period. This relaxation period corresponds to the time spent removing calcium from the sarcoplasm, sequestering it back in the sarcoplasmic reticulum. Just as in the electrical activity discussed in Chapter 8, the all-or-none principle applies here. This contraction will be either as forceful as this cell is capable of making it, at this time, or it will not occur at all (think back to the toilet analogy). Note that I said "as this cell is capable of making it *at this time.*" I state it that way because, if we apply repeated stimuli in rapid succession (Figure 9.7b), the force of each of the first few contractions will increase, one after the next. This phenomenon, called treppe, is caused by increases in the amount of calcium available in the sarcoplasm during each successive contraction, and by the generation of heat by the contractions and its effect on subsequent contractions. This is one of the reasons that athletes warm up before performing their athletic feats.

Now, how about if we wanted a sustained contraction from this muscle fiber? Is that possible? You may recall the absolute refractory period seen in our discussion of action potentials (Chapter 8). It obviously would apply here. There is a refractory period of about 5 milliseconds after the initial stimulus, during which a second stimulus will not cause a second contraction. The cell is simply too busy with the first action potential to initiate a second one. However, if we initiate a second action potential after the refractory period, but before the cell has had a chance to relax, we can develop a sustained contraction. This is called tetany. Complete tetany involves applying stimuli at a rate that does not allow the cell any relaxation between subsequent contractions (Figure 9.7c). If, on the other hand, the stimuli are applied at a slightly slower rate, a slight relaxation will occur between contractions (Figure 9.7d). This relaxation will not allow the cell to relax completely between contractions, however. This is called incomplete tetany. We use tetany to generate sustained contractions in individual muscle fibers.

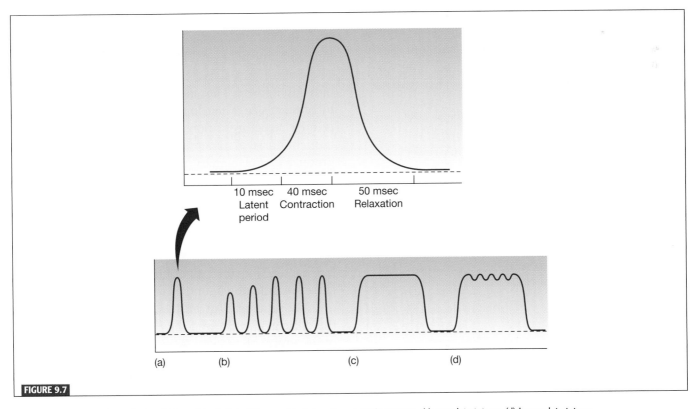

10 msec   40 msec   50 msec
Latent   Contraction   Relaxation
period

(a)   (b)   (c)   (d)

FIGURE 9.7

Muscle contraction in an isolated fiber: (a) a twitch, (b) several twitches demonstrating treppe, (c) complete tetany, (d) incomplete tetany.

■ Contractions Involving Multiple Muscle Fibers

We have been discussing the actions of individual muscle fibers, as we would find them isolated in laboratory experiments. We know, however, that while this helps us understand what goes on in our bodies, we are generally using multiple muscle fibers at once. This is necessary to generate the force needed to perform work. The nerve cells that innervate our muscle fibers, called motor neurons, innervate multiple muscle fibers. They do this by having individual axon terminals (see **FIGURE 9.8**) that extend to individual muscle fibers. In this way, when one motor neuron is stimulated, it will, in turn, stimulate multiple muscle fibers. The number of muscle fibers innervated by one motor neuron varies. Where great force must be generated with each contraction, such as in your thigh muscles, one neuron will innervate many muscle fibers. Where minute control must be applied to contractions, such as in your fingers, one motor neuron will stimulate very few muscle fibers. This allows you to successively contract very few, slightly more, or many more muscle fibers, as required. The process of contracting more and more muscle fibers as needed is called recruitment. All of the muscle fibers that are innervated by the same motor neuron must contract at the same time, however. It is as if they are all on the same switch. Hit the switch and they all come on. A motor neuron and all of the muscle fibers it innervates act as one unit, and this unit is called a motor unit.

To develop sustained contractions without overly fatiguing individual motor units, our motor units share the responsibility for the contraction. That is to say,

one motor unit will briefly contract, using tetany of course. As it fatigues, it will relax and another will take over. The work is shared by many motor units, just as work may be shared by people in a group. In this way, muscles involved in posture can continue to work all day without fatigue. These muscles are obviously not fully contracted at any one time. By that I mean that they do not have all of their motor units contracted at the same time. They are, instead, contracting only a small portion of their motor units at any one time. Even though the muscle fibers in those motor units are fully contracted (all-or-none principle applies), the muscle itself has only a partial contraction. We refer to this partial contraction of the whole muscle as muscle tone.

The Types of Skeletal Muscle Fibers

We have several different types of muscle fibers that also play a role in determining the type of activity that suits a muscle best. Type One fibers are seen in muscles that provide posture. They are very resistant to fatigue but contract only slowly. Type Two B fibers fatigue easily but allow fast contractions. We see these in our arms and legs. Type Two A fibers can be developed by endurance training, as fibers are able to switch types over time. These fibers can contract rapidly and resist fatigue. Unfortunately, they are relatively rare.

In addition to allowing us to switch types, exercise builds our muscles. It may cause a slight increase in the number of fibers in our muscles by causing longitudinal splitting of fibers. That is, however, a minor effect. The major effect of exercise is to cause hypertrophy of individual fibers. That means that the individual fibers increase in size. They do this by developing more intracellular structures: more contractile machinery, more mitochondria to generate energy, more ribosomes to produce that machinery, more nuclei to run the protein syntheses. Exercise increases the production of organelles in your muscle cells. There, aren't you glad you know about organelles?

■ Energy for Contraction and Relaxation

In Chapter 3, we discussed aerobic and anaerobic cellular respiration at length. If you cannot recall the details of these processes (glycolysis, the transition reaction, the citric acid cycle, and the electron transport chain), please review them now. Here, we will just look at their role in muscle contraction and relaxation.

Muscle fibers need energy for contraction and for relaxation, and that energy is in the form of ATP. But how long can we exercise our muscles by using the

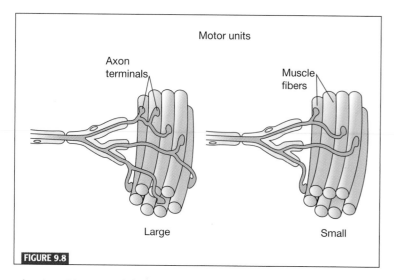

Motor units

Axon terminals

Muscle fibers

Large   Small

FIGURE 9.8

A motor unit is composed of a motor neuron and all of the muscle fibers it innervates.

ATP stored in them? Only a few seconds. That's right, a few seconds. Not too good, huh? Well, we have a backup system. Phosphocreatine, also stored in muscle cells, can be broken down into creatine and phosphate, releasing energy. This energy can be used to generate a little more ATP. How long can we run our muscles on this? Again, not too long. Together, these two systems are called the phosphagen system and can run the exercising muscle cell for about 15 seconds. O.K., so we can take it easy after 15 seconds. Not very likely, you say. What's next?

Glucose is next. You remember glucose, a nice little hexose monosaccharide from Chapter 2? Stored in glycogen, released as needed? I am sure you remember this, but if not, a review of the carbohydrate section of Chapter 2 is essential. We can break down glucose in a process called glycolysis to fuel exercising muscle (this was presented in great detail in Chapter 3). Glucose is broken down to two pyruvic acids, and the released energy is used to generate a small amount of ATP. This occurs in the cytoplasm. If oxygen is present, the pyruvic acids can enter aerobic metabolism. In this way, they enter the mitochondria and are broken down into carbon dioxide and water, and the resulting energy is used to generate much more ATP. If insufficient oxygen is present, the pyruvic acids can only be broken down to lactic acid and generate a little more ATP. This is called anaerobic metabolism. The lactic acid acidifies the exercising muscle and must be carried away by the blood. Also, the carbon dioxide must be carried away by the blood and released into the external environment in the lungs. The lungs must oxygenate the blood in an attempt to stave off anaerobic metabolism. Do you now see why you breathe heavily during exercise? Despite the best efforts of your cardiovascular and respiratory systems, the buildup of lactic acid and carbon dioxide, and the depletion of oxygen and ATP result in muscle fatigue. Ultimately, this fatigue requires you to cease your activity. The heavy breathing that continues after the exercise is necessary to return the tissues and the blood to the proper pH, to get rid of excess carbon dioxide, to reoxygenate the blood and the tissues, and to return ATP stored in the cells to pre-exercise levels. We are, in effect, paying back an oxygen debt. Please review the detailed section on ATP production in Chapter 3 if these processes are not clear to you.

One last comment on a muscle fatigue-related topic before we move on. Did you ever experience painful cramping of your muscles after exercising, especially if you were performing an exercise to which you were not accustomed? Even vigorous note taking during an especially exciting anatomy and physiology lecture can result in muscle fatigue (writer's cramp). Recall from our discussion of the sliding filament theory that it is necessary for ATP to bind to the myosin side arm for that side arm to release actin. If ATP is not present, actin and myosin remain bound together. If they do not release, the muscle cannot relax. This is the cause of that painful, sustained contraction we call a cramp. The lack of ATP also blocks the removal of calcium from the cytoplasm back to the terminal cisterns, exacerbating this problem (see the "Breaching Homeostasis" section on rigor mortis that follows. These cramps are, in part, a similar phenomenon).

9.4 Making the Leap to the Gross Anatomy of Muscles

We will discuss the gross anatomy of individual muscles and of this system in our next chapter. We will learn how muscles work together in groups and how they oppose each other. We will also learn how they are named and the names of some of our muscles. To make the leap from considering single cells to discussing the structure of an entire muscle, we must first think about how individual muscle fibers fit into that larger structure. Muscles are not simply random collections of individual fibers; they have internal organization. Muscle fibers are arranged into bundles called fascicles (**FIGURE 9.9**). Within fascicles, individual muscle fibers are surrounded by a fine network of connective tissue called endomysium. Fascicles are, in turn, surrounded by a slightly heavier network of connective tissue called perimysium. The entire muscle is also surrounded by connective tissue, called epimysium. It may appear, from these descriptions or the figure, that these connective tissues are separate, distinct structures. That, however, is not the case. The endomysium, perimysium, and epimysium are all interconnected and part of a continuous network. By connecting together all of the fibers within a muscle, the contraction of individual fibers results in the application of force to the entire muscle. The contraction of a small number of fibers in a muscle might not result in shortening of the muscle. Instead, the tension developed may only stretch these connective tissues, making the muscle more rigid. We will learn more about this phenomenon in our next chapter.

Although our discussion of the physiology of individual muscle fibers has ended, we still have plenty of work to do in this system. Be sure to look over "What You Should Know" and "What Did You Learn?" to assess your mastery of this chapter before proceeding.

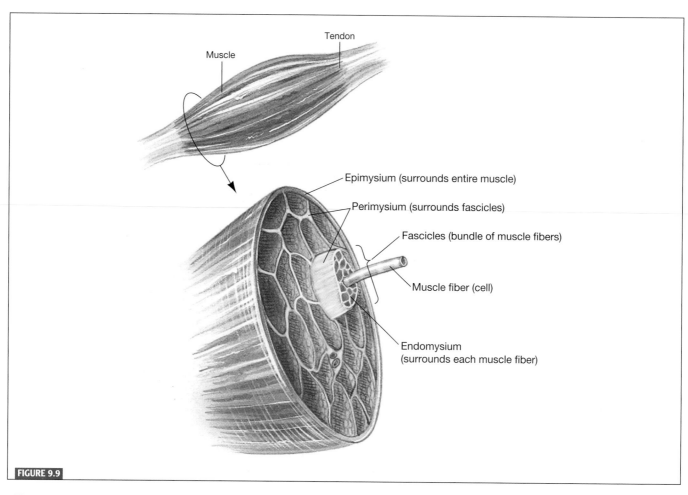

FIGURE 9.9

The connective tissue associated with a muscle. Note that muscle fibers are bundled into fascicles.

Breaching Homeostasis . . . When Things Go Wrong

Postmortem Changes: What Happens to Your Cells After Death

So, just how wrong can things go? The ultimate in "gone wrong" must be death. We know that death can result from a severe breach of homeostasis, or a long-lasting less severe breach. In either event, we reach the point where the body no longer can maintain life. Do all chemical activities stop at the time of death? The answer must be no. If all chemical activities stopped at death, the fixatives we learned about in our earlier "Breaching Homeostasis" section that dealt with preparation of tissues for histologic examination would be unnecessary. This is a good time to think about postmortem changes (changes occurring after death).

The enzymatic degradation of cells and tissues due to the action of enzymes present in them is called autolysis. It is not to be confused with putrefaction, the degradation of tissues due to the action of saprophytic bacteria (bacteria that live and grow in dead tissue). Putrefaction results in the production of gasses, odor, bloating, and discoloration that make dead bodies such unpleasant companions.

Algor motris is the loss of body heat that occurs after death. Although it varies with ambient temperature and other environmental factors, it is generally about one degree per hour. Palor mortis, or paleness after death, occurs as a result of the loss of blood circulation in the subcutaneous tissues. Livor mortis, the seepage of blood from the vasculature into dependent tissues (those in a lower position), begins 2–3 hours postmortem. This can sometimes be used to determine whether a body has been moved after death (is the blood pooled in tissues that are dependent in the position in which the body was found?).

Finally, rigor mortis, the postmortem change that relates to the topic we have been discussing in this chapter. The term *rigor mortis* comes from the Latin words for "rigidity" (rigor) and "death" (mortis). This is the rigidity, or muscle contraction, that occurs after death. We are all somewhat aware of this from dead animals we have seen at the side of the road, or even from horror movies, but what causes it? You already have the tools to figure out the answer to that question.

Following an action potential in a muscle fiber, what actually triggers the thick and thin myofilaments to slide along each other? If you said "the release of calcium from the terminal cisterns," good for you! You know that calcium is sequestered in the terminal cisterns, away from the myofilaments, until a muscle contraction is needed. The release of the calcium results in the contraction of the muscle fiber. You also know that energy in the form of ATP is required to run the Ca^{++}ATPase that pumps the calcium out of the sarcoplasm, into the terminal cisterns. So, what happens when muscle cells run out of ATP? The Ca^{++}ATPase can no longer function. Because of this, and the loss of membrane polarization caused by the same lack of ATP (the Na^+K^+ATPase can't function either), the muscle cells in the dead body can no longer keep the calcium in the terminal cisterns. As calcium leaks into the sarcoplasm, the muscle fibers begin to contract. In the human body, this generally occurs about 6–8 hours after death, beginning with the facial muscles and moving in an inferior direction.

Rigor mortis begins to dissipate 16–24 hours after death; the muscles again relax. This is due to autolysis occurring in the muscle fibers: the contractile machinery is being broken down enzymatically. Muscles relax in the order in which they contracted, from the face down. Refrigeration will slow down rigor mortis, as well as many of the other changes that occur after death.

What You Should Know

1. The functions of the muscle system include movement, posture, a role in breathing, and generation of heat.

2. Three types of muscle exist: smooth, skeletal, and cardiac.

3. Smooth muscle cells lack striations; are fusiform with single, central nuclei; and are capable of slow, involuntary contractions.

4. Skeletal muscle fibers have striations; are long, cylindrical syncytia with many peripheral nuclei; and are capable of voluntary, quick, forceful contractions.

5. Cardiac muscle cells have striations, are irregular in shape, and some are branched, have one or two central nuclei, and are capable of involuntary rhythmic contractions.

6. Many features of muscle fibers have special names and special characteristics. The cytoplasm is called sarcoplasm, the sarcolemma (plasmalemma) is polarized and has special invaginations called T-tubules, and the sarcoplasmic reticulum (smooth endoplasmic reticulum) ends in terminal cisterns that are modified for the storage and release of calcium.

7. Skeletal muscle fibers contain myofibrils made up of thick and thin myofilaments.

8. Thick myofilaments are composed mainly of myosin, which, under appropriate conditions, binds actin, cleaves ATP, and is capable of a major conformational change (change in shape).

9. Thin myofilaments have a backbone of tropomyosin that is decorated with actin and troponin. Actin is a myosin-binding molecule, and troponin is a calcium-binding molecule that influences the confirmation of tropomyosin.

10. The sliding-filament theory explains how the thick and thin myofilaments move along each other to produce the forceful contractions we observe in muscles.

11. The release of calcium from the terminal cisterns, in response to an action potential, triggers muscle contraction.

12. A single action potential affecting a single muscle fiber induces a single short-term contraction called a twitch.

13. Increased sarcoplasmic calcium content caused by multiple action potentials in rapid succession results in increased forces of contraction in the initial few contractions. This phenomenon is called treppe.

14. Repeated stimuli resulting in either limited or no relaxation between contractions in a single muscle fiber is called tetany. Tetany may be complete or incomplete.

15. A single motor neuron and all of the fibers it innervates is called a motor unit.

16. Three types of skeletal muscle fibers exist and these differ in their rate of contraction and resistance to fatigue. Through exercise, one type can sometimes be transformed into another.

17. Aerobic and anaerobic metabolism provide the ATP necessary to power the contraction and relaxation of muscle fibers.

18. Muscle fibers are arranged into fascicles.

19. Muscle fibers within fascicles are surrounded by endomysium, fascicles are surrounded by perimysium, and the entire muscle is surrounded by epimysium.

What Did You Learn?

Multiple choice questions: choose the best answer.

1. Which of the following is not a function of the muscle system?

   a. Movement

   b. Posture

   c. Movement of substances along the small intestine

   d. Production of heat

   e. All of the above are functions of the muscle system

2. All of the following groupings are correct except:

   a. Cardiac, striated, voluntary

   b. Skeletal, striated, voluntary

   c. Smooth, nonstriated, involuntary

   d. All of the above are correct groupings.

   e. None of the above are correct groupings.

3. If a muscle tissue has cells with striations and one or two nuclei per cell, the nuclei would be:

   a. Central

   b. Peripheral

   c. They may be in either location.

   d. No such tissue exists.

What Did You Learn? (continued)

4. The cells of which type of muscle are true syncytia?
   a. Skeletal
   b. Smooth
   c. Cardiac
   d. None of the above

5. Striations are present in which of the following:
   a. Cardiac muscle
   b. Smooth muscle
   c. Both of the above
   d. Neither of the above

6. Which of the following is the term for the muscle cell membrane?
   a. Sarcoplasm
   b. Sarcoplasmic reticulum
   c. Motor endplate
   d. Sarcomere
   e. Sarcolemma

7. In a sarcomere, which of the following is found in the H zone?
   a. Thick myofilaments
   b. Thin myofilaments
   c. Both of the above
   d. Neither of the above

8. Identify the name of the feature indicated:
   a. I band
   b. H zone
   c. A band
   d. Z line

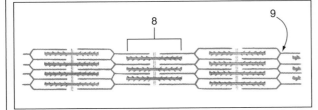

9. Identify the name of the feature indicated:
   a. I band
   b. H zone
   c. A band
   d. Z line
   e. M line

10. Identify the feature indicated:
    a. Thick myofibril
    b. Thick myofilament
    c. Thin myofibril
    d. Thin myofilament

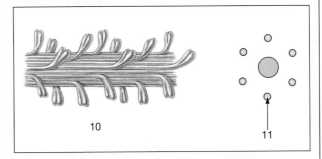

11. Identify the feature indicated:
    a. Thick myofibril
    b. Thick myofilament
    c. Thin myofibril
    d. Thin myofilament

12. The striations of skeletal muscle result from:
    a. The myosin cross bridges
    b. The alignment of sarcomeres throughout the fiber
    c. Intercalated disks
    d. The sarcoplasmic reticulum

13. Terminal cisterns are part of what organelle?
    a. T-tubules
    b. Sarcolemma
    c. Nucleolus
    d. Golgi apparatus
    e. None of the above

14. As you begin to exercise, the phosphagen system provides energy for the initial _____ of muscle contractions.
    a. Fifteen seconds
    b. Fifteen minutes
    c. Fifteen hours
    d. None of the above is correct. The phosphagen system provides as much energy as is required for any amount of contraction and relaxation.

15. The functions of myosin include:
    a. Actin binding
    b. ATPase activity
    c. Both of the above
    d. Neither of the above

What Did You Learn? (continued)

16. What is stored in terminal cisterns?
    a. Sodium
    b. Calcium
    c. Potassium
    d. Magnesium
    e. None of the above

17. When a skeletal muscle fiber is at rest:
    a. Calcium is bound to troponin.
    b. Calcium is bound to tropomyosin.
    c. Calcium is bound to the myosin side arm.
    d. Calcium is bound to actin.
    e. None of the above is correct.

18. The binding of neurotransmitter to receptors in the motor endplate:
    a. Opens sodium channels in the receptor
    b. Closes sodium channels in the receptor
    c. Opens calcium channels in the receptor
    d. Closes calcium channels in the receptor
    e. None of the above is correct.

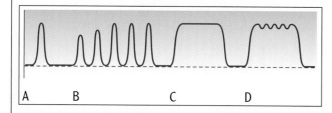

19. Which panel best demonstrates incomplete tetany?
    a. A
    b. B
    c. C
    d. D

20. Which panel best demonstrates treppe?
    a. A
    b. B
    c. C
    d. D

Short answer questions: answer briefly and in your own words.

1. If a weight lifter began to train as a marathon runner, what change would be likely to occur in the types of fibers of which her muscles are composed?

2. During a weight-lifting competition, you observe an athlete warming up before her big lift. What principle might she be taking advantage of here? Please explain your answer.

3. Indicate what happens during each of the stages of the contraction of a muscle fiber, as described by the sliding filament theory.

4. Where does the energy come from for muscle contraction and relaxation? Is energy required for relaxation? Please be specific in your answers.

5. Please name and describe the connective tissue that organizes the fibers of a muscle. You may draw a diagram and label it, if you choose.

6. If an athlete who is used to training at a low altitude (on the beach in Maine, for example) engages in a competition at a high altitude (the Colorado Rockies, for example), would you expect to see a change in that athlete's performance? What change would you expect? What are the physiologic causes for this change?

Your Body in Motion: The Gross Anatomy of Your Muscle System

What You Will Learn

- The names of the attachments of muscle to bone.
- The ways in which multiple muscles participate to produce the movements desired.
- The characteristics used to name skeletal muscles.
- Tips to help you memorize the names and locations of muscles.
- The names, locations, and actions of the superficial muscles.

We have been discussing the finer aspects of your muscles: the activities of individual muscle fibers. Here we will discuss the gross aspects of this system, that which you can see with the naked eye. We will begin with the gross anatomy of an individual muscle and then discuss how muscles work together. Next, we will move on to how muscles are named, and finish with a small atlas of the superficial muscles of your body.

10.1 The Parts of an Individual Muscle

Of course, everything in the body has a name. The parts of muscles are no exception (**FIGURE 10.1**). These names are useful; they help us to identify the location of the muscle and to figure out its function. In our last chapter, we learned that muscles have connective tissue within them that organize muscle fibers into fascicles and connect the fascicles into one unit. This connective tissue does not stop at the margins of the muscle. It continues beyond the muscle to attach the muscle to bones. Muscles need strong attachments to bones to perform their functions. Bones act as levers in the body, and joints act as the fulcrums on which those levers pivot. Muscles provide the force that moves the levers, doing the work necessary to move our bodies or parts of our bodies. Tendons are the connective tissue structures that attach muscles to bones. Tendons are extensions of epimysium (which, as you know, are continuous with perimysium and endomysium). Do you remember what the tissue that covers and surrounds bones is called? Recall that on the superficial surface of bones, we have a two-layered covering. The outer layer of this covering is made of dense connective tissue. I hope you remember that this covering is called periosteum (if not, please review this material in Chapter 6). The fibrous layer of the periosteum is

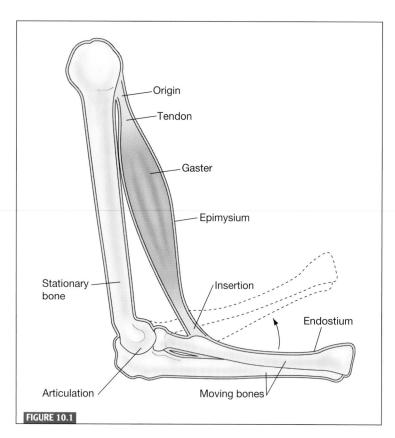

FIGURE 10.1

The parts of a muscle. The actual origin of the muscle shown is the scapula. Origin on humerus is shown for clarity.

continuous with tendons. Since the tendons are continuous with the connective tissues within our muscles, the entire connective structure is one unit. That makes for a very strong structure, indeed. Now, can you figure out which type of connective tissue makes up the tendons? Let's make this multiple choice: are they loose connective tissue, dense regular connective tissue, or dense irregular connective tissue? Recall our discussion of these tissues in Chapter 4. If you said dense regular connective tissue, you are correct (sorry, no prize giveaways here; it is only a book, after all). It must be dense regular connective tissue: it needs great strength (hence, dense connective tissue, lots of collagenous fibers), and all of the force it encounters is along one plane, directly between the muscle and the bone (hence, the regular type of dense connective tissue, with all fibers parallel).

Depending on which end of the muscle they are on, we have different names for the tendons that attach muscles to bones. Hold your arm straight out to your side. That's right, go ahead and do it; no one is looking. Now, bend your arm at your elbow so your forearm is at a 90° angle to your upper arm. You have just flexed your elbow joint. Extending your elbow would be the opposite movement (recall these movements from Chapter 7). Notice that when you flexed your elbow, only your forearm moved; your upper arm did not move. This move-

ment was caused by contraction of your biceps brachii. The biceps brachii is attached on one end to your scapula. It actually makes two attachments to the scapula (hence, the name *bi*ceps), but both are on the same end of the muscle. The other end of this muscle is attached to your radius. As this muscle contracts, your radius moves but your scapula does not. That is the way most muscles work. The bone attached to one end of the muscle moves as the muscle contracts; the bone attached to the opposite end of the muscle does not move. The attachment of the muscle to the bone that does not move is called the *origin* of the muscle. The attachment of the muscle to the bone that does move is called the *insertion* of the muscle. The origin and the insertion of a muscle tell us its location and its action. Some muscles have multiple origins or insertions. It merely has to do with the shape of the muscle, which we will discuss shortly. The portion of the muscle that is between the origin and the insertion and is mainly composed of muscle fibers is called the belly or gaster of the muscle.

10.2 How Your Muscles Cooperate to Move You: Group Actions

Working together in a group makes a lot of things easier, doesn't it? Wouldn't that also be true in the body? Your muscles are arranged to work together in groups. Your complex movements require the interaction of numerous muscles in a coordinated fashion, and your muscles are arranged in groups to allow that coordination. The topic we are considering here is called muscle group actions (**FIGURE 10.2**). It implies that our muscles are arranged in groups and that each member of the group has a particular job to do for each movement in which it is involved. A moment ago, we discussed a motion that flexed your elbow. The muscle responsible for that motion is the biceps brachii. When the biceps brachii contracts, your elbow flexes. Therefore, your biceps brachii is the prime mover of that motion. The prime mover is the muscle in a group that, when it contracts, provides the force for the desired motion. *Agonist* is another term for prime mover.

If instead you wanted to move your forearm in the opposite direction, that is to say you wanted to extend your elbow, you would have to contract a different muscle. You would have to contract your triceps brachii to perform this motion. The triceps brachii would be the prime mover for extension of your elbow. However, what must your triceps brachii do if you are to flex your elbow? Think about this; your biceps brachii flexes your elbow, your triceps brachii extends your elbow. The triceps brachii would have to relax to allow the elbow to flex when the biceps brachii contracts. That makes the triceps brachii the antagonist for that movement. The

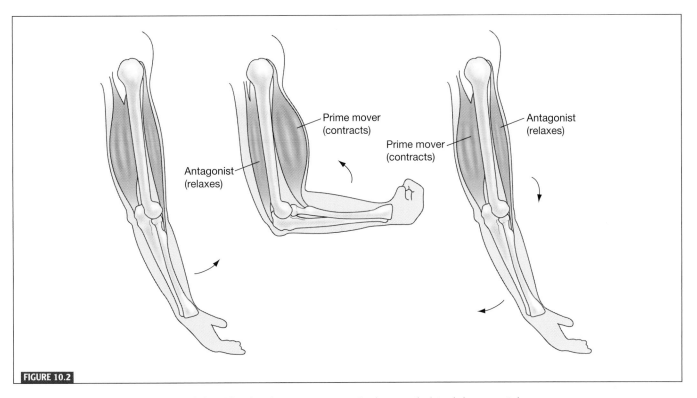

FIGURE 10.2

Muscle group actions. The muscles identified as either the prime mover or antagonist change as the intended movement changes.

antagonist in a muscle group is the muscle that opposes the action of the prime mover. The antagonist must relax to allow the prime mover to produce the desired motion. If a muscle is a prime mover for one movement, it is the antagonist for the opposite movement.

In most cases, there are additional muscles involved in movement. These muscles are called synergists. Synergists aid the prime mover in a variety of ways. They may provide additional force for the prime mover. They often make motion smoother and more efficient. They may also stabilize the origin of the prime mover so the origin does not move as the contraction occurs. When they stabilize the origin of the prime mover, they are called fixators.

10.3 Naming the Muscles

■ How Skeletal Muscles Are Named

Like most things in life, there is a system to the naming of skeletal muscles. The names of the muscles have meanings to them, and you can often figure out which muscle is being referred to by knowing these meanings. Otherwise, all you can do to learn the muscles is to use rote memorization. That gets a little dull, not to mention being rather a difficult task. Here we will discuss how skeletal muscles are named.

Various characteristics of a muscle are used to name that muscle. These include features such as where the muscle is located, what the muscle looks like, and what

work the muscle performs. **TABLE 10.1** lists the characteristics used to name muscles, representative names that are based on those characteristics, and examples of muscles named in that way. Remember, these are only examples to show you how these names are generated. Look for similar meanings in the muscles you are learning. A good medical dictionary might help you in this endeavor. If you do not have a medical dictionary, you might find it a useful addition to your personal and professional library (for example, *Essential Medical Terminology, Second Edition*, by Peggy S. Stanfield, published by Jones and Bartlett Publishers, Inc.). You can also spend time using a medical dictionary in the library, if you choose. That has the advantage of letting you determine how useful it is to you before parting with your money for one.

■ How to Know the Muscles: A Strategy for Learning

There are over 600 muscles in the human body. I do not give an exact figure here because, like many things people do, anatomists can't agree on how some of them should be counted. You have your "lumpers," who join some muscles together into one and have a lower count, and you have your "splitters," who count each possible muscle separately and have a higher count. Maybe you will go on to become a great anatomist and find a new way of counting the muscles that will put this burning controversy to rest. In the meantime, we have some muscles to learn.

Table 10.1   Naming of Skeletal Muscles

Characteristic	Example Terminology	Meaning	Examples
Direction	Rectus	Parallel to the midline (like a sagittal section)	Rectus femoris
	Transversus	Perpendicular to the midline (like a transverse section)	Transversus abdominis
	Oblique	Diagonal to the midline	External oblique
Location	Tibialis	Near the tibia	Tibialis anterior
	Anterior	Toward the anterior surface	Tibialis anterior
	Lateralis	Located laterally	Vastus lateralis
	Medialis	Located toward the midline	Vastus medialis
Shape	Deltoid	Triangular	Deltoid
	Rhomboid	Diamond shaped	Rhomboideus
	Serratus	Saw toothed (like a serrated knife)	Serratus anterior
	Platysma	Flat	Platysma
Relative size	Maximus	Largest	Gluteus maximus
	Minimus	Smallest	Gluteus minimus
	Major	Large	Teres major
	Minor	Small	Teres minor
	Longus	Longest	Peroneus longus
	Brevis	Shortest	Peroneus brevis
Location of attachments	Sterno-	Sternum	Sternocleidomastoid
	Cleido-	Clavicle	Sternocleidomastoid
	Mastoid	Mastoid process (of temporal)	Sternocleidomastoid
	Brachio	Upper arm	Brachioradialis
	Radialis	Radius	Brachioradialis
Number of origins	Biceps	Two origins	Biceps femoris
	Triceps	Three origins	Triceps brachii
Action	Levator	Elevates	Levator scapuli
	Flexor	Flexes	Flexor carpi ulnaris
	Extensor	Extends	Extensor digitorum

How many of them should we learn about here? That is a tough question to answer. It is like one of those desert island games. (If you were to be trapped on a desert island and could only take 15 things with you, what would you bring?) To expect you to learn all 600 muscles is well beyond the scope of this text. The goal of this text is to help you develop a basic understanding of the human body. That understanding should be deep enough that you could use this information and these concepts in your daily life and build on them in the future. If you are given too little information, no real understanding can develop. If you are given too much information, you may become overwhelmed and not actually gain as much understanding as is possible.

Here, you will learn the names, locations, and actions of mainly the superficial muscles of the body.

These are the muscles you can generally see or palpate (feel) in a living person. These are the muscles you would see in a dissection specimen once you removed the skin and underlying connective tissue. Many additional muscles lie deep to these muscles; if you are interested, you can look into an atlas of the muscles that will show these. Many good atlases are available. Several deep muscles are presented; these are muscles that are important for you to know. These muscles are generally important for your understanding of some of the topics we will discuss later on in this text.

So, we have about 60 muscles to learn; how should we go about doing this? First of all, don't panic when you look at the first couple of diagrams. **FIGURE 10.3** shows many of the muscles you will learn at this time. Do not start by trying to learn them from this figure.

Like so many jobs, learning the muscles is much easier when you break it down into manageable units. The next figure (**FIGURE 10.4**) shows the muscles of the anterior trunk and face. **TABLE 10.2**, which accompanies Figure 10.4, lists the origin, insertion, and action of each of these muscles. Work with this figure and table until you know this information. Be very careful not to simply memorize the order or placement of the muscle names on the diagram. We are learning anatomy here, not only the diagram. You need to be able to recognize these muscles in settings other than this diagram, so learn where the actual muscles are.

Also, when you are working on the names of the muscles, recall what you have just learned about how muscles are named. Don't just look at the names as some unrecognizable syllables; try to find terms you know in the names. This often will help you to learn to associate the name with the location or action of the

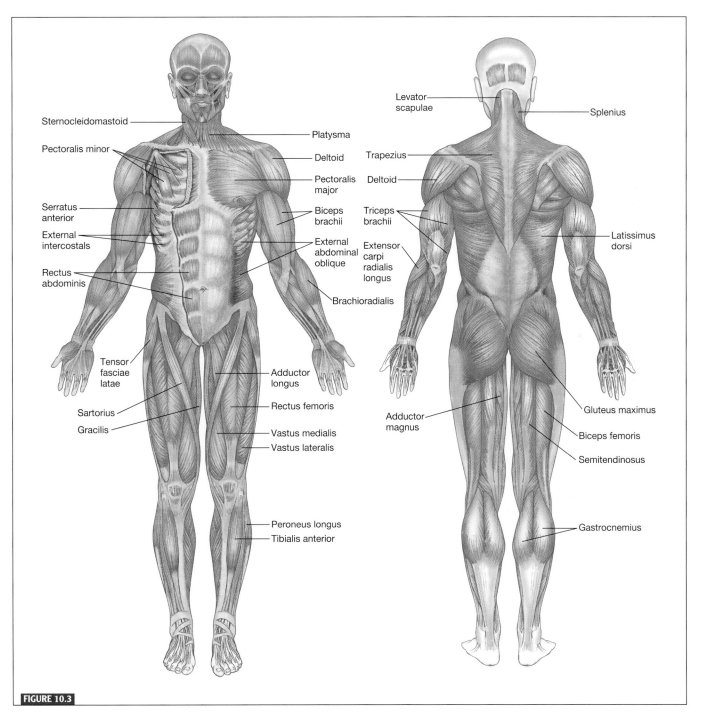

FIGURE 10.3

The anterior (left) and posterior (right) superficial muscles.

muscle. Try to say the names out loud. By saying them and hearing yourself say them, you activate different areas of your brain. This will help you to get the information into your memory more efficiently.

As you learn the origin and insertion of each muscle, use your knowledge of the skeletal system to visualize the location of the muscle and reason out what would happen if that muscle were to contract. This will make learning the actions of the muscles easier. Ideally, you will not have to memorize these actions. If you learn the locations well enough and gain an understanding of how the muscles work, you may be able to figure out the actions on your own, as you need them. As you learn these muscles, move onto the next figure. You will find that some of the muscles appearing in the next figure are muscles you have already learned. By learning the muscles presented on one figure at a time, you will be done sooner and have less frustration than you would think possible.

Test yourself as you move through the figures. It is easy to kid ourselves into thinking we know something that we do not really know. By seriously testing yourself, you will overcome any possible self-deception and identify the areas that need work. This too makes your work more efficient. The flashcards available with your text are very useful for this self-testing process. Have someone go through these cards with you, quizzing you as you go. A classmate who is also learning this information might make a good study partner in this way. Just remember, pay special attention to be sure you are staying focused on the subject and not drifting off into other conversations. The goal is to spend your time learning. Carry these flashcards with you and try to find moments during your day when you can look through them, even very briefly. Every minute you can work on this subject will be beneficial to you.

10.4 An Atlas of the Superficial Muscles

With this, we have finished our discussions of the muscle system, and our section dealing with support and motion. Much of what you have learned here will be revisited in some form, as we delve into other areas of anatomy and physiology. Please be sure you have learned what you need to know by using the "What You Should Know" and "What Did You Learn?" features of these chapters. Hopefully, you have found these topics useful and exciting. We will next begin to learn about how your body is regulated, including how homeostasis is monitored and maintained.

Table 10.2   The Superficial Muscles of the Face and Anterior Trunk

Name	Origin	Insertion	Action
External abdominal oblique	Inferior 8 ribs	C.T.* of anterior midline and lateral posterior ilium	Depresses ribs, compresses abdomen, flexes spine
External intercostals	Inferior surface of each rib	Superior surface of each rib	Moves ribs superiorly and anteriorly
Internal intercostals	Superior surface of each rib	Inferior surface of each rib	Moves ribs inferiorly and posteriorly
Levator palpebrae superioris	Sphenoid superior to eye	Upper eyelid	Elevates upper eyelid (opens eye)
Masseter	Lateral zygomatic	Lateral mandible	Elevates mandible
Orbicularis oculi	Medial wall of orbit	Skin around eye	Closes eyelid
Orbicularis oris	C.T. around mouth	Lateral margins of mouth	Closes and moves lips anteriorly
Pectoralis minor	Ribs 3–5	Scapula	Protract and move shoulder inferiorly, rotate scapula inferiorly, elevate ribs
Platysma	C.T. of shoulder	Mandible and C.T. of face	Depresses mandible and lower lip, moves lower lip posteriorly
Rectus abdominis	Anterior, superior pubis	Inferior costal cartilage and xiphoid	Depresses ribs, flexes vertebral column
Risorius	C.T. of lateral face	Lateral margins of mouth	Moves margin of mouth laterally
Scalenes (group of 3)	Cervical vertebrae	Superior surfaces of ribs 1 and 2	Elevate ribs, flex neck, rotate head
Serratus anterior	Anterior, superior surfaces of ribs 1–9	Anterior medial scapula	Protract shoulder
Sternocleidomastoid	Medial clavicle and manubrium	Temporal	Flex neck, laterally flex and rotate head
Zygomaticus major	Zygomatic	Lateral margins of mouth	Elevates and retracts lateral margins of mouth
Zygomaticus minor	Zygomatic	Superior lip	Elevates and retracts superior lip

*In each of the tables, C.T. indicates an attachment to connective tissue instead of bone.

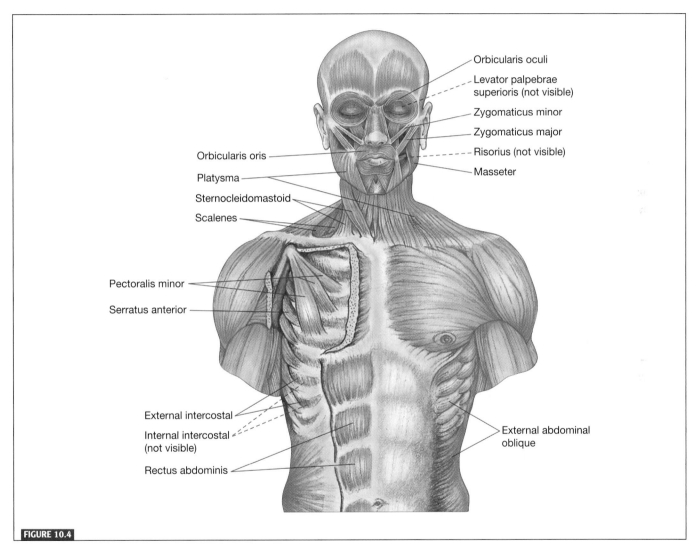

FIGURE 10.4

The superficial muscles of the face and anterior trunk.

Table 10.3   The Superficial Muscles of the Anterior Shoulder and Arm

Name	Origin	Insertion	Action
Biceps brachii	Two sites on scapula	Proximal anterior radius	Flex elbow
Brachialis	Anterior distal humerus	Proximal ulna	Flex elbow
Brachioradialis	Distal lateral humerus	Distal lateral radius	Flex elbow
Deltoid	Clavicle and scapula	Lateral humerus	Abduct shoulder
Flexor carpi radialis	Distal medial humerus	Metacarpals #2 and #3	Flex and abduct wrist
Flexor carpi ulnaris	Distal medial humerus and medial proximal ulna	Pisiform, hamate, and metacarpal #5	Flex and adduct wrist
Hypothenars (group of 3)	Pisiform, hamate and carpal tendons	Medial proximal phalanx of little finger and metacarpal #5	Abduct, flex, and oppose little finger
Palmaris longus	Medial distal humerus	C.T. of palm	Flex wrist
Pectoralis major	Gladiolus, inferior medial surfaces of ribs 2–6	Proximal humerus	Flex, adduct, and rotate shoulder medially
Thenar (group of 4)	Scaphoid trapezium, trapezoid, carpal tendons	Lateral metacarpal #1, lateral medial proximal phalanx of thumb	Flex, adduct, and oppose thumb

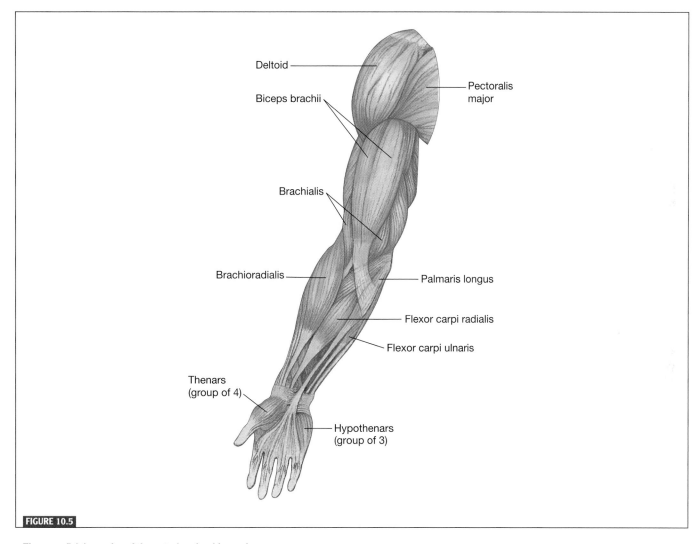

Deltoid

Biceps brachii

Pectoralis major

Brachialis

Brachioradialis

Palmaris longus

Flexor carpi radialis

Flexor carpi ulnaris

Thenars (group of 4)

Hypothenars (group of 3)

FIGURE 10.5

The superficial muscles of the anterior shoulder and arm.

Table 10.4   The Superficial Muscles of the Posterior Trunk, Shoulder, and Arm

Name	Origin	Insertion	Action
Anconeus	Distal lateral humerus	Proximal posterior ulna	Extension of elbow
Extensor carpi radialis brevis	Distal lateral humerus	Metacarpal 3	Extend and abduct wrist
Extensor carpi radialis longus	Distal lateral humerus	Metacarpal 2	Extend and abduct wrist
Extensor carpi ulnaris	Distal lateral humerus and posterior ulna	Metacarpal 5	Extend and adduct wrist
Extensor digitorum	Distal lateral humerus	Distal and middle phalanges of fingers	Extend fingers and wrist
Infraspinatus	Posterior scapula	Proximal posterior humerus	Rotate shoulder laterally
Latissimus dorsi	Inferior T* and all L* vertebrae and ribs	Proximal anterior humerus	Extend, adduct, and rotate shoulder medially
Levator scapuli	Vertebrae C* 1–4	Medial scapula	Elevate scapula
Rhomboideus (group of 2)	Vertebrae C7 and T1–5	Medial scapula	Adduct and rotate scapula inferiorly
Splenius (group of 2)	Vertebrae C7–T6	Occipital, temporal, vertebrae C1–4	Extend, flex, and rotate head
Supraspinatus	Posterior scapula	Proximal posterior humerus	Abduct shoulder
Teres major	Inferior scapula	Proximal anterior humerus	Extend, adduct, and rotate shoulder medially
Teres minor	Lateral scapula	Proximal lateral humerus	Rotate shoulder laterally
Trapezius	Occipital and vertebrae C7, T1–12	Clavicle and scapula	Multiple movements of clavicle, scapula, and neck
Triceps brachii	Scapula and humerus	Proximal posterior ulna	Extend elbow

*The following abbreviations apply to all tables: C means cervical, T means thoracic, L means lumbar.

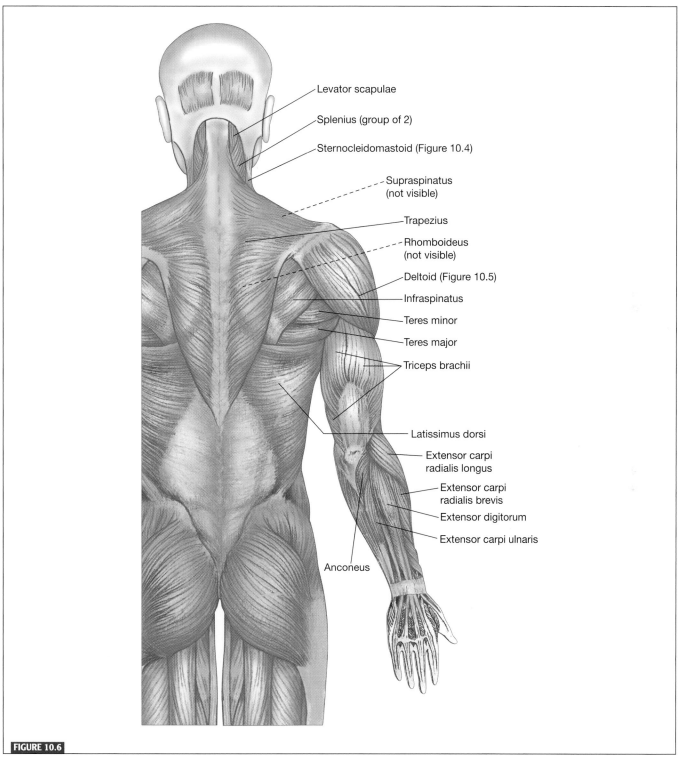

Levator scapulae

Splenius (group of 2)

Sternocleidomastoid (Figure 10.4)

Supraspinatus
(not visible)

Trapezius

Rhomboideus
(not visible)

Deltoid (Figure 10.5)

Infraspinatus

Teres minor

Teres major

Triceps brachii

Latissimus dorsi

Extensor carpi
radialis longus

Extensor carpi
radialis brevis

Extensor digitorum

Extensor carpi ulnaris

Anconeus

FIGURE 10.6

The superficial muscles of the posterior trunk, shoulder, and arm.

Table 10.5   The Superficial Muscles of the Anterior Hip and Leg

Name	Origin	Insertion	Action
Adductor longus	Medial pubis	Posterior femur	Adduct, flex, and rotate hip medially
Adductor magnus	Pubis and ischium	Posterior femur	Adduct, flex, and rotate hip medially
Gracilis	Inferior pubis	Proximal medial tibia	Adduct, flex, and rotate hip medially
Iliopsoas (group of 2)	Lateral vertebrae and ilium	Proximal medial femur	Flex trunk, flex hip, and rotate laterally
Pectineus	Superior pubis	Proximal medial femur	Flex, adduct, and rotate hip medially
Peroneus longus	Proximal lateral tibia and proximal fibula	Metatarsal #1 and #1 cuneiform	Plantar flex ankle, evert foot, support arch
Rectus femoris	Lateral anterior ilium	Proximal anterior tibia	Flex hip and extend knee
Sartorius	Lateral anterior ilium	Medial anterior tibia	Flex knee, flex, and rotate hip laterally
Tensor fasciae latae	Lateral ilium	Lateral tibia	Flex and abduct hip
Tibialis anterior	Lateral proximal tibia	Metatarsal #1 and #1 cuneiform	Dorsiflex ankle invert foot
Vastus lateralis	Lateral proximal femur	Anterior proximal tibia	Extend knee
Vastus medialis	Posterior femur	Anterior proximal tibia	Extend knee

Table 10.6   The Superficial Muscles of the Posterior Hip and Leg

Name	Origin	Insertion	Action
Biceps femoris	Posterior lateral ischium and posterior femur	Proximal fibula and tibia	Flex knee, extend and rotate hip laterally
Gastrocnemius	Distal femur	Posterior calcaneus	Plantar flex ankle, invert and adduct foot, flex knee
Gluteus maximus	Posterior lateral coxal, sacrum, coccyx	Posterior femur	Extend and rotate hip laterally
Gluteus medius	Posterior lateral coxal	Proximal femur	Abduct and rotate hip medially
Peroneus brevis	Fibula	Metatarsal #5	Plantar flex foot and ankle, evert foot
Plantaris	Distal femur	Posterior calcaneus	Plantar flex ankle, flex knee
Popliteus	Distal lateral femur	Proximal posterior tibia	Rotate tibia medially
Semimembranosus	Posterior ishium	Proximal medial tibia	Flex knee, flex and rotate hip medially
Semitendinosus	Posterior ishium	Proximal medial tibia	Flex knee, flex and rotate hip medially
Soleus	Proximal posterior fibula and tibia	Posterior calcaneus	Plantar flex ankle

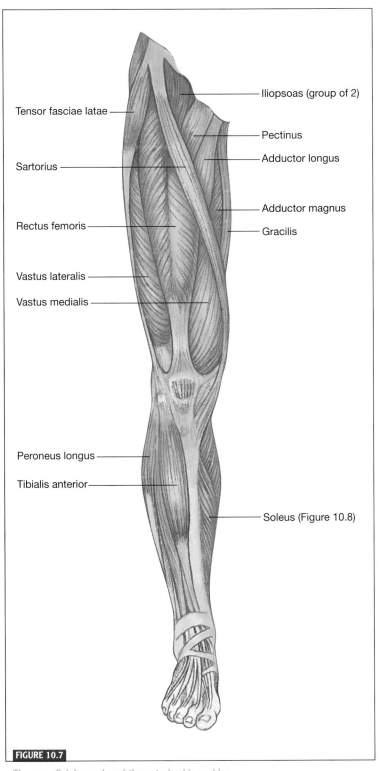

Tensor fasciae latae

Sartorius

Rectus femoris

Vastus lateralis

Vastus medialis

Peroneus longus

Tibialis anterior

Iliopsoas (group of 2)

Pectinus

Adductor longus

Adductor magnus

Gracilis

Soleus (Figure 10.8)

FIGURE 10.7

The superficial muscles of the anterior hip and leg.

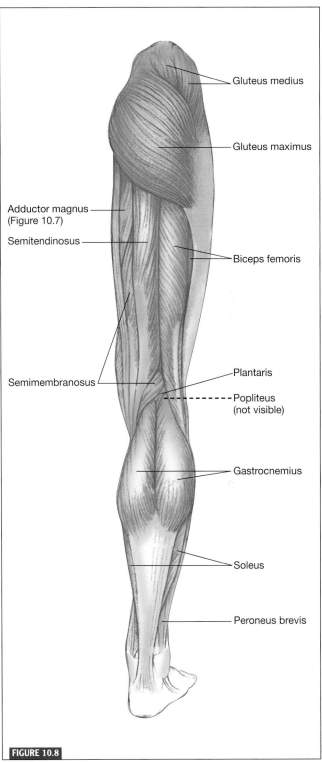

Adductor magnus
(Figure 10.7)

Semitendinosus

Semimembranosus

Gluteus medius

Gluteus maximus

Biceps femoris

Plantaris

Popliteus
(not visible)

Gastrocnemius

Soleus

Peroneus brevis

FIGURE 10.8

The superficial muscles of the posterior hip and leg.

What You Should Know

1. Tendons are made of dense regular connective tissue that is continuous with the epimysium, perimysium, and endomysium, as well as the periosteum.

2. The end of a muscle that attaches to a bone that does not move as the muscle contracts is that muscle's origin.

3. The end of a muscle that attaches to a bone that does move as the muscle contracts is that muscle's insertion.

4. Muscles work together in groups to produce the movements you desire. This is called group action.

5. The muscle that produces the actual desired movement as it contracts is the prime mover.

6. The muscle that opposes the action of the prime mover, and must relax to allow the desired movement, is the antagonist.

7. Synergists aid the prime mover, making the movement smoother and more efficient.

8. One type of synergist, called fixators, stabilizes the origin of the prime mover as it contracts.

9. We name skeletal muscles in a variety of ways. By learning the meanings of some of the muscle names, you can more easily learn their locations.

10. You must know the names, locations and actions of the superficial muscles.

What Did You Learn?

Multiple choice questions: choose the best answer.

1. Which of the following best defines the origin of a muscle?
   a. The attachment of the muscle to a bone that moves as the muscle contracts
   b. The attachment of the muscle to a bone that does not move as the muscle contracts
   c. The distal attachment of the muscle
   d. The proximal attachment of the muscle

2. Tendons are composed of:
   a. Dense irregular connective tissue
   b. Dense regular connective tissue
   c. Loose connective tissue
   d. Cartilage

3. Which of the following is continuous with a tendon?
   a. Epimysium
   b. Periosteum
   c. Both of the above
   d. Neither of the above

4. The muscle that directly causes the desired movement as it contracts is the:
   a. Antagonist
   b. Prime mover
   c. Synergist
   d. Fixator

5. A muscle that stabilizes the origin of the prime mover is:
   a. A fixator
   b. A synergist
   c. Both of the above
   d. Neither of the above

6. Muscles may be named according to their:
   a. Direction
   b. Location
   c. Shape
   d. Relative size
   e. All of the above

7. Which of the following is the best example of a muscle being named according to its location?
   a. Gluteus maximus
   b. Deltoid
   c. Platysma
   d. Tibialis anterior

8. The name triceps tells us that this muscle has:
   a. Two origins
   b. Two insertions
   c. Three origins
   d. Three insertions
   e. Three horns on its nose

What Did You Learn? (continued)

9. Identify the muscle indicated in the accompanying diagram.

   a. Masseter

   b. External abdominal oblique

   c. Orbicularis oris

   d. Platysma

   e. Serratus anterior

10. Identify the muscle indicated in the accompanying diagram.

    a. Masseter

    b. External oblique

    c. Orbicularis oris

    d. Platysma

    e. Serratus anterior

11. Identify the muscle indicated in the accompanying diagram.

    a. Masseter

    b. External oblique

    c. Orbicularis oris

    d. Platysma

    e. Serratus anterior

12. Identify the muscle indicated in the accompanying diagram.

    a. Masseter

    b. External oblique

    c. Orbicularis oris

    d. Platysma

    e. Serratus anterior

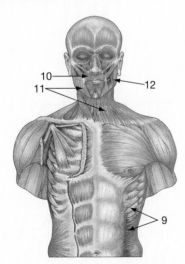

13. Identify the muscle indicated in the accompanying diagram.

    a. Hypthenars

    b. Deltoid

    c. Flexor carpi radialis

    d. Pectoralis minor

    e. Pectoralis major

14. Identify the muscle indicated in the accompanying diagram.

    a. Hypthenars

    b. Deltoid

    c. Flexor carpi radialis

    d. Pectoralis minor

    e. Pectoralis major

15. Identify the muscle indicated in the accompanying diagram.

    a. Hypthenars

    b. Deltoid

    c. Flexor carpi radialis

    d. Pectoralis minor

    e. Pectoralis major

16. Identify the muscle indicated in the accompanying diagram.

    a. Hypthenars

    b. Deltoid

    c. Flexor carpi radialis

    d. Pectoralis minor

    e. Pectoralis major

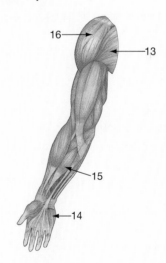

17. Identify the muscle indicated in the accompanying diagram.

    a. Adductor magnus

    b. Peroneus longus

    c. Sartorius

    d. Tibialis anterior

    e. Vastus lateralis

18. Identify the muscle indicated in the accompanying diagram.

    a. Adductor magnus

    b. Peroneus longus

What Did You Learn? (continued)

c. Sartorius

d. Tibialis anterior

e. Vastus lateralis

19. Identify the muscle indicated in the accompanying diagram.

   a. Adductor magnus

   b. Peroneus longus

   c. Sartorius

   d. Tibialis anterior

   e. Vastus lateralis

20. Identify the muscle indicated in the accompanying diagram.

   a. Adductor magnus

   b. Peroneus longus

   c. Sartorius

   d. Tibialis anterior

   e. Vastus lateralis

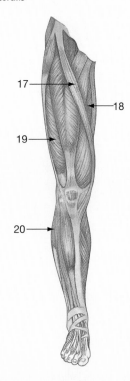

Short answer questions: answer briefly and in your own words.

1. Discuss what is meant by "muscle group actions." Please include in your discussion the terms for each of the muscles in a group, and indicate what they do (for example, prime mover).

2. List five characteristics that are used in naming muscles and an example term for each characteristic.

3. List the origin and insertion for each muscle indicated.

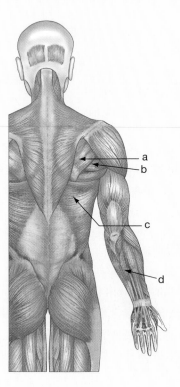

4. List the action for each of the muscles indicated.

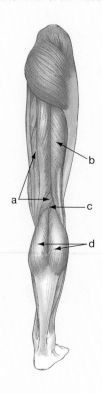

Regulating Your Body

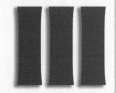

PART III

The Nervous and Endocrine Systems: Two Great Systems That Go Great Together

What is the underlying theme of physiology? Homeostasis! And what is homeostasis? Homeostasis is the constant state of conditions that our body attempts to maintain in its internal environment. These conditions include the concentrations of numerous chemicals, a variety of pressures, and physical parameters such as pressures and temperature. There is a vast array of conditions that must be held in a relatively narrow range for life to continue. It would actually be a little frightening to think about, if not for the fact that our bodies are so good at maintaining homeostasis.

So, if we are to use the systems of our bodies to keep all of these parameters within a narrow range, we must somehow monitor these conditions and coordinate all of the activities aimed at maintaining them. Something must be "minding the store." Which systems perform these regulatory functions? We learned in Chapter 5 that the nervous system and the endocrine systems are the regulators of homeostasis. In this section, we are about to learn how these systems function. Remember, the nervous system is the fast-acting regulator of homeostasis and it works primarily through electrical means. The endocrine system is the slow-acting regulator of homeostasis; it acts through the use of chemical messengers called hormones.

We will spend more time learning about these two systems than on any other systems. This is in part due to their importance and in part due to their complexity. Be sure to work carefully and understand the concepts of each chapter before moving on, as this material is very important and builds from one section to the next. Relax a little, too, as you are about to learn about some of the most fascinating aspects of the human body.

11 Your Neurons and their Electrical Activity

What You Will Learn

- The cells that make up the parenchyma and the stroma of the nervous system.
- The parts of a neuron.
- The characteristics of the neuron cell body, dendrites, and axon.
- How substances are transported in axons.
- The definition of a nerve fiber.
- The importance of myelination and the cells responsible for it.
- How conduction differs between myelinated and nonmyelinated fibers.
- A simple classification scheme for neurons.
- More detail about synapses.
- The types of glial cells, which are the stroma of the nervous system.

11.1 Your Fascinating Neurons

As we begin our discussion of the nervous system, we must get to know the cells that are found in this system. You may recall that we had two categories into which we could place the cells of any organ. One category included the cells that perform the actual function of that organ; the other category included the cells that support the cells that do the work of that organ. Does this sound familiar (hint: think back to Chapter 4)? The cells that perform the function of an organ are that organ's paren-

chyma. The cells that support the parenchyma are the stroma. We must begin by learning about the parenchyma of the nervous system: neurons (**FIGURE 11.1**). Neurons are fascinating cells. Think about it. We could not think about neurons without using our neurons. We are using our neurons to learn about our neurons. I have to stop this train of thought before we hurt ourselves.

Anyway, neurons are fascinating cells. Neurophysiologists spend all of their time studying neurons and they never get bored. In fact, they have given the various parts of neurons specific names. They have even given special

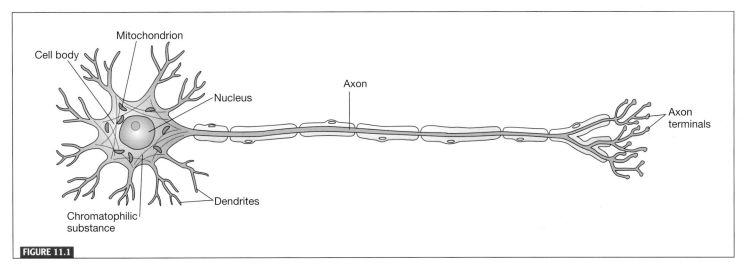

Cell body
Mitochondrion
Nucleus
Axon
Axon terminals
Dendrites
Chromatophilic substance

FIGURE 11.1

A typical neuron.

names to things in neurons that exist in other cell types. We are about to learn some new names (bet you can hardly wait). Let's start in the part of the cell that we think of as its central region, the place where we find the nucleus.

The Neuron Cell Body

This central region of a neuron is called the cell body, perikaryon, or soma. I do not mean to imply here that this part of the cell is in the geographic middle of the cell; rather, the other parts of the cell extend outward from here. The cell body varies in diameter (5–135 µm) and contains a single large nucleus. It also contains most of the typical organelles we would expect to find in a cell. Notably absent are the centrioles. Most neurons lack centrioles. This renders them unable to divide. Although it has been widely accepted that neurons are incapable of division, recent research seems to indicate that in some very limited fashion, some division may occur. Whether these dividing cells are mature neurons or members of a limited stem cell population remains to be determined. This is a fascinating field of research that could potentially provide important new therapies for people suffering stroke, traumatic injury, and other serious conditions (see the "Breaching Homeostasis" section of Chapter 12).

Rough endoplasmic reticulum is abundant and is referred to as chromatophilic substance, or Nissl bodies, in neurons. The intermediate filament type is neurofilament (NF). In some neurons, such as those of the hippocampus (Chapter 12), we may find cytoplasmic inclusions composed of lipofuscin. This varies with the type of neuron and with the age and condition of the person whose neurons we are considering. It seems to have little if any effect on the neurons' functioning. Mitochondria are present in large numbers due to the high level of metabolic activity carried out in neurons.

The Dendrites

Cytoplasmic extensions reach out from the cell body like arms. One type of extension is called dendrites. The term *dendrite* means "branches," as in a tree. This is because dendrites are often very numerous and highly branched. Some neurons may have several hundred highly branched dendrites. These cell extensions contain the full array of cellular organelles, such as mitochondria, chromatophilic substance, and ribosomes. Large amounts of intermediate filaments are present to give these very fine structures strength.

The most notable feature you must keep in mind about dendrites involves their electrical activity. Their electrical impulses, called graded potentials, are similar to the action potentials discussed in Chapter 8 (please review Chapter 8 if you are unsure of this material). One difference between graded potentials and action potentials is that graded potentials are local events; although they may involve a large area of membrane, they do not travel as a wave of depolarization and repolarization. Action potentials, you may recall, spread across the entire excitable membrane as a wave of depolarization followed by a wave of repolarization. Another difference is that action potentials adhere to the all-or-none principle, while graded potentials can have varying degrees of depolarization or hyperpolarization. Recall that the all-or-none principle tells us that when the membrane reaches threshold, an action potential will be generated. A subthreshold stimulus (less than threshold) will not generate an action potential, and a larger than threshold stimulus will generate the same-sized action potential as a threshold stimulus. The neuron is capable of generating only one size of action potential. Graded potentials come in different sizes (varying degrees of depolarization or hyperpolarization).

Graded potentials arise in the dendrites or in the cell body as a result of various stimuli and are instrumental in initiating action potentials in neurons. Action potentials are initiated when a graded potential depolarizes an excitable area of membrane to threshold. Since graded potentials can result in hyperpolarization, they may also render a cell unable to generate an action potential. As the graded potential passes through the cell body, it may initiate an action potential at the base of another cytoplasmic projection, the axon.

■ The Axon

Unlike dendrites, axons are single. Although the structure of axons may vary, and distally they may be branched, each neuron has only one axon. Axons can be quite long, however, sometimes reaching over a meter in length. They begin in a raised region of soma called the axon hillock (small hill). The plasma membrane of an axon is called axolemma; its cytoplasm is called axoplasm. Unlike dendrites and soma, no chromatophilic sub-

stance is found in axons. This important fact will be revisited in a few moments.

Distally, axons may branch into axon terminals, also called telodendria. These end in sacks called synaptic end bulbs. Synaptic end bulbs are parts of synapses or neuroeffector junctions, which were described in Chapter 8 and are diagrammed in **FIGURE 11.2**. Synapses between neurons may be axodendritic, axosomatic, or axoaxonic. Also note in **FIGURE 11.3** that structural variation exists among different types of neurons.

Axons carry action potentials away from the perikaryon (toward the synaptic end bulbs), and these action potentials require the axolemma to have many integral proteins in the form of voltage-gated ion channels (described in Chapter 8). These action potentials result in the release of neurotransmitters from synaptic vesicles into the synaptic cleft. Remember that there is no chromatophilic substance (rough endoplasmic reticulum) in axons, and axons may be as long as 1 meter; do you see the need for transport systems to move substances up and down the axon? It makes sense, doesn't it, that the axon must need membrane proteins and other products of chromatophilic substance? The problem of what to do with worn-out organelles, such as mitochondria, so far from the cell body, also presents a challenge. Fortunately, our neurons are up to these problems; transport mechanisms are present in axons.

Picture a slow-moving river (**FIGURE 11.4a**). Like water in a slow-moving river, axoplasm flows very slowly down axons (away from the cell body). If you were on the

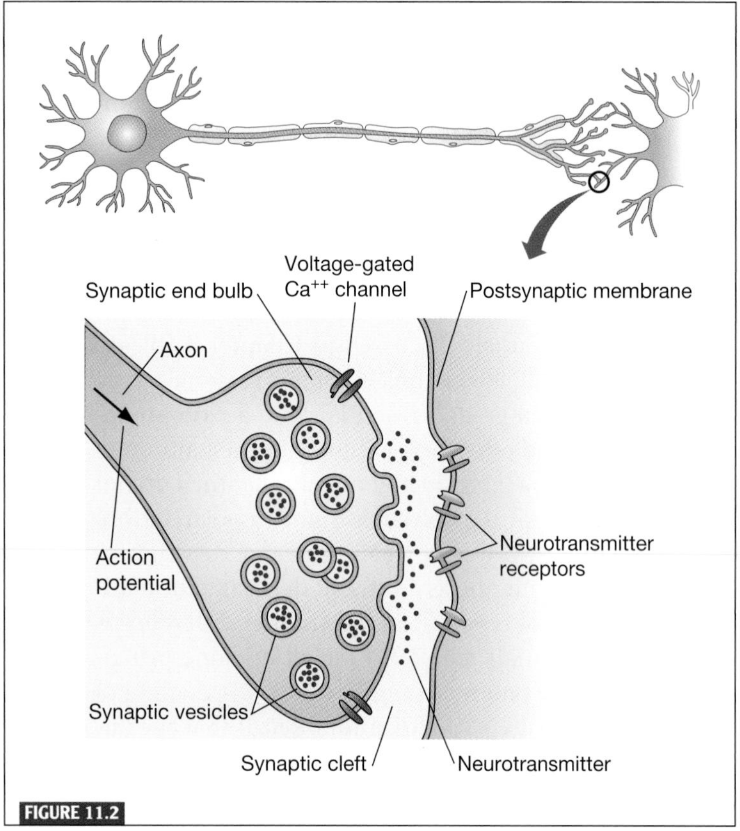

FIGURE 11.2

A chemical synapse.

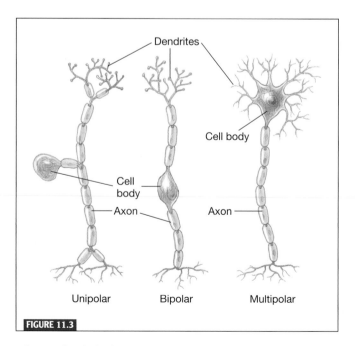

FIGURE 11.3

Structural variation in neurons.

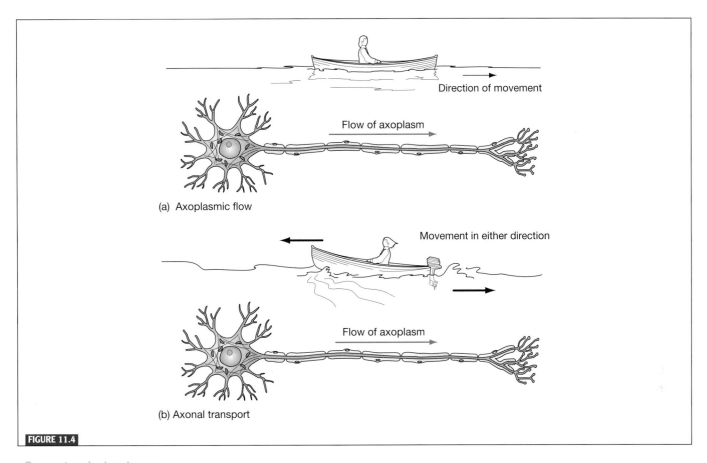

(a) Axoplasmic flow

(b) Axonal transport

FIGURE 11.4

Transport mechanisms in axons.

banks of a slow-moving river and wanted to go downstream, couldn't you simply jump into a canoe and drift along until you reached your destination? No energy would have to be exerted; you could simply drift in the slow-moving current. Well, the same situation exists in the neuron. The flow of axoplasm down the axon is called axoplasmic flow (catchy term, huh?). Substances that are needed in the axon can simply be released by the cell body into the axoplasm, and they will slowly (1–5 mm per day) travel to their destination. New axoplasm is supplied in this way.

What about if you needed to move down the river more quickly, or if you needed to get back up the river? Could you still simply drift along? Of course not. Now you need to exert some energy; perhaps you even need to use an outboard motor. Again, a parallel situation exists in the axon. Axonal transport is a mechanism of active movement in the axon (Figure 11.4b). It expends energy to move substances bidirectionally in the axoplasm at a rate of about 300 mm per day. This mechanism involves the cytoskeleton (mostly microtubules) almost like a monorail, and is used to deliver organelles, such as mitochondria, down the axon, and wastes, such as worn out mitochondria, back to the cell body.

■ Nerve Fibers

Axons or dendrites are collectively called nerve fibers. Axons and dendrites sometimes have additional layers surrounding them, sort of like insulation. This insulation, myelin, is also part of a nerve fiber. So, nerve fibers are axons or dendrites and the myelin that surrounds them, if it is present. Now that we have a working definition of a nerve fiber, we must discuss myelin, its functions, and the cells that provide it.

Myelination

The term *myelination* may indicate either the myelin sheath or the process of producing that sheath. In either event, the cells responsible for this activity are oligodendrocytes in the brain and spinal cord and neurolemmocytes (Schwann cells) elsewhere in the body. The brain and spinal cord are collectively called the central nervous system (CNS). Nervous tissue elsewhere in the body is part of the peripheral nervous system (PNS). We will learn about these two components of the nervous system in our next chapter. For now, you must learn that different cells are responsible for myelination in these two locations. Oligodendrocytes and neurolemmocytes are two types of stromal cells of the nervous system. We will learn more about this stroma in a few moments.

Let's first think about myelination in more detail. We will begin in the PNS with neurolemmocytes. Let's picture a balloon and a ballpoint pen for a moment. Imagine that you had the balloon, only partially inflated, in one hand. In the other hand you held a ballpoint pen. You could carefully take the end of the balloon and wind it around the pen, adding a layer of balloon membrane

to the outside of the pen with each rotation (**FIGURE 11.5a**). If you think of the balloon as a neurolemmocyte and the pen as a nerve fiber (axon or dendrite), you can begin to picture how myelin is added to a nerve fiber. The neurolemmocyte wraps layers of its membrane (plasmalemma) around the axon or dendrite until 20 to 30 layers have built up. These layers of phospholipid are the myelin sheath. Then, the neurolemmocyte takes one more step. It wraps its cell body, cytoplasm and all,

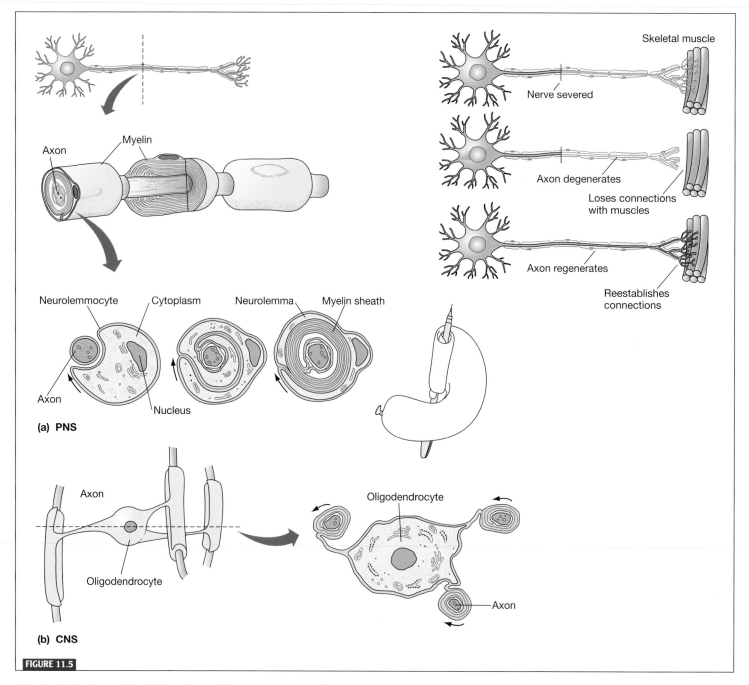

FIGURE 11.5

Myelination in the peripheral (a) and central (b) nervous systems. In the peripheral nervous system, the cells responsible for myelination also provide neurolemma. Neurolemma aids regeneration of axons following injury.

around the myelin sheath as a structure called a neurolemma (hence, the name neurolemmocyte). In this way, each neurolemmocyte myelinates and provides neurolemma to about 1 millimeter of the nerve fiber. Neurolemmocytes line up along the fiber, leaving only small gaps between them that remain unmyelinated. These gaps are called neurofibral nodes, or nodes of Ranvier. We will discuss the function of the myelin sheath in a moment; for now, however, let's think about the role of the neurolemma.

The neurolemma provides support to the axon or dendrite. This support becomes especially important when the fiber is injured. After injury, such as a cut through the nerve fiber, the fiber distal to the injury dies. The only way to renew the connection that was made by that fiber would be to regrow the axon to its original location. After injury, neurolemmocytes hypertrophy (become larger) and proliferate (become more numerous) to provide a tube indicating the former route of the axon. The axon can regrow (regenerate) down this tube and, in that way, be directed to its former connection (see Figure 11.5).

Perhaps at some time you have cut your finger and, as a result, noted a loss of sensation in that finger. Over a long period of time (weeks to months), feeling may have been restored to the affected finger. If so, you have experienced nerve fiber regeneration aided by neurolemmocytes.

We now need to consider myelination in the CNS. Here, myelin is provided by oligodendrocytes. The term *oligo-* indicates "few;" the term *–dendro* indicates "branches" (remember dendrite?). So, oligodendrocyte indicates "few branch cells." They are called this because they have fewer branches than another member of the nervous system stroma, to which they are compared. We'll get back to that.

Oligodendrocytes provide myelin to nerve fibers in the CNS in much the same way that neurolemmocytes provide myelin in the PNS (Figure 11.5b). There are a couple of notable differences, however. Oligodendrocytes do not wrap their cell bodies around the myelin sheath. In other words, these cells do not provide neurolemma. Because of this, regeneration of damaged nerve axons in the CNS is generally ineffective. Also, each oligodendrocyte wraps portions of its membrane around several nerve fibers, as many as 15 fibers per oligodendrocyte. These extensions of the cell, reaching out to the various fibers, are the "few branches" of the oligodendrocyte.

In either case, nonmyelinated fibers are supported by oligodendrocytes or neurolemmocytes. In the PNS, neurolemmocytes provide neurolemma to fibers, even in the absence of providing myelin. In fact, one neurolemmocyte can provide neurolemma to multiple nonmyelinated fibers. In the CNS, oligodendrocytes merely line up along nonmyelinated fibers.

Conduction in Nerve Fibers: Donkeys or Kangaroos?

So, what's the point of all this myelination anyway? Let's think for a moment about a race between a donkey and a kangaroo (**FIGURE 11.6**). I realize that this is a very unlikely match, but never-the-less, it could happen. If we were to choose a donkey and a kangaroo of about the same size, which would you guess would be faster? Think about how they move. The donkey runs along the ground, essentially covering all of the ground in its path. The kangaroo springs along, only touching the ground at distant intervals. This should make the kangaroo much faster.

A similar situation exists in nerve fibers. Think for a moment about the action potential traveling down a nonmyelinated fiber. As we have discussed, it travels like a wave along the fiber. All portions of the membrane of this fiber undergo the depolarization and repolarization. Now think about the structure of the myelinated fiber. Every millimeter or so, there is a gap in the myelin sheath or "insulation" surrounding the fiber. These gaps, the neurofibral nodes (nodes of Ranvier), are the only places that completely undergo this depolarization and repolarization. The action potential skips along the fiber just like a kangaroo travels across the land. This results in the movement of fewer ions (therefore, it is more efficient) at a faster rate. The action potential travels faster in a myelinated neuron. That is the purpose of myelination.

Conduction in the nonmyelinated fiber is called continuous conduction; conduction in the myelinated fiber is called saltatory conduction. Other factors influencing the rates of conduction in nerve fibers include diameter and temperature. The larger the diameter of the fiber, the faster the rate of conduction will be. Increased temperature raises the rate of conduction; hence, application of ice reduces pain after injury. Pain impulses travel along the sensory nerve fibers at a slower rate when the fiber is cooled so that the brain receives fewer impulses and perceives less pain.

■ Classification of Neurons

There exist several classification schemes for neurons. Most are based on the structure of the neuron, such as the position of the perikaryon relative to the axon. One such scheme was depicted in Figure 11.3, and you may want to refer back to that diagram now. Here we are going to use only the simplest of classification schemes.

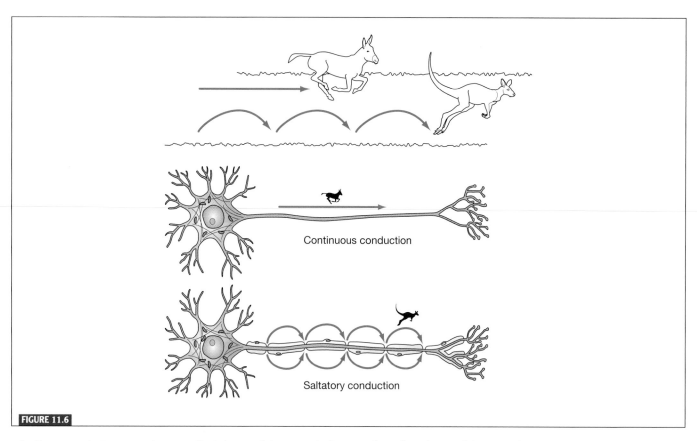

FIGURE 11.6

Continuous conduction occurs in nonmyelinated axons. Saltatory conduction occurs in myelinated axons. Saltatory conduction is faster and more efficient than continuous conduction.

It is useful for you to know that neurons do have a variety of morphologies and that they can be classified based on that characteristic.

Neurons that are carrying impulses toward the CNS are called sensory neurons. The fibers of sensory neurons are referred to as afferent fibers. Sensory neurons travel from some sensory receptor (receptors for our senses) to the CNS for interpretation.

Those neurons carrying impulses away from the CNS (toward an effector) are called motor neurons. Efferent fibers are the fibers of motor neurons. Remember, "e" for "efferent" and "effector." If that doesn't work for you, think "e" for "efferent" and for "export." These fibers export impulses from the CNS.

Interneurons or association neurons are present in the CNS and interconnect with other neurons in the CNS. They are neither carrying impulses toward nor away from the CNS, as they are already there. Association neurons are generally present between sensory neurons and motor neurons. They are important in interpreting the information carried by the sensory (afferent) neurons and signaling the appropriate response to motor (efferent) neurons. Association neurons are by far the most numerous.

11.2 Synapses Revisited: Interconnections Between Neurons

Synapses have been described in several places in this book (Chapters 8 and 9, as well as elsewhere in this chapter). It may seem like overkill to present them again, but you have more information available to you than you did before, so we will look at them once again to make sure you have a full understanding of their structure and function.

You know that an action potential travels away from the soma via the axon. You also know that this impulse must ultimately travel to either another neuron or an effector of some type (muscle or gland). For clarity, here we will limit our discussion to the interactions between two neurons. The interaction between a neuron and an effector cell is similar to the interaction between two neurons.

There are actually two types of synapses found between neurons (**FIGURE 11.7**). Electrical synapses are very rare in mature individuals; they are more prominent

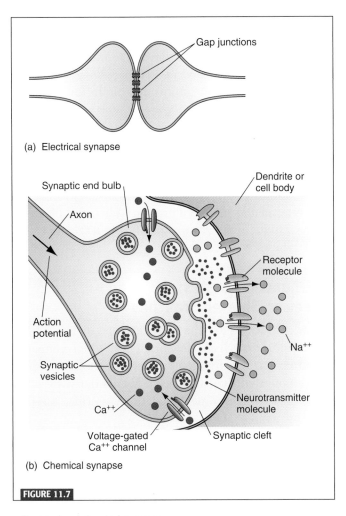

(a) Electrical synapse

(b) Chemical synapse

FIGURE 11.7

Electrical and chemical synapses.

during development of the nervous system. In electrical synapses, there is no synaptic cleft. Instead, the presynaptic and postsynaptic membranes are in direct contact with each other, and small pores called gap junctions interconnect the two neurons. Ions are able to pass through these pores, allowing the effect of an action potential to pass directly from one neuron to the next. As indicated, these are very rare in adult humans.

Chemical synapses are those with which you are now somewhat familiar. Here, when the action potential reaches the synaptic end bulb of the presynaptic neuron, it must be changed into a chemical message to traverse the synaptic cleft and reach the postsynaptic neuron. These two neurons are not in direct contact with each other, and, therefore, the action potential can not simply pass from one neuron to the next. Instead, the action potential opens voltage-gated calcium channels in the presynaptic membrane. This allows calcium to rush into the axoplasm (by diffusion); this, in turn, causes synaptic vesicles to fuse with the presynaptic

membrane. This releases neurotransmitters into the synaptic cleft. These neurotransmitters are the chemical messengers that diffuse across the synaptic cleft and induce changes in the postsynaptic membrane.

In our previous discussion about this topic (Chapter 8), we discussed the chemically gated channels in the neurotransmitter receptors and learned that this can trigger an action potential if threshold is reached. Now you know a little more about what actually happens. The neurotransmitter binds to its receptor. Different neurotransmitters exist, and these work through two major mechanisms. They generally either open a chemically gated ion channel or work through an indirect (second-messenger) system that we have not yet discussed. But what they actually induce in the postsynaptic membrane is a graded potential. You know that action potentials are always of the same amplitude (size) in a given neuron. You also know that the binding of neurotransmitter to its receptor may or may not get the postsynaptic membrane to threshold; therefore, the actual effect caused by the neurotransmitter is a graded potential, not an action potential.

So, what about this potential in the postsynaptic membrane? How can its response to neurotransmitters vary? One way that it varies is determined by the class of neurotransmitter released into the synaptic cleft. Some neurotransmitters are excitatory. These are the ones that cause a threshold stimulus (under appropriate conditions) and, therefore, induce an action potential. Other neurotransmitters are inhibitory. Inhibitory neurotransmitters cause a graded potential that hyperpolarizes the postsynaptic membrane rather than depolarizing it. This renders the postsynaptic neuron unable to generate an action potential. The importance of this will become apparent in Chapter 12; however, you can imagine instances in which you would not want a particular muscle to contract. To keep these muscles from contracting, the motor neuron to these muscles must be inhibited from generating an action potential. Inhibitory neurotransmitters are released into synapses on these neurons rendering them inactive. Although these two classes of neurotransmitter (excitatory and inhibitory) seem very different from each other, it is important to realize that the receptors are responsible for the differences, not the neurotransmitter itself. In Chapter 12, we will examine quite a few different neurotransmitters. By then we will know enough about the nervous system to make more sense of where different neurotransmitters are located. For now, however, be aware that there are neurotransmitters that may be excitatory in one location and inhibitory in another location. The difference in neurotransmitter effect is caused by differences between the neurotransmitter receptors present in the two locations. When activated, one causes depolarization while the other causes hyperpolarization.

All this time, we have been primarily discussing the parenchyma of the nervous system. We must now shift to the stroma.

11.3 Glia: The Stroma of the Nervous System

Like organs throughout the body, the tissues that make up the nervous system are composed of both parenchyma and stroma. Up to this point, we have mainly discussed the nervous system parenchyma, neurons. Now we will spend some time on the stroma of the nervous system. This stroma is collectively called glia. *Glia* means "glue," a fitting term when you think about how the glia holds the nervous system together. That does not nearly begin to cover the many functions that the glia provides the nervous system, however.

Please look over **TABLE 11.1**. The types of glia are presented in this table. You may recall from our discussion in Chapter 4 that glia is one of the five classes of tissue found in your body. Here we are using the term *glia* more inclusively. **FIGURE 11.8** presents diagrams and photomicrographs of the various glia. You will want to refer to that illustration as you read this section.

■ Astrocytes: Genuine Glia

Note in Table 11.1 that the first cell type presented is the astrocyte. These are by far the most numerous of our glial cells. The term *astrocyte* means "star cell." This is a fitting term because these cells have a stellate or star-shaped appearance. There are actually many types of astrocytes. Astrocytes perform a great many functions in our CNS, the only place they are found. They form a supporting network, giving structure to our nervous systems. They play an important role in formation of the blood-brain barrier, a topic to which we will devote quite a bit of time in our next chapter. They aid in the removal of wastes, errant neurotransmitters, and debris from our CNS. Each of these functions becomes much more critical after injury. Please note that only astrocytes contain GFAP (glial fibrillary acidic protein) as their intermediate filament protein. When we talk about glia as a tissue type, we are specifically referring to the many types of astrocytes.

■ Oligodendrocytes: Fewer, Shorter Branches

Oligodendrocytes are the next cell type in Table 11.1. Oligodendrocytes have "few branches" when compared to astrocytes. You are already aware of their functions. Please note that they are mesenchymal derivatives because they express vimentin as their intermediate filament protein.

■ Microglia: Macrophages of the CNS

Microglia are a fascinating cell type. Originally thought to be specific for the CNS, we now know that they are, in fact, cells in the monocyte-macrophage lineage and have the ability to move into and out of the CNS throughout our lives. Their function, like resident macrophage populations in our other organs, is to phagocytize debris. They are especially important after injury.

Table 11.1 Glia: Stroma of the Nervous System

Cell Type	IF	Nucleus	Description	Function
Astrocyte	GFAP	Large, spherical light staining	Stellate	Form supporting network, role in BBB formation
Oligodendrocyte	Vimentin	Small, round darkly staining	Stellate, fewer shorter branches	Myelination in CNS, support for nonmyelinated fibers
Microglia	Vimentin	Small, elongated darkly staining	Monocyte/macrophage lineage	Phagocytosis
Ependyma	Keratin	Low cuboidal-ciliated columnar epithelium	Low cuboidal-ciliated columnar epithelium	Line ventricles and central canal of spinal cord, form and circulate CSF
Neurolemmocytes	Vimentin	PNS only		Myelination in PNS, support for nonmyelinated fibers

IF = intermediate filaments, GFAP = glial fibrillary acidic protein, BBB = blood-brain barrier, CNS = central nervous system, CSF = cerebrospinal fluid, PNS = peripheral nervous system.

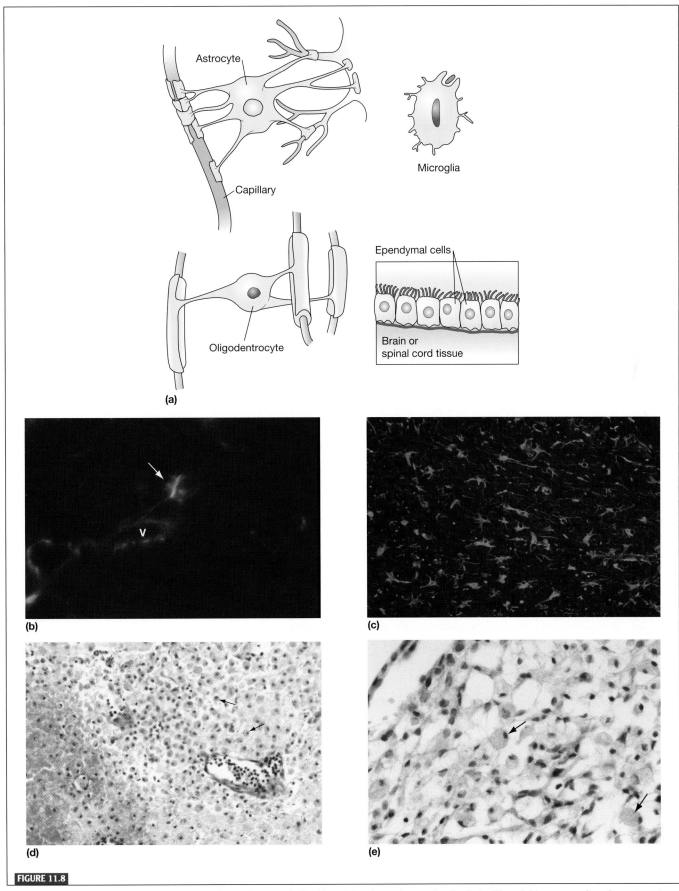

FIGURE 11.8

Glia, stroma of the central nervous system, shown diagramatically (a) and by photomicrographs (b–e). In (b) and (c), we are observing astrocytes. Immunofluorescence is used to identify the astrocytes in normal brain tissue (b). This astrocyte (*arrow*) sends a branch to a blood vessel (v) and brain tissue 24 hours after a stroke (c). Notice how the astrocytes become larger and more numerous in response to this injury. Panels (d) and (e) show brain tissue 5 days (d) and 15 days (e) after a stroke. Notice the microglia (*arrows*) phagocytizing debris.

■ Ependyma: True Epithelia

Next there are ependyma. These are the only true epithelial cells found as glia. Ependymal cells line ventricles (cavities) within the brain, as well as the central canal of the spinal cord. Their function is to produce and circulate cerebrospinal fluid (CSF). CSF is a topic we will examine in our next chapter.

■ Neurolemmocytes: Not Really Glia at All

Strictly speaking, neurolemmocytes are not glia. Glia is only found in the CNS and, as you know, neurolemmocytes are PNS cells. They are included in Table 11.1 to give you the opportunity to review them and to make sure you are aware of their role in the nervous system.

Please look at the photomicrographs shown in Figure 11.8. This figure is one of the few found in this text of injured tissue. This is because the workload of our glia increases greatly after injury. Injury causes glia to become more active and more numerous. We can, therefore, get a better idea of what glia look like after injury than at other times. This injury will be explained more fully in the "Breaching Homeostasis" section at the end of Chapter 12.

This completes our discussion of nervous tissue. You will need this information to understand the material presented in the next chapter. Be certain to use the "What You Should Know" and "What Did You Learn?" features before proceeding. I hope you have enjoyed learning about these fascinating cells. In Chapter 12, you will have the opportunity to apply what you have learned.

What You Should Know

1. Neurons make up the parenchyma of the nervous system.
2. Neurons have a cell body, also called a perikaryon or soma, from which cellular extensions arise.
3. Rough endoplasmic reticulum in a neuron is called chromatophilic substance or Nissl bodies.
4. Neurons generally lack centrioles and are usually incapable of division.
5. Neuronal dendrites are usually numerous and branching.
6. Dendrites carry graded potentials.
7. Axons begin in an axon hillock, are single, and may reach more than 1 meter in length.
8. Axons branch distally into axon terminals or telodendria.
9. Axons carry action potentials away from the cell body.
10. Substances may be moved in the axon by: (a) axoplasmic flow, which is unidirectional and slow but does not require energy; or (b) axonal transport, which is bidirectional and fast but requires energy.
11. Nerve fibers are axons or dendrites and their myelin sheath, if they are myelinated.
12. Myelination is provided in the CNS by oligodendrocytes and in the PNS by neurolemmocytes.
13. Neurolemmocytes also provide neurolemma, useful during nerve fiber regeneration.
14. Oligodendrocytes do not provide neurolemma.
15. Myelination enables saltatory conduction to occur. Saltatory conduction is much faster than the continuous conduction of nonmyelinated fibers.
16. In saltatory conduction, only the neurofibral nodes (of Ranvier) completely depolarize.
17. Afferent neurons are sensory: they carry action potentials toward the CNS.
18. Efferent neurons are motor: they carry action potentials away from the CNS.
19. Interneurons are association neurons: they interconnect other neurons.
20. Electrical synapses are rare; they lack a synaptic cleft and allow ions to move between two neurons.
21. Chemical synapses rely on neurotransmitters to conduct a signal between two neurons.
22. Glia, the stroma of the nervous system, is made up of a variety of cell types.
23. Astrocytes form a supporting network and play a role in the formation of the blood-brain barrier.
24. Microglia are the resident macrophages of the CNS.
25. Ependyma line ventricles and other spaces within the CNS.

What Did You Learn?

Multiple choice questions: choose the best answer.

1. Neurons are the _____ of the nervous system.
   a. Parenchyma
   b. Stroma
   c. Both of the above
   d. Neither of the above

2. Nissl bodies is another name for _____ in neurons.
   a. Rough endoplasmic reticulum
   b. Chromatophilic substance
   c. Both of the above
   d. Neither of the above

3. Soma is another name for _____ in neurons.
   a. Cell body
   b. Perikaryon
   c. Both of the above
   d. Neither of the above

4. _____ are usually numerous and branching.
   a. Axons
   b. Dendrites
   c. Both of the above
   d. Neither of the above

5. Electrical activity in dendrites is in the form of _____.
   a. Action potentials
   b. Graded potentials
   c. Both of the above
   d. Neither of the above

6. An individual neuron can have _____ of different sizes.
   a. Action potentials
   b. Graded potentials
   c. Both of the above
   d. Neither of the above

7. Axons transmit action potentials:
   a. Toward the cell body
   b. Away from the cell body
   c. In either direction
   d. Action potentials don't occur in neurons, only in muscle

8. To transport a wornout mitochondrion from the distal end of an axon to the cell body for autophagy, your neuron would use:
   a. Axonal transport
   b. Axoplasmic flow
   c. Either of the above
   d. UPS

9. An axon or dendrite plus its myelin sheath, if it is myelinated, is called _____.
   a. A telodendrion
   b. An axon terminal
   c. A nerve
   d. A nerve fiber

10. Which of the following is faster?
    a. Continuous conduction
    b. Saltatory conduction
    c. They are equally fast
    d. Their speeds are both quite variable

11. Saltatory conduction occurs in:
    a. Myelinated fibers
    b. Nonmyelinated fibers
    c. Both of the above
    d. Neither of the above

12. The structure of _____ aids in axonal regeneration.
    a. Neurolemmocytes
    b. Oligodendrocytes
    c. Both of the above
    d. Neither of the above

13. Which of the following is found in the PNS?
    a. Neurolemmocytes
    b. Oligodendrocytes
    c. Both of the above
    d. Neither of the above

14. _____ carry action potentials toward the CNS.
    a. Efferent neurons
    b. Afferent neurons
    c. Interneurons
    d. AT&T long distance

15. Which of the following are the most numerous?
    a. Efferent neurons
    b. Afferent neurons
    c. Interneurons
    d. They are present in approximately equal numbers

16. Gap junctions are part of:
    a. Electrical synapses
    b. Chemical synapses
    c. Both of the above
    d. Neither of the above

What Did You Learn? (continued)

17. Neurotransmitters are used in:

    a. Electrical synapses

    b. Chemical synapses

    c. Both of the above

    d. Neither of the above

18. Hyperpolarization of a postsynaptic membrane is caused by:

    a. Inhibitory neurotransmitters

    b. Excitatory neurotransmitters

    c. Either of the above

    d. Neither of the above

19. Which of the following is not included in the glia of the CNS?

    a. Astrocytes

    b. Oligodendrocytes

    c. Microglia

    d. Neurolemmocytes

    e. All of the above are glia of the CNS

20. Which of the following is not true of astrocytes?

    a. They express GFAP as their intermediate filament protein

    b. They have small elongated, darkly staining nuclei

    c. They form a supporting network in the CNS

    d. They play a role in the formation of the blood-brain barrier

    e. All of the above are true

21. Which of the following is in the monocyte-macrophage lineage?

    a. Astrocytes

    b. Oligodendrocytes

    c. Microglia

    d. Neurolemmocytes

    e. Ependymal cells

22. Which of the following is epithelial?

    a. Astrocytes

    b. Oligodendrocytes

    c. Microglia

    d. Neurolemmocytes

    e. Ependymal cells

Short answer questions: answer briefly and in your own words.

1. Please draw and label a typical neuron, showing the special features and organelles of this cell. If a particular feature has more than one name, please use as many names as you know.

2. Describe myelination in the CNS and PNS, indicating the responsible cells. Please include any differences between the activities of these cells, and how these differences alter the abilities of the fibers they myelinate.

3. Please indicate how continuous conduction and saltatory conduction differ. Where would we find these two types of conduction? You may use a diagram as part of your answer, if you would like.

4. How do chemical and electrical synapses differ? Which is the more common of these two types of synapses?

5. Make a list of the stromal cells of the CNS. Describe how we could distinguish among them in histologic sections. Also, list their functions.

6. Imagine that an individual has suffered a brain injury. What cells are involved in limiting and repairing the damaged brain tissue? What are the roles of these individual cell types?

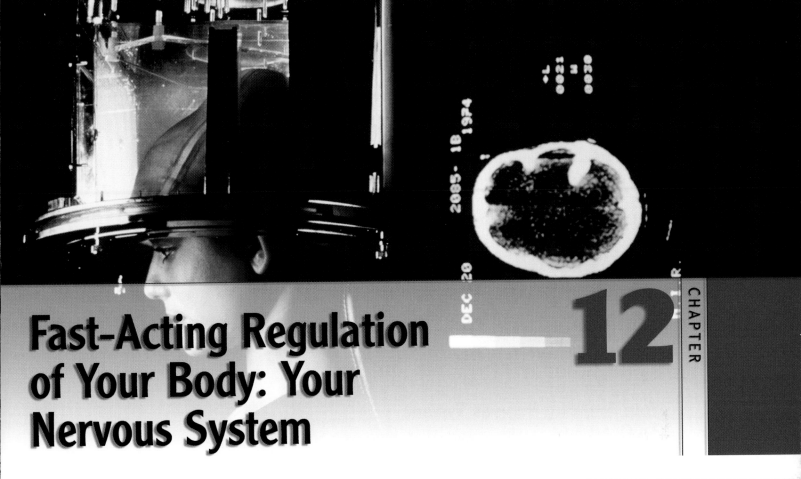

Fast-Acting Regulation of Your Body: Your Nervous System

A Brief Organizational Note

This is a very long chapter, but don't panic! Sometimes students find the nervous system a little daunting. Just looking at the extreme length of this chapter can be a little intimidating. Don't be intimidated; our study of the nervous system is broken down into smaller, more "digestible" units. These units are not based on any biologically sound subdivisions; they are devised only for your convenience. In this way, you can stop and take a breather now and again as you go through this system. You can also review your knowledge with the "What You Should Know" and "What Did You Learn?" features placed at the end of each section, rather than wait until the distant time when you will emerge victorious from this entire chapter.

I have not broken this chapter into separate chapters because I did not want you to be misled into thinking that the nervous system is divided into biologically separate entities. It is easy to start to think of the central nevous system (CNS) and the peripheral nervous system (PNS) as distinct organ systems. This is not the case: the nervous system is one organ system.

Begin your study of the nervous system knowing that you can achieve your goal of understanding it. Take your time and read carefully, pausing frequently to consider what you have read; you will find this an enjoyable system to study.

12A
Your Amazing Nervous System

What You Will Learn

- How the nervous system can be subdivided based on anatomic and functional considerations.
- The basic functions of the nervous system.
- How your nervous system is protected and supported.
- The structure and function of the meninges.
- The role of cerebrospinal fluid in the maintenance of homeostasis in your CNS.
- How the extracellular environment of your CNS differs from the extracellular environment in your other organs.
- The role of your blood-brain barrier.
- How capillaries in your CNS differ from those in your other organs.

12.A1 Your Amazing Nervous System: An Overview

Whether viewed from a structural or functional standpoint, your nervous system is truly amazing. Your more than 20 billion neurons perform functions ranging from regulating your cardiac and respiratory rates, to interpreting the sights and sounds around you, to allowing you to recall the name of the carpal bone in the distal row, nearest the thumb. This range of functions gives you some idea of the complexity of this system.

Keep in mind that, as we consider the physiology of this system, we are examining its role in the maintenance of homeostasis. It is the fast-acting regulator of homeostasis. It works together with the endocrine system to monitor the internal and external environments to assure that conditions within our body remain compatible with life.

12.A2 Subdivisions of Your Nervous System: Structural and Functional

Many schemes have been proposed for dividing the nervous system into its component parts. If you examine a few textbooks, you will find that each author has an opinion on the best way to divide this system for ease in understanding it. I will present a simple, basic scheme here that will enable you to understand this system. If you choose to continue your reading in more advanced textbooks, and I hope you will, you will easily adapt your knowledge to the schemes used by those authors.

Our first level of dividing the nervous system is purely anatomical (**FIGURE 12.1**): CNS versus PNS. The CNS includes the brain and the spinal cord. The PNS includes all other nervous tissue. If a structure is composed of neurons and is located anywhere in the body except the brain or spinal cord, it is part of the PNS.

To understand our next level of subdivision, we must consider some physiology. The activities of our nervous system can be divided into three functions (**FIGURE 12.2**). First, we have the sensory functions. These are the activities that sense our internal and external environment and convey this sensory information. We have a vast array of sensors that allows us to gather lots of data about conditions around and within ourselves. We will discuss these sensory receptors later in this chapter. All of the data collected by these receptors must be conveyed to locations where it can be interpreted.

Second, we have integrative functions. Integrative functions are those functions that interpret the information collected and conveyed through the sensory functions. This interpretation includes making "go, no-go" decisions based on this information. All of our higher intellectual functions also fall within this integration category.

Our third group is motor functions. Would it do us any good to be able to sense our environment and make the interpretative decision that an adjustment must be made if we could not, in fact, make that adjustment? Our nervous system's motor functions involve conveying information from the centers involved in integration to effectors capable of making the required changes.

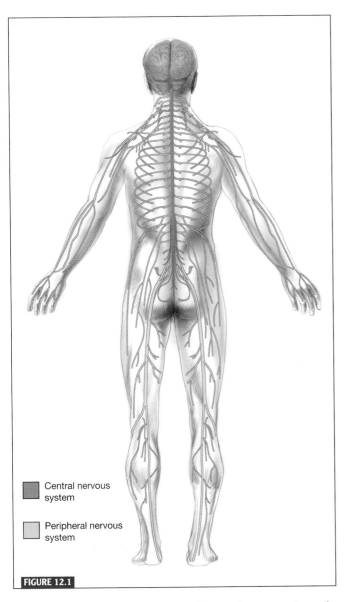

FIGURE 12.1

Central nervous system

Peripheral nervous system

The nervous system can be divided into the central nervous system and peripheral nervous system.

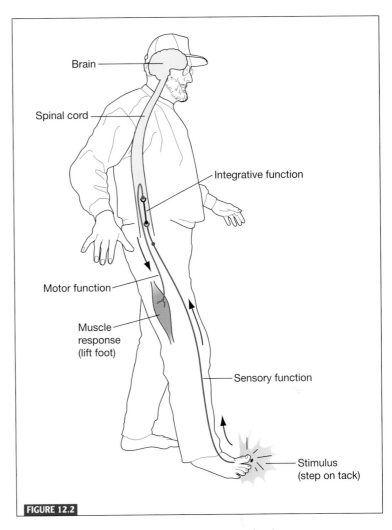

Brain

Spinal cord

Integrative function

Motor function

Muscle response (lift foot)

Sensory function

Stimulus (step on tack)

FIGURE 12.2

The nervous system has sensory, integrative, and motor functions.

These effectors include the three types of muscle and glands.

With that in mind, how can we further divide our nervous system? We can start to think about where these functions are performed. The integrative functions are the easiest. Integration is carried out only in the CNS.

How about the sensory function? Since it involves gathering information and conveying it to where it can be interpreted, and we must collect that information in a great many internal and external locations, sensory functions must be carried out by the PNS.

Motor functions involve conveying information from our integrative centers (CNS) to effectors located throughout our bodies. Again, sounds like the PNS, huh?

So let's put it all together. Integration occurs in the CNS, which is composed of the brain and spinal cord. The PNS has two functional subdivisions: a sensory subdivision, which uses sensory receptors to collect data from the internal and external environment, and conveys that information to the CNS, and a motor subdivision, which carries the responses signaled by the CNS to effectors throughout the body.

Now, as if that is not complex enough, there are two subdivisions within the motor subdivision of the PNS. The motor subdivision of the PNS is divided into the somatic nervous system and the autonomic nervous system (**FIGURE 12.3**). The term *somatic* refers to "body." The somatic nervous system includes the motor components, which have skeletal muscle as their effector. Therefore, although some reflex activities exist, these effectors are generally under voluntary control.

The term *autonomic* basically means "automatic or self-regulating." The functions regulated by the autonomic nervous system were originally thought to occur

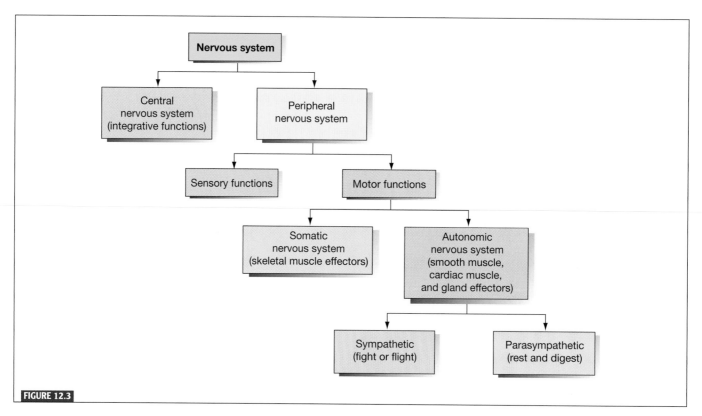

FIGURE 12.3

Major subdivisions of the nervous system.

automatically without nervous system involvement, or with the involvement of a component of the nervous system entirely independent of the rest of the nervous system. We now understand that they are under the control of the autonomic nervous system and that there is interaction between the autonomic and somatic components. The autonomic nervous system, again a subdivision of the motor component of the PNS, includes motor control of all activities in which the effectors are smooth muscle, cardiac muscle, or glands.

As they say on the television advertisements "Wait, there's more!" We have one more level of division to consider. The autonomic nervous system is further divided into the sympathetic and parasympathetic nervous systems. The autonomic nervous system supplies its effectors with dual innervation. Think of it like the accelerator (gas pedal) and brake pedal in your car. Step on the gas pedal and it increases the activity of your car. Step on the brake pedal and it inhibits the activity of your car. In effectors with dual innervation, one component of the autonomic nervous system is like that accelerator; it increases their activity. The other component of that system will have the opposite effect; it will inhibit that effector's activity. In this way, you are able to increase or decrease the activity of each of these involuntary effectors (smooth muscle, cardiac muscle, or

glands) by balancing the activities of these two antagonistic components of the autonomic nervous system.

At this stage in the game, you are probably wondering, "Is the sympathetic nervous system the accelerator and the parasympathetic nervous system the brake pedal or vice versa?" That varies, depending on what effector we are considering. For some, the sympathetic nervous system increases activity; for others it decreases activity. We will cover this in greater detail later in this chapter.

The organizational arrangement of the nervous system is presented in Figures 12.1 through 12.3. Please look them over to be certain that you are comfortable with this material.

12.A3 Support and Protection for Your Central Nervous System

The continuous, effective functioning of your brain and spinal cord are absolutely essential to your ongoing survival. Sure, in today's world, many people do quite well after severe injury to the brain or spinal cord, even if that injury is irreparable. However, that has not always been the case. Historically, before the advent of our understanding of these organs and the development of the tremendous medical technology currently available, even minor injuries to these structures often meant certain death.

So, doesn't it make sense that our bodies would have strong safety features in place to protect these vital organs? We certainly do have such life-saving features. Think about how the brain and spinal cord are both encased within a strong, protective bony fortress (**FIGURE 12.4**). The skull is a veritable built-in helmet. Without it, any of the minor bumps our heads have all experienced could easily have destroyed this delicate organ. The bones that surround the brain include the frontal, parietal, occipital, temporal, sphenoid, and ethmoid bones. Collectively, these bones are called the cranium. The top of our skulls consists of the frontal, parietal, and occipital bones and is called the calvarium. The calvarium really does have the appearance of the proverbial helmet mentioned earlier.

The spinal cord is similarly protected within the vertebral column. As we have already learned, the structure of that column allows us great flexibility, even as it gives our spinal cord that protection.

■ Your Meninges

Deep to these bones, membranes surround and protect the brain and spinal cord (**FIGURE 12.5**). These membranes, called meninges, are composed of three layers. The most superficial of the three is the dura mater. *Dura* means "tough" and *mater* means "mother": the dura mater is a tough protective layer consisting of two layers of fibrous connective tissue. The more superficial of the two is called the periosteal layer, because it is actually continuous with the fibrous layer of the periosteum of your cranium. The deep layer of the dura mater is called the meningeal layer. The dura mater gives the meninges an attachment to the bones of the cranium, anchoring these membranes firmly in place.

The intermediate layer of the meninges is called the arachnoid mater. *Arachnoid* means "spiderlike." The arachnoid mater is composed of delicate fibrous connective tissue that has extensions to the deep layer of the meninges. These extensions result in a small space between these two layers called the subarachnoid space.

The deep layer of the meninges is the pia mater. *Pia* means "delicate." The pia mater is very thin and adheres tightly to the surface of the brain and spinal cord. It has the appearance of a thin layer of clear plastic wrap covering these organs. In fact, wherever blood vessels, which travel in the subarachnoid space, penetrate the brain or spinal cord, pia mater extends into the nervous tissue separating the vasculature from the tissue of these organs.

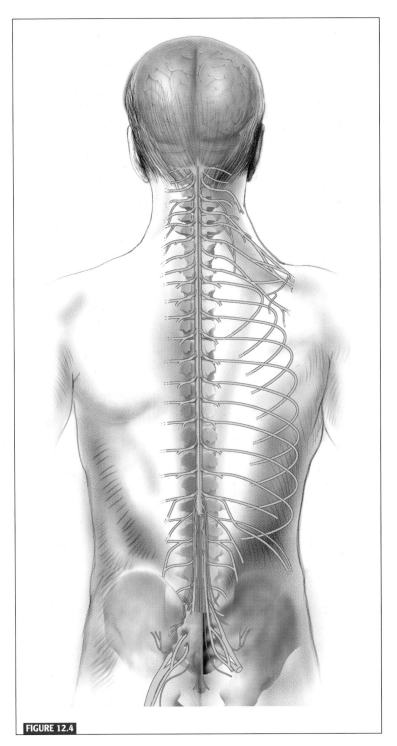

FIGURE 12.4

The central nervous system is protected by the skull and the vertebral column.

■ Your Cerebrospinal Fluid

We learned earlier that one important tool in the maintenance of homeostasis is the use of moving fluids. One such moving fluid was interstitial fluid, which bathes the tissues of our organs. That is, it bathes the tissues of most of our organs. The CNS requires a slightly different fluid. This fluid also serves the brain

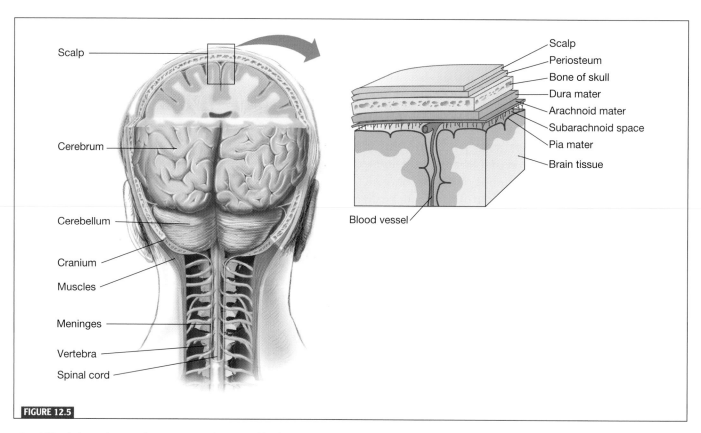

FIGURE 12.5

In addition to bone, the central nervous system is protected by the meninges.

in ways that interstitial fluid does not serve the organs of the body.

Are you hungry? Let's prepare some hard-boiled eggs. When you cook a few hard-boiled eggs, could you toss the eggs into the pan and then add the water? If you do it that way, you had better place the eggs in very gingerly. If you put the water in the pan first, you do not have to be nearly as careful when you place the eggs into the pan. The water will cushion the eggs so they do not break.

Think about your brain, a relatively soft organ, sitting within your cranium, a very hard structure. Now, picture your brain as you dance to a fast tune. As your head whips around, your brain is at risk of damage on the walls of the cranium. What protects it from being dashed to bits by these bones? The cerebrospinal fluid (CSF) cushions the brain like the eggs floating in the pan of water. The brain is actually floating in this fluid.

Have you ever gone swimming with another person and noticed that you can easily lift him while he is in the water, even if you cannot lift him on land? That is because the water is buoying him up, partially floating that person. The brain is partially floating in CSF (**FIGURE 12.6**). If we were to remove your brain and weigh it, it would weigh about 1,360 grams. If we were then to place your

brain and the balance in CSF, so that the brain was partially afloat, its apparent weight would be about 50 grams. For comparative purposes, if we did a similar experiment with a whole person and reduced the person's weight to the same extent, a 165-pound person would have an apparent weight of about 6 pounds. You can see that the brain is well cushioned by the CSF.

But what about CSF's other roles in the CNS? If it serves as interstitial fluid for the brain, why must it be different from interstitial fluid? Recall that interstitial fluid carries nutrients and gasses to cells and carries away wastes. Think about the electrical activity of neurons. In particular, think about activities at synapses. The electrical activity of the CNS requires a different extracellular environment than that of other organs. Some substances found in normal interstitial fluid would be toxic if they were present in the CNS in a similar concentration. For example, the amino acids glutamic acid, aspartic acid, and glycine are neurotransmitters within the CNS, but are present in interstitial fluid. If they were in the "interstitial fluid" of the CNS, the synapses in which they act as neurotransmitters would continuously be stimulated. This would result in uncontrolled neuronal activity and ultimately death of those neurons due to excitotoxicity (overstimulation).

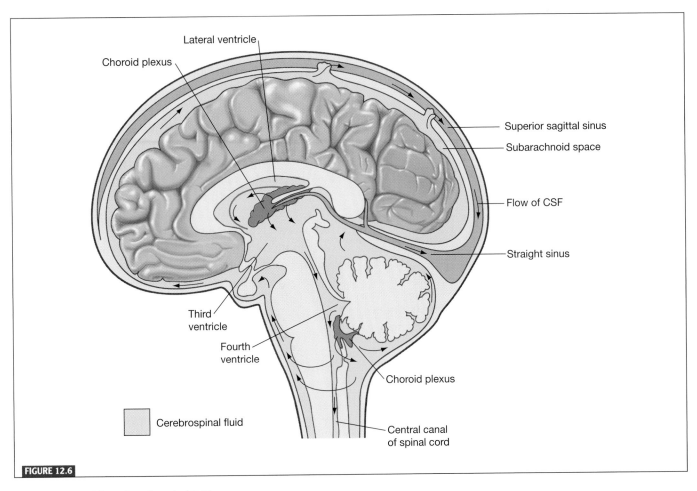

FIGURE 12.6

The location and flow of cerebrospinal fluid.

We have discussed what CSF is and what it does, but we have not yet discussed where it comes from and where it goes. CSF is present in cavities in the brain called ventricles. We have two lateral ventricles that are separated from each other by the septum pellucidum (meaning transparent wall), a third ventricle, and a fourth ventricle. From the fourth ventricle, CSF travels into the subarachnoid space and the central canal of the spinal cord. Ultimately, this fluid is passed into the blood in the superior sagittal sinus, a large venous structure. Please familiarize yourself with the anatomy of this pathway as diagrammed in **FIGURE 12.7**.

Cerebrospinal fluid is made in a number of locations in this pathway. Ependymal cells (see the glia section in Chapter 11) wrapped around capillaries in small feathery structures called the choroid plexus are located within the ventricles. The choroid plexus produces some of the CSF. Cerebral spinal fluid is also produced by ependymal cells throughout this pathway. These cells select which substances do and do not make it into the CSF. The total capacity of these spaces is about 130 ml. Approximately

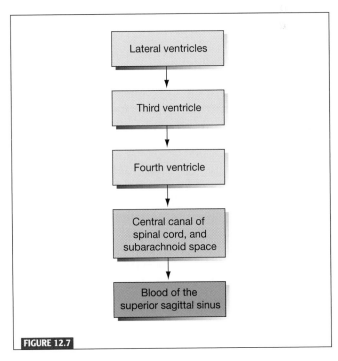

FIGURE 12.7

The pathway of cerebrospinal fluid.

500 ml of CSF is produced per day. This fluid is continuously being produced, circulating through these spaces, and returning to the blood.

The Blood Supply of Your Brain

We have already learned that neurons are highly metabolically active and that active cells need a constant blood supply. In fact, although the brain comprises only about 2 percent of our entire mass, it requires about 20 percent of our blood supply. Even with that requirement, the blood must be kept separate from the brain tissue. The mechanism used to do this is called the blood-brain barrier. This barrier is really quite fascinating. We will discuss its composition and implications now.

Your Blood-Brain Barrier

To understand the blood-brain barrier, we have to understand the typical blood vessels through which exchange occurs in tissues throughout the body. Capillaries are our smallest blood vessels. They are the vessels that act as the

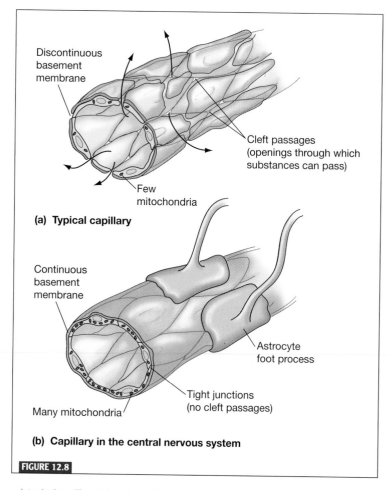

(a) Typical capillary

Discontinuous basement membrane

Cleft passages (openings through which substances can pass)

Few mitochondria

(b) Capillary in the central nervous system

Continuous basement membrane

Astrocyte foot process

Tight junctions (no cleft passages)

Many mitochondria

FIGURE 12.8

A typical capillary (a) and a capillary in the central nervous system (b). The special features of capillaries in the central nervous system result in the blood-brain barrier.

"business districts" of our circulatory system. Their walls are generally only one cell thick. That cell, the endothelial cell, is very thin as well. **FIGURE 12.8a** shows a diagram of a typical capillary, such as we would find in most tissues throughout the body. Variations do exist, but the capillary represented here is pretty typical. Note that openings are present between the endothelial cells that allow substances to pass through the vessel wall quite easily. Also note the discontinuous basement membrane and the fact that relatively few mitochondria are present.

Now, let's examine a capillary typical of those in the CNS (Figure 12.8b). Instead of openings, we find tight junctions. Tight junctions are special features of the plasma membrane that seal cells together, like the zipper in resealable plastic bags (refer to Chapter 4). The basement membrane of these endothelial cells is continuous, and they have many mitochondria. The increased mitochondria indicate that this cell is much more active metabolically and, therefore, may have increased duties, such as active transport. Note also the astrocyte foot processes surrounding the endothelial cells. These are shown in Figure 12.8b.

It was at one time thought that the blood-brain barrier was a direct result of these astrocyte foot processes. This was a reasonable conclusion based on the phenomenon that occurs when the CNS is injured. The barrier may be dropped for some hours in the region of injury. During this time the foot processes retract from the endothelial cells. When the differences between endothelial cells within and outside the CNS were noted by electron microscopy, it was concluded that there may be different types of endothelial cells in these two locations. Now it is known that endothelial cells co-cultured (grown together in culture) with astrocytes will appear like those of the CNS regardless of their non-CNS origin; CNS endothelial cells cultured without astrocytes will resemble those from elsewhere. The bottom line here is that astrocytes in the CNS influence endothelial cells to take on characteristics that are responsible for the blood-brain barrier.

Given that, what do you think is able to make it through the barrier? Since the barrier is made up of cells and since cells have a phospholipid bilayer as their membrane, anything that cannot pass through that membrane has trouble getting into the CNS. Anything that is lipid soluble can pass right through, however. Also, any molecule for which these endothelial cells have a specific carrier can make it through. Examples of substances for which these cells have a carrier include glucose and some amino acids. Examples of substances that can pass through due to their solubility include oxygen, carbon dioxide, and drugs such as anesthetics (lipid soluble) and alcohol (equally soluble in water and lipids). This helps our understanding of how alcohol has its CNS effects.

There are certain locations in the CNS where a blood-brain barrier does not exist in this form. These places include the choroid plexus and hormonally ac-tive regions, such as the hypothalamus and the posterior pituitary. In these regions, some access to the blood must be maintained (for production of CSF and secretion of hormones). Specialized cells are responsible for the blood-brain barrier in these structures.

What You Should Know

1. The nervous system is the fast-acting regulator of homeostasis.

2. The central nervous system (CNS) includes the brain and spinal cord; all other components of the nervous system are in the peripheral nervous system (PNS).

3. The sensory function of the nervous system includes our ability to collect information about our internal and external environments, and convey that information to the CNS.

4. The nervous system's integrative functions are those activities that interpret and make decisions about the information conveyed through the sensory functions.

5. Integration is carried out only in the CNS.

6. The motor functions of the nervous system are those activities that convey information from the centers involved in integration to effectors that allow us to act on that information. These effectors include the three types of muscle and glands.

7. The motor subdivision of the nervous system can be further subdivided into somatic and autonomic components.

8. The somatic nervous system includes those motor components that have skeletal muscle as their effectors. These are generally under voluntary control.

9. The autonomic nervous system includes those motor components that have smooth muscle, cardiac muscle, or glands as their effectors. These are under involuntary control.

10. The autonomic nervous system is further divided into two antagonistic components, the sympathetic and parasympathetic nervous systems.

11. The cranial bones and vertebral column protect our CNS from trauma.

12. The CNS is surrounded by membranes called meninges. These support and protect the brain and spinal cord.

13. The meninges are composed of three layers: the dura mater (most superficial), the arachnoid mater, and the pia mater (deepest).

14. The ventricles, subarachnoid space, and the central canal of the spinal cord are filled with cerebrospinal fluid (CSF).

15. Cerebrospinal fluid cushions the CNS and acts as an intermediary between the vasculature and tissues of the brain.

16. The blood-brain barrier determines which substances can move from the blood into the CNS. This is important because the special functions of these organs would be disrupted by many substances present in the blood.

17. Astrocytes cause changes in the structure of endothelial cells, resulting in the blood-brain barrier.

18. Several regions of the CNS are protected by mechanisms other than the typical blood-brain barrier. These regions are the locations where the CSF is produced and hormonally active structures.

What Did You Learn?

Multiple choice questions: choose the best answer.

1. The nervous system is our:
   a. Fast-acting regulator of homeostasis
   b. Slow-acting regulator of homeostasis
   c. Our only regulator of homeostasis
   d. Not involved in the regulation of homeostasis

2. Our PNS contains our:
   a. Brain
   b. Spinal cord
   c. Both of the above
   d. Neither of the above

What Did You Learn? (continued)

3. The integrative functions of our nervous system include:
   a. The ability to sense our internal and external environments
   b. The ability to interpret sensory input and make decisions about the need for a response
   c. The ability to transmit information to effectors
   d. All of the above
   e. None of the above

4. Skeletal muscle is the effector for the _____ component of the nervous system.
   a. Somatic
   b. Autonomic
   c. Both of the above
   d. Neither of the above

5. The sympathetic and parasympathetic nervous systems are components of the _____ nervous system.
   a. Somatic
   b. Autonomic
   c. Both of the above
   d. Neither of the above

6. The frontal, parietal, and occipital bones are part of the:
   a. Cranium
   b. Calvarium
   c. Both of the above
   d. Neither of the above

7. Place the following in their proper order from most superficial to most deep:
   1. Arachnoid mater
   2. Dura mater
   3. Pia mater
   a. 2,1,3
   b. 2,3,1
   c. 3,1,2

   d. 3,2,1
   e. 1,2,3

8. The choroid plexus produces:
   a. The meninges
   b. PBS
   c. CNS
   d. CSF
   e. BBB

9. Modified endothelial cells are responsible for the blood-brain barrier. Which cell type causes them to form this barrier?
   a. Astrocytes
   b. Oligodendrocytes
   c. Microglia
   d. Neurolemmocytes
   e. No other cell type; they produce the blood-brain barrier on their own.

10. Which of the following can readily cross the blood-brain barrier?
   a. Lipid-soluble substances
   b. Water-soluble substances
   c. Both of the above
   d. Neither of the above

Short answer questions: answer briefly and in your own words.

1. Draw and explain a flow chart demonstrating the functional subdivisions of the nervous system.

2. List and describe the layers of the meninges.

3. Why is CSF necessary? How does it differ from the interstitial fluid seen elsewhere in the body?

4. Draw and label cross sections through: (a) a capillary in the CNS and (b) a typical capillary elsewhere in the body. Be sure to indicate the differences between these two structures.

5. You are a scientist working on a cure for a degenerative brain disorder. What characteristic must you design into the drug you are developing to assure it will gain access to the diseased neurons? Why is this necessary?

The Structure and Function of Your Brain

What You Will Learn

- The structure and function of your brainstem.
- The structure and function of your diencephalon.
- The structure and function of your cerebrum.
- The structure and function of your cerebellum.
- The activities of your limbic system.
- How your autonomic nervous system works.
- The anatomic arrangement of the motor pathways in your somatic and autonomic nervous systems.
- The locations, names, and functions of your cranial nerves.
- The neurotransmitters that are present in your chemical synapses and their activities.

We are now ready to begin our exploration of the brain. This fascinating organ can be divided into the following structures: the brain stem, the diencephalon, the cerebrum, and the cerebellum. This is the order in which we will proceed. First, look at **TABLE 12.1** for some definitions you will need.

12B.1 Your Brainstem

The brainstem is the most inferior portion of your brain (**FIGURE 12.9**). In fact, the brainstem directly connects to your spinal cord. Your brainstem is composed of three parts. The most inferior portion is the medulla oblongata. The intermediate portion is the pons or pons Varolii. The most superior structure is the midbrain. We will discuss each component in turn.

Your Medulla Oblongata

The medulla oblongata is the most inferior portion of the brain. It is approximately 2.5 centimeters (about 1 inch) long and lies between the spinal cord and the pons. The main component of the medulla is white matter: ascending (sensory), descending (motor), and transverse (interconnecting the medulla and the cerebellum) tracts.

On the ventral side of the medulla, there are two triangular structures called pyramids. These contain the largest motor tracts, coming from the cerebral cortex. These motor tracts cross from one side to the other within the medulla. This crossing over is called the decussation of pyramids and results in each side of your brain controlling motor activity on the contralateral (opposite) side of your body.

Ascending (sensory) tracts are found on the dorsal side of the medulla. Sensory tracts do not all cross over from one side to the other in the same location. Some sensory tracts cross over in the brainstem; others cross over in the spinal cord. Two prominent sensory nuclei are also found here.

Oval projections (swellings) called olives are present on the lateral surfaces of the medulla. The olives contain nuclei that function with the cerebellum to control the efficiency and precision of movement, equilibrium, and posture.

Three vital reflex centers reside in the medulla: the cardiac center, the medullary rhythmicity area, and the vasomotor center. The cardiac center sets the rate and force of the heart's contractions. The medullary rhythmicity area works together with two areas in the pons to control the rhythm of breathing. This fascinating topic will be covered in detail in Chapter 17. The vasomotor area controls blood flow in your body through vascular tone. Vascular tone is the degree to which the smooth muscle in your muscular arteries and arterioles is contracted. This is the basic mechanism used to direct blood flow to where it is needed and to maintain blood pressure by restricting blood flow where it is not needed. The vasomotor area controls this vital function (see Chapter 16 for more information).

Several nonvital reflex centers are also present in the medulla. For example, centers for swallowing, coughing, sneezing, and vomiting are found here. You might think you would be better off if you did not have a reflex center for vomiting. In fact, this is a very important safety feature. Haven't we all eaten something at some point that

Table 12.1   A Few Important Definitions

Term	Definition
Nerve fiber	An axon or dendrite and its myelin (if it is myelinated)
Tract	A bundle of nerve fibers in the CNS
Nerve	A bundle of nerve fibers in the PNS
Nucleus	A group of neuron cell bodies in the CNS
Ganglion	A group of neuron cell bodies in the PNS
Gray matter	Tissue composed mainly of neuron cell bodies
White matter	Tissue composed mainly of nerve fibers

CNS = central nervous system, PNS = peripheral nervous system.

"didn't agree with us" and ended up vomiting it back up? Depending on the toxin ingested, you might have become much more ill or even died if your body did not have the ability to reject that toxin in that manner. So, perhaps you are thinking that reflexes such as swallowing and vomiting should be considered vital reflexes. The term *vital reflex* is reserved for those reflexes that, if interfered with, could lead to our immediate demise. Of course, we could die if we were unable to swallow, but death would not be immediate. Interference with any of the vital reflex centers listed in the previous paragraph could result in immediate death. This is why traumatic damage to the brain stem can be life threatening.

■ Your Pons

The pons, or pons Varolii, is immediately superior to the medulla oblongata, lying between the medulla and the midbrain and is about 2.5 centimeters long. The term

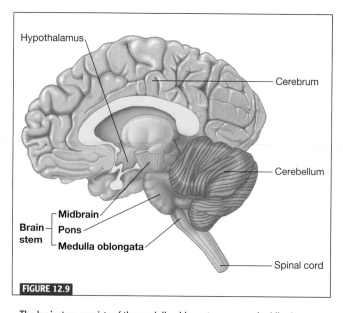

Hypothalamus

Cerebrum

Cerebellum

Midbrain
Brain- Pons
stem Medulla oblongata

Spinal cord

FIGURE 12.9

The brainstem consists of the medulla oblongata, pons, and midbrain.

pons means "bridge," and this region is mainly composed of tracts. Longitudinal tracts are present, conveying sensory and motor fibers between the medulla and the midbrain. Transverse tracts are also present, carrying fibers to and from the cerebellum.

Two important nuclei are present. The pneumotaxic area and the apneustic area work with the medullary rhythmicity area to control respiration. These will be discussed in Chapter 17.

■ Your Midbrain

The midbrain, also called mesencephalon, which means middle brain, is the most superior region of the brainstem. It extends from the pons to the diencephalon. It is about 2.5 centimeters long, and the cerebral aqueduct (aqueduct of Sylvius) passes through it. Again, as in other regions of the brainstem, tracts make up much of the midbrain. Longitudinal and transverse tracts are present, as are nuclei, to control reflex movement of the skeletal muscles.

If something were to flash by the window of the room you are in right now, at the very margin of your field of vision, what would you do? The chances are that you would quickly turn your eyes and maybe more of your body toward that direction to see what it was. This would be a reflex movement on your part. You would not have made a conscious, voluntary effort to turn. In fact, you might have turned before you were even consciously aware of why you were turning.

Reflex centers in the midbrain control that type of reflex movement. These are protective mechanisms, meant to help you to avoid injury. These centers include one for movement of the eyeballs, head, and neck in response to a variety of stimuli, and for movement of the head and trunk in response to auditory stimuli. That second reflex is the one that would cause you to turn quickly toward an unexpected noise, such as in response to a classmate dropping a book during lecture.

Now we can begin our discussion of the diencephalon.

12B.2 Your Diencephalon

The diencephalon is our next higher region of the brain (**FIGURE 12.10**). The term *diencephalon* means "between brain or inter brain." The diencephalon is composed of three parts, two of which are more important to our discussion. We will spend the majority of our time on the thalamus and the hypothalamus. There is also an epithalamus. The epithalamus includes the roof of the third ventricle, the choroid plexus of the third ventricle, and the pineal gland. The pineal gland is an endocrine gland that will be discussed in Chapter 13.

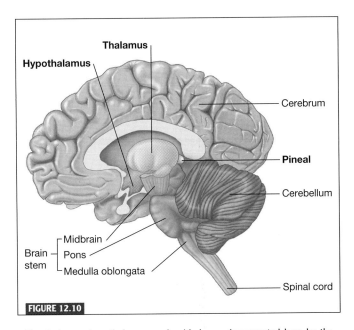

FIGURE 12.10

The thalamus, hypothalamus, and epithalamus (represented here by the pineal gland) are included in the diencephalon.

Your Thalamus

The term *thalamus* comes from a root meaning chamber. This is the largest component of the diencephalon and is located inferior to the lateral ventricles and lateral to the third ventricle (see **FIGURE 12.11**). Two oval masses of gray matter connected by the massa intermedia (intermediate mass) make up the thalamus. It is superior and medial to the internal capsule, which we will discuss with the cerebrum. The thalamus has several important functions. It contains synapses for neurons conveying sensory impulses to the cerebrum for all senses except smell. Integration (interpretation) of senses such as light touch, pressure, temperature, and pain occur here. Perhaps at some time you noticed, on touching some object briefly, that you knew it was either very hot or very cold, but were not sure which. Or perhaps you felt pressure at some point, but it took a moment to be sure that it hurt. This is the region of the brain that makes those decisions. It also contains synapses for voluntary movement.

Your Hypothalamus

The term *hypothalamus* indicates the location of this structure below the thalamus. It is much smaller than the thalamus, but is a very important region of the brain. It makes up the inferior portion of the walls and the floor of the third ventricle, and overlies the sella turcica. Quick, of what bone was the sella turcica a feature, and what is enclosed within the sella turcica?

There are four regions of the hypothalamus. Moving from anterior to posterior they are the preoptic,

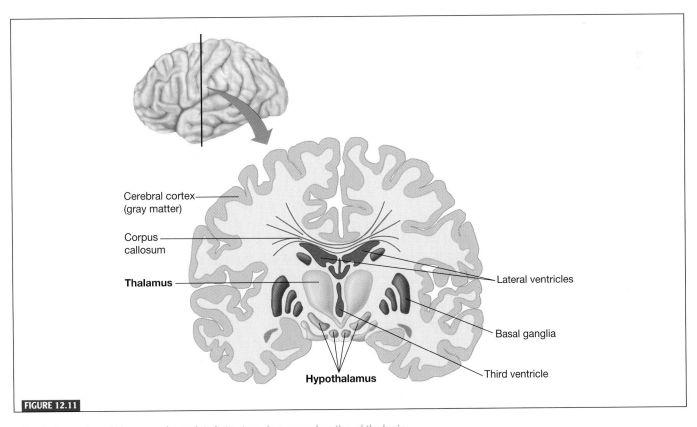

FIGURE 12.11

The thalamus, hypothalamus, and associated structures in a coronal section of the brain.

supraoptic, tuberal, and mammillary. The terms *preoptic* and *supraoptic* refer to positions relative to the optic chiasma, part of the second cranial nerve (later in this chapter). The tuberal region includes the infundibulum, which connects the pituitary gland to the hypothalamus. The mammillary bodies (*mammillary* refers to their appearance like little breasts) are involved in our sense of smell.

The functions of the hypothalamus are many and complex. Some texts list a relatively large number of functions; others combine functions and create a smaller list. Here, I will not combine functions, but will instead list eight functions for clarity. Some of these functions will seem to overlap other functions. If some functions seem redundant to you, you are doing well at making connections: good for you.

1. The hypothalamus controls the autonomic nervous system and, therefore, controls the internal organs (the viscera). You should remember what the effectors of the autonomic nervous system are and should conclude that these are under involuntary control. Remember the hypothalamus when we discuss the autonomic nervous system later in this chapter.

2. Interpretation of sensations from internal organs. Why isn't this included in control of the autonomic nervous system? If you answered that the autonomic nervous system is motor, not sensory, you are correct. Interpretation of sensory input from the viscera is necessary for the autonomic nervous system to function. Here is where that interpretation takes place.

3. Coordination of the body's two principle regulators of homeostasis. Think of it; we have two systems regulating homeostasis. If these two systems did not coordinate their activities, they might work against each other, causing major disruptions in homeostasis. Although it is in the nervous system, the hypothalamus has nervous and endocrine functions, and acts as intermediary between these two systems. We will learn more about this in Chapter 13.

4. Control of our reactions to sudden threats and fear. This function overlaps with the previous one. Emotions such as rage are controlled by the hypothalamus. The hypothalamus also controls the activities of the adrenal medulla. The adrenal medulla is a gland that straddles the border between the endocrine system and the nervous system. The responses of the endocrine and nervous systems to sudden fear, rage, and related emotions come together in the adrenal medulla. That gland is controlled by the hypothalamus. It, therefore, plays a major role in our ability to survive a wide range of sudden attacks. More on this topic later on in this chapter.

5. Control of thirst and hunger. The thirst center of the hypothalamus monitors our need for water. When our fluid volume is low, it gives us the sensation of "being thirsty" and triggers endocrine activities that conserve water. Our drive to eat is triggered by the feeding center of the hypothalamus. Our sense of fullness is triggered by the satiety center of the hypothalamus. Some people have malfunctioning satiety centers, which can lead to problems with obesity. We have come to understand that their difficulty in limiting their eating does not come merely from a "lack of will power," as was previously thought, but from the inability of their satiety center to send the appropriate signals for them to feel full. This knowledge may lead to the development of pharmaceutical agents beneficial to these people. In the meantime, this knowledge should lead to better public understanding of their problems.

6. Control of waking, sleep, and related cycles. Our waking and sleep cycles are incredibly complex activities involving a number of regions of the brain. Much of this control lies in the hypothalamus. Using input from the eyes, the hypothalamus regulates the release of melatonin from the pineal gland, helping to regulate our ability to sleep and wake up. Many similarly complex cycles exist in our bodies. For instance, growth hormone is released in a complex, daily cyclical manner, as controlled by the hypothalamus. We will discuss these topics further in Chapter 13, but again be aware of how this places the hypothalamus at the interface between the nervous and endocrine systems.

7. Control of the sexual response. The sexual response is very important to our species, not just from a psychosocial standpoint, but from the standpoint of the actual continuation of our species. No sexual response would result in no human beings in a very short time. Our response to sexual stimuli and even the characteristic movements associated with sexual activity are controlled by the hypothalamus.

8. Control of the body's temperature. Your body's thermostat is located in the hypothalamus. This is where the decision to shiver or sweat, and to direct blood to the body's surface or restrict it to the core, is made.

This concludes our discussion of the hypothalamus and the diencephalon. Some of this information may not be entirely clear to you. That is because you are looking at a partially completed puzzle. Some of what we have just discussed requires prior knowledge of topics we have not yet discussed for complete clarity. Don't worry; we are moving toward discussions of overlapping topics. Our next region of the brain is the cerebrum.

12B.3 Your Cerebrum: Its Anatomy and Physiology

Now here is a major topic. In humans, the cerebrum makes up nearly seven eighths of the brain (**FIGURE 12.12**). It is far smaller in most other animals. For instance, in sheep the cerebrum is quite small. Have you ever noticed what sheep do all day? They eat grass. That's about it. They just eat grass. They do not write novels or symphonies. They do not build cathedrals or monuments. They have not developed automobiles or spacecraft. This is because they do not have well developed cerebrums. We do all of those things and, not coincidentally, we do have well-developed cerebrums. Get it? This is where our creative, intellectual, and scientific abilities reside! This is an amazing region of the brain.

Cerebral Gray Matter

As we look at the surface of your cerebrum, and certainly we have all seen one somewhere, even if in a horror movie, the most distinguishing characteristic we notice is its many folds (**FIGURE 12.13**). The surface of the cerebrum has a highly folded morphology. There is a very good reason for this.

Let us suppose for a minute that you collected art (and maybe you actually do). You have a one-room art gallery in which you keep your art (even though you could "live with it" more fully if you spread it throughout your home). What do you do when all of the walls in this room are covered and you have purchased some more great artwork? No, you can't build another room or

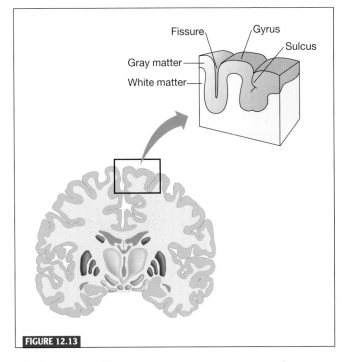

Surface features of the cerebrum.

move to another gallery; you have this one room and that's all. O.K., you could add additional wall space if you built folds in the outer walls of the room (**FIGURE 12.14**). These folds in the wall would allow you to hang more artwork in the same size room because the room would now have more surface area.

Now, back to the cerebrum. The surface of the cerebrum, that is to say the outer layer of the cerebrum, is called the cerebral cortex (**FIGURE 12.15**). The term *cortex* means "bark" or "rind" and is often used to describe the outer portion of an organ. The cerebral cortex contains gray matter. Gray matter is made up of neuron cell bodies and associated stroma. These neuron cell bodies give the cortex its gray color. We need to have a lot of neurons in our cortex, because of the many important functions of the cerebrum. If the surface of our cortex was smooth, we would have less room for these cell bodies. By throwing it into folds, the volume of the cortex increases greatly. The cortex is actually a highly structured area organized into six layers, based on the morphology of the neurons found there.

These folds (the bulging parts) are called gyri (gyrus is singular). Between them we find shallow grooves called sulci (sulcus is singular). Very deep grooves are called fissures. Notice in Figures 12.13 and 12.15, for example, the longitudinal fissure that separates the two hemispheres of the cerebrum. Notice also the central sulcus, which is a major landmark in the brain, separating the precentral gyrus and the postcentral gyrus (Figure 12.16).

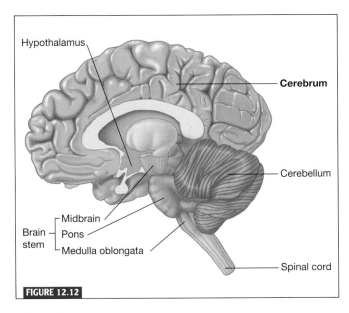

The cerebrum.

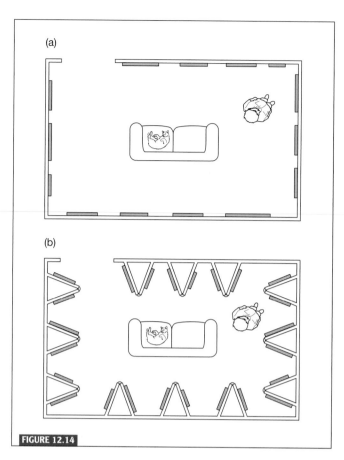

FIGURE 12.14

As seen in this art gallery, a structure of flat surfaces (a) has less surface area than a structure of folded surfaces (b). Folds on the surface of the cerebrum increase the area we have for gray matter.

While looking at the surface of the brain (**FIGURE 12.16**), we can also identify the lobes of the cerebrum. Note that the names of the lobes match the names of the overlying bones, which you already know. Note also that the frontal and parietal lobes are separated by the central sulcus and that the frontal and temporal lobes are separated by the lateral cerebral sulcus. The parieto-occipital sulcus separates the parietal and occipital lobes. There is one more component of the cerebral cortex that is somewhat hidden. A deeper fold of cortex, deep to the temporal lobe, called the insula, adds additional volume to the cortex. If you think back to the art gallery analogy, it would be as if you built a small room within the gallery, as an extension of the existing wall of your gallery (see Figures 12.14 and 12.15). The posterior border of the cerebrum is marked by the transverse fissure that separates the cerebrum from the cerebellum.

■ Cerebral White Matter

Cerebral white matter lies deep to the gray matter. This design makes perfect sense from a structural standpoint, as the white matter is made up of nerve fibers connecting the cerebral cortex with parts of the CNS. If the gray matter was deep and the white matter was superficial, the fibers would have to pass through the gray matter to make these connections.

We can classify the fibers of the cerebral white matter into three categories, based on what they connect (**FIGURE 12.17**). Association fibers connect one gyrus to another or one lobe to another within the same hemisphere. Commissural fibers interconnect the right and left hemispheres. There are three important structures containing commissural fibers. The largest of the three is the corpus callosum, which is indicated in **FIGURE 12.18**. The term *corpus callosum* means "hard body," and in any dissection of the brain, it is easy to pick out because of its firm texture. It is located anterior and superior to the lateral ventricles.

The anterior commissure is in the anterior wall of the third ventricle, and the posterior commissure is in the posterior wall of the third ventricle (don't you like it when names make sense?). These are the other two structures composed of commissural fibers.

The third type of fiber in the cerebral white matter is the projection fiber. Projection fibers are composed of ascending and descending tracts, interconnecting higher and lower structures in the brain. The internal capsule is an example of a structure composed of projection fibers. The internal capsule was named in the time before the functions of nervous tissue were understood. Anatomists dissecting the brain found a firm area along which it was easy to separate brain tissue and decided that it was some form of a capsule. Since it was within brain tissue, it was called the internal capsule. We now know that it is no capsule at all, but is instead ascending and descending tracts. Superiorly, the internal capsule splits into a fan shape called the corona radiata. This area of deep cortex, containing the internal capsule, is called the corpus striatum (striped body) because of its striped appearance.

The corpus striatum also contains several pockets of gray matter called basal ganglia. By our definitions, you know that these are not ganglia at all, but nuclei. The basal ganglia are involved in coordinating some of the subconscious contractions of skeletal muscle (i.e., swinging your arms when you walk).

■ The Functional Areas of the Cortex

The history of our knowledge of cortical function in particular, and brain function overall, is long and fascinating. Before the 19th century, the brain was thought to be a glandular organ. The tissue of the brain was believed to be a syncytium, cells fused together into one giant cell with lots of nuclei. Nerves were considered to be tubes that carried the secretions produced by the

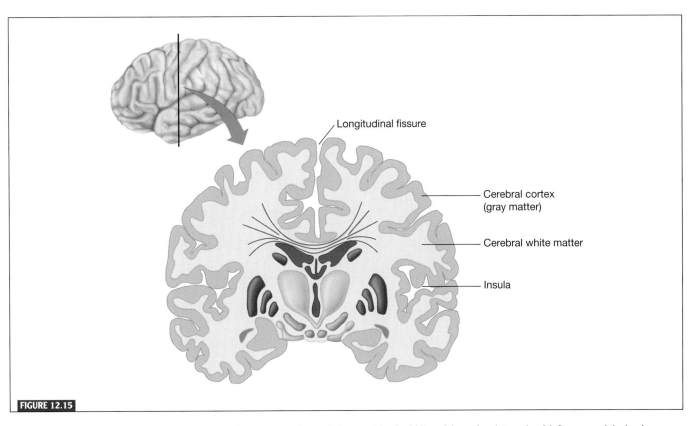

FIGURE 12.15

A coronal section through the cerebrum. The area for gray matter is greatly increased by the folding of the surface into gyri, sulci, fissures, and the insula.

brain to other regions of the body. During the 19th century, scientists figured out that the brain is composed of many individual cells and that some of these cells have electrical activity.

After these discoveries were made, the role of the brain in determining behavior was an area of intense investigation. For a time, people thought that the shape of the brain was directly related to personality and that individual regions on the surface of the brain were responsible for specific behaviors. Exhibiting these behaviors led to increasing the size of the centers that controlled those behaviors, and that led to bumps on the skull. Based on that belief, the now discredited "science" of phrenology involved describing a person's behavior by interpreting the bumps on that person's skull.

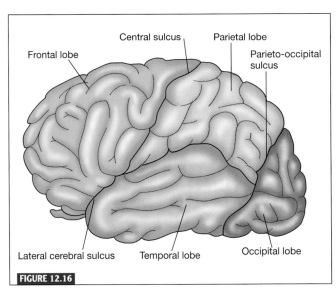

FIGURE 12.16

The lobes of the cerebrum.

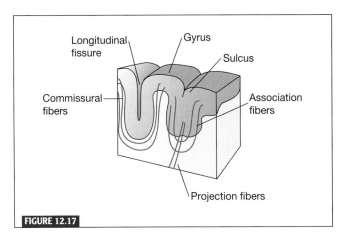

FIGURE 12.17

Three categories of cerebral fibers.

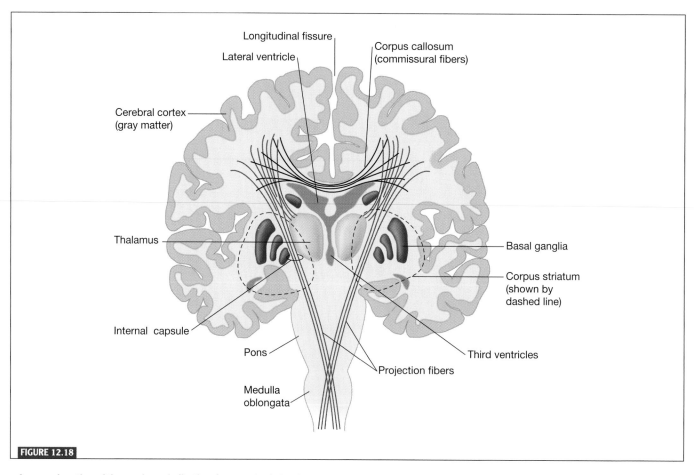

A coronal section of the cerebrum indicating deep cerebral structures.

During the 19th and early 20th centuries, scientific opinion vacillated back and forth between whether individual regions of the brain controlled specific activities or whether the entire brain controlled these activities as a unit. Problems with the design of experiments meant to answer these questions prolonged the time necessary to develop an accurate understanding. Experiments involving individuals with brain lesions (injuries) in areas that process language led to later work with improved technologies for detecting the level of activity in specific areas of the brain. These studies have greatly enhanced our understanding of brain function. A detailed explanation of the activities of specific areas of the brain is beyond the scope of this book. **FIGURE 12.19** shows the functional areas of the cerebral cortex, however. Examine that figure carefully and you will see how cerebral functions are distributed. Note that the frontal lobe (and particularly the precentral gyrus) is the primary motor area of the cerebrum. The parietal lobe (and particularly the postcentral gyrus) is the primary sensory area. Note also the location of areas primarily responsible for sight (occipital lobe), hearing, and smell (temporal lobe). Individual emotional states also involve specific areas of

the cerebrum. Anxiety and panic involve the temporal lobes, for example.

Many good advanced texts are available to guide you to further understand this topic, should you desire. As in other topics, I encourage you to continue to advance your study of neuroanatomy and neurophysiology after completing your current study.

We will, however, discuss some additional aspects of anatomical neurophysiology here. First of all, we need to consider the split brain concept, which tells us that, although the two hemispheres of the cerebrum are anatomically somewhat symmetrical, functionally they are not symmetrical. Most people are right handed. Since the cerebrum exercises contralateral control over the body (remember the decussation of pyramids), the left side of the brain controls the right side of the body. The left side of the brain is, therefore, dominant in most people. If you are left handed, however, your right hemisphere is more likely to be dominant. The left hemisphere of the cerebrum is more logical and reason oriented. It is the side that determines mathematical skills, memorization skills (i.e., memorizing the bones and muscles), and language skills. Interestingly, the left hemisphere is

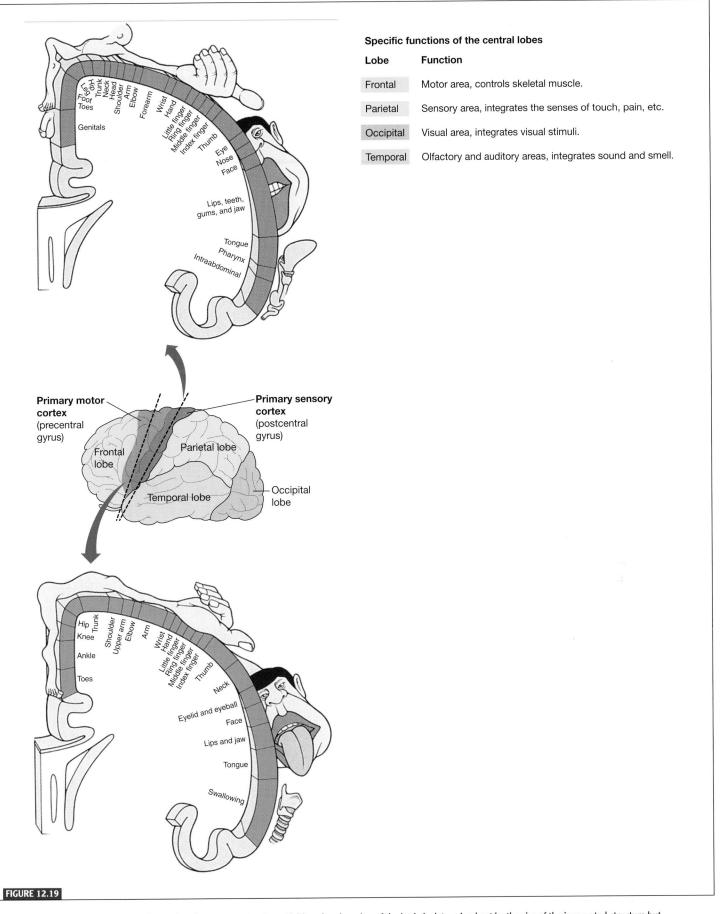

Specific functions of the central lobes

Lobe	Function
Frontal	Motor area, controls skeletal muscle.
Parietal	Sensory area, integrates the senses of touch, pain, etc.
Occipital	Visual area, integrates visual stimuli.
Temporal	Olfactory and auditory areas, integrates sound and smell.

FIGURE 12.19

The volume of the cerebrum that is devoted to the sensory or motor activities of each region of the body is determined not by the size of the innervated structure but by the needs of that location. Here, the body has been drawn beside a representation of the precentral gyrus (primary motor area) and postcentral gyrus (primary sensory area). The relative size of each drawn structure represents the amount of cerebrum dedicated to that structure.

responsible for spoken, written, and sign language skills, but different areas of this hemisphere are stimulated by reading, listening to, speaking, and thinking about language. This is one reason why you will learn best when you combine different forms of studying; reading quietly, listening to lectures, writing notes, and discussing what you are learning with others.

The right hemisphere is the emotional side in most people. Its responsibilities include mental imaging and visual-spatial skills (i.e., eye-hand coordination, computer games), artistic and musical creativity and the creative use of language (poetry), the recognition of faces and the emotions expressed by those faces, intuition, insight, and the ability to interconnect areas of knowledge.

Even though it is interesting to ascribe discrete activities to individual hemispheres of the cerebrum, it is important to note that the hemispheres do not act independently. The commissural fibers carry information between the hemispheres, keeping both sides in continuous contact with each other. In this way, both sides are involved at some level in all cerebral functions.

12B.4 Your Cerebellum: Its Anatomy and Physiology

■ A Brief Word of Caution

We need to start this discussion with a note of caution. Notice how similar the word *cerebellum* (from the Latin for "little brain") is to the word *cerebrum* (Latin for "brain"). Sometimes after an anatomy and physiology exam, a student will come to me, greatly upset, and tell me that he or she got a few questions wrong because he or she thought the word in those questions was cerebellum when it was actually cerebrum (or vice versa). I hate to see students lose points because of misreading a word when they knew the information all along. Please don't make that mistake. As similar as these words look now, when you are calmly reading your text, the emotional stress of an exam will make them look even more similar and you may confuse them. Be careful when you see either word on an exam. Look at the letters and make sure it is the word you think it is!

■ The Gross Anatomy of Your Cerebellum

Now, about the cerebellum. The cerebellum is the second largest component of your brain (**FIGURE 12.20**). It is in an inferior and posterior position, lying posterior to the brainstem and inferior to the occipital lobe of the cerebrum. It is separated from the cerebrum by the transverse fissure and a heavy fold of meninges found in that fissure.

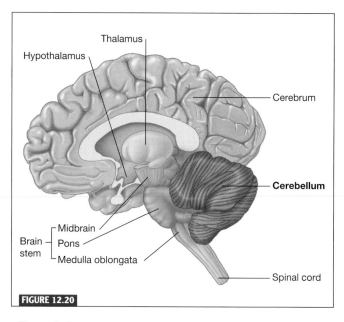

FIGURE 12.20

The cerebellum.

The cerebellum has two hemispheres connected by a structure called the vermis (**FIGURE 12.21**). The term *vermis* means "worm," and the reason for this rather unflattering name is apparent when you examine the cerebellum. When you look at the dorsal surface of the cerebellum, you see two fan-shaped hemispheres with a constricted area between them. To the anatomist who named the vermis, the cerebellum looked like a butterfly with two lateral wings (hemispheres) and a central body (the worm or vermis).

■ Cerebellar Gray and White Matter: Leaves on the Trees

The gray matter is superficial in the cerebellum, just as in the cerebrum (Figure 12.21). Here also it is thrown into gyri, but these are much finer and are called folia (as in foliage or leaves on trees). The white matter lies deep to the gray matter. In section, it has a shape reminiscent of a small, tortured tree, like you would see growing on a high rocky mountain or in a Japanese bonsai garden. This white matter is called arbor vitae (tree of life), which is fitting because of its shape and the presence of the folia.

■ Functions of Your Cerebellum

So, what does the cerebellum do? It can be thought of as our body's center for quality control of movement. It is primarily a motor area that works with the basal ganglia to control the subconscious movement of skeletal muscle. It also fine tunes the movements generated by the primary motor areas of our cerebrum. The cerebel-

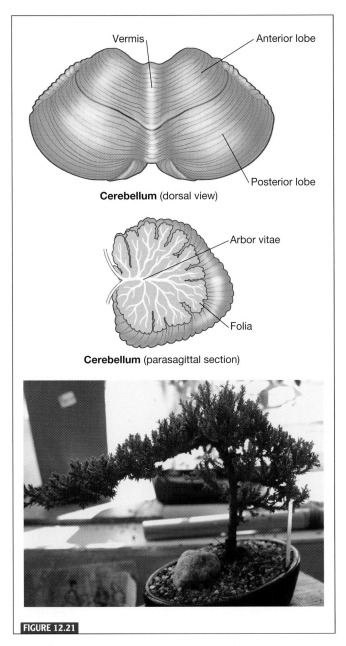

Vermis

Anterior lobe

Posterior lobe

Cerebellum (dorsal view)

Arbor vitae

Folia

Cerebellum (parasagittal section)

FIGURE 12.21

The cerebellum in dorsal view and parasagittal section. The shape of the cerebellar white matter (arbor vitae) resembles that of a bonsai tree.

lum compares the location, speed, and direction of our limbs during movement with the intended target of that movement, and makes subtle corrections so that we end up with the movement we actually intended. This involves proprioception, the ability to sense the three-dimensional location of our limbs. Think about how you reach for a glass of water. It is very complex. First, you accelerate the arm toward the target (the glass). As it nears the glass, it must decelerate and stop in precisely the right spot. Only then can the hand close around the glass so you can pick it up. If the motion stops too soon, you will miss the target. If it stops too late, you will

knock the glass over, spilling the contents. The cerebellum makes certain our motions are what we intend them to be. That is quality control for movement. It also plays a role in posture and equilibrium, along with other regions of the brain.

12B.5 Your Limbic System: Emotion and Memory

What were we talking about? I forgot for a moment. Boy, forgetting like that makes me angry. Ah yes, memory, what every student of anatomy and physiology needs in abundance. Let's talk about the limbic system.

The limbic system is composed of structures found at the border between the diencephalon and the cerebrum. In fact, the term *limbic* means "border." These structures include the cingulate gyrus (cingulated means girdle), the dentate gyrus (*dentate* means tooth), the hippocampus (refers to seahorse), the amygdala (almondlike), the olfactory bulbs (smell), and parts of the thalamus and hypothalamus. These structures are shown in **FIGURE 12.22**.

The limbic system plays a major role in emotions. Working together with the cerebral cortex, it allows us to interpret the emotions of others and to be aware of our own emotions. It also allows us to express our emotions or to suppress them when expression is inappropriate.

Parts of this system (especially the hippocampus and amygdala) are involved in memory. Many parts of the cerebral cortex are involved in memory. Memories are stored in areas of the cortex near where the memories are generated or used. The hippocampus is important, however, in converting short-term memories into long-term memories. The amygdala plays a role in memories involving multiple senses (the smell, taste, and texture of your favorite foods) and emotions (who prepared that food for you when you were young and how you felt about that person). When you consider that the limbic system is involved in both emotion and memory, it is easy to understand how we are able to remember details of a day in which something of great emotional importance occurred (the birth of a loved one), even if it happened a long time ago, but are not able to remember the details of a day in which not much occurred, even if it was only a couple of days ago (or for that matter, where you put your car keys 10 minutes ago).

12B.6 Your Autonomic Nervous System

AHHH RUN AWAY!!! THERES AN ALLIGATOR RIGHT BEHIND YOU!!! There, that got your attention, didn't it?

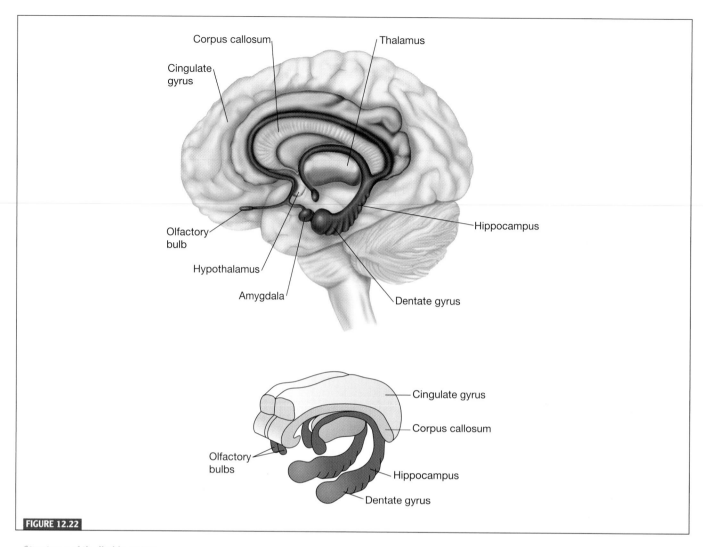

FIGURE 12.22

Structures of the limbic system.

Why would the thought of an alligator right behind you seem more immediately important than the limbic system functions we were just discussing? Simple, because an alligator can kill you, but the limbic system can't. So, here's where the autonomic nervous system comes in.

You already know that there are two components to the autonomic nervous system: the sympathetic nervous system and the parasympathetic nervous system. You also know that these two systems are antagonistic to each other. Let's now consider how they are antagonistic.

■ Two Antagonistic Components: One Caveman

Let's think about a caveman for a minute (**FIGURE 12.23**). Here he is at the end of his long caveman day, sitting by his caveman fire outside of his cave (he is a caveman after all). He's munching on a nice little barbequed dinosaur (O.K., so cavemen, dinosaurs, and barbeque sauce didn't

all co-exist; it's my story and I'll tell it as I like) that he prepared for supper. He's very relaxed. Should he have a high heart rate or a low heart rate? How about his respiration rate? Should his gastrointestinal (G.I.) tract be active or inactive? How about other internal organs like his kidneys? Does he need a lot of blood flow to his skeletal muscles? What determines all of these things? The autonomic nervous system does. Under these circumstances (relaxing, eating, taking life easy), the parasympathetic nervous system is in charge. For this reason, it is called the energy conservation and restoration system ("rest and digest"). Our caveman is resting, conserving energy with a slow heart and respiration rate. His G.I. tract is active (energy restoration), as are his kidneys. He does not need to have very much blood flowing through his relaxing skeletal muscles. These are the effects of the parasympathetic nervous system.

Now wait a minute, what does he hear coming up behind him? Big foot steps; very big foot steps. It's the

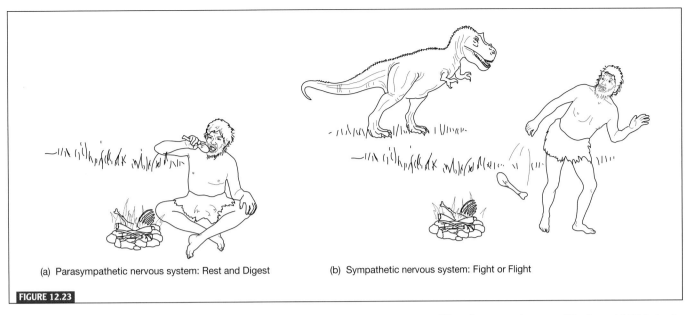

(a) Parasympathetic nervous system: Rest and Digest   (b) Sympathetic nervous system: Fight or Flight

FIGURE 12.23

Activities of the parasympathetic and sympathetic subdivisions of the autonomic nervous system. OK, so dinosaurs and cavemen did not co-exist; think about what would have happened if they did and you will have a useful framework for considering the activities of these antagonistic systems.

momma of the little dinosaur he's eating! Does he still want slow heart and respiration rates? Does he still need an active G.I. tract? Does he need to get the heck out of there? Now the activity of the sympathetic nervous system kicks in and dominates over the effects of the parasympathetic nervous system. This results in increased cardiac and respiration rates; increased blood flow to skeletal muscle; decreased blood flow to the kidneys, G.I. tract, and other internal organs; and increased sweating. These are the changes that will enable him either to run away from this danger or to stand and fight it. The sympathetic nervous system is also called the fight-or-flight system. When we perceive danger, the sympathetic nervous system increases its activity and the parasympathetic nervous system decreases its activity. Conditions in the body alter from those of energy conservation and restoration to those that prepare the body to flee or fight.

You should now see that these two antagonistic systems have different effects, depending on what organ we consider. The parasympathetic nervous system stimulates the G.I. tract, while inhibiting cardiac activity. The sympathetic nervous system inhibits G.I. activity, while stimulating cardiac activity. Face it, if our caveman does not get away from that dinosaur, it is of little importance whether he is able to digest his dinner!

O.K., so he does get away, or so he thinks. He ran off into the forest and now is leaning on a tree trying to catch his breath. He is pretty sure he got away, but he can't be completely certain. Should he now go immediately back to the energy conservation and restoration state, or should he maintain an increased state of alert-

ness and readiness to run or fight? He probably should remain at that heightened state of preparedness, listen for footsteps, and be ready to run again (she might still be out there). For this reason, the activity of the sympathetic nervous system is global and long lasting. When it kicks in, the entire body gets ready to fight and stays ready for some time. The global (systemic) and long-lasting nature of this system has to do with the activity of the adrenal medulla. This endocrine gland is actually part of the sympathetic nervous system as well as the endocrine system. The hormones it secretes are the neurotransmitter norepinephrine and the closely related epinephrine (adrenalin), used in the sympathetic nervous system. By releasing them into the blood, the norepinephrine and epinephrine travel throughout the body and are available for a longer period of time than they would be if they were only released in synapses.

The activities of the parasympathetic nervous system are discrete and short acting. That means that they can involve individual parts of the body and they can be shut down instantly when danger approaches. This makes sense; to get ready to run or fight, we cannot wait for the parasympathetic nervous system to shut off. Danger often approaches very rapidly. Any delay might result in our death. Think about the times something has scared you: perhaps a near-miss with an accident in your car, or someone startling you while you were out walking in the dark. Didn't you instantly feel the effects of the sympathetic nervous system, even if you were very relaxed beforehand? Didn't it take some time to again become relaxed, even after you were sure the danger had passed? If so, you have experienced the qualities of these systems that we have just discussed.

12B.7 The Anatomic Arrangement of Your Motor Nerves

We need now to think about the anatomic arrangement of the motor nerves of the somatic and autonomic nervous systems. In the somatic nervous system (remember, the effector is skeletal muscle), there is a single motor neuron extending from the CNS to the muscle fiber (**FIGURE 12.24a**). The cell body of that neuron is within the CNS; only its fiber travels in the PNS. We refer to this as a single motor neuron pathway.

The motor nerves of the autonomic nervous system have a very different arrangement (Figure 12.24b). We begin with one motor neuron in the CNS, which sends its fiber out into the PNS. This fiber synapses with a second motor neuron within a ganglion. Remember what a ganglion is? It is a collection of neuron cell bodies in the PNS. The autonomic nervous system contains ganglia. The second motor neuron sends its fiber from the ganglion to the effector, which may be smooth muscle, cardiac muscle, or glands. This is a two-motor neuron pathway.

There is also an interesting difference in the ways in which these two systems inhibit the activity of an effector. If we need to inhibit the activity of an effector in the somatic nervous system (remember, we may need to keep an antagonist from contracting to allow the prime mover to work), inhibition cannot be at the level of the effector. In the somatic nervous system, inhibition is always at the level of the motor neuron. A neuron that precedes the motor neuron in its pathway releases an inhibitory neurotransmitter, where it synapses with the motor neuron. This inhibits the motor neuron from generating an action potential, effectively keeping the effector from becoming activated.

In the autonomic nervous system, inhibition is at the level of the effector. We have dual innervation using two antagonistic systems. When we need to inhibit the activity of an autonomic effector, we merely fire the motor neuron that inhibits the activity of that effector.

To help you to understand this phenomenon, think about driving your car. Assuming you have an automatic transmission, you have two pedals: the gas pedal speeds the car up, and the break pedal slows the car down. The car is the effector. When you are operating the car like the somatic nervous system, you use only one leg (the motor neuron), and it is attached to the gas pedal. When you want to increase the activity of the effector (go faster), you stimulate the motor neuron (your leg) and press down on the gas pedal. When you want to go slower, you have no mechanism at the effector (car) to do this. You simply inhibit your leg from stepping on the gas pedal, and the car slows down.

When you drive your car like the autonomic nervous system, you use both legs. One will stimulate the activity of the car (it is attached to the gas pedal); the other will inhibit the activity of the car (it is attached to the break pedal). That is dual innervation, as seen in the autonomic nervous system.

12B.8 Your Cranial Nerves

There are 12 pairs of nerves that arise not from your spinal cord, but from your brain (**TABLE 12.2**). It is important to know something about the cranial nerves, as damage to them resulting in functional deficits sometimes occurs because of illness or injury. The following table concisely lists the name and number of each nerve pair, as well as where the nerve originates in the brain and the functions of that nerve. A mnemonic device such as "Only on overcast Tuesdays, Tom and Frank visit grand Victorian antique homes" will help you to memorize the order of the names.

12B.9 Your Neurotransmitters

Now that we have studied neuron physiology and the brain, we are ready to consider the various chemicals used as neurotransmitters. Since we have already discussed how neurotransmitters work, we can learn this information most readily from a table. **TABLE 12.3** lists the

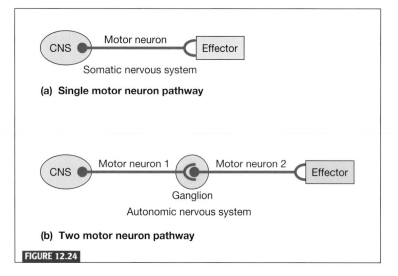

FIGURE 12.24

Compare the structure of a single motor neuron pathway (a) in the somatic nervous system to that of a two motor neuron pathway (b) in the autonomic nervous system.

Table 12.2   Your Cranial Nerves

Name and Number	Origin	Function
I. Olfactory	Cerebral cortex	Sense of smell
II. Optic	Thalamus	Sense of sight
III. Oculomotor	Midbrain	Eye movement, focusing, and pupil diameter
IV. Trochlear	Midbrain	Eye movement
V. Trigeminal	Pons	Sensation from head, face, and mouth, and chewing
VI. Abducens	Pons	Eye movement
VII. Facial	Pons	Facial sensation and expression, taste (anterior two thirds of tongue), tear secretion, and salivation
VIII. Vestibulocochlear	Pons & medulla oblongata	Hearing, balance, and equilibrium
IX. Glossopharyngeal	Medulla oblongata	Swallowing, taste (posterior one third of tongue), salivation, sensation from soft palate and pharynx, blood pressure, and dissolved blood gas concentration
X. Vagus	Medulla oblongata	Activity and sensation for parts of ear, diaphragm, pharynx, respiratory tract, G.I. tract (esophagus through colon), and heart
XI. Accessory	Medulla oblongata	Head movement, voluntary component of swallowing, control of vocal cords
XII. Hypoglossal	Medulla oblongata	Voluntary tongue movements, speech, and swallowing

G.I. = gastrointestinal.

Table 12.3   Your Neurotransmitters

Neurotransmitter and Class	Location and Features of Interest	Effect
Choline Derivatives		
Acetylcholine	Brain, spinal cord, neuroeffector junctions, autonomic preganglionic fibers, parasympathetic postganglionic fibers.	Direct, excitatory
Amino Acids		
Glutamic and aspartic acids	Brain. These neurotransmitters play a major role in injury to the brain after crossing the blood-brain barrier as a consequence of stroke or head trauma.	Direct/indirect, excitatory
Glycine	Spinal cord: this neurotransmitter is the smallest amino acid.	Direct, inhibitory
GABA	Brain. Increased activity of this unusual amino acid is a probable mechanism of action of antianxiety drugs (e.g., diazepam).	Direct/indirect, inhibitory
Amines	All major psychedelic drugs resemble these tyrosine/tryptophan derivatives. Amine neurotransmitters are decreased in people suffering from depression.	
Dopamine	Brain. Role in emotional responses, subconscious movement of skeletal muscle, separation of real from imagined. Decreased in Parkinson's disease; may be increased in schizophrenia. Some antipsychotic drugs block dopamine receptors; cocaine and amphetamines may reduce removal of dopamine from synapses.	Indirect/direct, inhibitory
Catecholamines (epinephrine and norepinephrine)	Brain. Postganglionic sympathetic neurons. Role in mood regulation, temperature regulation, and dreaming.	Indirect, excitatory
Serotonin	Brain. Potent vasoactive compound. Role in sleep, sensory perception, mood, temperature regulation, cerebral blood flow. LSD inhibits serotonin activity. Prozac inhibits serotonin inactivation (increasing its effect). Possible role in appetite regulation; some appetite suppressants stimulate serotonin. Also thought to be deficient in people with ADHD.	Indirect, excitatory
Neuropeptides	These are not true neurotransmitters; they modulate the effects of neurotransmitters.	
Opiods (enkephalins, endorphins, dynorphins)	Brain and spinal cord. Major activity is inhibition of pain perception by inhibiting release of substance P. Roles also in sexual activity, learning, and temperature regulation. Involved in depression and schizophrenia.	
Substance P	Sensory nerves, spinal cord, brain. Role in perception of pain.	

GABA = gamma amino butyric acid, LSD = lysergic acid diethylamide, ADHD = attention deficit hyperactivity disorder.

neurotransmitters, their chemical class, example locations, and their effects. Effects listed include whether they are excitatory or inhibitory, but please keep in mind that this difference is determined by the neurotransmitter receptor, not the neurotransmitter itself. Effects listed also include whether this activity is direct, meaning that it opens a chemically gated channel in the receptor, or indirect, meaning that it works through a second-messenger system (to be covered in Chapter 13). Interesting facts are also included about some of the neurotransmitters.

This ends our discussion of the brain. We are now ready to turn our attention to the spinal cord. Remember, the spinal cord is still part of the CNS.

What You Should Know

1. A bundle of nerve fibers in the CNS is a tract; in the PNS, it is a nerve.
2. A group of neuron cell bodies in the CNS is a nucleus; in the PNS, it is a ganglion.
3. Your brainstem is directly superior to your spinal cord and consists of the medulla oblongata, pons, and midbrain.
4. The functions of the medulla oblongata include conveying ascending and descending tracts; a role in movement, posture, and equilibrium; and the location of several vital and nonvital reflex centers.
5. The pons is directly superior to the medulla oblongata, conveys ascending and descending tracts, and contains nuclei involved in respiration.
6. The midbrain is the most superior structure of your brainstem, and contains numerous tracts and several reflex centers.
7. The diencephalon consists of the thalamus, the epithalamus, and the hypothalamus.
8. The thalamus is an important sensory structure.
9. The hypothalamus has many complex and important functions, including control of the autonomic nervous system and coordination of the activities of the nervous and endocrine systems.
10. The cerebrum is by far the largest portion of the human brain and is the structure that gives us our creative, intellectual, and scientific abilities.
11. In the cerebrum, the gray matter is superficial to the white matter.
12. The arrangement of gyri and sulci give the cerebral cortex much more room for gray matter.
13. The cerebral white matter is made up of association, commissural, and projection fibers.
14. Basal ganglia are actually nuclei found within cerebral white matter. They influence the motor activities.
15. Specific functions can be ascribed to discrete areas of the cerebrum.
16. The cerebellum is the second largest component of your brain and is located in an inferior and posterior position.
17. The gray matter of the cerebellum is superficial and is called the folia.
18. The white matter of the cerebellum is deep to the gray matter and is called the arbor vitae.
19. The cerebellum is your body's quality control center for movement.
20. Your limbic system, located at the border of your diencephalon and cerebrum, is involved in interpretation and expression of emotions and in conversion of short-term memory to long-term memory.
21. Your sympathetic and parasympathetic nervous systems are two components of your autonomic nervous system and are antagonistic to each other.
22. The sympathetic nervous system controls the fight-or-flight response. Its activities are global and long lasting.
23. The parasympathetic nervous system controls the energy conservation and restoration response. Its activities are discrete and short acting.
24. The somatic nervous system uses a single motor neuron pathway. The autonomic nervous system uses a two motor neuron pathway that, therefore, contains ganglia.
25. In the somatic nervous system, inhibition is at the level of the motor neuron; in the autonomic nervous system, inhibition is at the level of the effector.
26. Your brain gives rise to 12 pairs of cranial nerves. You must know their names, locations, and functions.
27. Neurotransmitters may be choline derivatives, amino acids, or amines. You must know examples of each of these.

What Did You Learn?

Multiple choice questions: choose the best answer.

1. Located in the medulla oblongata, the decussation of pyramids is the place where _____ tracts cross over.
   a. Sensory
   b. Motor
   c. Both of the above
   d. Neither of the above

2. Which of the following is not a vital reflex center of the medulla oblongata?
   a. The cardiac center
   b. The medullary rhythmicity area
   c. The vasomotor center
   d. All of the above are vital reflex centers
   e. None of the above is a vital reflex centers.

3. Integration of the senses of light touch, pressure, temperature, and pain occurs in the:
   a. Pons
   b. Midbrain
   c. Thalamus
   d. Hypothalamus

4. Which of the following coordinates the activities of the nervous and endocrine systems?
   a. Brainstem
   b. Thalamus
   c. Hypothalamus
   d. Cerebrum
   e. Cerebellum

5. The sensations of thirst and hunger are controlled by:
   a. Brainstem
   b. Thalamus
   c. Hypothalamus
   d. Cerebrum
   e. Cerebellum

6. The _____ is the largest portion of the human brain.
   a. Brainstem
   b. Thalamus
   c. Hypothalamus
   d. Cerebrum
   e. Cerebellum

7. In the cerebrum, the _____ is superficial.
   a. Gray matter
   b. White matter
   c. Blue-green matter
   d. Doesn't matter

8. A very deep fold into the surface of the cerebrum is a _____.
   a. Gyrus
   b. Fissure
   c. Sulcus
   d. Foramen
   e. None of the above

9. Which of the following connects together the two cerebral hemispheres?
   a. Corpus callosum
   b. Massa intermedia
   c. Both of the above
   d. Neither of the above

10. The internal capsule of the cerebrum is composed of _____.
    a. Projection fibers
    b. Association fibers
    c. Commissural fibers
    d. Long stringy fibers

11. The postcentral gyrus is the primary _____ area.
    a. Motor
    b. Sensory
    c. Gustatory
    d. Speech
    e. All of the above

12. The _____ is your quality-control center for movement.
    a. Cerebrum
    b. Cerebellum
    c. Brainstem
    d. Diencephalon
    e. None of the above

13. It is important for people to be able to express and interpret emotions appropriately. We use the _____ to do this.
    a. Precentral gyrus
    b. Diencephalon
    c. Limbic system
    d. Cerebellum
    e. None of the above

14. Increased activity of your sympathetic nervous system would cause:
    a. An increased heart rate
    b. Increased gastric activity

What Did You Learn? (continued)

c. Both of the above

d. Neither of the above

15. The activity of the parasympathetic nervous system is:

   a. Discrete and long lasting

   b. Discrete and short acting

   c. Global and long lasting

   d. Global and short acting

16. Which of the following uses a two-motor neuron pathway?

   a. The somatic nervous system

   b. The autonomic nervous system

   c. Both of the above

   d. Neither of the above

17. Inhibition in the autonomic nervous system is at the level of the _____.

   a. Effector

   b. Motor neuron

   c. Both of the above

   d. Neither of the above

18. Name the third cranial nerve.

   a. Optic

   b. Oculomotor

   c. Trochlear

   d. Glossopharyngeal

   e. Vagus

19. Glycine is a (an) _____ neurotransmitter.

   a. Choline derivative

   b. Amine

c. Amino acid

d. It's not a neurotransmitter, it's a neuropeptide

20. The effect of serotonin is:

   a. Indirect and excitatory

   b. Direct and excitatory

   c. Indirect and inhibitory

   d. Direct and inhibitory

Short answer questions: answer briefly and in your own words.

1. Damage to the brainstem can be immediately fatal. What activities of the brainstem make this a possibility?

2. Your body has two main regulators of homeostasis. Please explain what part of the brain coordinates the activities of these regulators and why this is necessary.

3. The surface of your cerebrum is highly folded. Why is this so? Please explain how this structural adaptation increases our intellectual abilities.

4. Which activities are centered in the right cerebral hemisphere? Does each hemisphere act independent of the other? What structures allow the two hemispheres to interact?

5. What effects might you observe in someone who has suffered damage to their cerebellum?

6. The anatomical arrangement of your autonomic nervous system differs from that of your somatic nervous system. What special abilities does this give to your autonomic nervous system? Consider the effectors that are innervated by the autonomic nervous system and explain why this arrangement is desirable.

Your Spinal Cord

What You Will Learn

- The structure and location of the spinal cord.
- The structure and anatomical arrangement of the spinal nerves.
- The cross-sectional anatomy of the spinal cord.

You are certainly aware of the importance of the spinal cord. Perhaps everyone has known or heard of someone who has suffered a spinal cord injury and the functional deficits that result from such an injury. You may not be as familiar with the anatomy of this fascinating structure. We will begin this section with a discussion of the gross anatomy and histology of the spinal cord.

12C.1 The Anatomy of Your Spinal Cord

The spinal cord is located in the vertebral canal, which is made up of the vertebral foramina of all the vertebrae (**FIGURE 12.25a**). Like the brain, the spinal cord is surrounded by meninges (Figure 12.25b). It is held in the middle of the vertebral canal by extensions of pia mater called denticulate ligaments. These connect directly to the dura mater like spokes of a wheel to hold the spinal cord away from the bony wall. The epidural space between the dura mater and the vertebrae contains adipose tissue to further cushion the cord.

Your spinal cord is anchored superiorly by its attachment to the brain stem. Its inferior end is anchored to your coccyx by strands of dense regular connective tissue called filum terminale (end threads). This is of great importance when you stand on your head.

Your Spinal Nerves

The spinal cord gives rise laterally to spinal nerves, which enter and exit the spinal cord as nerve roots. The posterior or dorsal nerve root is purely sensory (afferent) and contains a ganglion (the dorsal root ganglion). The anterior root is purely motor and contains no ganglion. The nerve roots join together to become spinal nerves. Spinal nerves are part of the PNS (remember, the CNS is made up of the brain and spinal cord only).

There are 31 pairs of spinal nerves; each one corresponds to one nerve segment. These correlate with the number of vertebrae, as shown in **TABLE 12.4**.

Note a few facts about the information in Table 12.4. First, note that the number of spinal nerve pairs corresponds to the number of vertebrae, except that in the case of the cervical vertebrae there is one extra pair of spinal nerves. We already know that the spinal nerves exit between the vertebrae (Chapter 7). In fact, you should remember that the spinal nerves pass through the intervertebral foramen between vertebrae (**FIGURE 12.26**). How do we account for the extra pair of spinal nerves? One pair exits superior to the first cervical vertebrae (the atlas). All others pass between vertebrae.

Now note that spinal nerves pass between all vertebrae all the way down to the first coccygeal vertebrae. But how far down the vertebral canal does the spinal cord extend? Note in Figure 12.25 that the tapered distal end on the spinal cord (the conus medullaris) is located at the border between the first and second lumbar vertebrae. How then do we have spinal nerves beyond the end of the spinal cord? Think about it for a minute and the answer becomes easy. Spinal nerves extend down the vertebral canal beyond the end of the spinal cord to exit at the proper intervertebral foramen. This bundle of spinal nerves that travels down the vertebral canal is called the cauda equina (meaning horse's tail). In fact, it does look like a horse's tail (Figure 12.25).

Your Spinal Cord in Cross Section

When we examine the spinal cord in cross section, we find that, unlike the cerebrum and cerebellum, the white matter is superficial and the gray matter is deep. Does this arrangement make sense? Sure it does; with spinal nerves entering and exiting the white matter, if the gray matter were superficial to the white matter, the nerve roots would have to pass through the gray matter.

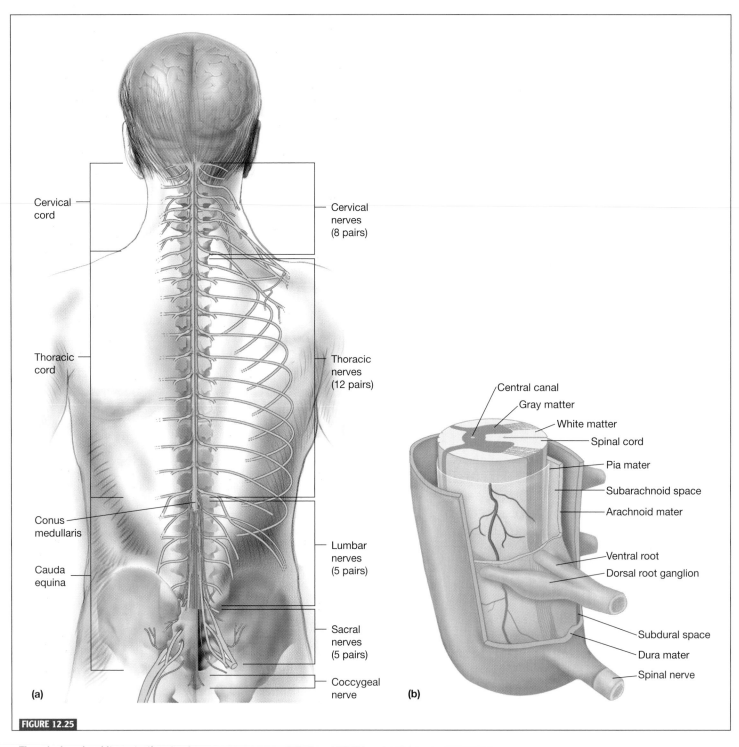

Cervical
cord

Cervical
nerves
(8 pairs)

Thoracic
cord

Thoracic
nerves
(12 pairs)

Conus
medullaris

Cauda
equina

Lumbar
nerves
(5 pairs)

Sacral
nerves
(5 pairs)

Coccygeal
nerve

(a)

Central canal

Gray matter

White matter

Spinal cord

Pia mater

Subarachnoid space

Arachnoid mater

Ventral root

Dorsal root ganglion

Subdural space

Dura mater

Spinal nerve

(b)

FIGURE 12.25

The spinal cord and its protective structures.

With the white matter superficial, this does not happen. Notice in **FIGURE 12.27** that the gray matter is in the shape of the letter "H." The regions of this gray matter are called horns. Note also that the central canal of the spinal cord is within the gray commissure (which is <u>not</u> made of commissural fibers). Cerebrospinal fluid flows within the central canal.

The regions of white matter are called columns, which makes sense, as the white matter tracts run longitudinally (up and down) the spinal cord. There are two grooves in the spinal cord, and it is useful to know their names. They are important landmarks that aid in locating regions of damaged tissue that might be seen in histologic sections. The posterior groove is shallow, so

Table 12.4 The Spinal Nerves

Region	Number of Vertebrae	Number of Spinal Nerve Pairs
Cervical	7	8
Thoracic	12	12
Lumbar	5	5
Sacral	5 (fused)	5
Coccygeal	Variable	1

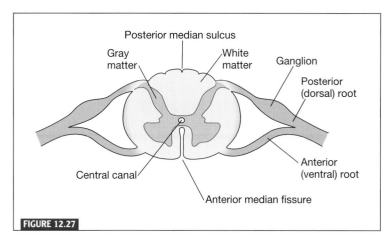

FIGURE 12.27

A transverse section of the spinal cord showing spinal nerve roots.

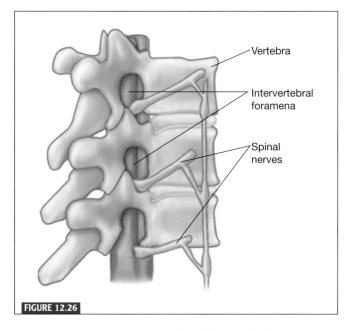

FIGURE 12.26

Spinal nerves exit between vertebrae, through intervertebral foramena.

it is a sulcus: the posterior median sulcus. The anterior groove is deeper, so it is a fissure: the anterior median fissure. It is easy to confuse which side has a sulcus and which has a fissure, so to keep them straight use the initials PMS (posterior median sulcus).

After the spinal nerves exit the vertebral canal, they divide into branches called rami (ramus is singular). These rami travel throughout the body and then form networks with rami from adjacent nerves. These networks are called plexuses (plexus is singular). The cross sectional anatomy of a nerve is similar to that of a muscle. Nerve fibers are surrounded by endoneurium (connective tissue) within fascicles, which are surrounded by perineurium. The entire nerve is surrounded by epineurium.

What You Should Know

1. The spinal cord is located within the vertebral canal.
2. Denticulate ligaments are extensions of pia mater that connect directly to the dura mater to hold the spinal cord in place.
3. The filum terminale attaches the distal end of the spinal cord to the coccyx.
4. Your spinal cord gives rise to 31 spinal nerve pairs.
5. Spinal nerves exit the vertebral canal between vertebrae through intervertebral foramina.
6. The attachment of the spinal nerves to the spinal cord is through roots. Each posterior (dorsal) root is sensory and contains a ganglion; each anterior root is motor and does not contain a ganglion.
7. The white matter of the spinal cord is superficial.
8. The gray matter of the spinal cord is in the form of the letter "H" with regions designated as horns and a commissure. The central region (the gray commissure) contains the central canal of the spinal cord.
9. An anterior median fissure and a posterior median sulcus can be identified on the surface of the spinal cord.
10. The branches of spinal nerves are called rami; these interconnect into networks called plexuses.
11. A nerve has an anatomical arrangement similar to that of skeletal muscle. Nerve fibers within fascicles are separated by endoneurium, perineurium surrounds the fascicles, and the entire nerve is surrounded by epineurium.

What Did You Learn?

Multiple choice questions: choose the best answer.

1. Extensions of pia mater that hold the spinal cord in the middle of the vertebral canal are called:
   a. Filum terminale
   b. Cordae tendineae
   c. Cauda equina
   d. Denticulate ligaments
   e. Conus medularis

2. What anchors the distal end of the spinal cord?
   a. Filum terminale
   b. Cordae tendineae
   c. Cauda equina
   d. Denticulate ligaments
   e. Conus medularis

3. The dorsal root of the spinal nerves is:
   a. Sensory
   b. Motor
   c. Mixed

4. Which root of a spinal nerve contains ganglia?
   a. Posterior
   b. Anterior
   c. Both of the above
   d. Neither of the above

5. How far down the vertebral canal does the spinal cord extend?
   a. All the way
   b. Through the end of the sacrum
   c. To the border of the fourth and fifth lumbar vertebrae
   d. To the border of the first and second lumbar vertebrae
   e. Only to the fifth thoracic vertebrae

6. The white mater of the spinal cord is:
   a. Superficial
   b. Deep
   c. Mixed with the gray matter
   d. There is no white matter in the spinal cord

7. A sulcus is found on the _____ surface of the spinal cord.
   a. Anterior
   b. Lateral
   c. Posterior
   d. Anterior and posterior

8. Branches of the spinal nerves are called:
   a. Plexuses
   b. Rami
   c. Filum terminale
   d. Cauda equine

Short answer questions: answer briefly and in your own words.

1. What are the consequences to a spinal nerve if an intervertebral disk were to be crushed? How does the anatomical arrangement of these two structures contribute to this risk?

2. Where is the distal end of the spinal cord located? What holds this end of the spinal cord in place? Do spinal nerves exit between inferior vertebrae? If so, how do they get there?

Reflexes and Senses

What You Will Learn

- What a reflex is and the components of a complete reflex arc.
- The anatomy and physiology of your eyes.
- The anatomy and physiology of your ears.
- How the senses of taste and smell work.

12D.1 Reflexes: Your Nervous System in Action

Reflexes are involuntary responses to stimuli and are usually very similar between individuals. They are so similar, in fact, that they are routinely used to determine whether neural pathways are intact or damaged. The complete functional unit of a reflex is called a reflex arc and consists of a receptor, a sensory nerve, a center, a motor nerve, and an effector (**FIGURE 12.28**). Various types of receptors exist, and we will discuss them briefly in our section on the senses. Sensory nerves, you already know about. The center of the reflex arc is where integration takes place. Integration is that go, no-go decision that must be made: to respond or not to respond to the sensory input being received. If the center is merely where a sensory neuron synapses with a motor neuron, the reflex arc is called monosynaptic. If one or more association neuron lies between the sensory and motor neurons, the reflex is polysynaptic.

Reflexes may be ipsilateral (sensory and motor activities on the same side) or contralateral (sensory and motor activities on opposite sides). Reflexes may be somatic (effector is skeletal muscle) or autonomic (effector is smooth muscle, cardiac muscle, or gland). They may be cranial or spinal, depending on where the center is located; the center is always within the CNS, however. They may also involve reciprocal innervation, meaning that in addition to exciting the motor neuron of the prime mover, the motor neuron of the antagonist must be inhibited from generating an action potential.

Somatic reflexes are those with which you may be the most familiar. Examples of somatic reflexes include the patellar (knee-jerk) reflex and the Achilles tendon reflex, both of which involve stretching a tendon by gently striking it. This stimulates receptors that, in turn, cause the characteristic response. Autonomic reflexes include the dilation and constriction of your pupils in response to light and the movement of substances in your digestive tract after a meal.

12D.2 Your Senses

We will briefly discuss several senses here. First we will consider sight, then hearing and balance. Afterward, we will consider receptors used in smell and taste.

■ Your Amazing Eyes

The eye is a truly amazing organ. It has the ability to convert a lighted image into electrical impulses that your brain can then interpret as the scene in front of you. Look at **FIGURE 12.29** (and note that it is your eyes that enable you to do this). The structures of the eye are organized into tunics. A tunic is a sheath or covering, and we can assign the components of the eye to three tunics.

The Anatomy of Your Eyes: A Tale of Three Tunics

The fibrous tunic contains the sclera, or white of the eye, and the cornea, or clear anterior part of the eye. The sclera provides shape and protection; the cornea also provides shape and protection, but it admits and refracts (bends) light as well.

The vascular tunic contains the choroid, the iris, and the ciliary body. The choroid is the vasculature at the back of the eye. This provides nourishment for the eye, but also absorbs scattered light. The reflection of excess light off the choroid is why a person's eyes often glow red in a photograph lighted by a flash bulb. The iris is the structure that contains the pupil, a hole in the iris through which light enters the eye. The iris regulates the amount of light entering the eye. In bright light, the iris constricts the pupil, effectively admitting less light. In dim light, the iris enlarges (dilates) the pupil to admit

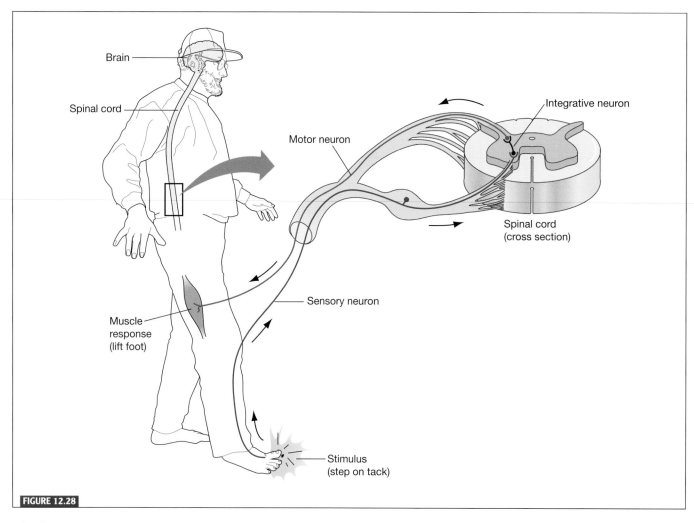

FIGURE 12.28

A reflex arc.

more of the available light. This is a reflex action. The ciliary body is composed of the ciliary muscle and the ciliary process. The ciliary muscle alters the shape of the lens to enable focusing on objects that are near or far. The ciliary process secretes aqueous humor into the anterior cavity (more on this in a moment).

The nervous tunic contains the retina. The retina converts light into receptor potentials (electrical impulses), which become the action potentials of the optic nerve (cranial nerve II) and transmit the image to the brain. Photoreceptive cells called rods and cones are primarily responsible for this amazing conversion. The approximately 100 million rods, which contain the photopigment rhodopsin, are responsible for black and white vision and vision in dim light. Images generated by rods tend to have low resolution; they are grainy and lack great detail. The approximately 30 million cones are for color vision. One region of the retina, called the macula lutea, contains most of the cones and no rods.

The highest concentration of cones is found in one area of the macula lutea, called the fovea centralis (central cup-like depression). The fovea centralis (Figure 12.29) is the region of the retina that develops the sharpest images. Each cone contains one of three different photopigments.

Each molecule of photopigment contains a glycoprotein, called an opsin, and retinal, a derivative of vitamin A (eat your carrots). Absorption of light by these molecules causes a conformational (shape) change in the opsin; this change starts the signal transduction process of converting light to a graded potential to initiate an action potential. This process involves the rod and cone cells, bipolar neurons (neurons with single axons and dendrites; to review, refer to Figure 11.3), and ganglion cells. The axons of the ganglion cells are bundled together as the second cranial nerve (optic nerve) and carry images to the optic regions of the cerebrum. Rhodopsin is best stimulated by blue to green light. The remaining three opsins are best stimulated

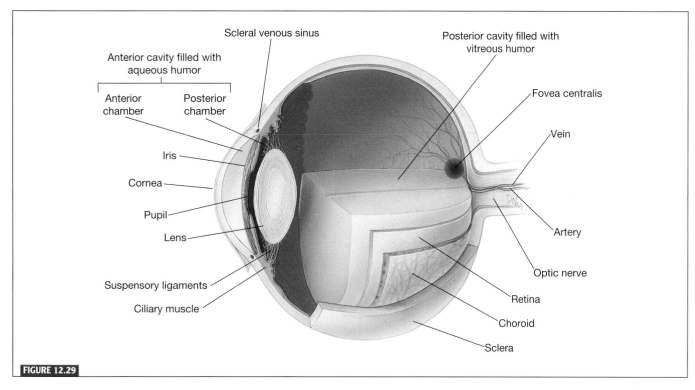

Scleral venous sinus

Anterior cavity filled with
aqueous humor

Anterior
chamber

Posterior
chamber

Iris

Cornea

Pupil

Lens

Suspensory ligaments

Ciliary muscle

Posterior cavity filled with
vitreous humor

Fovea centralis

Vein

Artery

Optic nerve

Retina

Choroid

Sclera

FIGURE 12.29

The eye.

either by blue light, green light, or red light. These three opsins allow us to see in color. Stimulation of combinations of cones allows us to see a great variety of colors.

The Cavities of Your Eyes

This figure also shows that the eye contains two cavities (Figure 12.29). The anterior cavity is made up of an anterior chamber and a posterior chamber. These chambers are separated by the iris. The ciliary body produces aqueous humor, the fluid found in the anterior cavity (both chambers). This fluid provides oxygen and nutrients to the lens and cornea, and carries away their wastes. It also maintains the shape of the anterior portion of the eyeball. It is produced at a rate that replaces it every 90 minutes. Aqueous humor leaves the anterior cavity through the scleral venous sinus (canal of Schlemm). Blockage of the scleral venous sinus results in the buildup of excess aqueous humor. This increases the pressure in the anterior cavity of the eye and is responsible for the disease glaucoma.

The posterior cavity contains a viscous (thick) fluid called the vitreous body or vitreous humor. This fluid is not replaced but remains throughout life. A thinner fluid, much like aqueous humor, is added to it and leaves by diffusing through the retina.

The two cavities of the eye are separated by the lens. Just like the lens of a magnifying glass, it is the lens of your eye that focuses the image you observe onto the retina. The shape of the lens is altered by contraction or relaxation of the ciliary muscles. This process is called accommodation. A rounder, thicker shape is necessary for near vision, while a flatter shape allows for far vision. In many people, the lens becomes less elastic with increased age, requiring the use of corrective glasses to allow for near or far vision, or perhaps for both.

■ Your Amazing Ears

Your ears, also called your vestibulocochlear organs, provide you with two very different senses. They allow you to hear, and they also provide you with a sense of balance. Two different structures in the ears are responsible for these activities. The structure of the ear is quite complex, as you can see in **FIGURE 12.30**.

The Three Components of Your Ears

We can divide the ear into three components: the external ear, the middle ear, and the inner ear. The external ear is composed of the pinna or auricle, the external auditory meatus, and the tympanic membrane or eardrum. The pinna is that flaplike structure we often think of as the ear. The pinna contains a core of elastic cartilage, which gives it its great flexibility (good for us, otherwise we would break them off!). The external

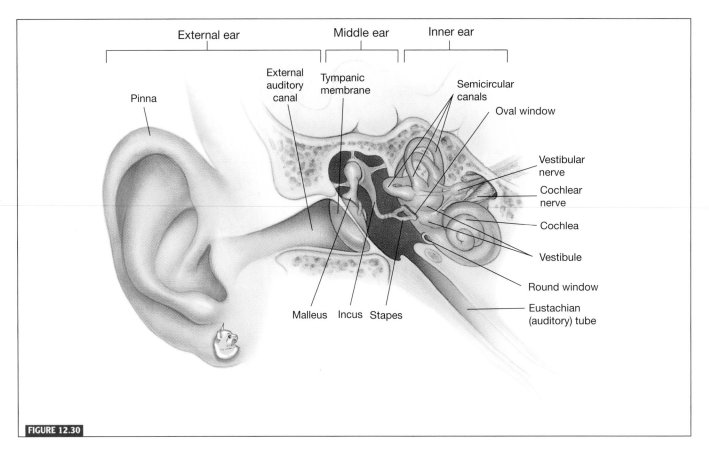

FIGURE 12.30

The ear.

auditory meatus is that passageway leading to the tympanic membrane (eardrum) that can become filled with cerumen (earwax). Cerumen is a fatty substance that is protective; it traps particulate matter and repels some insects. The tympanic membrane is covered externally by a thin layer of stratified squamous epithelium and internally by simple cuboidal epithelium. A thin layer of connective tissue rich in elastic and collagenous fibers is found between these two epithelia. The purpose of the external ear is to funnel vibrations in the air to the tympanic membrane, which, in turn, will also vibrate.

Your Middle Ear

The middle ear is also called the tympanic cavity. It is a chamber within the temporal bone and begins at the tympanic membrane. It communicates with the pharynx through the pharyngotympanic tube. This tube has alternately been called the auditory tube and the Eustachian tube. The walls of the pharyngotympanic tube are usually compressed together, leaving no lumen. When we move our pharynx in certain ways (swallowing, yawning, exaggerated depression of our mandible), we open this tube, allowing air to pass through it. This is important, as it is the only way we can balance the pres-

sures on either side of the tympanic membrane. You understand how important this is if you have ever flown or traveled in the mountains when your pharyngotympanic tubes have been blocked by a head cold. The middle ear also contains three bones: the malleus (hammer), incus (anvil), and stapes (stirrup). (I'll bet you thought you were done learning the names of bones). The malleus is partially inserted into the tympanic membrane. It articulates with the incus, which also articulates with the stapes. The stapes is partially embedded in the oval window at the start of the internal ear. These bones articulate with each other in synovial joints, allowing them free movement. When the tympanic membrane vibrates, due to the reception of sound (vibrations in air), these bones move against each other transmitting those vibrations to the oval window. If you have ever been on a rocky beach in a storm and noticed how waves could set stones in motion against each other, you will have a pretty good idea of how these bones move in response to sound.

Two of these bones (malleus and stapes) provide the insertions for the tensor muscles. These muscles contract when we experience loud, harsh sounds, thus tightening the tympanic membrane and oval window. This diminishes their vibrations and serves as a protective mechanism, reducing the amount of damage these sounds do to our hearing. Note that this mechanism only reduces the damage but does not eliminate it. Keep that in mind, and wear hearing protection when needed.

Your Inner Ear

The inner ear, or labyrinth (maze), is composed of two major parts: the osseous (bony) labyrinth and the membranous labyrinth. These are a series of fluid-filled cavities and tubes within the temporal bone, posterior to the eye sockets. These fluids are important for both the transmission of vibrations generated by sound and the movements important to our sense of balance. The fluid of the osseous labyrinth is called perilymphatic fluid (perilymph) but is actually CSF. The bony labyrinth is in direct communication with the subarachnoid space.

The fluid of the membranous labyrinth is called endolymphatic fluid or endolymph. It is modified interstitial fluid, having more potassium (K^+) than normal interstitial fluid. Much of the membranous labyrinth is a series of membrane-bounded tubes containing endolymph, floating in the perilymph of the osseous labyrinth.

The osseous labyrinth is composed of three main structures: the vestibule, the semicircular canals, and the cochlea. At specific locations, the simple squamous epithelium of the inner ear is modified into special sensory receptor cells, important in the generation of graded receptor potentials for hearing and balance. The vestibule contains the saccule and the utricle of the membranous labyrinth. The saccule and utricle contain motion-sensitive balance-receptor membranes called maculae. There are three semicircular (half-round) canals, each of which has a different orientation. They contain the membranous labyrinth semicircular ducts and are important in balance. The cochlea (meaning land snail) resembles a coiled snail shell with two and one half turns. The cochlea is compartmentalized longitudinally into three chambers. The vestibular duct and the tympanic duct contain perilymph. The cochlear duct, which is situated between the other two, contains endolymph. In its membrane, the cochlear duct contains the organ of Corti, the site of the cochlear hair cells. Cochlear hair cells possess large stereocilia on their apical (superficial) surfaces and serve as receptors for sound. Stereocilia are not actually cilia; they are long microvilli that move readily when exposed to vibrations.

Hearing: Vibrations Become Action Potentials

Vibrations in the air (sound) are converted into action potentials (described in Chapter 8) in the following way. Sounds set the tympanic membrane vibrating, which causes the bones of the middle ear to vibrate, which causes the oval window to vibrate. This causes the vestibular perilymph to vibrate, which causes the endolymph within the cochlear duct to vibrate. The cochlear hair cells also vibrate. This moves their stereocilia, which opens pressure-sensitive (gated) ion channels in the plasmalemma of the hair cells. This generates graded (receptor) potentials, which are transmitted to neurons of cranial nerve VIII (vestibulocochlear nerve). If threshold is reached, an action potential is generated in these neurons, which is transmitted to the auditory portions of the cerebrum. Higher pitched (shorter wavelength) sounds cause these vibrations to occur in the proximal region of the cochlear duct (nearer to the oval window), while lower (longer wavelength) sounds cause the vibrations to occur more distally. It is in this way that we perceive pitch.

Balance

Balance involves the vestibule and semicircular canals of the inner ear. Fluid moving within the structures of the inner ear signals information about movement and the position of the head and body. Within the saccule and utricle of the vestibule, the maculae contain hair cells. These hair cells are surrounded by a gel-like liquid containing calcium carbonate crystals called statoconia. Movement of your head causes changes in the pressure applied by the statoconia to the hair cells. This information is relayed to the cerebrum via the eighth cranial nerve and indicates the angle of your head.

The semicircular canals have widened regions called ampullae. Within the ampullae, cristae or cristae ampullaris are located. The cristae contain hair cells and are also covered by a gel-like liquid. Movement of the head causes the endolymph in the semicircular canals to flow. This alters the pressure on the gel covering the hair cells. This affects the graded potential generated by these cells. The graded potentials may initiate or inhibit action potential generation in neurons of the eighth cranial nerve. As the three semicircular canals exist in three different planes, the cerebrum can interpret the information received from this organ as information about the direction and rate of movement of the head.

■ Your Senses of Taste and Smell

Imagine your world without your senses of taste and smell. It would certainly be a less enjoyable place. It would also be a much less safe place. Our smell and taste senses lead us to food and encourage us to eat. They warn us when our food or drink is tainted or unsafe. Smell in particular also warns us of environmental dangers. How often are people saved from death in a fire because someone smelled smoke? Although related, these senses have certain anatomical and functional differences. We will begin by considering the sense of taste.

You must have at some point heard of taste buds, even if it was during an advertisement for some packaged foods. To understand how our sense of taste works, we must understand the taste buds. The vast majority of taste buds are located on the tongue. A smaller number are found on the walls of your oral cavity (your cheeks), esophagus, pharynx, and epiglottis, and even in your stomach.

A Quick Look at Your Tongue

On your tongue, taste buds are mainly found in two types of papillae: vallate and fungiform. Vallate papilla, also called circumvallate, have an interesting structure. *Vallate* means "wall"; *circum* means "around." Circumvallate papillae have a form somewhat reminiscent of a castle surrounded by a moat. A central raised structure is surrounded by a trench. It is within this trench that we find the taste receptors.

Circumvallate papillae can easily be seen on your tongue by examining it in the mirror (**FIGURE 12.31**). If you look toward the posterior aspect of your tongue, you will notice a "V"-shaped, double row of round structures. You will need a flashlight to see that far back, and it may be easier to look at someone else's tongue. These structures are the circumvallate papillae. They

are found just anterior to the sulcus terminalis, a line that separates the body of the tongue from its root. Fungiform papillae, as their name implies, resemble mushrooms. They are much more widely distributed on the tongue. In either case, these papillae contain layered structures that are the actual taste buds. Taste buds are found on the walls of circumvallate papillae and on the tops of fungiform papillae.

Taste receptor cells are present in taste buds. They line a pit in the taste bud and send fine processes called taste hairs into the pit. These taste hairs are not actual hairs at all, but are extensions of the cell, much like long microvilli. Taste receptor cells are actually only one of three cells in this parenchymal lineage (remember our terminology: the parenchyma are the cells that do the actual work of the organ; stroma are the cells that support parenchyma). Basal cells are the stem cells of this lineage. These give rise to supporting cells, which are not stroma, as we usually think of supporting cells, but actual members of the parenchymal lineage. Supporting cells differentiate into taste receptor cells. The difficult lives these cells lead (think of how we scald them, abrade them, and otherwise abuse them) makes their lives rather short; hence, we need to continually replace them.

The Primary Tastes

We have the ability to sense at least five primary tastes: acid, bitter, salty, sweet, and umami. Perhaps you have

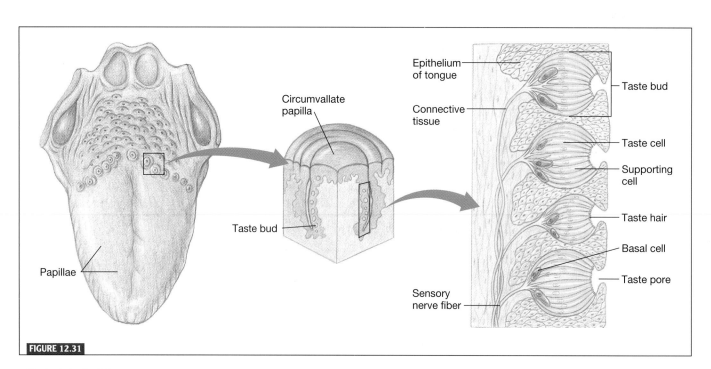

FIGURE 12.31

The taste buds of the tongue.

not heard of umami before; it has only been described recently. Umami is the flavor that makes meat appealing and is sometimes referred to as savory. Some researchers claim an additional "taste" to be that of water; we are able to sense the presence of water much the way we taste other substances.

These tastes are detected through the binding of ligand (the substance being tasted) to receptors present on the taste hair. This affects ion channel receptors, which generate graded (receptor) potentials and causes release of neurotransmitters from the receptor cells. This generates action potentials in adjacent neurons, transmitting this taste toward the brain via cranial nerve VII and IX. (Quick, what are the names of these two nerves?) The vagus (X) nerve may also transmit the sense of taste, but its role is very minor.

And Now Your Nose: It's How You Smell

Now, how about smell? Smell is pretty interesting also. Smell works in a manner very similar to taste. We have olfactory (smell) receptor cells in our olfactory epithelium, which is a pseudostratified columnar epithelium, in the following locations: the roof of the nasal cavity, the superior nasal conchae, and the nasal septum. This epithelium has a brownish to reddish-gray color because of the pigment in some of the cells. We have approximately 500 square millimeters of this epithelium. This sounds like a lot until you consider that some species of animals that have a much greater sense of smell have an area of olfactory epithelium similar to the entire surface area of their bodies!

Our olfactory receptor cells are highly modified neurons. One unique feature of these neurons is that they have a stem cell population and are replaced throughout our lifetime. Again, think about how we abuse these cells (pumped any gas lately?) and you will see why they need frequent replacement.

The olfactory receptor cells send a dendrite to the surface of the nasal cavity, where it ends in an olfactory vesicle. The olfactory vesicle is a modified region at the distal end of the dendrite, which contains several extremely long, nonmotile cilia. The internal structure of these cell extensions matches that of cilia, at least at their base, but they are nonmotile nonetheless. These cilia possess receptors for ligands called odorants. Odorants are the substances we can smell. Some researchers believe that there may be 7 to 10 primary odorants. When an odorant binds to an odorant receptor, a second messenger system is activated. We have not yet examined those systems, but you will recall that second messenger systems are one way in which neurotransmitters work (the indirect method). We will discuss second-messenger systems in our next chapter.

Activation of the second-messenger system leads to the opening of ion channels in these neurons and the generation of an action potential. These potentials travel via the olfactory nerve (cranial nerve I), through the olfactory bulbs, which lie in the cribriform plates of the ethmoid bone, superior to the nasal cavity, to the brain. Within the brain, the impulses pass from the olfactory bulbs along the olfactory tracts to reach the temporal lobes of the cerebrum.

12D.3 Take Some Time to Comprehend the Beauty of Your Nervous System

Wow, we have just finished the nervous system. That is certainly not all there is to the nervous system (not by a long shot), but it is enough for you to develop a basic understanding of how this fascinating system functions. I hope you have enjoyed learning about your nervous system. If you have not, think about going back over it again. Sometimes this system can be a little daunting, and only on the second or third time through can you relax enough to see its real beauty. The simplicity of the individual cellular activities, the complexity of their interactions, and the vast amount of which this system is capable truly are inspiring and elegant concepts.

Be sure to use the "What You Should Know" and "What Did You Learn?" features of this chapter. They are there to help you. If you do not use them, you will not become aware of what you need to work on, until perhaps it is too late (do I detect an exam coming on?). You will find many of the concepts contained in this chapter useful in our next chapter, "Slow-Acting Regulation of Your Body: Your Endocrine System."

What You Should Know

1. Reflexes are involuntary responses to stimuli and are used by health-care providers to determine the functional status of the nervous system.

2. A reflex arc is the functional unit of the nervous system; it consists of a receptor, a sensory nerve, a center, a motor neuron, and an effector.

3. Reflexes exist in different forms, including ipsilateral or contralateral, somatic or autonomic, cranial or spinal, and may or may not involve reciprocal innervation.

4. Your eyes convert light energy into electrical impulses for interpretation by your brain.

5. The structure of your eyes can be defined by three tunics: the fibrous tunic, consisting of the sclera and the cornea; the vascular tunic, consisting of the choroid, iris, and ciliary body; and the nervous tunic, consisting of the retina.

6. Photoreceptive cells (rods and cones) present in the retina use light-reactive molecules (photopigments) to convert light to a graded potential. These graded potentials trigger action potentials, which are carried to the optic regions of the cerebrum by the second cranial nerve (the optic nerve).

7. The lens separates your eye into an anterior cavity and a posterior cavity. The anterior cavity of your eye is separated into an anterior chamber and a posterior chamber by the iris.

8. The anterior cavity of your eye contains aqueous humor, which is produced by the ciliary body and is drained from this cavity by the scleral venous sinus (the canal of Schlemm).

9. The posterior cavity of your eye contains the vitreous body, a viscous fluid.

10. Your ears or vestibulocochlear organs provide you with two senses: hearing and balance.

11. Three structures make up your ears: the external ear, middle ear, and inner ear.

12. Your external ear is composed of a pinna or auricle, an external auditory meatus, and a tympanic membrane or eardrum.

13. Your middle ear or tympanic cavity is a chamber in the temporal bone that extends from the tympanic membrane to the oval window. It contains three bones: the malleus, incus, and stapes. When sound causes the tympanic membrane to vibrate, these bones transmit those vibrations to the oval window.

14. Your inner ear or labyrinth consists of an osseous labyrinth and a membranous labyrinth, fluid-filled cavities, and tubes within the temporal bone.

15. A series of fluid-filled tubes makes up much of the membranous labyrinth. These tubes float in the fluid of the osseous labyrinth.

16. The osseous labyrinth is composed of a vestibule, three semicircular canals, and the cochlea. This is where information regarding posture and movement, and vibrations generated by sound are converted into graded potentials, which may generate action potentials in cranial nerve VIII (vestibulocochlear) for interpretation by the cerebrum.

17. The senses of taste and smell are important survival mechanisms.

18. Taste buds are distributed mainly on your tongue, but are also on the walls of your oral cavity (cheeks), esophagus, pharynx, epiglottis, and stomach.

19. On your tongue, taste buds are found on raised structures called vallate and fungiform papillae.

20. Taste receptor cells are present in taste buds. They detect the five primary tastes, converting this information into graded potentials. These potentials may generate action potentials in cranial nerves VII (facial), IX (glossopharyngeal), and, to a lesser degree, X (vagus) for interpretation in the cerebrum.

21. Olfactory receptor cells present in our nasal cavities are receptors for molecules called odorants. The binding of odorants to these receptors leads to the generation of action potentials in cranial nerve I (olfactory) for interpretation by the cerebrum.

What Did You Learn?

Multiple choice questions: choose the best answer.

1. Place the components of a reflex arc in the order in which they would become active, if you were to touch a hot surface.

    1. A motor nerve
    2. A sensory nerve
    3. A receptor
    4. A center
    5. An effector

    a. 3,1,4,2,5
    b. 3,2,4,1,5
    c. 3,4,2,1,5
    d. 5,1,4,2,3
    e. 5,4,2,3,1

2. If the receptor is on the left side of the body and the effector is on the right side, the reflex is:

    a. Ipsilateral
    b. Contralateral
    c. Somatic
    d. Autonomic
    e. Monosynaptic

3. If smooth muscle is the effector, the reflex is:

    a. Ipsilateral
    b. Contralateral
    c. Somatic
    d. Autonomic
    e. Monosynaptic

4. The iris is part of the:

    a. Fibrous tunic
    b. Nervous tunic
    c. Vascular tunic
    d. None of the above

5. Rods are responsible for:

    a. Color vision
    b. Low light vision
    c. Both of the above
    d. Neither of the above

6. The scleral venous sinus drains the:

    a. Anterior chamber
    b. Posterior chamber
    c. Both of the above
    d. Neither of the above

7. Which structure is between the middle ear and the inner ear?

    a. Tympanic membrane
    b. Eardrum
    c. Either of the above
    d. Neither of the above

8. Which of the following bones is not partially embedded in either the tympanic membrane or the oval window?

    a. Stapes
    b. Malleus
    c. Incus
    d. None of the above are partially embedded in these membranes

9. Which of the following fluids is found in the membranous labyrinth?

    a. Perilymphatic fluid (perilymph)
    b. Endolymphatic fluid (endolymph)
    c. Both of the above
    d. Neither of the above

10. Which of the following fluids is continuous with the CSF?

    a. Perilymphatic fluid (perilymph)
    b. Endolymphatic fluid (endolymph)
    c. Both of the above
    d. Neither of the above

11. Taste buds are not found on which of the following?

    a. Esophagus
    b. Pharynx
    c. Epiglottis
    d. None of the above contain taste buds
    e. All of the above contain taste buds

12. Which type of papilla is arranged in a "V" pattern where the root and body of your tongue meet?

    a. Circumvallate
    b. Fungiform
    c. Both of the above
    d. Neither of the above

13. Your sense of taste is transmitted through the _____ cranial nerve.

    a. VII
    b. IX
    c. X
    d. All of the above
    e. None of the above

What Did You Learn? (continued)

14. Your sense of smell is transmitted through cranial nerve _____.

   a. I

   b. II

   c. Both of the above

   d. Neither of the above

Short answer questions: answer briefly and in your own words.

1. You are walking on the beach and you step on a sharp shell. Diagram and describe the activities that take place in the reflex arc that helps you to avoid injury.

2. In the scenario described in the previous question, you can imagine that while lifting your foot off of the sharp shell, you must maintain your balance. Please describe that process as well.

3. As you read this question, your eyes and brain are working together to form an image that you can interpret. How do they do this? What structures are involved in this process? Please follow the process through from the question before you on the page to the answer you will write. Explain what steps must occur and how they occur.

Breaching Homeostasis . . . When Things Go Wrong

Stroke

Certainly you have heard the term *stroke* and, in fact, may know someone who has suffered one of these debilitating and sometimes fatal events. But what actually is a stroke? This is the topic of this chapter's "Breaching Homeostasis" section.

Stroke is a clinical term, applied when a patient has sudden onset neurological deficits resulting from a localized brain lesion of vascular origin. Simply put, an artery in the brain either becomes blocked or bleeds, resulting in neural tissue damage. Our discussion will focus mainly on the type of stroke more precisely called cerebral infarction. An infarction occurs as a result of focal ischemic damage: loss of blood flow to a specific area, resulting in cell death.

Cerebral infarctions are quite common in Western society. People in these cultures frequently suffer from atherosclerosis (the topic of Chapter 16's "Breaching Homeostasis" section). When atherosclerosis occurs in cerebral arteries, such as the internal carotid arteries, the vertebral arteries, and their tributaries, the risk of stroke greatly increases. Atherosclerotic lesions may cause gradual narrowing of an artery; more commonly as a cause of stroke, the surface of these lesions rupture and a thrombosis (clot within a vessel) develops. These thromboses may completely block (occlude) the artery, leading to a lack of blood flow downstream. Alternately, atherosclerosis and subsequent thrombosis elsewhere in the body may cause fragments of a clot to travel in the bloodstream (thromboemboli). A thromboembolus may lodge in a cerebral artery, occluding the artery and causing a stroke.

Think back to the "Breaching Homeostasis" section in Chapter 3. There we learned that either the lack of some necessary substance or the presence of some toxic substance can lead to cell death. Both mechanisms play a role in neuronal death after stroke. Obviously, when the blood supply to cells as metabolically active as neurons becomes blocked, these cells rapidly become injured because of oxygen deficiency. We typically think of cell death after stroke as resulting from oxygen depletion, but that is not the whole story. Neurons continue to die over a period of several days after the initial occlusive event. Some of these neurons die because of the presence of substances toxic to them. Remember the blood-brain barrier? After cerebral ischemia, the blood-brain barrier goes down (the barrier becomes permeable) in the region surrounding the lesion. This allows substances such as glutamic acid and aspartic acid to enter the brain from the blood. Some of these substances are used as neurotransmitters; their uncontrolled presence causes overstimulation of the neurons that have receptors for them (excitotoxicity), leading to death of these neurons. Alternatively, some of the substances released by inflammatory cells responding to the injury kill neurons as innocent bystanders (see Chapter 21).

So, let's think about the course of events that occurs once the artery becomes occluded. Initially (within minutes), neurons that relied on that artery for their blood supply begin to die. This triggers acute inflammation (Chapter 21). Neutrophils are the first responders to this type of emergency, and they begin to arrive within the first 12 hours (within minutes if reperfusion of the occluded artery occurs). Although some glia in the affected area

Breaching Homeostasis . . . When Things Go Wrong

may also die, these stromal cells are more resistant to injury than are the neurons. Glia survive and become more active, at least in the periphery of the lesion. Over the next few days, neutrophils accumulate and begin the emergency clean-up process. Microglia and monocytes migrate into the lesion and become activated (gaining phagocytic ability and becoming macrophages). Thus, macrophages become abundant in the 3- to 5-day time period and may increase in numbers for some time. Astrocytes also become more numerous and active surrounding the lesion.

Over a time course that varies greatly, depending on the size of the lesion and whether bleeding has occurred, the necrotic tissue is removed by phagocytosis, leaving a fluid-filled cyst in its place. The margins of this cyst are walled off by astrocytes. Astrocytes perform the functions a scar would perform outside of the CNS.

So, what are the sequelae of stroke (what happens following stroke)? The loss of brain tissue is an obvious outcome. People lose different abilities depending on where the brain tissue is lost. That is directly dependent on which artery becomes blocked. An artery that has become occluded can also reperfuse if the blockage fragments or dissolves. This can transform an ischemic stroke into a hemorrhagic stroke, bleeding into the cranium, potentially with more serious consequences. Even if reperfusion does not occur, the tissue damage and inflamma-

tion may lead to swelling of the affected hemisphere. Remember that the brain is held within the skull and no room is available for expansion. Swelling, therefore, presents a major risk for further damage; herniation of brain tissue into a ventricle or through the foramen magnum.

Despite all of this, many people do survive strokes and, in fact, with medical intervention and therapy, they minimize their neurological deficits and regain much of what was lost. Necrotic brain tissue cannot be regenerated: a fluid-filled cyst will always be present where there was formerly brain tissue. Abilities return as the brain finds new ways to perform lost functions, such as rerouting messages around the injured area.

How can we avoid strokes? We can minimize our risk of stroke by limiting our risk factors. Many risk factors (such as our underlying genetics and advancing age) cannot be controlled. Other risk factors, such as smoking, obesity, hypertension, and uncontrolled diabetes, can be reduced or eliminated. Transient ischemic attacks (TIA or "ministroke") often precede an actual stroke. Transient ischemic attacks are ischemic events of limited duration that do not leave permanent deficits. Many people ignore these brief episodes of strokelike symptoms. Like a tremor before an earthquake, they are, in fact, often warnings of the stroke to come and should never be ignored. Medication after a TIA can reduce the risk of a subsequent stroke. Be sure to talk to your health-care provider about limiting your risk of stroke.

13 Slow–Acting Regulation of Your Body: Your Endocrine System

What You Will Learn

- The manner in which the endocrine and nervous systems interact in the regulation of homeostasis.
- The organs that make up the endocrine system.
- The difference between endocrine and exocrine glands.
- The types of chemicals that are used as hormones.
- What determines which cells respond to a specific hormone.
- The ways in which hormone-receptor binding causes cells to respond.
- How second-messenger systems work.
- How the release of hormones is controlled.
- The ways in which hormones interact with each other in the regulation of homeostasis.
- The structure and function of portal systems.
- The anatomy and physiology of each of your endocrine glands.
- The activities and release mechanisms for each of your hormones.

We have just finished learning about one of the two systems responsible for regulating homeostasis. In that system, the body is regulated through the use of sensory and motor electrical messages. This is a very rapid means of moving information and, therefore, regulating the body's internal environment. Now we must think about another system of regulation. In this system, we are not as concerned with the instant-to-instant regulation but rather regulation with a slightly longer time window. This is not meant to imply that the endocrine system cannot adjust to rapidly changing conditions; it can. This is meant more as a framework for thinking about the balance between the two systems.

13.1 Two Regulatory Systems: The Body As a Department Store

Think of it this way. The body is like a large department store. Homeostasis, from the perspective of the store, involves things like what merchandise is on hand to be sold, how it is displayed, what is on order for the next season, and similar issues. One group of people is responsible for keeping the shelves and hangers stocked and looking good (**FIGURE 13.1**). Their work is a moment-to-moment job; as customers sort through, rumple, and purchase merchandise, they have to continually restock, straighten, and sort out the merchandise for effective sales. These people are like the nervous system of the store. Even while the customers are in the store and considering purchases, they are at work keeping it all in proper order.

Another group of people is thinking about inventory strategy two or three seasons ahead. They are preparing for upcoming seasons, ordering merchandise, making sure the store is ready for the larger trends in the marketplace, rather than what went out the door yesterday and what to put on the shelves this afternoon. These people are the endocrine system of the store. Both systems are important, and both have to coordinate their efforts or the store will go out of business. This is how our nervous and endocrine systems function in our bodies.

13.2 The Endocrine Glands: A Few Quick Questions and Answers

So, what makes up the endocrine system? What organs do we find in this system and where are they? How exactly do they work, anyway? These are the questions we will consider in this chapter. The first portion of the chapter will provide a basis for understanding the endocrine system as a whole; the second portion of the chapter will involve considering the organs of this system individually.

The term *endocrine* comes from roots that mean "internal" (*endo-*) and "to secrete" (*krinen* or *-crine*). We are talking about glands that secrete some substance within the body. The substances they secrete are called hormones. The term *hormone* comes from the Greek word *hormone*, which means "urging on." These secretions cause or urge changes in body functions.

So, the endocrine system is made up of organs that produce secretions within the body: endocrine glands (**FIGURE 13.2**). These must be contrasted with another type of gland. We can contrast them with exocrine glands. Exocrine glands include salivary glands, sweat glands, and other glands that secrete their products to an external surface of the body. Keep in mind, however, that the lumen of the alimentary canal (digestive tract) is considered an external surface. To secrete to a surface, exocrine glands secrete their products through ducts. The

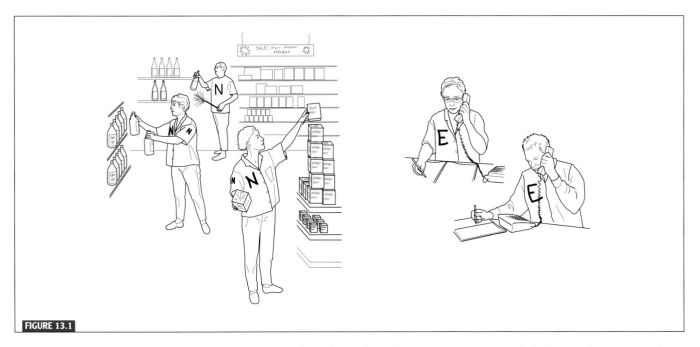

FIGURE 13.1

The nervous system, our fast-acting regulator of homeostasis, generally regulates body activities on a moment-to-moment basis. The endocrine system, our slow-acting regulator of homeostasis, generally regulates body activities over a longer time frame. See how these two systems compare to employees in a department store.

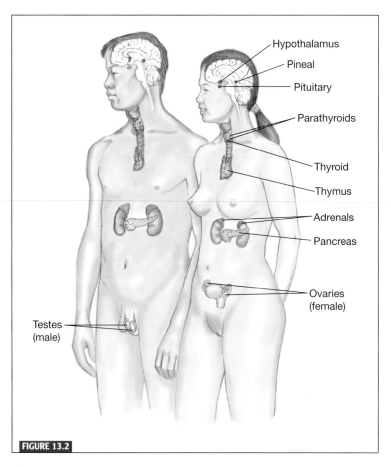

FIGURE 13.2

The organs of the endocrine system: the endocrine glands.

cells of endocrine glands generally release their secretions into the interstitial space; these secretions are then taken up by blood vessels. Therefore, the characteristics that distinguish exocrine glands from endocrine glands are that exocrine glands have ducts and secrete their products to a surface, and endocrine glands have no ducts and secrete their products (hormones) internally. Interestingly, many glands have both an endocrine and an exocrine function. For example, one component of the pancreas secretes the hormones insulin and glucagon directly into the bloodstream; therefore, the pancreas is an endocrine gland. However, another component of the pancreas secretes digestive enzymes such as pancreatic lipase and chymotrypsin through a duct into the small intestine; therefore, the pancreas must be exocrine. In this chapter, we will learn about the endocrine functions of mixed (heterocrine) glands; in later chapters, we will consider their exocrine functions.

In most cases, the method of secretion used by endocrine glands, essentially secreting directly into the bloodstream, ensures whole-body (systemic) distribution of hormones. Unlike the nervous system, where individual fibers travel to individual cells within effectors,

in the endocrine system, systemic distribution results in altered activity in cells, which may be widely distributed in the body. In a few moments, we will discuss what determines which cells respond to any specific hormone. What are the effectors of the endocrine system? Virtually all cells in the body are affected by some hormone. Many cells respond to many different hormones. As we proceed in this chapter, we will see that the effects of hormones may be many and varied. Since distribution is systemic, the effects tend to be long lasting. Unlike a neurotransmitter, which must be removed only from a synapse, a hormone must be removed from the blood.

13.3 Classes of Hormones: Some Simple Chemistry

Chemically, hormones come in three categories (**FIGURE 13.3**). Some are proteins or glycoproteins, some are amines, and some are steroids. We will consider each class individually.

The concept of proteins as hormones should not be difficult for you to grasp. Just think back to Chapter 2, where we learned that proteins are chains of amino acids and that there are 20 different amino acids used for this purpose. The order of individual amino acids in a protein determines what protein we have, just as the letters we use to spell a word determine what word we have. Some hormones are made from a large number of amino

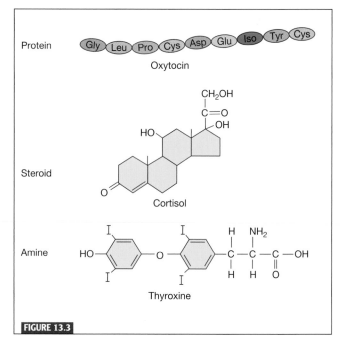

FIGURE 13.3

Three chemical classes of hormones. Only the primary structure (order of amino acids) is shown for the protein hormone. Compare the thyroxine to the tyrosine in Figure 2.11.

acids; others, from very few. The hormone oxytocin contains only nine amino acid residues (we refer to the number of amino acids in a protein as residues). Insulin contains 51 amino acid residues, distributed in two chains. Insulin makes an interesting example of how proteins are synthesized and will be discussed briefly in our next chapter. While not an extremely large protein hormone (growth hormone and prolactin each have nearly 200 amino acid residues), it is an interesting one because of its two chains. For now, suffice it to say that insulin begins as a much larger molecule (somewhere over 115 amino acid residues) and is successively modified (cleaved) down to the active form, with 51 residues.

Glycoprotein hormones are similar to protein hormones, except that they also contain a carbohydrate moiety. The carbohydrate is generally added, as you recall from Chapter 3 in the Golgi apparatus. Note that since proteins are hydrophilic (water loving), protein hormones can travel easily in an aqueous environment like blood. They are not lipid soluble, however, and, therefore, cannot cross the plasma membrane of their target cells.

Amine hormones are produced through modifications to the amino acids tyrosine or tryptophan. As such, they are relatively small molecules. The catecholamines (epinephrine and norepinephrine) and the thyroid hormones (T_3 and T_4) are tyrosine derivatives. Melatonin is a tryptophan derivative. Whether amines are hydrophilic or hydrophobic (water hating) depends on what modifications have been performed. If they are hydrophobic, they must be transported in the blood (an aqueous environment) while bound to a protein carrier. When they reach the plasma membrane, they can pass straight through because they are lipid soluble.

Steroid hormones are multi-ringed cholesterol derivatives. By that I mean that some of the carbons of these lipids make up the form of rings. You will recall that lipids like these are made in the smooth endoplasmic reticulum. Some also are produced in the mitochondria. Testosterone, aldosterone, cortisone, and progesterone are examples of steroid hormones. All are hydrophobic, indicating that they are transported in blood by carrier proteins, but cross the cell membrane readily to exert their effects within their target cells.

13.4 Target Cells Are Like Students with Radios

So, what is a target cell and how do these hormones work anyway? A target cell is a cell that responds to a particular hormone. Essentially, all cells are target cells for some hormone, and most are target cells for multiple hormones. The ability of a cell to respond to a particular hormone is dictated by whether or not that cell has a receptor for that hormone. No receptor, not a target cell: it is that simple. Want it a little simpler? Here we go.

You are in class one day and in walks your instructor, smiling widely, carrying a big box. In that box are many radios. Your instructor is in a very good mood, based on the recent excellent results your class has achieved on exams. Your instructor has decided to celebrate by buying gifts for the students in your class. This instructor doesn't have much of a budget, however (teaching salaries being what they are), so these radios are economy models.

As they are being passed out, a couple of deficiencies become apparent. First, there are no knobs on these radios; they can't be tuned to different stations, and the volume can't be adjusted. The first two rows of students are quick to determine that their radios receive only the local classical station; the next two rows determine that their radios only receive the local jazz station. Unfortunately, that is where the radios run out: the remaining students receive no radios at all.

The first row of students happens to love classical music. When the harmonious strains of a Rachmaninoff concerto come through their speakers, they get up and dance. The second row hates classical music, however, and the Rachmaninoff puts them to sleep. The third row (receiving jazz), gets up and dances to the enchanting melodies of Marian McPartland. The fourth row doesn't like jazz and goes to sleep. The remaining students do not know what all the fuss is about and go about their business as if the radios were not there at all.

This complicated tale is exactly how hormones affect their target cells. Notice that the radio stations, like endocrine glands, distribute their product (radio waves or hormones) globally; they're everywhere. But only people with radios specific for their radio wave can receive them. Only the first two rows of students are even aware that the classical music waves are present. This is exactly how it is with the endocrine system (**FIGURE 13.4**). If a cell has a receptor for a particular hormone, it is a target cell; otherwise, it won't even notice the hormone. Notice also that some people are reacting one way to the classical music they are receiving and some are acting another way, even though they have the same receptor (radio). That too is the way it is with target cells and hormones. The intracellular processes to which the receptor is connected will determine how the cell responds when the hormone binds to the receptor. Two cells may have the same receptor for the same hormone, but may react differently to it, if it is connected to different machinery within the cell.

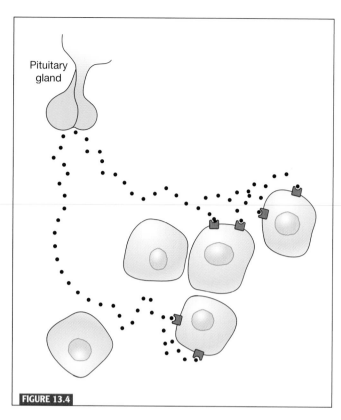

The presence or absence of specific receptors determines which cells are target cells for each hormone.

Recall that these students do not have the ability to increase or decrease the volume of these radios (no volume knob). If a student wanted to hear the music at a higher volume, the only solution would be to obtain additional radios. This is how cells alter their responsiveness to hormones. Target cells have the ability to upregulate (increase) receptor numbers or downregulate (decrease) receptor numbers, and thereby control their sensitivity to the presence of a particular hormone.

Mechanisms of Receptor Activity

So, since we know that the presence of a receptor for a particular hormone makes that cell a target cell for that hormone, perhaps we need to think a little about these receptors and how they work. Receptors can be either within the cell or on the cell surface. Think for a moment about what characteristics of a hormone make either of these two locations more suitable for its receptor. Think about a protein hormone for a moment. Would you expect to find its receptor on the cell surface or within the cell? Can this hormone cross the cell membrane readily? If not, perhaps its receptor should be on the surface rather than within the cell. How about a steroid? Steroids are hydrophobic and, therefore, can easily pass through the phospholipid bilayer. Why would you expect to find

its receptor on the cell surface if the cell membrane is not a barrier for it? So, hydrophobic hormones, such as steroids and some amines, usually have their receptors within the target cells, often within the nucleus of these cells. Hydrophilic hormones, such as proteins and glycoproteins, do not cross the cell membrane and, therefore, have their receptors on the cell surface.

Cell-Surface Receptors and Second-Messenger Systems

Have you ever been in a classroom and had someone come to the door with a message? Perhaps the instructor went to the door and took the message and then passed it on to the student to whom it was addressed. The person in the hall was the first messenger; the instructor was the second messenger. This is how cell-surface receptors work. We call this mechanism a second-messenger system. The hormone is the first messenger; it brings the message from the endocrine gland to the target cell. Another form of the message is generated on the inner surface of the cell membrane and brings the message in to where it is needed, within the cytoplasm. It is a lot like the old Mousetrap game where one thing causes another thing to happen, which causes another thing to happen, and so on. Mechanisms that work in this way are called cascade mechanisms. Second-messenger systems are one example of a cascade mechanism. Here is how one such system works.

The cyclic adenosine monophosphate (cAMP) second-messenger system is commonly linked to cell-surface hormone receptors. There are other second-messenger systems, but this one makes a good example to study (**FIGURE 13.5**). When the hormone binds to the receptor, it causes a conformational change (change in shape) in the receptor. Since the receptor is an integral protein, this conformational change shows up across the cell membrane. Linked to the receptor, on the inner surface of the membrane, is a G-protein. This G-protein is activated by this change and, in turn, activates the enzyme adenylate cyclase. Adenylate cyclase is an enzyme that cleaves ATP into cAMP. Remember from Chapter 2 that ATP (adenosine triphosphate) has three phosphate groups, and when two are removed it becomes adenosine monophosphate (AMP). When AMP has a cyclic shape, it is called cyclic AMP (cAMP). So the G-protein activates adenylate cyclase, which produces lots of cAMP. The cAMP is the second messenger. The presence of cAMP activates protein kinases. Protein kinases are enzymes that phosphorylate specific proteins, meaning they add phosphate groups (PO_4^{3-}) to these proteins. Phosphorylation determines the activity of many proteins, so they may be turned on or off by phosphorylation. This is ultimately

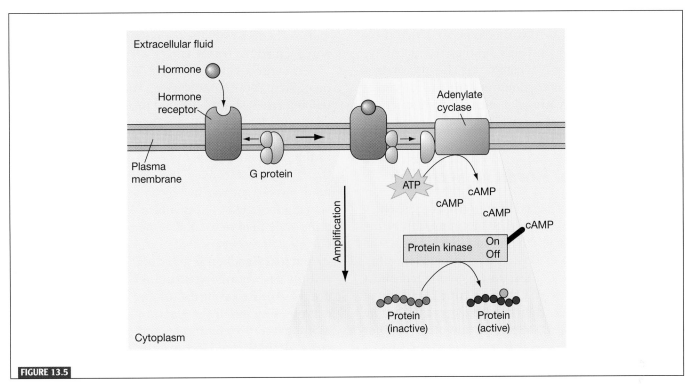

FIGURE 13.5

Second-messenger systems such as the cAMP second-messenger system (shown here) are cascade mechanisms that involve amplification.

the effect of the hormone on the target cell. This second messenger is ultimately turned off when another enzyme, phosphodiesterase, cleaves cAMP to AMP (removes the bond that makes it cyclic), inactivating it.

Amplification: It's Like a Good Mood

One key feature of this mechanism is amplification (Figure 13.5). The binding of one molecule of hormone to one receptor results in the generation of lots of second messenger (cAMP), which activates lots more protein kinases, which phosphorylates lots more proteins. Let me explain amplification a little further here.

You walk into class and are in a very good mood, so you turn to your classmate and hand her a quarter. That puts her in a good mood, so she turns to two classmates and hands each of them 50 cents. That puts each of them in a good mood, so they each turn to three more classmates and hand each of them a dollar (Hey, this is starting to get expensive!). Do you get the point? Amplification is when a little change leads to bigger changes in a stepwise manner. Cascade mechanisms often involve amplification. Second-messenger systems are cascade mechanisms with amplification.

Another common second-messenger system involves G-proteins that open calcium channels, using calcium as the second messenger. In this case, calcium binds to the calcium-binding protein calmodulin, which then activates or inactivates other enzymes.

Intracellular Receptors

Lipid-soluble hormones have direct access to the inside of the cell, including the inside of the nucleus and mitochondria. Just like a ghost in the cartoons, the hormone passes through the plasmalemma as if it were not there (**FIGURE 13.6**). This is particularly true of steroids and some amines. When they enter the nucleus, they bind to genes, or proteins interacting with the genes,

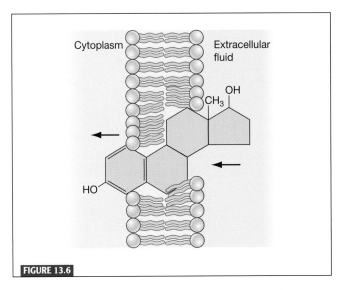

FIGURE 13.6

Lipid soluble hormones pass through the cell membrane to interact with receptors within the cell.

and trigger the activation of specific genes. This causes the synthesis of specific proteins to occur. Often these proteins are enzymes, and once synthesized, they have their effects on the cell's metabolism. These hormones may also enter the mitochondria and cause changes there, including increasing the rate of ATP production, thereby increasing the energy available to the cell.

13.5 Control of Hormone Secretion

So, what determines when endocrine glands secrete hormones? Do they all secrete their hormones all of the time? Well no, that would not be any good at all. If the endocrine system is to be effective in regulating homeostasis, the release of these potent compounds must be tightly linked to need. Our endocrine glands must only release hormones when they are needed and in the amount that is needed. Release in any other manner would push our bodies away from homeostasis, not toward it. In fact, much of what we know about hormones is knowledge gained from studying people with endocrine diseases. Many hormones were discovered by studying people with diseases caused by either overproduction or underproduction of those hormones.

So, how do our bodies determine when to release hormones? There are three principle mechanisms that control hormone release. They are direct innervation, indirect nervous system involvement, and direct endocrine control (no nervous system involvement). We will consider each of these now.

Direct innervation as a method of controlling hormone release means, in effect, that the endocrine gland is an effector and that an action potential in a motor pathway triggers release of the hormone. That is actually a slight oversimplification, but we will see how it works when we examine the posterior pituitary and the adrenal medulla (**FIGURE 13.7a**).

In indirect nervous system involvement, the nervous system determines when an endocrine gland will or will not release hormones, but that gland is not directly controlled by motor fibers. There are simply no nerve fibers routed to conduct the order to secrete directly to the hormone-producing cells. The nervous system, therefore, must convey that message through some other means. The way in which the message is conveyed actually more closely resembles the activities of endocrine cells than neuron. The nervous system releases chemical messengers that travel through the bloodstream to the endocrine gland and act on the endocrine cells just as a hormone would act on a target cell (Figure 13.7b). Releasing factors or hormones from the nervous system tell the gland to secrete hormone; inhibiting factors or hormones stop such release. The anterior pituitary gland is controlled by the hypothalamus in this way (more on that in a moment).

In our first two cases (direct innervation and indirect nervous system involvement), the nervous system monitors the internal (and perhaps external) environment and determines when the release of a particular hormone is needed. In our third mechanism, the nervous system is not involved. Direct endocrine control is a mechanism that involves direct monitoring of the internal environment by the endocrine gland itself: the endocrine gland determines when to secrete or withhold its hormones (Figure 13.7c). Insulin and glucagon release by the pancreas are controlled in this way. Pancreatic cells monitor blood glucose and determine when to release which hormone. This truly is an autonomous mechanism that does not involve the nervous system. Early scientists who did

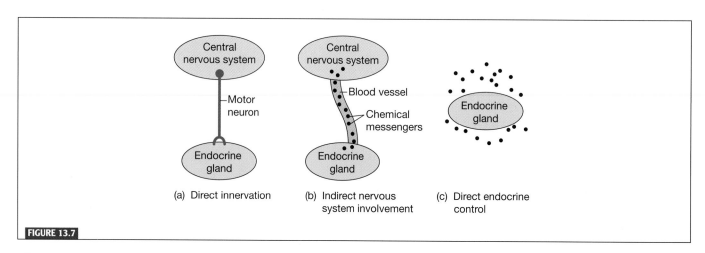

(a) Direct innervation

(b) Indirect nervous system involvement

(c) Direct endocrine control

FIGURE 13.7

Three mechanisms control hormone secretion.

not know about the autonomic nervous system thought essentially all internal functions were controlled in this way. They would be pleased to know that some endocrine glands actually do work this way.

One crucial point to recall is that of negative feedback. Hormone release, like most things in the body, is under the control of negative feedback. We release a hormone when it is needed. It does its job and is no longer needed; its release is shut off. Great system, huh? Except that there are three examples of positive feedback in the endocrine system. Two involve the hormone oxytocin; the third involves luteinizing hormone. We will look at those fascinating "exceptions to the rule" in this chapter and in Chapter 15.

Please keep in mind that hormones must also be removed from circulation if we are not to become overwhelmed by them. Hormones may be removed or inactivated by their target cells. They also may be removed or degraded by cells in the liver, lungs, and kidneys.

13.6 Hormone Interactions

One last topic to consider before we start discussing specific endocrine glands is that of how hormone activities overlap, how hormones interact with each other. They must interact with each other, right? After all, they are all released into the blood, and many cells are target cells for more than one hormone. So, let's think about the ways in which they might interact.

One way is immediately obvious. Some hormones have opposite effects. We say that they are *antagonistic* for each other. This is similar to the way that the sympathetic and parasympathetic nervous systems work against each other. Glucagon and insulin are examples of two antagonistic hormones. Glucagon is released when the blood glucose levels are low. It raises blood glucose levels. When blood glucose levels are high, insulin is secreted and it lowers blood glucose. We will learn about these and other examples later in this chapter.

Another way in which hormones interact involves a phenomenon you have certainly observed. We have all, at some point, noticed that a young person we know has suddenly grown inches, seemingly overnight. What has happened in those cases? Well, that young person has probably just hit puberty. Before puberty, that child was growing, as stimulated by growth hormone (abbreviated hGH for human growth hormone). When he or she reached puberty, sex hormones began to be released. The combination of sex hormones (estrogens and testosterone) and hGH causes much more rapid growth than hGH alone, or the sex hormones alone, for that matter.

Their effects are not merely additive; when present together, their effects are compounded. This is called synergistic effects. The term *synergistic effect* implies that the effect of two hormones together is greater than simply the sum of the two hormones' individual effects. It is as if two plus two now equals five. Incidentally, how were the bones of that young person able to increase in length, as they must have to result in this growth spurt? Think back to our discussion on the lengthwise growth of long bones for the answer. Also, note that the growth spurt stops with closure of what structure?

This leaves us with our last type of hormone interaction. We will soon learn that the hormone prolactin causes lactation, the production of milk in the mammary glands. Oxytocin causes milk letdown, the release of milk by the mammary glands. Considering that effect only (oxytocin does have other effects), could oxytocin have its effect without the prior exposure of mammary tissue to prolactin? No, of course not. Without prolactin to cause milk production, there is no milk present for oxytocin to release. This is referred to as permissive effect. The term *permissive effect* indicates that for one hormone to exert its effect, some other hormone must have already prepared the tissue for this effect. We will see other interesting examples of this in Chapter 15.

We have now completed the background work necessary to understand the individual organs of the endocrine system. The rest of this chapter will be devoted to moving through this system one gland at a time. In some cases, we will complete our discussions of the gland and its products. In other cases, we will lay the groundwork for information to be presented in later chapters. Let us now begin examining the endocrine glands.

13.7 Your Endocrine Glands: Their Anatomy and Physiology

■ Your Pituitary Gland

What a neat organ! The pituitary is quite small, about the size of the distal portion of your little finger, yet it is actually two organs in one structure. It is so important to homeostasis that some call it the master gland. We will learn that it is actually not the master of anything, but that its functions are tightly regulated. Let's start by considering its structure.

The pituitary (**FIGURE 13.8**), also called the hypophysis, hangs from the hypothalamus on a stalk called the infundibulum (which means funnel). It sits in a bony nest called the sella turcica (Quick, of what bone is the sella turcica a feature?). From structural, functional, and

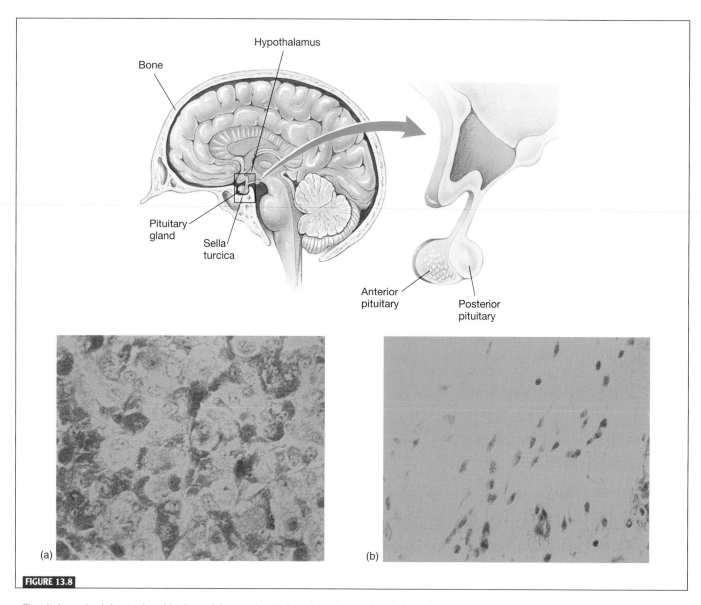

Hypothalamus

Bone

Pituitary gland

Sella turcica

Anterior pituitary

Posterior pituitary

(a)

(b)

FIGURE 13.8

The pituitary gland. Insets show histology of the anterior pituitary (a) and posterior pituitary (b).

developmental standpoints, it is actually two distinct glands. The portion nearest the infundibulum is called the posterior pituitary, posterior lobe of the pituitary, or neurohypophysis. This is because it is the most posterior portion of this gland and is actually composed of modified nervous tissue. The anterior portion of this gland, called the anterior pituitary, anterior lobe of the pituitary, or adenohypophysis, is constructed of very different tissue. The term *adeno-* means "gland." Well, you might ask, isn't the whole organ a gland? It is, but the term *adeno-* is applied here because the anterior pituitary has a glandular appearance histologically (more on this in a moment), as opposed to the neural appearance of the posterior pituitary (Figure 13.8 insets a and b). These two portions of the pituitary produce different hormones

and are controlled by different mechanisms. They just happen to be located together.

Your Posterior Pituitary: Neurohypophysis

The posterior pituitary is by far the smaller portion of this gland, making up only about 25 percent of its mass. Its modified nervous tissue composition gives it the alternative name neurohypophysis (Figure 13.8 inset b). The neurohypophysis is a highly unusual endocrine gland because, strictly speaking, it produces no hormones. It only stores and releases the hormones oxytocin and antidiuretic hormone (ADH) that are actually produced by the hypothalamus. Modified nerve cell bodies in the hypothalamus produce hormones that are transported down modified fibers extending into the posterior pituitary. These fibers store their hormones until their release is triggered by action potentials.

The functions of oxytocin are related to the reproductive system. The principle activities of this hormone are related to childbirth and breastfeeding. During the early stages of labor, the uterine cervix is stretched by the baby's head. The posterior pituitary releases oxytocin in response to this stretching. Oxytocin causes the smooth muscle of the uterus to contract, pushing on the baby, causing more stretching of the cervix. This causes more oxytocin release, which causes more contraction, which causes more stretching, and so on. This is one of our examples of positive feedback. It is limited by the birth of the child. Once the child is born, the stretching ends, and so does the oxytocin release.

The second major activity of oxytocin is now ready to begin. The sensation of the infant suckling on the nipple causes oxytocin release. Oxytocin causes ejection of milk from the nipple, called milk letdown. This encourages more suckling by the infant, then more nipple sensation and more oxytocin release; again, this is an example of positive feedback. This process too is self-limiting. Once the infant is full, the suckling stops, ending the sensation and oxytocin release. Oxytocin affects the CNS to encourage development of the mother-infant bond.

Oxytocin is also instrumental in the human sexual act. It is released during the later stages of intercourse in both males and females. In males, it contributes to the smooth muscle contractions of ejaculation, which propel the sperm and seminal fluid from the urethra. In the female, uterine contractions that accompany orgasm play a role in moving the seminal fluid higher into the reproductive tract, increasing the likelihood of fertilization. These contractions are, in part, due to oxytocin release.

Antidiuretic hormone, also called vasopressin, is released in response to dehydration. Osmoreceptors in your hypothalamus monitor the osmotic pressure of your blood. This pressure varies with your state of hydration. When you begin to become dehydrated, your blood osmotic pressure increases. In response, your hypothalamus causes your posterior pituitary to release ADH. Antidiuretic hormone has two main effects.

First, it causes your kidneys to remove water from the urine they are producing and return that water to the blood. Similar changes also occur in the water content of your perspiration. Your urine and perspiration are made more concentrated, and the blood is made more dilute. This raises blood volume, thereby increasing blood pressure.

Second, ADH is a potent vasoconstrictor, hence the alternate name, vasopressin. When blood volume is low,

blood pressure is low (explained in Chapter 16). By constricting the small arteries and arterioles that supply the capillaries in your body, blood flow is reduced through these capillaries. This, in turn, raises blood pressure. This is similar to the way that water pressure in a garden hose increases if you put your thumb over the end of the hose. Antidiuretic hormone is "putting its thumb" over your vascular garden hose! The maintenance of blood pressure is crucial to the maintenance of homeostasis.

Insufficient secretion of ADH causes the disease diabetes insipidus. This is described in our "Breaching Homeostasis . . ." feature at the end of this chapter.

Your Anterior Pituitary: Adenohypophysis

The adenohypophysis was given that complex moniker due to its histologic appearance. The prefix *adeno* is applied to tissues that appear glandular in histologic sections. For instance, you may have heard of someone having an adenoma (benign glandular tumor) or an adenocarcinoma (malignant glandular tumor). Glandular tissue typically has cells organized in ball, sack, or tubular arrangements. We would certainly expect to see a glandular histology when looking at the pituitary, but as we just learned, the posterior pituitary does not fit this pattern. If you examine Figure 13.8 inset a, you will see that the anterior pituitary does fit this pattern. You will also notice its highly vascular nature. This is characteristic of endocrine glands, as the vasculature is necessary to carry away the hormones produced in the gland.

Secretion of hormones by the anterior pituitary is under the control of the hypothalamus, but in a very different way than the hypothalamic control of the posterior pituitary. There are no nerve fibers extending from the hypothalamus to the anterior pituitary. The hypothalamus secretes releasing and inhibiting hormones (or factors) that travel in the blood to the adenohypophysis and stimulate or inhibit the release of specific hormones. Again, we see the hypothalamus on that interface between the nervous and endocrine systems. Let's think about how those releasing and inhibiting factors could best be delivered to the anterior pituitary.

Portal Systems: Interoffice Mail

Being really impressed with your class, your instructor might want to send a letter to the head of your school, bragging about you. This letter could be placed in the mail picked up by the U.S. Postal Service, mixed with other mail, brought to a post office, sorted out of the other mail, and brought back to your school for delivery to the school's chief administrator. That doesn't sound too efficient, though. Instead, your instructor might place it in the interoffice mail. It would then go directly to the chief administrator's office without being mixed with other mail, transported all over the place, and then brought back to the proper office. That's a much better system. That's exactly the type of system used to deliver the releasing and inhibiting factors to the anterior pituitary. It's called a portal system.

In the general scheme of things, blood leaves your heart and travels through successively smaller arteries, then an arteriole, and then through a capillary bed (**FIGURE 13.9a**). The capillary bed is where exchange takes place. (Remember our discussion of this in Chapter 12? We will also discuss it in detail in Chapter 16.) Capillaries have very thin, somewhat porous walls, allowing easy diffusion of substances into and out of the blood. Blood leaves the capillaries and travels through venules to successively larger veins, where the cycle starts over again. Now, if that were the only arrangement, blood leaving the hypothalamus, carrying releasing and inhibiting factors for the anterior pituitary, would have to travel all through the body and get mixed in with all the other blood to get where it needs to go. That's not good.

Instead, there is a portal system in place (Figure 13.9b). A portal system is one in which the blood leaves one capillary bed, travels through portal veins to a second capillary bed, before traveling again through veins, back to the heart. The value of this is that substances (such as hypothalamic releasing and inhibiting factors) can diffuse in, in the first capillary bed (in the hypothalamus), and back out from the second capillary bed (in the anterior pituitary). No need to distribute these things throughout the body; it's just like having an interoffice mail system traveling between these two locations. We will learn about another portal system later in this text (Chapter 18).

So, what hormones are produced and secreted by the anterior pituitary? There are seven that we need to learn about, and we will consider them one at a time (mostly). However, let's take the first two together.

The Gonadotropins

Two hormones make up the category called the gonadotropins. They are called this because of their effects on the gonads (testes and ovaries). They are luteinizing hormone (LH) and follicle- stimulating hormone (FSH). Gonadotropin-releasing hormone (GnRH) from the hypothalamus stimulates their release. They have a variety of effects that we will consider in detail in Chapter 15, but for now, let's briefly consider their chief effects. Follicle-stimulating hormone causes development of the gametes (sperm and ova). In females, it causes development of the ovarian follicles that contain the ova, hence its name. Luteinizing hormone causes release of the sex hormones from the gonads. The male sex hormones are called androgens (the major one is testosterone) and are released by cells called interstitial endocrinocytes. This gives LH its alternate name, interstitial cell-stimulating hormone (ICSH). The female sex hormones are the estrogens (actually several related hormones) and progesterone. These are released in response to LH, but in a cyclic manner, as part of the menstrual cycle. We will

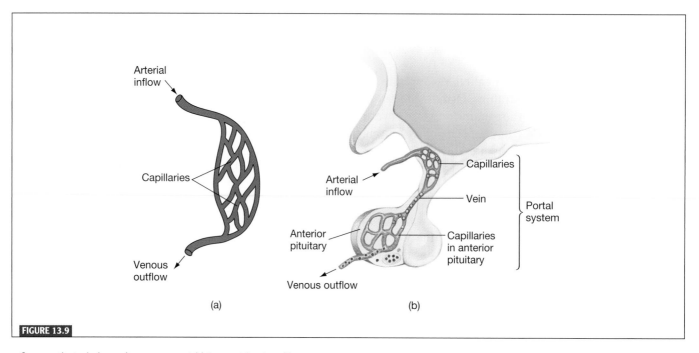

FIGURE 13.9

Compare the typical vascular arrangement (a) to a portal system (b).

learn their individual roles and the timing of their release later on. Let's now think about how their release might be controlled based on what we know about negative feedback. Gonadotropin-releasing hormone (from the hypothalamus) causes release of LH and FSH (from the anterior pituitary). Follicle-stimulating hormone and LH cause release of estrogens, progesterone, and androgens (from the gonads). When the levels of estrogens or androgens are sufficient, they have a negative feedback effect on GnRH, shutting off its release. This causes the GnRH levels to drop, which causes levels of FSH and LH to drop, which causes levels of estrogens or androgens to drop, which eliminates the negative feedback and allows GnRH to again be released. Phew, that seems like a lot of interactions. But think carefully about it, and you will see that it makes perfect sense. In Chapter 15, we will learn about a positive feedback loop that is also involved in this process, but let's wait until we get there (can you handle the suspense?).

Prolactin

Prolactin stimulates milk production in mammary glands. Obviously, this is necessary for breastfeeding and can only occur in mammary glands that have been prepared for this purpose by the combined and sequential actions of estrogens, progesterone, placental hormones, and prolactin. In males, prolactin may play a role in stimulating testosterone production by interstitial endocrinocytes. Prolactin release is triggered by prolactin-releasing factor (PRF) and is inhibited by prolactin-inhibiting hormone (PIH). Prolactin-inhibiting hormone has now been identified as the neurotransmitter dopamine. During the menstrual cycle, PIH is released, inhibiting the release of prolactin. Late in the cycle, however, progesterone levels fall, triggering menstruation. This drop in progesterone can cause a decrease in PIH production, leading to release of prolactin in some women. This accounts for the breast tenderness and swelling seen in some women at that time. During breastfeeding, oxytocin release stimulates PRF release and inhibits PIH release, causing prolactin release.

Let me give a brief word of caution here. Don't get too caught up in the "factor" versus "hormone" terminology used in these regulating substances. Generally, if the substance has been identified and characterized, it is called a hormone. If we only know about the activity, but need to do more work on the substance's identification, it is a "factor." Obviously, the terminology evolves as our knowledge grows.

Growth Hormone

Growth hormone (abbreviated hGH, with the small "h" indicating "human"), has been a subject of great interest to the press in recent years. Its many desirable effects include increased protein synthesis, increased muscle mass, increased breakdown of lipids, and increased blood sugar. These effect can be stimulated in older adults by pharmacologic administration of hGH. This has led some to irresponsibly tout it as a wonder drug or fountain of youth. Over the years, many hormones have fallen under this aura of fashion and popularity, and certainly many do have beneficial effects when used pharmacologically, in suitable patients, and under appropriate medical supervision. No hormone, however, is without deleterious side effects when mishandled, and the popular press is not the place to find reliable information on the safe use of these compounds. Please think about the words of caution in Chapter 1 on how to find reliable medical information.

So, what does hGH do? It does have the effects previously listed, and it does stimulate growth in young people; most notably the lengthwise growth of long bone and increased muscle mass. After closure of the epiphyseal plates at age 20 or so, the lengthwise growth of long bone cannot occur. These, however, are generally not the direct effects of hGH itself. This hormone has, as its target cells, a number of cell types throughout the body. These cells, in response to hGH, produce insulinlike growth factors (IGFs), which produce the effects we ascribe to growth hormone. Therefore, the effects with which we credit hGH are actually indirect effects.

Growth hormone is released in response to growth hormone-releasing hormone (GHRH), and inhibited by growth hormone-inhibiting hormone (GHIH). These factors are released by the hypothalamus in a complex cycle throughout the day and night, giving the timing of hGH release a similarly complex cycle.

Insufficient secretion of hGH during childhood results in a condition called pituitary dwarfism or pituitary growth failure. Untreated, this condition results in insufficient growth at the epiphyseal plates and extremely short stature. Fortunately, the effects of this disorder are limited by administration of hGH.

Excessive hGH secretion in childhood (before closure of the epiphyseal plates) results in gigantism. Currently, in the United States, this condition rarely goes untreated. Before the availability of such treatment, these individuals would commonly exceed 8 feet in height, with proportional enlargement of all parts. This led to the early development of arthritis and other signs of premature aging. Excessive hGH secretion in adulthood leads to acromegaly, a condition characterized by enlargement of the face, hands, and feet. No increase in height occurs, as the epiphyseal plates have already closed.

Thyroid-Stimulating Hormone

Thyroid-stimulating hormone (TSH) does exactly what its name implies. It stimulates the release of thyroid hormones T_3 and T_4 from the thyroid. We will learn about their effects shortly. Thyrotropin-releasing hormone (TRH) stimulates its release, and it is controlled by a simple negative feedback mechanism.

Adrenocorticotropic Hormone

Adrenocorticotropic hormone (ACTH) sure has a long name, but it accurately describes its function. It is obviously involved with the adrenal cortex: *adrenocortico-* refers to the "adrenal cortex," a gland we will learn about very soon. *Tropic* comes from the Greek word indicating a "turn" or to turn toward or away from something. It is used to indicate hormones that have a stimulating effect on some other tissue. So, adrenocorticotropic hormone must be a hormone that stimulates the adrenal cortex. In fact, only one region of the adrenal cortex is targeted by this hormone: the region that produces hormones called glucocorticoids. Adrenocorticotropic hormone release is stimulated by corticotropin-releasing hormone (CRH) from the hypothalamus. Corticotropin-releasing hormone release is stimulated by stress, especially of a more chronic nature (prolonged illness, job-related stress, the approach of final exams, etc.). Adrenocorticotropic hormone is also released in response to interleukin-1 (Il-1), which is produced by macrophages. The reason for this will become apparent when we study the glucocorticoids.

Melanocyte-Stimulating Hormone

Do you know what the role of melanocyte-stimulating hormone (MSH) is in the mature human? If not, you are in good company. Melanocyte-stimulating hormone increases skin pigmentation in numerous animals, including fish, amphibians, and reptiles. It does this by stimulating melanocytes, the cells responsible for skin pigmentation. It also has that effect in humans under specific circumstances, such as early in life and in women during pregnancy. It will darken the skin of people into whom it is injected, but this is not a good experiment for determining its physiologic function, as the conditions under which it is given vary greatly from how the body naturally makes it. In fact, adult humans do not make it in any measurable quantity. The jury is still out on this one; we are not certain of its function in humans. It may have a role in the CNS.

So, that's it for the pituitary. Look over **TABLE 13.1**, which summarizes pituitary function before moving on to your next endocrine gland.

■ Your Adrenal Gland: Two Glands in One

We will next consider the adrenal, or suprarenal, gland. This is my personal favorite endocrine gland (everyone should have a favorite endocrine gland; choose one as your own!) because of its interesting internal architecture and its diverse functions. Let's start with its structure.

The adrenal glands are immediately superior to the kidneys; that is to say, they sit on top of the kidneys like a hat on a head. They are somewhat flattened and somewhat triangular. If you would cut one open, you would see that it has a central region that is a different color from the outer region. The outer region, or cortex (meaning rind, as on a fruit), is a distinctly different gland than its middle, the medulla. They are simply located together. We will consider the adrenal cortex first (why not work from the outside in?).

Table 13.1   The Hormones of Your Pituitary Gland

Region	Hormone	Function
Posterior pituitary	Oxytocin	Stimulates uterine contraction during labor, stimulates the milk letdown reflex, and may play a role in promoting fertility
	Antidiuretic hormone	Increases water resorption by the kidneys, and elevates blood pressure by increasing blood volume and vascular tone
Anterior pituitary	Gonadotropins (FSH and LH)	Stimulates sperm and ova development and stimulates secretion of sex hormones
	Prolactin	Stimulates mammary gland development and milk production
	Growth hormone	Stimulates growth, protein synthesis, and lipid degradation
	Thyroid-stimulating hormone	Stimulates the secretion of T_3 and T_4 from the thyroid
	Adrenocorticotropic hormone	Stimulates secretion of glucocorticoids from the adrenal cortex
	Melanocyte-stimulating hormone	Role is obscure, but can stimulate melanocytes to darken skin

FSH = follicle-stimulating hormone; LH = luteinizing hormone.

Your Adrenal Cortex: Like a Ball of Yarn

What a neat organ! Your adrenal cortex is a three-layered structure. These layers are only apparent histologically, and it may take some imagination to see them that way, but they are structurally distinct and do produce different hormones (**FIGURE 13.10**).

Take a ball of yarn and, while standing up, unroll some of the yarn so that there is a disorganized pile of yarn at your feet. You now have a model of the adrenal cortex. The outer (most superficial) region of the adrenal cortex is called the zona glomerulosa, meaning zone of little balls. If you had numerous balls of yarn to go with the one in your hand, it would mimic the balls of cells in the zona glomerulosa. The straight cord of yarn extending from this ball to the floor represents the intermediate (middle) zone of the adrenal cortex, the zona fasciculata. *Fasciculata* means "bundle," like a bundle of sticks. The cords of cells in the zona fasciculata give this zone its name. The disorganized net of yarn at your feet resembles the zona reticularis, which means net or network. This is the deepest part of the cortex, lying alongside the medulla.

The zona glomerulosa produces mineralocorticoids, the major one of which is aldosterone. Aldosterone is produced in response to low blood pressure, through a really interesting mechanism involving the kidneys. The kidneys have cells that monitor blood pressure. We will learn about them when we study the kidneys. In response to low blood pressure, they release an enzyme called renin into the blood. Renin reacts with a protein called angiotensinogen, which is produced by the liver and is always present in the blood. Angiotensinogen is cleaved by renin, thereby producing angiotensin I. Both angiotensinogen and angiotensin I are inactive. Angio-tensin I is then cleaved to angiotensin II, mainly in the lungs, by angiotensin-converting enzyme (ACE). You may have heard of people with hypertension (high blood pressure) taking drugs called ACE inhibitors; this is the enzyme they inhibit. Angiotensin II is the active compound in this cascade. Angiotensin II causes aldosterone release (that's why we're discussing it here). It also increases blood pressure by causing vasoconstriction (contraction of smooth muscle in artery walls).

So, aldosterone is released when blood pressure is low. What does aldosterone do? Aldosterone increases resorption of sodium by the kidneys. Resorption means that as urine is being formed, sodium is taken out of it and added back to the blood. By osmotic effect, water follows the sodium, thereby increasing blood volume and increasing blood pressure. Also, chloride ions and bicarbonate ions follow the sodium. The movement of bicarbonate into the blood increases the blood pH (makes it less acidic), which is also a good thing. Aldosterone also causes the kidneys to remove potassium and hydrogen ions from the blood and dump them into the urine. The removal of hydrogen from the blood further elevates blood pH, and decreases urine pH. Excess potassium in the blood can directly trigger aldosterone release.

The zona fasciculata (that middle zone) produces glucocorticoids. The glucocorticoids include cortisol (hydrocortisone), corticosterone, and cortisone. Are these names familiar to you? They may be, because of their anti-inflammatory effects. They are often used pharmacologically in either cream or injectible forms to decrease inflammation. Their effects are all related to helping us to endure prolonged stress. They elevate our blood glucose levels, which give us the energy needed to stay alert and fight or run, as required. They make

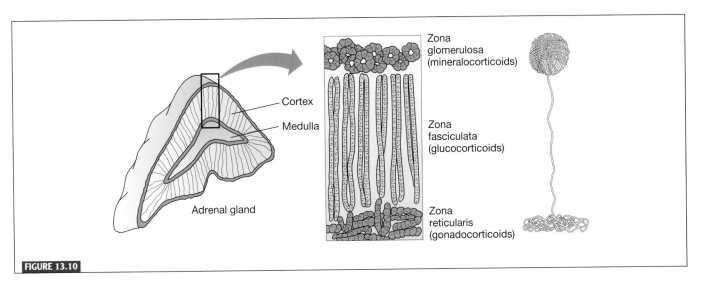

Zona glomerulosa (mineralocorticoids)

Zona fasciculata (glucocorticoids)

Zona reticularis (gonadocorticoids)

Cortex

Medulla

Adrenal gland

FIGURE 13.10

The adrenal cortex.

our blood vessels more responsive to the body's vaso-constrictors. This elevates blood pressure to ensure blood flow to vital organs and muscle; this also increases our ability to stop blood loss, should we become injured. The anti-inflammatory effects already noted also enable us to fight off stress. Inflammation is the body's non-specific response to any form of injury (covered in detail in Chapter 21). Anything from a bee sting to a splinter to a gun shot wound will cause inflammation in any vascularized tissue (tissue supplied with blood vessels). The signs of inflammation are redness, swelling, heat, pain, and loss of function. The pain and loss of function are generally good things, as they inform us of the injury and cause us to rest the affected body part to allow it to heal. Without this, we might injure it further.

By limiting inflammation, the glucocorticoids allow us to function when injured. This may delay healing, but may also save our lives. Remember our caveman running from the dinosaur (back in the autonomic nervous system section of Chapter 12)? What would happen if he were to twist his ankle? Could he explain to the dinosaur that he is injured and that inflammation is forcing him to stay off of his ankle? Dinosaurs don't generally care about that; our caveman would be lunch. Glucocorticoids allow people who are under stress to delay the rest needed for healing until the stress diminishes. Although they may become more seriously injured by this delay, it may allow them to survive long enough to have the opportunity to heal.

Stress causes the hypothalamus to release CRH, which causes the pituitary to release ACTH, which acts on the zona fasciculata, causing release of glucocorticoids. Also, during inflammation, generally late in that process, macrophages (inflammatory cells) release interleukin I (Il-1). Interleukin I is an intercellular communication molecule used by white blood cells. Interleukin-I causes ACTH release and, subsequently, glucocorticoid release, thereby reducing the inflammation. Again we see a nice example of negative feedback.

Hyposecretion of glucocorticoids results in Addison's disease, a condition characterized by an inability to tolerate stress, mobilize energy reserves, and maintain normal glucose levels in the blood. Hypersecretion of glucocorticoids results in Cushing's disease, characterized by unusual patterns of adipose tissue deposition, generalized weakness, and emotional instability.

The zona reticularis secretes gonadocorticoids. In both males and females, androgens (male hormones like testosterone) and estrogens (female hormones) are released. They are necessary for a variety of reasons, although we are not really sure what all of those reasons may be. In females, the androgens may increase libido (sex drive). This may be necessary for continuation of our species (no libido: no offspring: no human beings). In both sexes, estrogen appears to be necessary for normal brain functioning (females have suspected this for some time). The zona reticularis is where the estrogens are produced in males. In females, the importance of the zona reticularis may increase after menopause.

Your Adrenal Medulla

O.K., that's it for the adrenal cortex. Now how about the medulla? You already know more about the medulla than you might suspect. Let's think back to the nervous system for a minute. What was the name for a group of neuron cell bodies in the PNS? Right, a ganglion. The autonomic nervous system had two neurons in its motor neuron pathway rather than one, as in the somatic nervous system. Remember? (If you don't remember this, you should review it in Chapter 12.) One autonomic motor neuron left the CNS and traveled to a ganglion, where it synapsed with a second motor neuron, which traveled to the effector. What would happen if we were to modify that second motor neuron so that instead of traveling to an effector, it simply released its neurotransmitter onto capillaries (into which it could then diffuse)? The neurotransmitter would have direct access to the blood. Sounds like the sympathetic nervous system, doesn't it? That is the structure of the adrenal medulla (**FIGURE 13.11**).

The adrenal medulla is a modified sympathetic ganglion that releases the neurotransmitters epinephrine (adrenalin) and norepinephrine (noradrenalin) directly into the blood as hormones (Figure 13.11). This interaction between the nervous and endocrine systems makes the effects of the sympathetic nervous system global (systemic) and long lasting. This is the "adrenalin rush" people talk about that occurs when a dinosaur suddenly jumps out at you from behind a bush. You may have also felt these effects when your instructor has handed out an unannounced pop quiz (that rat!).

Be sure to examine **TABLE 13.2** for a summary of the hormones produced in the adrenals. Also study Figure 13.11 to learn the structure of this complex gland.

■ Your Pancreas

Your pancreas is one of those organs that acts as both an endocrine gland and an exocrine gland. Here, we will consider only its endocrine components. This organ is located near the proximal region of your small intestines, inferior to your stomach (**FIGURE 13.12**). Its exocrine components (acini) make up about 99 percent of its mass (**FIGURE 13.13**). Its endocrine components consist of about 1 million small clusters of cells called pancreatic islets, or islets of Langerhans. (Good name, huh? Sounds like

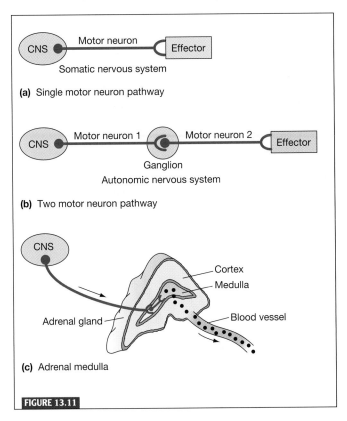

(a) Single motor neuron pathway

(b) Two motor neuron pathway

(c) Adrenal medulla

FIGURE 13.11

The adrenal medulla is a modified sympathetic ganglion. Notice how a single motor neuron pathway of the somatic nervous system (a) compares to the two motor neuron pathway of the autonomic nervous system (b) and how the adrenal medulla (c) is a modification of that pathway (the effector has been removed from the pathway).

somewhere exotic you could go on a cruise). When seen histologically, these cell clusters do look somewhat like small islands distributed through a sea of acini.

Pancreatic Islets and Their Hormones

The islets are made up of three parenchymal cell types (**TABLE 13.3**). Alpha cells produce glucagon, beta cells produce insulin, and delta cells produce growth hormone–inhibiting hormone (GHIH). We will consider each of these in turn. You may be puzzled by the presence of GHIH here. Don't be concerned about the GHIH; it

has a special function here in the pancreas and we will discuss it momentarily.

Glucagon is produced by the alpha cells of the pancreas in response to low blood sugar. It causes an increase in blood sugar through several mechanisms. It promotes glycogenolysis (the breakdown of glycogen to release glucose) in the liver. Recall that glycogen is the storage form of glucose: large branching chains of this simple sugar. When we need increased glucose in the blood, enzymes are activated that cleave off glucose, releasing it into the blood. Glucagon promotes that activity. It also promotes gluconeogenesis. Gluconeogenesis is the production of glucose, using noncarbohydrate sources for the carbon, hydrogen, and oxygen that make up this sugar. The sources used in gluconeogenesis are proteins and fats. Therefore, glucagon also promotes fat and protein catabolism (breakdown).

Insulin is produced by the beta cells of the pancreas in response to high blood sugar. It promotes glucose uptake by cells, thus reducing blood glucose and making glucose available for storage as glycogen. Insulin, therefore, also promotes glycogenesis (the production of glycogen). The liver is a major site of this function. Insulin and glucagon are antagonistic to each other.

Insulin exerts its effects in part by promoting the translocation of glucose transporter molecules (GLUTs) from the Golgi apparatus into the cell membrane. Recall that glucose cannot cross the cell membrane unaided; it is transported into and out of the cell by facilitated diffusion. The carriers for this molecule are called GLUTs. By inserting more GLUTs into cell membranes, the cells can take up glucose more rapidly and blood sugar levels are lowered. An inability of insulin to exert its functions because of either a lack of insulin or a lack of receptor sensitivity results in diabetes mellitus. We will discuss this condition in the "Breaching Homeostasis . . ." feature at the end of this chapter.

Growth hormone–inhibiting hormone is produced by the delta cells of the pancreas. It exerts its effect locally, not in the pituitary. Growth hormone–inhibiting

Table 13.2	The Hormones of Your Adrenal Gland	
Location	**Hormone**	**Effect**
Cortex, zona glomerulosa	Mineralocorticoids (aldosterone)	Increased renal resorption of sodium, bicarbonate, and water. Renal dumping of potassium and hydrogen. Elevation of blood pH
Cortex, zona fasciculata	Glucocorticoids (e.g., cortisol)	Increased stress tolerance and blood glucose, decreased inflammation
Cortex, zona reticularis	Gonadocorticoids (androgens and estrogens)	Provide each sex with the benefits of the hormones of the opposite sex
Medulla	Catecholamines (epinephrine and norepinephrine)	Makes the effects of the sympathetic nervous system global (systemic) and long lasting for ensured survival during immediate and extreme stress

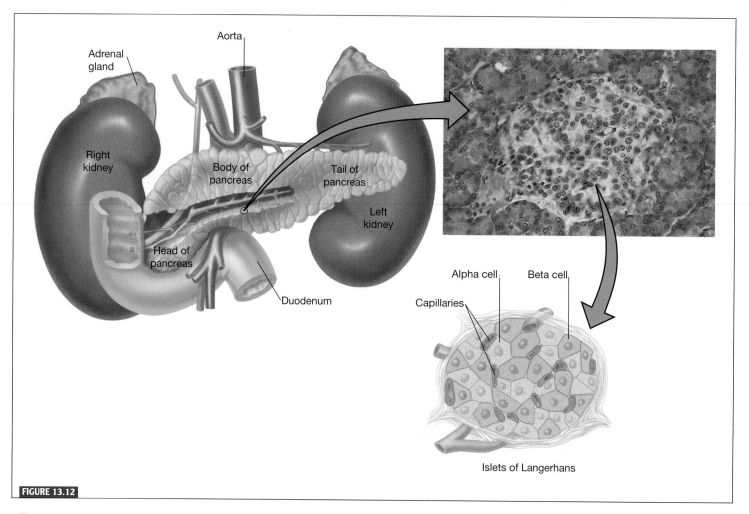

FIGURE 13.12

The pancreas.

hormone in the pancreas inhibits production of both insulin and glucagon. This is important, as the pancreas could begin a weapons race, producing ever increasing quantities of these two antagonistic hormones without a system to keep them in check.

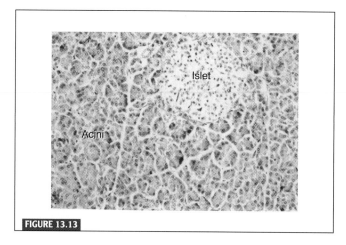

FIGURE 13.13

Histology of the pancreas.

■ Your Thyroid

Your thyroid gland is located anterior and lateral to your larynx and trachea in your throat. It has an "H"-shaped appearance, with one lobe on each side of your trachea, and an isthmus connecting the two lobes (**FIGURE 13.14**). In some individuals, a small fingerlike projection extends superiorly from the isthmus. This is called the pyramidal lobe. The shape of the thyroid does vary somewhat from individual to individual, and the size varies according to its level of activity.

Table 13.3 Hormones of Your Pancreas

Cell Type	Hormone	Effect
Alpha	Glucagon	Increases blood glucose levels
Beta	Insulin	Decreases blood glucose levels
Delta	GHIH	Inhibits secretion of glucagon and insulin

GHIH = growth hormone-inhibiting hormone.

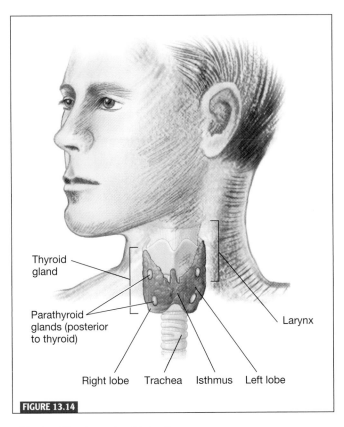

FIGURE 13.14

The thyroid and parathyroid glands.

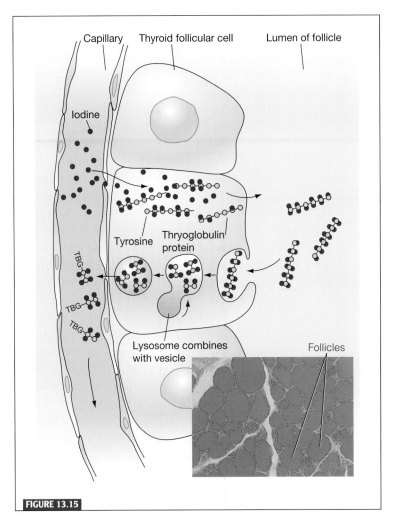

FIGURE 13.15

Production, storage, and secretion of the thyroid hormones.

This is a very interesting gland. Its microscopic structure is very different from the other endocrine glands we have examined (**FIGURE 13.15**). When examined histologically, the thyroid is seen to be composed of numerous small chambers called follicles. These follicles are filled with a protein-rich, gel-like substance called thyroid colloid. Thyroid colloid is the storage form of the thyroid hormones T_3 (triiodothyronine) and T_4 (thyroxine). T_3 and T_4 are produced by the cells that line the follicle, called follicular cells (good name, huh?). An additional parenchymal cell type is the parafollicular cell. Parafollicular cells are larger than follicular cells and do not reach the follicle lumen. They produce the hormone calcitonin, which is not stored in follicles. We will consider calcitonin after we have discussed T_3 and T_4.

Production, Storage, and Secretion of Thyroid Hormones

T_3 and T_4 are collectively known as "thyroid hormone," even though the thyroid makes another hormone as well. They are derivatives of the amino acid tyrosine and, as such, they are amines. Tyrosine is altered through the addition of iodine in the production of these hormones. Figure 13.15 demonstrates this process. It works as follows. The follicular cells of your thyroid take up iodide (the ionic form of iodine) from your blood. In fact, so

important is this iodide to the maintenance of homeostasis that table salt has iodide added (iodized salt). For this reason, people in Western societies rarely suffer from an iodine deficiency. Unfortunately, this is not consistently true throughout the world. Iodide is a necessary ingredient in the production of thyroid hormone.

The follicular cells produce a protein called thyroglobulin. The "globulin" portion of its name tells us that it is a globular protein (a protein with a bulging, complex three-dimensional shape). This protein contains numerous tyrosine residues. The iodide is combined to these paired tyrosines at a rate of one or two iodides per tyrosine. This is the basis for the thyroid hormones. Each molecule of hormone consists of parts of two molecules of tyrosine, with a total of either three iodides (T_3) or four iodides (T_4) bound to them.

The thyroglobulin containing the thyroid hormone is transported into the follicle lumens and stored as thyroid colloid. Your thyroid stores these hormones in this way so that if your diet should become deficient in iodide for a period of time, thyroid hormone would still be available. This was very important historically, when peoples' diets consisted of what was available locally and varied with the season. Vegetables grown in iodine-rich soil and seafood are good sources of iodine. These have not always been readily available in all places, and may still not be in many parts of the world.

When called on to secrete thyroid hormone, the thyroid colloid is taken up by the follicular cells through endocytosis. Follicle lumens, therefore, serve as warehouses of stored product that can be shipped out as needed. The thyroid hormones are removed from the thyroglobulin by lysosomal enzymes and the thyroid hormones diffuse out of the cell. As hydrophobic amines, these hormones pass readily through cell membranes but do not "travel well" in the aqueous environment of the blood. They are, therefore, transported bound to carrier proteins. Most is transported by the protein thyroxin-binding globulin (TBG). Circulating TBG is sometimes referred to as protein-bound iodine (PBI) in clinical blood tests. More T_4 is produced than T_3; however, T_3 is more potent than T_4. T_4 may be converted to T_3 in several organs throughout the body.

Secretion of thyroid hormones is stimulated by TSH from the anterior pituitary. The uptake of iodide by follicular cells is also stimulated in this way. This results in increased thyroid hormone synthesis. So it can be said that TSH stimulates synthesis and secretion of T_3 and T_4.

Effects of Thyroid Hormones

Thyroid hormone can easily access the interior of the cell, as it is hydrophobic and readily crosses the cell membrane. The receptors for this hormone, therefore, are found within the cell; specifically, they are found in the cytoplasm, in mitochondria, and in the nucleus. Mitochondrial receptors cause an increase in ATP production through carbohydrate and lipid degradation. This raises the basal metabolic rate (BMR) of the body; that is the amount of energy expended while you are awake but resting. An increased BMR requires increased energy levels and results in an increased body temperature. Blood flow and blood pressure are increased through more forceful cardiac contractions. The increased energy levels also result in increased alertness.

During fetal and early childhood development, thyroid hormones work synergistically with hGH to promote growth. Thyroid hormone is also necessary for development of the nervous system, including increases in neuron number and proper myelination of nerve fibers. Lack of iodine in the prenatal and postnatal diet can result in a condition called cretinism, profound mental and physical retardation, and deafness with mutism.

If experienced later in life (childhood or adulthood), hypothyroidism (insufficient secretion) results in myxedema, which is characterized by lethargy, lack of energy, cold intolerance, and edema (excessive interstitial fluid in the tissues). Several different conditions are associated with hyperthyroidism, excessive secretion of thyroid hormone (i.e., Grave's disease and Plummer's disease). These conditions are generally characterized by nervousness, rapid pulse, muscle weakness, weight loss (despite sufficient diet), prominence of the eyes and thyroid (goiter), and high temperature and basal metabolic rate.

Calcitonin

The other hormone produced by the thyroid is calcitonin. Calcitonin, a protein hormone, is produced by parafollicular cells and is not stored within the follicles. Its release is controlled independent of the nervous system; the parafollicular cells directly determine need and release calcitonin accordingly. Thyroid-stimulating hormone does not cause calcitonin release. The main target cell of calcitonin is the osteoclast. Do you remember what osteoclasts do (Chapter 6)? Were osteoclasts directly related to the other cells of bone? As you recall, they were not; they are in the monocyte-macrophage lineage. They are the giant cells that degrade bone during remodeling. You should also recall that osteoclasts dissolve the mineral salts of bone through the use of acids. These mineral salts diffuse into the blood, allowing the bone matrix to serve as a reservoir for these minerals. The main mineral salts of bone are calcium carbonate and calcium phosphate. Since calcitonin decreases osteoclast activity, it decreases the calcium content of the blood. This is its main function: regulation of blood calcium. In that regard it works antagonistically to parathyroid hormone, which we will learn about in a moment. Calcitonin also decreases blood phosphate levels, again by decreasing its removal from bone.

■ Your Parathyroid Glands

Your parathyroid glands (note the plural) are found posterior to the two lateral lobes of your thyroid gland (Figure 13.14). They are generally present as four very small round or oval masses of cells (two on each side); however, their number and structure vary among individuals. They are located outside of the thyroid capsule and are not a part of the thyroid, but are separate glands.

They produce parathyroid hormone (another catchy name), a protein hormone involved in the regulation of blood calcium levels. Opposite of its antagonist calcitonin, parathyroid hormone increases osteoclast activity. Release of parathyroid hormone is dependent on blood calcium levels, as determined by the cells that produce the hormone.

Even though osteoclast activity and blood calcium levels increase in response to parathyroid hormone, blood phosphate levels actually decrease overall as a result of this hormone's effect. This probably seems contrary to what you would surmise, based on what you already know. Think about it: osteoclast activity increases, releasing calcium salts into the blood. One of the main calcium salts is calcium phosphate; therefore, you might assume that blood phosphate would also increase. This is not the case, however, as parathyroid hormone also has target cells in the kidneys. These cells remove phosphate from the blood and excrete it into the urine in response to parathyroid hormone. Incidentally, they remove calcium from the urine they are producing and add that back to the blood. So, although more phosphate is being released from bone matrix, an even larger amount is being dumped into the urine; hence, there is a net reduction in blood phosphate. It is sort of like when you get a 20 dollar raise in salary, but your rent goes up 30 dollars, so you have less money left than you had to start with before the raise.

So, to be sure you get it, let's recap this parathyroid hormone/calcitonin thing. Parathyroid hormone and calcitonin are antagonistic for each other regarding osteoclast activity and blood calcium levels, and the level of calcium in the blood determines which will be released. Parathyroid hormone, released in response to low blood calcium, increases blood calcium levels mainly by increasing osteoclast activity. Calcitonin, on the other hand, is released when the blood calcium level is high; it decreases blood calcium levels by decreasing osteoclast activity. These two hormones are not antagonistic for each other regarding blood phosphate levels, however. Both of them reduce blood phosphate levels, but they use different mechanisms. Calcitonin decreases osteoclast activity, while parathyroid hormone promotes renal dumping of phosphate.

■ Your Pineal Gland

Here's an interesting little gem. Again we are at the interface between two systems. The pineal gland, which is part of the epithalamus and located superior to the third ventricle, is in many ways a nervous system structure (**FIGURE 13.16**). Overall, however, we will consider it as an endocrine gland. While it contains neurons and glial cells, it also contains secretory cells called pinealocytes. Pinealocytes are in contact with postganglionic sympathetic fibers.

Melatonin is the hormone produced by the pineal gland. Melatonin is produced by altering the neurotransmitter serotonin (a tryptophan derivative) and is

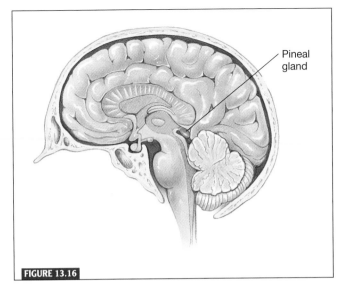

FIGURE 13.16

The pineal gland.

released in response to darkness. Many functions have been attributed to melatonin. One function that has been popularized in recent years is its role in promoting sleep. Some people have promoted the use of melatonin capsules or tablets as a sleep aid, as melatonin does induce sleep. The long-term safety of this approach is still unproven. Why not try a more natural approach?

Melatonin secretion is stimulated by darkness and inhibited by light. This worked great during the pre-electricity phase of human development. Now, what do we often do? We go into a brightly lit bathroom to get ready for bed. This light theoretically can diminish melatonin production, therefore reducing our ability to get to sleep. By limiting the amount of light entering our eyes for a period of time before bed, we may induce melatonin production and thereby promote sleep without the need for exogenous sleep aids.

Another interesting aspect of melatonin is its potential role in the etiology (cause) of seasonal affective disorder (SAD). Seasonal affective disorder is a disorder seen in northern regions, during the dark months of winter. It is characterized by depression, altered sleep patterns (less sleep), and an inability to concentrate and be productive. Seasonal affective disorder may be caused by the increase in melatonin secretion brought on by the seasonal lack of daylight.

■ Other Endocrine Glands

Some additional organs have, as a primary function, endocrine activity. The testes and ovaries are prime examples. Because of their specialized activities in other systems, they will be discussed in the chapters dealing with those systems. Other organs have endocrine activities as secondary activities related to their primary functions. The thymus and the small intestine are prime examples. These organs are also best left for the discussions of their systems. This now ends our discussion of the endocrine system. Remember the concepts you learned here so you will be able to apply them in our later chapters. Also make certain that you know the necessary information by going over the "What You Should Know" and "What Did You Learn?" features before continuing to your next section.

Breaching Homeostasis . . . When Things Go Wrong

Diabetes

In this "Breaching Homeostasis" section, we will discuss diabetes. The term *diabetes* is applied to multiple disorders; we will focus primarily on diabetes mellitus.

Let's start with a few definitions. The term *diabetes* comes from a Greek term meaning "passing through." This is because two common symptoms of diabetes are polydipsia (excessive thirst) and polyuria (excessive urine volume). The "water" is "passing through." With that in mind, we must distinguish diabetes mellitus from diabetes insipidus, the other major form of diabetes. *Mellitus* comes from the Greek word for honey or sweet. *Insipidus* means "without flavor." With those two terms, can you guess how early medical practitioners used to distinguish between these two forms of diabetes? When patients would present with polyuria and polydipsia (and other related symptoms), the physician (or more likely, his student) would taste the urine. If a sweet flavor was detected, diabetes mellitus would be diagnosed; if no sweetness was detected, diabetes insipidus would be diagnosed. Sooner or later it was also learned that the diabetes mellitus patients' urine would attract ants, while the diabetes insipidus patients' urine would not. My guess is that some of those "urine tasters" were pouring out their important medical sample and discovered that phenomenon serendipitously.

So, why the difference in urine taste? The presence or absence of glucose in the urine is the culprit. The reasons for the excessive urination (and, hence, excessive thirst) are different in the two diseases. In diabetes insipidus, insufficient secretion of ADH causes excessive urine volume. Without ADH, diuresis (high urine volume) ensues due to the lack of water resorption in the kidneys. A lack of ADH secretion from the neurohypophysis is the cause of diabetes insipidus.

Diabetes mellitus is caused by an inability to regulate blood glucose levels. Without the ability to control blood glucose, blood glucose levels rise too high (hyperglycemia). When this happens, the kidneys cannot resorb glucose from the urine they are producing. Normally there is no glucose in the urine, but high blood glucose levels leads to glucose "spilling" into the urine. The presence of glucose in the urine, where it does not belong, alters the osmotic balance in the kidneys, leading to an inability to resorb water from the urine (hence, polyuria). The glucose gives the urine its characteristic flavor. The actual mechanism for water resorption in urine production will be presented in Chapter 19.

So, why can't these patients regulate their blood glucose levels? That answer is related to the hormone insulin. There are two major forms of diabetes mellitus: Type I, also called insulin-dependent diabetes mellitus (IDDM); and Type II, or non-insulin-dependent diabetes mellitus (NIDDM). In Type I, auto-immune destruction of beta cells in the pancreatic islets leads to a lack of insulin production and secretion. These people must administer insulin to themselves daily to regulate their blood sugar level. Type II diabetes mellitus does not involve beta-cell destruction and these people continue to produce insulin. Insulin levels in people with Type II diabetes mellitus may be normal or increased: the target cells have become insensitive to insulin due to either destruction of insulin receptors or loss of the intracellular response to insulin. The underlying etiology of either form remains elusive but seems to involve genetic and environmental components.

Type I diabetes mellitus makes up only about 10 percent of diabetes mellitus cases. Onset of the illness is almost always before age 40 and usually before age 20. It may present with an acute onset, and aberrant glucose metabolism may result in weight loss, weakness, and fatigue. Type II diabetes, on the other hand, usually develops insidiously in people in their middle years. Most often, these patients are obese.

In either case, control of blood glucose levels in diabetes mellitus patients is absolutely necessary. An inability to control this disorder (regardless of the type) will result in pathologic changes in blood vessels, nerves, and kidneys. These changes can lead to an inability to heal wounds in the extremities (sometimes resulting in the need for surgical amputation), loss of sensation, loss of sight, and the need for renal dialysis or transplantation. All of these changes greatly impact the quality of life and ultimately become life threatening. Diabetes mellitus is the seventh leading cause of death in the United States.

What You Should Know

1. The nervous and endocrine systems work together to regulate homeostasis.

2. The endocrine system is the slow-acting regulator of homeostasis; the nervous system is the fast-acting regulator of homeostasis.

3. Endocrine glands lack ducts and secrete their products (hormones) into the interstitial space for transportation in the blood.

4. Exocrine glands secrete their products through ducts to some body surface.

5. Many glands have exocrine and endocrine components.

6. Hormones may be protein or glycoprotein, amine, or steroid.

7. For a cell to be a target cell for a particular hormone, it must have a receptor for that hormone.

8. Hormone receptors may be located on the surface of the cell or within the cell, typically in the nucleus.

9. Hormone receptors on the cell surface work through second-messenger mechanisms.

10. Second-messenger systems provide amplification of the signal that hormone is bound to the receptor.

11. Hormone release may be controlled by direct innervation, indirect nervous system involvement, or directly by the endocrine gland, with no nervous system involvement.

12. Hormones interact with each other in several ways. Their interactions may be antagonistic, synergistic, or permissive.

13. You must know the activities of each of the hormones named in the remainder of this section.

14. The pituitary gland is actually two independent glands attached together: the posterior pituitary or neurohypophysis, and the anterior pituitary or adenohypophysis.

15. The posterior pituitary is composed of modified nervous tissue. It does not make hormones; it stores and releases hormones made in the hypothalamus.

16. The hormones of the posterior pituitary include oxytocin and ADH.

17. Action potentials trigger release of hormones from the posterior pituitary.

18. Release of hormones from the anterior pituitary is controlled by releasing/inhibiting factors and hormones from the hypothalamus. These are delivered to the anterior pituitary through a portal system.

19. The anterior pituitary is composed of glandular tissue.

20. Hormones of the anterior pituitary include the gonadotropins FSH and LH, prolactin, hGH, TSH, ACTH, and MSH.

21. Your adrenal gland is actually two independent glands attached together: the adrenal cortex and the adrenal medulla.

22.   Your adrenal cortex is constructed in three layers, each of which produces a different category of hormones. The superficial layer, the zona glomerulosa, produces mineralocorticoids such as aldosterone. The intermediate layer, the zona fasciculata, produces the glucocorticoids such as cortisol. The deepest layer, the zona reticularis, produces the gonadocorticoids such as the androgens and estrogens.

23. Your adrenal medulla is a modified sympathetic ganglion acting as an endocrine gland. It produces the catecholamines epinephrine and norepinephrine.

24. Your pancreas is both an endocrine gland and an exocrine gland.

25. The endocrine portion of your pancreas is composed of pancreatic islets. Alpha cells in these islets produce glucagon, beta cells in these islets produce insulin, and delta cells in these islets produce GHIH.

26. Your thyroid gland produces and stores the thyroid hormones T_3 and T_4. It also produces (but does not store) calcitonin.

27. Your parathyroid glands are small structures attached to your thyroids. They produce parathyroid hormone.

28. Your pineal gland is made of modified nervous tissue and releases melatonin in response to darkness.

What Did You Learn?

Multiple choice questions: choose the best answer.

1. The ____ system is the body's slow-acting regulator of homeostasis.
   a. Nervous
   b. Endocrine
   c. Both of the above
   d. Neither of the above

2. Which of the following secrete their products through ducts?
   a. Endocrine glands
   b. Exocrine glands

What Did You Learn? (continued)

c. Both of the above

d. Neither of the above

3. Which of the following produce hormones?

   a. Endocrine glands

   b. Exocrine glands

   c. Both of the above

   d. Neither of the above

4. Which of the following can readily cross the plasma membrane to bind receptors within the cell?

   a. Protein and glycoprotein hormones

   b. Steroids

   c. Both of the above

   d. Neither of the above

5. The presence of a receptor for a specific hormone:

   a. Means that cell produces the hormone

   b. Means that all of the activities of that cell will be stimulated by that hormone

   c. Makes that cell a target cell for that hormone

   d. All of the above are correct

   e. None of the above is correct

6. Second-messenger systems are commonly associated with:

   a. Cell-surface receptors

   b. Intracellular receptors

   c. Both of the above

   d. Neither of the above

7. Which of the following is a common second messenger?

   a. G-proteins

   b. Adenylate cyclase

   c. ATP

   d. Protein kinases

   e. None of the above

8. Place the following in the order that they occur in the cyclic AMP (cAMP) second-messenger cascade.

       1. Adenylate cyclase

       2. Protein kinases

       3. cAMP

       4. Hormone-receptor binding

       5. G-proteins

   a. 1,4,2,3,5

   b. 4,5,1,3,2

   c. 4,2,3,1,5

   d. 4,1,5,2,3

   e. 5,4,2,1,3

9. What role does the CNS play in the regulation of hormone release?

   a. It directly controls hormone release through the use of action potentials

   b. It indirectly controls hormone release through chemical mechanisms

   c. Hormone release is independent of the nervous system

   d. All of the above are true, depending on the hormone under consideration

10. One hormone requires the prior activity of another hormone in order to exert its effect. This interaction is:

    a. Antagonistic

    b. Permissive

    c. Synergistic

    d. None of the above

11. The posterior pituitary produces:

    a. Oxytocin

    b. ADH

    c. Both of the above

    d. Neither of the above

12. Control of the activity of which of the following involves a portal system?

    a. The adenohypophysis

    b. The neurohypophysis

    c. Both of the above

    d. Neither of the above

13. Release of which of the following is controlled through a positive feedback mechanism?

    a. ADH

    b. Glucagon

    c. Insulin

    d. Oxytocin

    e. None of the above

14. Which of the following is a potent vasoconstrictor?

    a. ADH

    b. Glucagon

    c. Insulin

    d. Oxytocin

    e. None of the above

15. Release of ACTH is stimulated by:

    a. CRH

    b. Il-1

    c. Both of the above

    d. Neither of the above

What Did You Learn? (continued)

16. The zona glomerulosa of your adrenal cortex produces:

  a. Glucocorticoids

  b. Mineralocorticoids

  c. Gonadocorticoids

  d. All of the above

  e. None of the above

17. Aldosterone is an example of a:

  a. Glucocorticoid

  b. Mineralocorticoid

  c. Gonadocorticoid

  d. All of the above

  e. None of the above

18. Activation of the renin-angiotensin system stimulates release of:

  a. Cortisol

  b. Androgens

  c. Aldosterone

  d. None of the above

19. If you were crossing the desert on foot and had finished the last of your water two days ago (see the vultures circling), your endocrine system would probably be releasing:

  a. Aldosterone

  b. ADH

  c. Both of the above

  d. Neither of the above

20. Three weeks ago, you stubbed your big toe and got a large splinter in it. Although you removed the splinter, the toe has been red, painful, and swollen this entire time. In response, your endocrine system is probably about to secrete:

  a. Cortisol

  b. Androgens

  c. Aldosterone

  d. hGH

  e. None of the above

21. _____ is a modified sympathetic ganglion.

  a. Zona reticularis

  b. Zona glomerulosa

  c. Zona fasciculata

  d. Adrenal cortex

  e. None of the above

22. _____ increases blood glucose levels.

  a. Insulin

  b. Glucagon

  c. Both of the above

  d. Neither of the above

23. You ate three candy bars on the way to class. Your pancreatic islets would have then secreted:

  a. Insulin

  b. Glucagon

  c. Both of the above

  d. Neither of the above

24. Which of the following is stored in thyroid colloid?

  a. Calcitonin

  b. T_3 and T_4

  c. Both of the above

  d. Neither of the above

25. Calcitonin and parathyroid hormone are antagonistic for each other regarding blood _____ levels.

  a. Calcium

  b. Phosphate

  c. Both of the above

  d. Neither of the above

Short answer questions: answer briefly and in your own words.

1. Describe the difference between a portal system and the usual vascular arrangement. Where in the endocrine system do we find a portal system and what is its purpose?

2. How does positive feedback play a role in oxytocin release? Please discuss how that feedback system works. Why is positive feedback not used in controlling the release of more hormones?

3. List the steps involved in the cAMP second-messenger system. Why are second-messenger systems necessary? How does amplification work?

4. Draw and label a diagram of the adrenal cortex and list the hormones produced by each layer. Also list the actions of these hormones.

5. The pancreas plays a major role in the regulation of blood glucose levels. What does it secrete if you have had a very busy day during which you simply have not had the time to eat? What will it produce after you finally stop and eat a large pizza at the end of the day? Please explain your answers.

6. Describe the production and storage of the thyroid hormones. What are the activities of these hormones? What common dietary supplement makes this storage scheme less important in our society than it was historically.

7. Describe the role of the pineal gland in inducing sleep. How might you personally benefit from this knowledge?

Reproducing Your Body

Reproduction is a basic function of all biological species for one very important reason: without it, that species would not exist. If humans, for example, did not have the ability and will to reproduce, there would be no one to write this text, never mind read it. We simply would have become extinct at the very beginning of our existence. Despite the basic need for this ability, it is one of the more remarkable things that biological beings do. To be able to reproduce generation after generation, to "make again" with defects occurring only rarely, requires such precision in the mechanism that even our most sophisticated human technologies pale by comparison. This is especially apparent when you consider the complexity of the beings that are undergoing reproduction.

In this section, we must first expand on the foundation laid in our earliest chapters. We must expand our discussion involving the genetic apparatus of our cells so we can understand the role of this amazing molecular machinery in the reproductive process. We will also examine the way in which our cells use this machinery as the blueprints of our proteins. Then we will move on to how our bodies are reproduced.

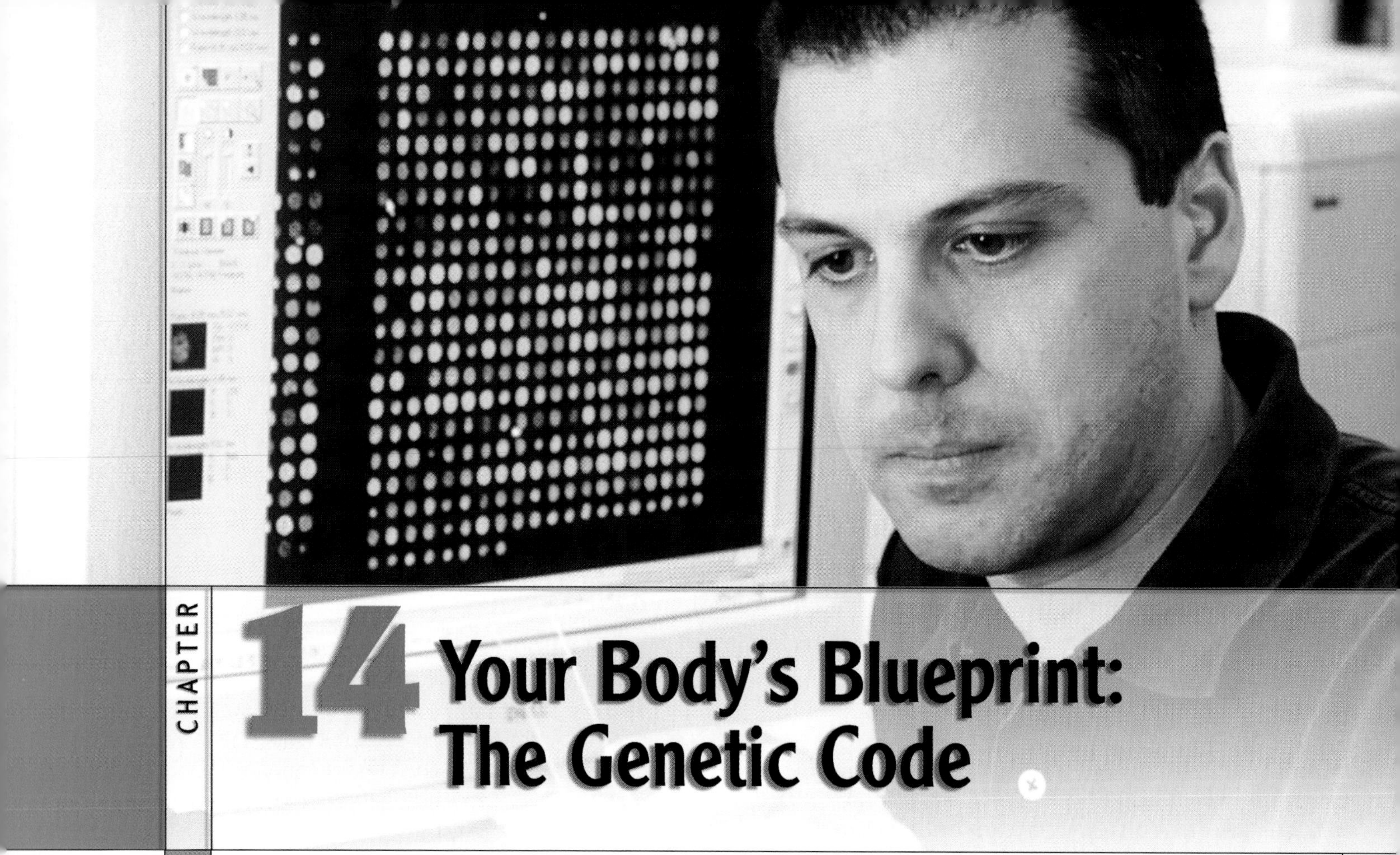

14 Your Body's Blueprint: The Genetic Code

What You Will Learn

- How complementarity determines which nucleotides bind together.
- The role of complementarity in DNA replication.
- How DNA is replicated.
- What is actually encoded in your DNA.
- The role of DNA in protein synthesis.
- Protein synthesis: transcription and translation.
- How meiosis enables the development of diversity through sexual reproduction.
- The stages of meiosis.

14.1 Let's Review

In Chapter 2, we learned about nucleic acids. We learned that nucleic acids are chains of nucleotides, and that nucleotides each contain a nitrogenous base, a pentose monosaccharide, and one or more phosphate groups. We noted that the pentose monosaccharide that is present in a nucleotide determines the class of that nucleotide. If the monosaccharide ribose is present in the nucleotides of a chain, we have a ribonucleic acid (RNA). If instead, deoxyribose is the monosaccharide, the nucleotide, and hence the chain, is deoxyribonucleic acid (DNA). We learned in Chapter 3 that DNA is primarily found in the nucleus, although some is also found in the mitochondria. We also learned about RNA in the nucleolus and ribosomes. In this chapter, we will learn what these nucleic acids are doing in those locations.

Back in Chapter 2 we also learned that the nitrogenous base that is present in a nucleotide gives that nucleotide its identity. Four different nitrogenous bases are used in DNA: adenine, thymine, guanine, and cytosine. In RNA, uracil is substituted for thymine; otherwise, the nitrogenous bases are the same.

We also learned that DNA exists in the nucleus in the form of a double chain, twisted into a spiral. This is called a double helix. To picture the double helix, imagine a ladder that is twisted into the shape of a spiral staircase (see **FIGURE 14.1**). If this seems like an awfully

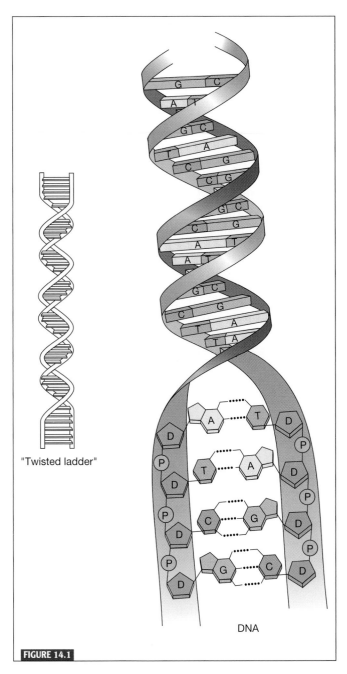

"Twisted ladder"

DNA

The structure of DNA. D indicates deoxyribose, A indicates adenine, T indicates thymine, C indicates cytosine, G indicates guanine, and P indicates a phosphate group.

complicated molecule to you, you are thinking about it correctly. It is complicated in a way, but when you see how it works, you will understand that within this apparent complexity is an elegant simplicity.

14.2 Complementarity: Like Singing in Harmony

Let's think about singing for a moment. You know the scale of notes that goes: do, re, mi, fa, so, la, ti, do. Imagine

singing a song with a friend. Initially, you each sing the same notes all of the time. Whenever one of you is singing a "do," the other is also singing a "do." After a while, you begin to experiment and you find that, but if one sings a "do" and the other sings a "re" it sounds sour, if one sings a "do" and the other sings a "mi," pleasant harmony develops. Now as you sing, whenever you sing a "do," your friend sings a "mi." Whenever you sing a "re," your friend sings a "fa." Whenever you sing a "mi," your friend sings a "do." Whenever you sing a "fa," your friend sings a "re" (see **TABLE 14.1**).

This works quite well, and in no time you and your friend are quite famous for your two-part harmony in songs with only four notes. And what a beautifully simple system you have here. Either of you can write the tune with these four notes and the other can fill in their part; it will always sound right. One advantage of this system is that whenever one of you makes a mistake, it's obvious. The note "do" always requires a corresponding "mi." The note "re" always requires a corresponding "fa." Mistakes are quickly identified and corrected.

That is exactly what happens in our DNA. Remember that our nucleotides are made with four different nitrogenous bases? Adenine and guanine have a form that classifies them as purines, nitrogenous bases with a double-ringed structure. Thymine and cytosine (and uracil, in RNA) are pyrimidines, nitrogenous bases with a single-ringed structure. Purines and pyrimidines in separate chains bind to each other. More specifically, the pyrimidine thymine always binds to the purine adenine in the corresponding chain. The pyrimidine cytosine always binds to the purine guanine in the corresponding chain. Nucleotides that bind together are said to be complementary for each other. This is no more confusing than the harmony notes indicated previously, only the words are changed. Look at **TABLE 14.2** for clarification.

Now, just like in the song, if one chain has adenine in the first position (the first note in the song), the other must have thymine in that position. If in the second position of the first chain you find guanine, the other chain must have cytosine in the corresponding position. If we assign a musical note to each of the nucleotides, we can actually sing the nucleotides, the genetic code,

Table 14.1 Simple Song Harmony

You Sing	Your Friend Sings
Do	Mi
Re	Fa
Mi	Do
Fa	Re

Table 14.2 Complementary Base Pairs

Chain One	Chain Two
Adenine	Thymine
Guanine	Cytosine
Thymine	Adenine
Cytosine	Guanine

in our DNA. We will find harmony between the two strands of DNA because that is how they are made.

Remember when you and your friend were thinking up melodies, one could think up a melody and the other would be able to match it with the harmonious notes because the system had regular rules: wherever one note was sung by you, the corresponding harmonious note was sung by your friend. The same rules apply here. If we know the order of the nucleotides in one chain, we can easily make the other chain.

14.3 DNA Replication: Like Teaching a Friend a Song

When you and your friend want to teach two others to sing like you do, you can each teach the rules to another person; then you can sing your tones and the new friend can sing the harmonious notes. In this way, you can get two pairs of singers quickly and easily. Each of the new singing pairs has one member of the first singing group (you or your initial friend) and one new singer (see **FIGURE 14.2**).

When we need to replicate our DNA (Remember in what phase of mitosis that occurs?), our DNA uncoils and the two chains separate from each other (Figure 14.2). This has the appearance of a zipper opening up, and exposes the binding sites between the two chains. Through the use of a series of enzymes, a new chain of nucleic acids is added to each of the two existing chains. This results in two double chains of DNA; each chain has one of the pre-existing chains and one newly synthesized chain. This is called semiconservative replication and is how our cells reproduce their DNA.

When you think about the great multitude of nucleotide pairs that must be reproduced because of the size of our genome, our genetic content, you soon realize that the S phase of the cell cycle, late in interphase (Remember this from Chapter 3?), would last forever if this were to be done only at one point per DNA chain (chromosome). So, it is actually occurring simultaneously at about 25,000 places in the genome. That's right, 25,000! Each

of these reproducing units consists of about 100,000 to 200,000 base pairs, and is referred to as a replicon.

What a great system this is! Just like when teaching your friend the song, any wrong notes will be recognized and corrected; incorrect nucleic acids are recognized and removed by enzymatic processes, giving highly accurate copies. When you consider the trillions of cells we have as an adult, never mind those that have been replaced over the years, and the fact that they all began from one cell that was reproduced over and over again, it is apparent why this high degree of accuracy in copying is needed. Add to this the fact that the genetic content of each cell contains about 3 billion pairs of nucleotides, and that mistakes, if they occur at crucial points in the code and at crucial points in development, could lead to death, birth defects, metabolic diseases, cancer, or other disturbances of homeostasis, and you see the need for accuracy in DNA replication. We generally consider an event that occurs "one in a million times" to be a rare event (think of the lottery system, or being hit by lightning). A "one in a million" error rate in DNA reproduction would result in 3,000 incorrect nucleotides per cell replication cycle. Since these mistakes would be compounded with each subsequent cell division, it is obvious that an error rate even far less than this would be lethal very quickly.

14.4 Your DNA Code: What It Actually Encodes

You have no doubt heard about the DNA code forever and have had everything from your blood type to your hair color attributed to it. But what does it actually encode and how does it do this? Think of your cells as protein factories, because that is the principle thing they are designed to do: cells make proteins. If cells are factories, they must have plans or blueprints for the things they make, right? If you had a furniture factory, you would have plans for chairs, tables, and other pieces of furniture that you would make. The DNA in the nucleus is the blueprint for the proteins the cell can make. That's all it is. Period. When people say that your genes, your DNA, encode your hair color, they are not being entirely accurate. Your DNA encodes the enzymes (proteins) that produce the pigment that is your hair color. The enzymes responsible for one hair color differ from the enzymes responsible for a different hair color. The enzymes are what is encoded by your DNA.

When people say that your blood type is encoded by your DNA, they are skipping a step. Blood group antigens (the molecules that confer blood type) differ in their carbohydrate moieties (what sugars they carry).

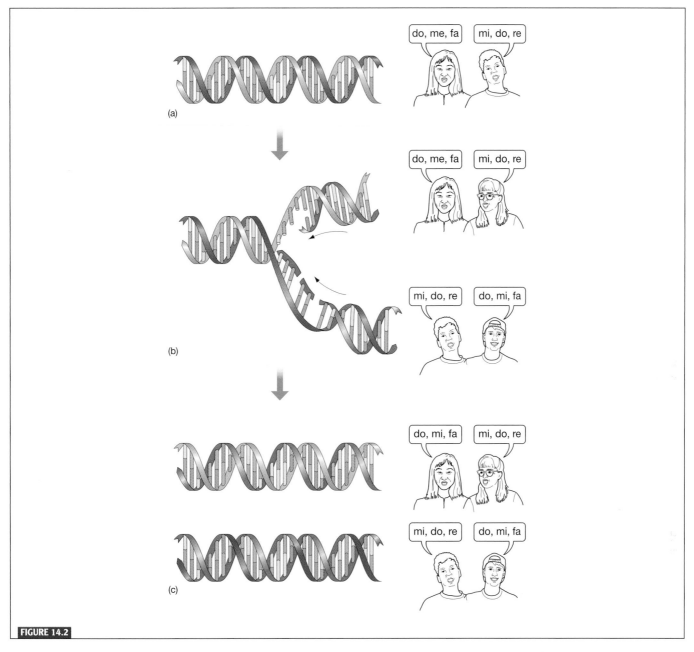

FIGURE 14.2

DNA synthesis. Complementarity of nucleotides makes semiconservative replication of DNA similar to using harmony when teaching a friend a song.

These carbohydrates are the products of enzymes that are encoded by your DNA. The DNA encodes the enzymes responsible for producing the carbohydrates that determine blood type. Bloodtyping is presented in greater detail in Chapter 16.

14.5 The DNA Code and Protein Synthesis

So, let's think about how the DNA can serve as the plans for proteins. You recall that we use 20 different amino acids to produce our proteins, and that we use these proteins much the way we use letters to write words. The order of the individual amino acids determines the protein. The DNA encodes the order of the amino acids in the proteins. If we can read off the order of the amino acids, we can produce the protein. The code that is used for this has been "cracked," and we can now look at a DNA sequence and determine what amino acids are being specified.

It works like this. Every three nucleotides in the chain specify one amino acid. It is important to know that only one of the two strands of DNA actually encode proteins; the other one is there so semiconservative replication can occur. The strand that is used in protein synthesis is called the template strand and is written in "anti-sense," which will be explained shortly (hold that thought). The encoding strand specifies one amino acid, every three nucleotides. These three nucleotides are called a codon. Codons are composed of three nucleotides and specify where to start protein synthesis, what amino acids to use, and where to stop protein synthesis. We must stop here before discussing the code fur-

ther because we are skipping one important step. Let's begin with that.

■ Transcription

Let's assume for a moment that you own a furniture factory (**FIGURE 14.3a**). This factory has been in your family for generations and now you run it. In fact, the furniture you make is the same as that made by your great grandfather; you have continued to use the plans you

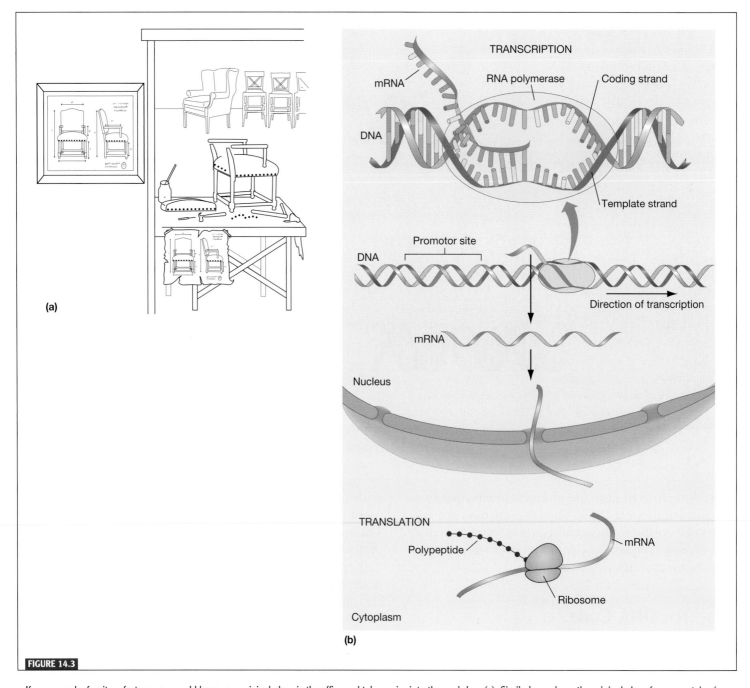

FIGURE 14.3

If you owned a furniture factory, you would keep your original plans in the office and take copies into the workshop (a). Similarly, we keep the original plans for our proteins (our DNA) in the nuclei of our cells. Transcription is the process we use to produce RNA copies of our DNA (b). These copies (mRNA) are used in the cytoplasm during translation.

inherited from him. When your workers are about to start production of a certain chair, would you allow them to take those precious plans out of the office into the shop where they are working? Of course not! You realize that anything could happen out in the shop. There's paint and varnish and glue and sharp tools and every other thing that could ruin those plans out there. Worse yet, if those plans are destroyed, you would not be able to make those chairs anymore, and they are crucial to the survival of your factory. You require your worker to copy the plans, and take the copy into the shop. The original plan must stay in the office.

Back to our cells (Figure 14.3b). The "office" of our protein factory is the nucleus. The original set of plans is the DNA. The DNA can not be taken out of the nucleus for use in the cytoplasm where proteins will be synthesized. The DNA must be copied into a form that can be removed to the cytoplasm so protein synthesis can occur.

The process of copying the DNA, the plan for our protein, for protein synthesis is called transcription. The DNA is transcribed into RNA for use within the cytoplasm. The particular form of RNA used this way is messenger RNA (mRNA). Messenger RNA is single-stranded RNA and is produced by RNA polymerase (an enzyme).

When a particular gene is to be transcribed, RNA polymerase moves along the DNA looking for a promoter sequence. This is essentially a sequence that tells the polymerase where to begin. The DNA must be in the proper form to allow this to occur: it must be single-stranded. Again an enzyme takes care of this, just as it does during DNA replication. The RNA polymerase uses the "template strand" to synthesize a complementary strand of RNA. The same base pairing that allows DNA synthesis to occur works here, except that we are now using ribonucleotides not deoxyribonucleotides, and uracil is substituted for thymine. There is no thymine in RNA; uracil is complementary to the adenine of DNA when synthesizing RNA.

The template strand of DNA is written in antisense. This means that its order of nucleotides does not encode amino acids; rather, the nucleotides that are complementary to its nucleotides encode amino acids. This is perfect, since the mRNA will consist of those complementary nucleotides and will be used in the cytoplasm as the plan to make the protein. Incidentally, the DNA strand not used for RNA transcription is called the coding strand and is written in sense. If we wish to know what amino acids are encoded by a gene, we look at the coding strand, not the template strand. We can read the coding strand, make sense of the code (it's written in sense), and know what amino acids are specified.

As it is producing RNA, the RNA polymerase watches for specific sequences to tell it where to stop transcription. The pieces of RNA generated in this way vary greatly in size. The average size at this point is around 5,000 nucleotides, but strands of up to 200,000 nucleotides have been observed. This variability makes sense, as the proteins encoded by these pieces of RNA also vary greatly in size. But that is not all there is to it.

This RNA must be processed further to become mature mRNA, ready for translation into the amino acids of protein. Only specific portions of the RNA encode amino acids. These are called exons (as in "expressed regions") or coding sequences. Exons must be retained in the processed mRNA. Other regions called introns (for 'intervening regions') are mixed in with the exons and must be cut out. Introns vary greatly in size and number. In some mRNA, the introns make up more of the strand than do the exons. We do not currently understand the role of the introns, but they must be removed for the mRNA to function.

Finally, our mRNA is mature and ready to serve as a blueprint for a protein. It's time for the next step.

■ Translation

First, we had to transcribe our DNA into a form that could be used as a plan for the protein we are synthesizing. Now it is time to produce the string of amino acids that will become the protein. This step is called translation: we are translating the genetic code from nucleotides (our mRNA) into amino acids (our protein). You already know a bit about this process. In what organelle does this occur? Remember, this organelle exists in two forms: one form for proteins to be used within the cell, the other for proteins that will be inserted into the cell membrane or exported from the cell. Ribosomes are the organelle that is the site of protein production. Recall that they can be either free ribosomes or bound ribosomes, which are located on the rough endoplasmic reticulum.

We need to think about how the mRNA serves as a blueprint for the protein. We already know that the nucleotides of the mRNA are ordered such that every three nucleotides (called a codon) specify one amino acid. This arrangement is referred to as a triplet code. Figure 14.4 diagrams the coding dictionary that indicates which codons specify which amino acids. Note that AUG is the start codon. Translation starts with this codon; therefore, the first amino acid in every polypeptide chain produced is a methionine.

The code continues one codon (three nucleotides) at a time. Amino acids are added sequentially until a stop codon is reached. The stop codons include the sequences UAG, UAA, or UGA. Any of these will cause termination of translation.

But what performs the actual translation and where does it occur? Well, we already decided that the ribosomes are the site of translation. They are composed of two subunits, each made up of ribosomal RNA (rRNA) and ribosomal proteins. They are constructed in the nucleolus, and although they are functional only when both subunits are together, they dissociate when not in use. Together they have two binding sites that are used in holding the amino acids in position as the polypeptide chain is constructed (Figure 14.5).

Transfer RNA (tRNA), small nucleic acid molecules, carries amino acids to the ribosome for assembly. They are composed of unusual nitrogenous bases that are mostly produced by modifying the more conventional bases. Transfer RNA contains, in a specific location, three nucleotides called the anticodon. The nucleotide sequence of the anticodon is complementary to the nucleotides of a codon on the mRNA. The same binding rules we learned about for DNA synthesis and RNA transcription apply here. Look at the coding dictionary (**FIGURE 14.4**) and determine what amino acid would be specified by the codon AAG. The tRNA that has an anticodon that is complementary to the codon AAG (what nucleotides would the anticodon contain?) would carry

the amino acid you just looked up. Let's try one more. The codon CGC specifies the amino acid arginine. The tRNA that carries arginine has the anticodon GCG.

Let's try to put it together now. To begin translation, the two subunits of the ribosome come together with mRNA. They align on one end of the mRNA (this is unidirectional) where the start codon AUG is located. The tRNA that carries methionine has the anticodon UAC. The UAC aligns with the AUG and transfers its amino acid to the ribosome. The ribosome moves to the next codon; we'll say it's CUA, but it could be almost anything. The tRNA with the anticodon GAU aligns itself with this codon and transfers the leucine it carries to the ribosome, which binds it to the methionine it already holds. The ribosome now moves to the next codon, which we'll say is ACC. The tRNA with the complementary anticodon (UGG) moves into position over the mRNA, next to the ribosome. It transfers its amino acid (threonine) to the ribosome, which binds it to the leucine, making three amino acids in our chain. This continues until a stop codon is reached. In this way, a polypeptide chain is formed. Look at **FIGURE 14.5** for another example.

Is this polypeptide chain our active protein? Usually the answer is no; post-translational modification of the polypeptide in the Golgi apparatus is usually necessary. Let's look at an example.

■ An Example of Protein Synthesis: Insulin

Insulin is an interesting example. Look at Figure 14.6 to see how insulin is translated and processed. Insulin is actually translated as preproinsulin, a very long polypeptide chain that is totally inactive. Initially, the beginning of this chain is cleaved off. This region, called the signal sequence, includes the methionine specified by the start codon. Once it is cleaved off, the remaining molecule is called proinsulin and is still inactive. Proinsulin consists of three subunits: the B chain has 30 amino acid residues, the C chain consists of 63 amino acid residues, and the A chain has 21 amino acid residues.

Now, think for a minute about something else. Did you ever make a model car, ship, or plane? When you opened the box, were the pieces all ready to be glued together? No, you had to separate them from some plastic that was used in the molding process during manufacture of the parts (**FIGURE 14.6**). This is very similar to the way in which the C chain is used in the manufacture of insulin. Together, the A and B chains are the actual insulin molecule. The C chain holds the A and B chains into position so they can be bound together. Once they are bound together, the C chain, used only in the "manufacturing" process, is cut out and discarded (broken down and recycled).

Second nucleotide in codon

		U	C	A	G	
First nucleotide in codon	U	UUU UUC Phe UUA UUG Leu	UCU UCC UCA UCG Ser	UAU UAC Tyr UAA Stop UAG Stop	UGU UGC Cys UGA Stop UGG Trp	U C A G
	C	CUU CUC CUA CUG Leu	CCU CCC CCA CCG Pro	CAU CAC His CAA CAG Gln	CGU CGC CGA CGG Arg	U C A G
	A	AUU AUC Ile AUA AUG Met	ACU ACC ACA ACG Thr	AAU AAC Asn AAA AAG Lys	AGU AGC Ser AGA AGG Arg	U C A G
	G	GUU GUC GUA GUG Val	GCU GCC GCA GCG Ala	GAU GAC Asp GAA GAG Glu	GGU GGC GGA GGG Gly	U C A G

Codon ⁄ Amino acid

FIGURE 14.4

The coding dictionary contains the code by which translation produces an amino acid sequence from the nucleotide sequence of mRNA.

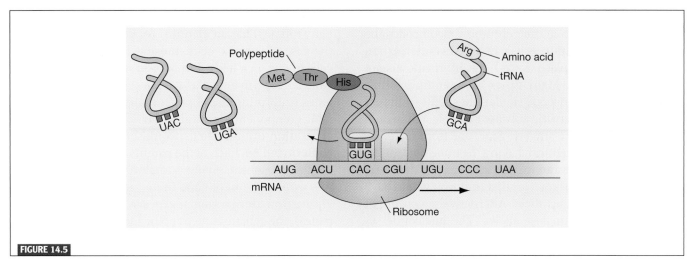

FIGURE 14.5

Translation.

The A and B chains, bound to each other, are the active insulin hormone. Without the C chain, they could not have been made, but the C chain had to be removed for them to become active.

That's it for protein synthesis. Now you see how our genetic apparatus specifies the characteristics that contribute to who we are. It is all done through proteins. Our DNA is the plan from which our proteins are made, and an intermediate plan, the mRNA, actually serves as the plan used out in our cells' "workshops."

One last topic we must consider before we move on to reproduction is where our genes come from and how

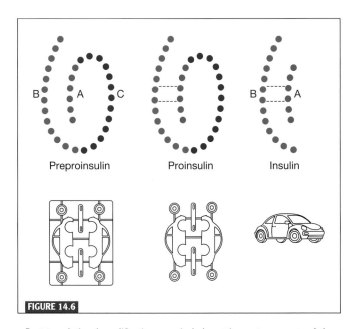

FIGURE 14.6

Post-translational modification may include cutting out segments of the newly formed polypeptide sequence and recombining the remaining pieces into the functional protein. Notice the similarity to model building.

genetic variability is maximized for the benefit of our species.

14.6 Meiosis: The Generation of Variability

We each have 46 chromosomes, or 23 pairs of chromosomes. Twenty-two of these are our somatic chromosomes, with the remaining pair being our sex chromosomes. This simply means that 22 pairs are not involved in sex determination, and one pair is. We refer to this full chromosomal compliment as being $2n$ or diploid, meaning that we have two sets of homologous pairs of chromosomes. Each pair of chromosomes is numbered: you have two chromosomes number one, two number twos, and so on. This means that we have two sets of chromosomes with each chromosome in a pair encoding the same type of information. The two chromosomes of the same number are referred to as a homologous pair. If, for example, we find the gene that encodes the enzyme pancreatic amylase on chromosome one, you actually have two copies of this gene, one on each of your two chromosomes number one (each member of the homologous pair). The one exception to this is the sex chromosomes. If you have a pair of X chromosomes, you are genetically female; if you have an unmatched pair of one X and one Y, you are genetically male.

How did you manage to get two sets of chromosomes, and are they identical to each other? You received one copy, one set of chromosomes, from each of your parents. One copy came in the spermatozoa from your father, and the other was in the ovum from your mother. When these two gametes fused and became the cell that would become you, you had 23 chromosomes from each parent: 23 pairs or two complete sets. Naturally, these sets are not identical. While each chromosome encodes the same type of information as its pair and that information is found in the same place (locus), the information is not necessarily identical. Many genes have multiple forms, called alleles, which encode similar but slightly different proteins. In our pancreatic amylase example, you would have two copies of the amylase gene, one from each parent. Both might be identical; having the same nucleotide, and, hence, the same amino acid sequence. In that case, you would be homozygous for that trait: you would have two copies of the same allele. Alternatively, you might have two different amylase alleles. The nucleotide sequence would be different between the gene received from your mother and that from your father. Both would be amylase genes, but the nucleotide sequence and potentially the resulting amino acid sequence of the two would differ. You would be heterozygous for this gene. Genotypic differences, differences in our genetic composition, might result in phenotypic differences, differences in actual traits we can measure or observe. These phenotypic differences might result from differences in the activity of the proteins specified by different alleles of the same gene; some might be more or less active, or even completely inactive or overly active. It is these differences in alleles that determine our individuality.

The facts that our parents each have two copies of each chromosome and that they donate to each of us one copy at the time of conception leads us now to a number of important questions. How do they give us only half of the genetic content of their cells? Do the chromosomes they pass on match the chromosomes they received from their parents, or is some further process leading to greater variability? We can answer both of these questions by learning about meiosis.

Remember mitosis, from Chapter 3? In discussing mitosis, we learned that to divide, our cells replicate their DNA and then split it so that each of their two daughter cells (or nuclei, if cytokinesis does not accompany mitosis) has an identical copy. This works great in the case of somatic cells, those cells that make up the cells of our own body. But how about our gametes? Our gametes (sperm and ova) are the cells that our body donates in forming the next generation. If they had a genetic component identical to our somatic cells, the next generation of individuals would not have a $2n$ genetic content, but $4n$. Each of the parents would have donated 46 chromosomes, giving a total of 92. As you can see, this would get out of hand in no time.

Instead, during gametogenesis (formation of the gametes), the genetic content of the forming sperm and ova is reduced by 50 percent. This condition is termed $1n$ or haploid: only one member of each of the original chromosome pairs is present. Rather than mitosis, meiosis is the form of nuclear division used. Meiosis is similar to mitosis in a many respects, but differs in some important ways. First, there are two nuclear divisions linked together in meiosis. Second, replication of DNA does not occur between the first and second meiotic divisions. Third, a reshuffling of genetic information occurs as part of this process. This reshuffling, called crossing over, ensures greater genetic variability between generations (**FIGURE 14.7**). The copy of any chromosome you receive from one of your parents does not match the chromosome they received from either one of their parents. Instead, it is a combination of the chromosomes from their parents (your grandparents). The steps of meiosis are shown in **FIGURE 14.8**. Please look this over and become familiar with the steps involved. Gametogenesis will be discussed in greater detail in Chapter 15.

Please also ensure your familiarity with this information by using the "What You Should Know" and "What Did You Learn?" features of this chapter before venturing on. This will help you to be certain you have laid the proper foundation for success in understanding reproduction.

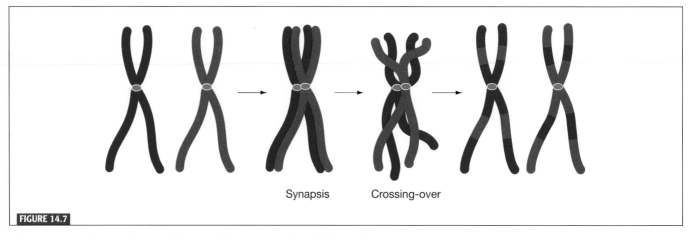

Synapsis   Crossing-over

FIGURE 14.7

Synapsis and crossing over during meiosis results in increased genetic variability in subsequent generations.

Stage	Description	Diagram

Meiotic Division I

Interphase — DNA replication occurs

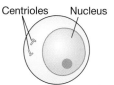

Centrioles   Nucleus

Prophase — As in mitosis except that chromosomes join together in homologous pairs. This pairing-up is called synapsis. Now portions of the homologous pairs are exchanged with each other. This is called "crossing-over" and maximizes genetic variability between generations.

Chromosomes

Metaphase — Chromosomes line up along the equatorial plane, similar to mitosis except that here the chromosomes are in their homologous pairs.

Anaphase — Homologous pairs, not individual chromatids, separate and move toward opposite poles. The centromeres do not split. This is a major difference from what we see in mitosis.

Telophase — As in mitosis, including the process of cytokinesis.

Meiotic Division II

Interphase — Is very brief or absent. Replication of DNA does not occur; hence these daughter cells begin this nuclear division with a $2n$ genetic content only.

Other phases — Exactly as in mitosis. Meiosis results in four daughter cells (from two successive divisions) with half the genetic content of the original parent cell. These daughter cells have an enhanced degree of genetic variability due to synapsis and crossing-over. As we will next learn, not all of the daughter cells may be viable.

FIGURE 14.8

Meiosis, the nuclear division of gametogenesis, results in daughter cells with a $1n$ genetic content.

Breaching Homeostasis . . . When Things Go Wrong

Genetic Mutations

When a system is as complex as the genetic code, it makes sense that things will sometimes go wrong. Mutations can occur during DNA replication. Most mistakes will be detected and corrected. Others may result in genetic mutations. If these mutations are present in the germ cells, they may be passed on to future generations. Spontaneous mutations occur during gameto-genesis at a rate of approximately one per 100,000 to 1 million gametes formed.

Several different forms of mutations can occur in this way. The easiest to imagine may be a point mutation or base substitution. In this form of mutation, one nucleotide is substituted for another during replication. These substitutions cause changes within one codon, which may result in the alteration of one amino acid in the ultimate product. This difference can have varying effects on the function of the encoded protein, ranging from increased activity to no activity at all. The result on the effected individual can range from no easily detectable difference to a lethal mutation (one not compatible with life). If the altered codon becomes a stop codon, larger changes to the gene product will follow. Sickle cell anemia is an example of a base substitution mutation. In that disorder, one nucleotide is substituted for another in the sixth codon of the gene encoding one of the hemoglobin chains. This alters the amino acid at that position from glutamic acid to valine. This seemingly small change alters the three-dimensional shape of the hemoglobin molecule, resulting in this debilitating inherited disease.

In another type of mutation, the insertion or deletion of one nucleotide puts the entire sequence of codons distal to that change off by one place. This results in major changes to the gene and its product. These are called frameshift mutations, as they result in a frameshift out of the reading frame. The extent of the effect on the encoded protein is dependent on where the frameshift occurs. If it occurs near the beginning of the gene, the effect on the protein it encodes will be drastic. If the frameshift is near the end of the gene, the effect may be minimal.

Larger mutations can also occur. One example is the loss of an entire codon. Several different mutations to the gene encoding a specific integral membrane protein called the cystic fibrosis transmembrane regulator (CFTR) each result in the disease cystic fibrosis. The most common of these mutations is a codon deletion eliminating a phenylalanine in the 508th position. Disruption in this protein's ability to transport the chloride ion (Cl^-) results in the viscous mucous secretions that block the airways and alimentary canal in these patients.

Another large alteration is that of the trinucleotide repeat. Trinucleotide repeats are insertion mutations: a triplet of nucleotides is repeated one or more times. Huntington's disease is an example of a disease caused by a trinucleotide repeat.

In some cases, these mutations have no effect on the individual; in other cases they are lethal. The multiple alleles we observe for many genes all apparently began as mutations to the original form of the gene, at some point in time. Mutations can result in beneficial biological diversity or in disease, depending on the gene and mutation involved.

What You Should Know

1. Base pair complementarity determines that, while any order of nucleotides can exist within a nucleic acid chain, the order of the nucleotides in one chain determines the order of nucleotides in its complementary chain.

2. Adenine and thymine are complementary; guanine and cytosine are complementary.

3. This complementarity allows highly accurate semiconservative replication of DNA.

4. The DNA in your nuclei act as permanent plans for the proteins your cells can synthesize: DNA encodes protein.

5. Three nucleotides (one codon) encode one amino acid.

6. Transcription is the process of copying our DNA code into a complementary strand of RNA for protein synthesis.

7. RNA does not contain thymine; in RNA, uracil is complementary for adenine.

What You Should Know (continued)

8. Once processed (modified in a variety of ways, including the removal of introns and the rejoining of exons), the RNA produced through transcription is called messenger RNA (mRNA).

9. In the cytoplasm, mRNA participates in translation, the next step in protein synthesis.

10. Translation is the process used to "translate" the genetic code from nucleic acids (mRNA) into the amino acids of protein.

11. Ribosomes (rRNA), messenger RNA (mRNA), and transfer RNA (tRNA) each play a role in the process of translation. Complementarity between nucleotides in the mRNA and the tRNA works to deliver the right amino acids in the proper order.

12. Meiosis is the form of nuclear division used during gametogenesis. It differs from mitosis in that meiosis results in daughter nuclei that have one half the genetic content of our somatic cells.

13. Nuclei with the full genetic content (46 chromosomes, 23 pairs of homologous chromosomes) are called diploid or $2n$. Nuclei after meiosis have 23 nonhomologous chromosomes, referred to as haploid or $1n$.

14. Meiosis involves two successive nuclear divisions with no DNA syntheses between the first and second meiotic division.

15. Crossing over, a process of genetic reshuffling, serves to increase the amount of genetic variability between individuals produced by sexual reproduction.

What Did You Learn?

Multiple choice questions: choose the best answer.

1. Complementarity in DNA dictates that adenine in one chain pairs with ___ in its complementary chain.
   a. Guanine
   b. Thymine
   c. Cytosine
   d. Uracil
   e. Adenine

2. During RNA synthesis, an adenine in the template strand results in a ___ nucleotide in the newly synthesized chain.
   a. Guanine
   b. Thymine
   c. Cytosine
   d. Uracil
   e. Adenine

3. Which nucleotide is not present in RNA?
   a. Guanine
   b. Thymine
   c. Cytosine
   d. Uracil
   e. Adenine

4. DNA <u>specifically</u> encodes:
   a. Blood type
   b. Hair color
   c. Protein structure
   d. Carbohydrate structure

5. Every _____ nucleotides encode one amino acid.
   a. Two
   b. Three
   c. Four
   d. Five

6. A group of nucleotides that encode one amino acid is called a:
   a. Replicon
   b. Codon
   c. Gyrase
   d. Aminicon
   e. None of the above

7. The template strand of DNA is written in:
   a. Sense
   b. Antisense
   c. Nonsense
   d. Horse sense
   e. Common sense

8. Messenger RNA is written in:
   a. Sense
   b. Antisense
   c. Nonsense
   d. Horse sense
   e. Common sense

What Did You Learn? (continued)

9. The step in protein synthesis in which the template strand of DNA is copied into RNA is called:

   a. Translation

   b. Transcription

   c. Transduction

   d. Transportation

10. AUG is the start codon. It specifies the amino acid _____.

    a. Glycine

    b. Glutamic acid

    c. Methionine

    d. Tyrosine

    e. None of the above

11. A stop codon specifies the amino acid _____.

    a. Glycine

    b. Glutamic acid

    c. Methionine

    d. Tyrosine

    e. None of the above

12. What carries amino acids to the ribosomes during translation?

    a. mRNA

    b. rRNA

    c. tRNA

    d. upsRNA

    e. None of the above

13. The multiple forms of a particular gene that might be found at a specific locus are called:

    a. Alleles

    b. Gyrases

    c. Options

    d. Replicons

14. Accurate replication of DNA is essential to our species. A simple substitution of one nucleotide in the DNA of a gamete can result in _____ in the resulting offspring.

    a. Disease

    b. A lethal mutation

    c. No change at all

    d. Any of the above

15. Crossing over occurs in:

    a. Mitosis

    b. Meiosis

    c. Both of the above

    d. Neither of the above

16. DNA replication occurs before (as part of):

    a. Meiotic division I

    b. Meiotic division II

    c. Both of the above

    d. Neither of the above

17. If our somatic cells have 23 pairs of chromosomes, our gametes have:

    a. Twenty-three pairs also

    b. Twenty-three unpaired chromosomes

    c. Forty-six pairs

    d. Forty-six unpaired chromosomes

18. The 1n genetic content of our gametes is also called:

    a. Haploid

    b. Diploid

    c. Triploid

    d. Tetraploid

    e. None of the above

Short answer questions: answer briefly and in your own words.

1. Define complementarity as it applies to nucleic acids. Which nucleotides are complementary for each other? How is complementarity used in DNA replication and protein synthesis?

2. Describe the process of DNA replication. What characteristics of this process contribute to its accuracy?

3. How does the DNA code actually specify the structure of proteins?

4. Describe the steps involved in protein synthesis, starting with those that occur in the nucleus and finishing with those that occur in the cytoplasm.

5. Why is meiosis necessary? What aspect of meiosis contributes to biological diversity?

6. What might happen if, during DNA replication, one nucleotide is substituted for another? Please explain your answer.

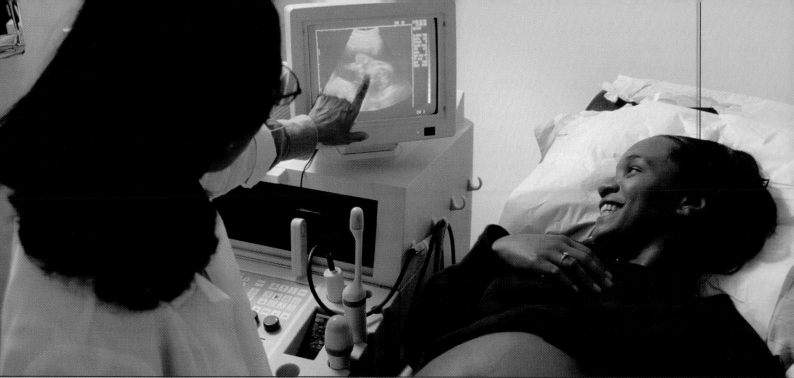

Your Reproductive System

What You Will Learn

- Which organs are primary sex organs and which are secondary sex organs.
- The functions, location, and internal structure of the testes.
- How and why the scrotum and associated muscles regulate the temperature of the testes.
- The types of cells that are found in and around the seminiferous tubules.
- The process of spermatogenesis and the structure of sperm.
- The structure of the ducts that convey sperm and associated fluids to the exterior of the body.
- The names, locations, and structures of the glands that make the fluid components of semen.
- How the male organ of copulation functions.
- The structure of the ovaries and the stages of ovarian follicle development.
- The steps involved in oogenesis.
- The hormones that regulate the activities of the female reproductive tract.
- The organs that convey the oocyte from the ovaries, provide the site for fertilization, support and nurture the developing embryo, and allow delivery of the baby at the end of gestation.
- The stages of the female reproductive cycle, including what happens at each stage, which hormones are responsible for that activity, and the timing of these stages.
- The structure and function of the mammary glands.
- How lactation is initiated and maintained, and the system that regulates release of milk from the mammary glands.

15.1 An Unusual System

This is truly an amazing system and highly unusual in that it exists in two forms, with approximately half of the population exhibiting each form. Together, the two forms of the reproductive system (the male and female genders) have enabled us to propagate this species for untold generations.

We will first consider the male reproductive system and then the female system. This will allow you to become familiar with several concepts in the "simpler" of the two systems before we study the more complex form.

The reproductive organs in each gender include a primary sex organ and several secondary sex organs. The primary sex organ is the one that produces the gametes of that sex: the sperm or ova. So, in the male, the primary sex organ is the testes. In the female, the primary sex organ is the ovary. The secondary sex organs are those that convey the gametes and associated secretions to the site of fertilization, or provide the site for development of the fetus, or provide for the passage of the fetus from the body. Please be careful not to confuse the secondary sex organs with the secondary sex char-

acteristics. The secondary sex characteristics are those features that are gender specific but are not necessarily essential for the reproductive process. They include the differences in physique, hair distribution, voice pitch, and other characteristics that we observe as generally being different between the two genders. For each gender, we will first consider the primary sex organ and then the secondary sex organs.

15.2 The Male Reproductive System

■ The Male Primary Sex Organ: The Testes

The male primary sex organ is the testicle (**FIGURE 15.1**) or testis (testes is plural). In males, this is the site of gametogenesis (production of gametes; since we're considering males, sperm). The testes are paired oval glands, weighing approximately 10–15 grams. They reside within the scrotum, an outpouching of the abdominopelvic cavity. The scrotum is separated by a connective tissue septum into two compartments, one for each testicle. Smooth muscle called dartos is found in this septum and in the subcutaneous tissues of the scrotum. It gives the skin of the scrotum a wrinkled appearance.

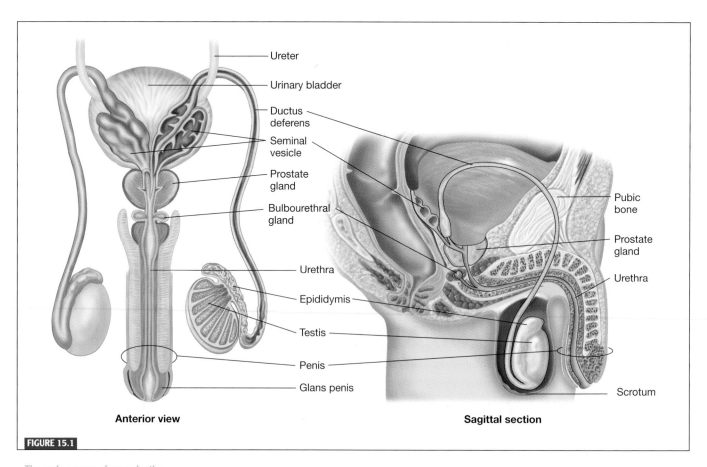

Ureter
Urinary bladder
Ductus deferens
Seminal vesicle
Prostate gland
Bulbourethral gland
Urethra
Epididymis
Testis
Penis
Glans penis

Pubic bone
Prostate gland
Urethra
Scrotum

Anterior view

Sagittal section

FIGURE 15.1

The male organs of reproduction.

The dartos and another smooth muscle structure called the cremaster muscle work together to elevate and lower the testes to maintain them at a specific temperature. The temperature of the body is approximately 3 degrees too warm to allow spermatogenesis (male gametogenesis, production of sperm). By housing the testes in a pouch outside of the main structure of the body and providing a mechanism that raises and lowers the testes based on temperature, the body is able to maintain a different temperature in the testes than in the rest of the body. It is sort of like the compartment that fancy refrigerators have for storing butter; it is part of the main structure, but somewhat separate, allowing separate temperature control.

The importance of this became apparent to many males during the 1970s, when an unusually high number of couples began complaining to their physicians about infertility problems. At that time it was the style for men to wear very tight pants, and this was defeating the temperature-controlling system of the scrotum by holding the testes tightly against the body wall. This created elevated temperatures in the testes and, subsequently, inadequate spermatogenesis. A simple change in clothing style corrected this sometimes-difficult medical problem for many couples at that time!

Within the scrotum, the testes are held within a pocket of peritoneum (called the tunica vaginalis) formed during the descent of the testes. During embryogenesis and fetal development, the testes arise in the abdominopelvic cavity and travel down into the scrotum. This is called the descent of the testes. The peritoneum forms a small pocket in the scrotum that makes this descent possible. In some cases, one or both testes may not descend properly. This condition, cryptorchidism (from the Greek *kryptos*, hidden; *orichis*, testes; and *ismos*, condition of), requires medical intervention.

The testes are tightly surrounded by a strong capsule (called the *tunica albuginea*). This capsule does not allow the testes to swell as they produce spermatozoa, forcing the sperm to travel out of the testes rather than being retained there. Unfortunately, this capsule also restricts the testes from distorting when being subjected to an impact, leading to great pain from even minor injury.

This capsule extends into the testes as septae (walls), dividing it into 200 to 300 lobules (**FIGURE 15.2**). These lobules each contain one to three highly coiled ducts called seminiferous tubules. It is within these tubules that spermatogenesis occurs.

Three major cell types are found in and around the seminiferous tubules. Within the tubules we find the germ cells (spermatogenic lineage) and the sustentacular cells. Lying between the tubules we find the interstitial endocrinocytes. We will discuss each of these in turn. Please refer to the illustration shown in Figure 15.2.

The Germ Cells and Spermatogenesis

The cell lineage that leads to the gametes (sperm in the male) is referred to as the germ cell lineage (in either sex),

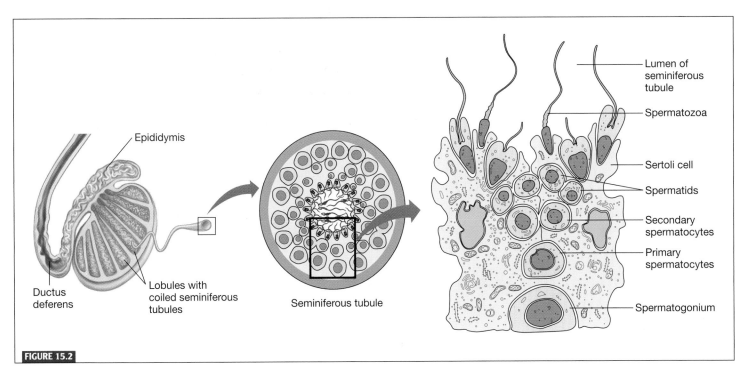

Lumen of seminiferous tubule

Spermatozoa

Sertoli cell

Spermatids

Secondary spermatocytes

Primary spermatocytes

Spermatogonium

Epididymis

Ductus deferens

Lobules with coiled seminiferous tubules

Seminiferous tubule

FIGURE 15.2

Internal structure of the testes.

or the spermatogenic lineage specifically in the male. The actual stem cell (the least differentiated cell, whose job it is to divide) of this lineage is the spermatogonium, which has a $2n$ (diploid) genetic content. Some of its daughter cells differentiate into primary spermatocytes, which begin meiosis (discussed in Chapter 14). After the first meiotic division, these become secondary spermatocytes. The second meiotic division results in spermatids with a $1n$ (haploid) genetic content. These differentiate further into spermatozoa. Spermatogenesis begins during puberty and continues throughout a man's lifetime.

To put this into some numerical perspective, approximately 300×10^6 (300 million) sperm are produced per day. In each milliliter of ejaculate (semen), there are $50–150 \times 10^6$ sperm. Ejaculate volumes are generally in the 1.5–5 milliliter range, giving a total of 75×10^6 to 750×10^6 (75–750 million) sperm per ejaculation. That may sound like an awful lot, when you consider that only one sperm fertilizes an ovum. High numbers of sperm are necessary, however, for the entry of one sperm into the ovum.

A mature sperm is shown in **FIGURE 15.3**. It is approximately 60 micrometers in length, most of which is tail. The acrosome, or acrosomal cap, is a modified lysosome that contains enzymes that break down the outer covering of the ovum. The acrosomal content of one sperm is not sufficient to break through this barrier. The combined contents of the acrosomes of many sperm are necessary.

The head of the sperm contains the nucleus. It carries the $1n$ (haploid) genetic content of this highly specialized cell. The midpiece contains the mitochondria that produce the energy needed to power the tail. The tail is actually a flagellum, a structure similar to a single cilia. It provides the propulsion needed to move the sperm far into the female reproductive tract where fertilization occurs. The life expectancy of a sperm after ejaculation into the female reproductive tract is 48–72 hours.

Sustentacular (Sertoli) Cells

Between the developing germ cells, but still within the seminiferous tubules, there are large cells called sus-

tentacular or Sertoli cells (Figure 15.2). These cells line the wall of the tubule and sit on the basement membrane of the tubule. Sustentacular cells organize and support the developing sperm cells. They control the position of the developing germ cells in the tubule, with the least differentiated toward the basement membrane and the most differentiated toward the lumen. Note in Figure 15.2 how the heads of the developing sperm are inserted into the sustentacular cells. They secrete the hormone inhibin, which regulates sperm production. In this way, sustentacular cells also control the release of spermatozoa from the testes. Inhibin is produced in response to FSH, the anterior pituitary hormone that stimulates sperm production. This is another example of negative feedback. Follicle stimulating hormone stimulates sperm production, but it also stimulates inhibin production. Inhibin inhibits sperm production; therefore, high levels of FSH cause inhibin to slow sperm production.

In keeping with their supporting role, sustentacular cells also phagocytize debris within the tubule.

Interstitial Endocrinocytes (Leydig Cells)

Do you remember, in Chapter 13, we discussed the fact that many glands have endocrine and exocrine functions. The testis is one such gland. The cells we have discussed thus far are those involved mainly with the exocrine function. The exocrine product is spermatozoa. The testis also produces androgenic (meaning male-producing) hormones, such as testosterone. Testosterone is necessary for spermatogenesis, for development of the male reproductive tract, and for development of the male secondary sex characteristics. Testosterone and related androgens are produced in response to luteinizing hormone (LH) from the anterior pituitary.

The cells that produce the androgens are aptly named interstitial endocrinocytes. The *interstitial* term refers to their position between the seminiferous tubules. The *endocrinocyte* term indicates that they are hormone-producing cells.

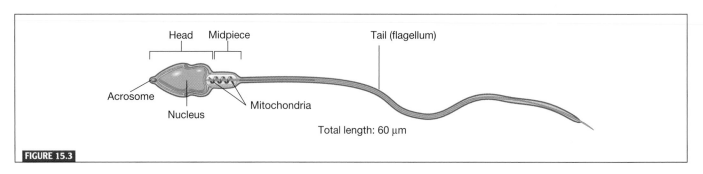

Head   Midpiece   Tail (flagellum)

Acrosome

Nucleus   Mitochondria

Total length: 60 μm

FIGURE 15.3

A mature sperm cell.

This ends our discussion of the cells of the testis. The developing sperm travel through the seminiferous tubules to exit this gland. They are not fertile when they leave the testis. Maturation must occur in the next structure in their path before they become fertile.

■ Secondary Sex Organs of the Male: Ducts for the Passage of Sperm and Fluids

Before we begin our discussion of the male secondary sex organs, please look again at Figure 15.1. This illustration depicts the male reproductive tract. Notice that you can follow a pathway through this system from the testes to the exterior of the body. This is the pathway that spermatozoa travel, and that we are about to "travel" as we learn about this system.

The Epididymis

The term *epididymis* is descriptive of the location of this structure. *Epi*-refers to being "upon," while the root of the term comes from the Greek word *didymos,* meaning testis. The epididymis sits on the testis, as a small, comma shaped structure. Note its location, shape, and relative size in Figure 15.1. It houses one highly coiled tubule that, if stretched out, would reach about 7 meters (approximately 20 feet) in length. It is necessary for sperm to mature for 10–14 days in the epididymis to become fertile. They may be stored here for 4 weeks, and if not used, are then reabsorbed.

The Ductus (Vas) Deferens

This duct of approximately 45 centimeters (18 inches) conveys sperm from the epididymis to the ejaculatory duct (Figure 15.1). It exits the scrotum as part of the spermatic cord. In addition to the ductus deferens, the spermatic cord contains the testicular artery, veins, lymphatic vessels, the cremaster muscle, and autonomic nerves. It travels from the scrotum into the actual pelvic cavity.

The walls of the ductus deferens are highly folded and lined with pseudostratified columnar epithelium. The walls also contain much smooth muscle, which contracts in peristaltic waves to propel sperm during ejaculation. As this duct ascends within the pelvic cavity, it loops over the lateral portion of the urinary bladder before ending with a dilated region called the ampulla (meaning "little jar").

Male surgical sterilization involves cutting the ductus (vas) deferens in a procedure called a vasectomy (*vas* means duct, *-ectomy* is from the Greek *ektome* meaning "to cut"). In this procedure, the normal pathway of the ductus deferens is interrupted by cutting and perhaps removal of a portion of this duct. After this procedure, ejaculation occurs as before, except that the semen no longer contains sperm. The "maleness" of the individual is absolutely unchanged; testosterone production and secondary sex characteristics remain as before. His semen simply does not contain sperm. This procedure must be considered permanent, however, due to the low success rate of reversal procedures.

The Ejaculatory Duct

This short duct (Figure 15.1) allows the mixing of sperm, coming from the vas deferens, with the secretion of the seminal vesicle (which we will learn about in a moment). The name "ejaculatory duct" is somewhat misleading. You might assume from its name that it provides some of the propulsive force for ejaculation; however, it lacks smooth muscle that would be required for that purpose. It merely is the site for mixing these secretions and connects those two structures to the urethra.

The Urethra

This is the final passageway for the exit of sperm from the body. It also carries urine and, thus, plays a role in two different organ systems. It is approximately 19 centimeters (8 inches or so) long and consists of three distinct regions. These regions are named for, and characterized by, the structures through which they pass.

The first region is the prostatic urethra and is only about 3 centimeters long. This section passes through the prostate (which we will consider in a moment) and is lined with transitional epithelium. Recall from Chapter 4 that this is the epithelium of the urinary bladder, which lies at its proximal end.

The membranous urethra is approximately 1 centimeter long and passes through the floor of the pelvis. The external urethral sphincter (a sphincter is a ring of smooth muscle) is part of this structure. The epithelium of the membranous urethra is columnar, of either the stratified or pseudostratified type. This is one of the rare places in which we may find stratified columnar epithelium.

The spongy urethra derives its name from the portion of the penis it traverses: the corpus spongiosum. It is about 15 centimeters long and is lined with stratified squamous epithelium. Mucous glands line this region of the urethra and are there to counteract the acidity of any urine residue that might remain and jeopardize the survival of passing sperm.

■ Secondary Sex Organs of the Male: Accessory Glands

We are still considering male secondary sex organs. We have followed the pathway of the genital tract all the way to its exit from the body at the tip of the penis. We now must consider several glands that deliver their secretions into this tract. These secretions are primarily the liquid component of semen, the fluid that contains sperm and is released during ejaculation. We will consider them in the order in which they enter this tract.

Seminal Vesicles

These paired glands of approximately 5 centimeters (2 inches) are located posterior and inferior to the bladder and lateral to the ductus deferens (Figure 15.1). Their importance lies in the fact that they produce 60 percent of the volume of semen. The thick, liquid secretion of the seminal vesicles is slightly alkaline to counteract the acidity of the vaginal environment and contains carbohydrates to nourish the sperm. Prostaglandins (recall prostaglandins from Chapter 2) are present to promote needed contractions in the male and female genital tracts. Fibrinogen, a coagulation protein (also found in blood), is present for reasons we will discuss in a moment. Smooth muscle in the walls of the seminal vesicles contributes to the propulsion of ejaculation.

The Prostate

This gland, slightly smaller than a golf ball, lies inferior to the urinary bladder and surrounds the prostatic urethra. It is divided into five distinct lobes and is actually a combination of approximately 50 separate glandular structures. Approximately 25 ducts link these glands to the urethra. The prostate is surrounded by a thick capsule of dense irregular connective tissue.

The prostatic secretion is added to semen during ejaculation by contraction of the abundant smooth muscle of this gland. Its thin secretion contributes fluidity to the semen, encourages sperm motility, and gives semen its characteristic odor. It also contains enzymes that first cause the semen to clot by activating the fibrinogen from the seminal vesicles, and later to regain fluidity by breaking down the clotted fibrin. This temporary clotting may contribute to fertility by first holding the semen in place within the vagina when the combined motion of the male and female participants might dislodge it; its later reliquefaction enables the sperm to more easily resume their journey into the female reproductive tract.

The prostate is a frequent site of medical problems in older men, ranging from benign hypertrophy (noncancerous enlargement of the prostate) to malignancy (prostatic carcinoma). As they age, men may develop trouble urinating; the flow of urine slows, and urine may be retained in the bladder. Retained urine increases the risk of bladder infections. Enlargement of the prostate restricts the lumen of the urethra, creating this reduced flow condition. Health-care providers can often

successfully treat this difficulty. The health status of this gland is easily monitored by a physician and should be regularly checked from midlife on.

The Bulbourethral Glands

Unlike the other glands we have discussed, the bulbourethral or Cowper's glands release the majority of their secretions during sexual arousal, before ejaculation. These pea-sized glands are inferior to the prostate and release their secretion into the proximal region of the spongy urethra. This secretion provides lubrication for the tip of the penis to assist in sexual intercourse. It also helps to raise the pH of the normally acidic urethra (from urine residue) and female reproductive tract, conditioning these structures to receive sperm.

■ Secondary Sex Organs of the Male: The Penis

If asked what their primary sex organ is, many men would probably respond: the penis. Its conspicuous appearance would lead many to think that. But, recall what the primary sex organ is, and you will see why this is a secondary sex organ.

The penis is a tubular organ that is actually made up of three cylindrical structures. Longitudinally, it has a root, made up of a bulb and two *crura* (crura means "legs"), then a body, and distally ends as the glans (**FIGURE 15.4**). In cross section (Figure 15.4), we see two corpora cavernosa and one corpus spongiosum. The bulb

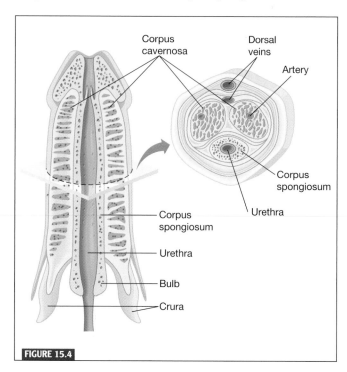

FIGURE 15.4

The penis.

of the root is the proximal portion of the corpus spongiosum. Each crus (singular form of crura) is the proximal portion of a corpus cavernosum. The glans is an enlarged portion of the distal end of the corpus spongiosum.

The corpora cavernosa are vascular structures, containing large vascular (blood-containing) sinuses, or collapsed veins. In their centers, they hold the deep arteries of the penis. The corpus spongiosum also is composed of vascular tissue, but has the spongy urethra at its core.

The penis has two functions: passage of urine (through the urethra) and copulation resulting in the delivery of semen into the vagina. To fulfill its second function, it must become erect. This is a vascular phenomenon, occurring as a result of sexual excitement.

Sexual excitement results in dilation of the arteries supplying blood to the penis. This engorges the sinuses in the erectile tissue of the corpora cavernosa and spongiosum. This engorgement results in compression of the veins that carry blood away from the penis, increasing pressure in the erectile tissue and further increasing the erection. This sounds like positive feedback, doesn't it? Further stimulation results in ejaculation. Erection is under the control of the parasympathetic nervous system, which makes perfect sense. Since activities of the sympathetic nervous system tend to be systemic, long lasting, and active during times of great stress and danger (for reasons discussed in Chapters 12 and 13), it would not be a good choice for controlling erection. If the sympathetic nervous system controlled penile erection, the fight or flight response would result in persistent erection. This would not serve the purposes that demand fight or flight. The parasympathetic nervous system is generally the more predominant system at times consistent with mating activity; therefore, it controls erection. Ejaculation, on the other hand, is a sympathetic response. Therefore, both branches of the autonomic nervous system are involved in sexual functioning.

15.3 The Female Reproductive System

■ "And Now for Something Completely Different . . ."

We are now going to discuss the other form of the human reproductive system. As you will learn, although there are fewer organs and structures to learn about in the female reproductive system, it is much more complex than the male system (**FIGURE 15.5**). This is true for several reasons, but the underlying one is that this system does not merely produce and deliver gametes; it provides the sites for fertilization and implantation, it nourishes and protects the developing embryo, and it delivers into the world the fully developed fetus.

As in the male counterpart, we will begin with the primary sex organ before moving on to the secondary sex organs. We will then discuss the mammary glands.

■ The Female Primary Sex Organ: The Ovary

As in the male, the female primary sex organ is the site of gamete production, which is here called oogenesis.

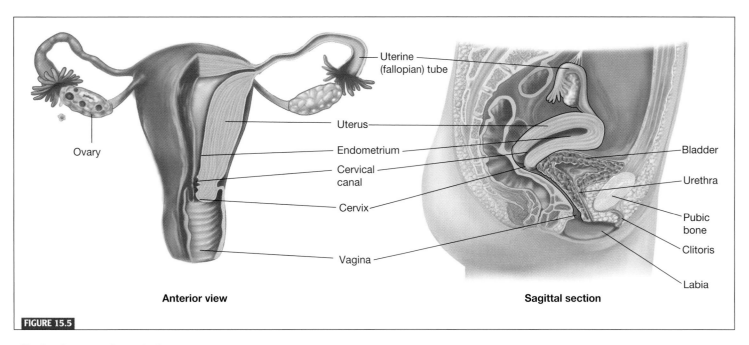

Ovary

Uterine (fallopian) tube

Uterus

Endometrium

Cervical canal

Cervix

Vagina

Bladder

Urethra

Pubic bone

Clitoris

Labia

Anterior view   **Sagittal section**

FIGURE 15.5

The female organs of reproduction.

Here, the primary sex organ is the ovary, and the gamete is the oocyte or ovum (**FIGURE 15.6a**). The ovaries are also responsible for the production of several important hormones. They are about the size and shape of an un-shelled almond: 5 centimeters long and about 1.5 cen-timeters thick. They are lateral to the uterus and are held in place by several ligaments. The ovarian liga-ment anchors the ovaries to the uterus. The suspen-sory ligament attaches the ovary to the pelvic wall. A fold of peritoneum (the lining of the abdominopelvic cavity) provides a route for blood vessels and nerves to reach the ovaries.

The outer layer of the ovaries is called the germinal epithelium. This is a misnomer that has carried over

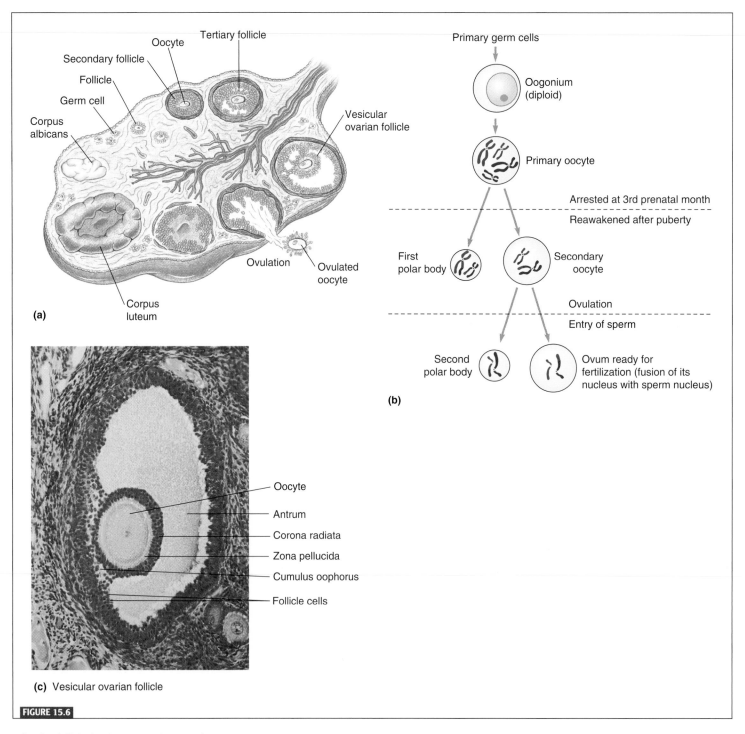

(a)

(b)

(c) Vesicular ovarian follicle

FIGURE 15.6

Ovarian follicle development and oogenesis.

from a time before the histophysiology of the ovary was understood. The germinal epithelium is merely the visceral fold peritoneum; it does not give rise to the germ cells, as the name implies. Deep to this, we find the tunica albuginea: the ovarian capsule. Made of connective tissue, the tunica albuginea is poorly defined (unlike the strong capsule of the testis).

Deep to the capsule, we find the ovarian follicles, which are the parenchyma of the ovaries. These are dispersed among a connective tissue stroma. We will spend some time on the ovarian follicles, as their fascinating development is linked to oogenesis and is crucial to understanding this reproductive system.

Oogenesis

The topic we are about to discuss is but one facet of the complex cycle that is the female reproductive cycle. This cycle begins at puberty and continues until menopause, in the meantime usually only interrupted by pregnancy or illness. By the end of this chapter, you will have a detailed understanding of this cycle. In the early stages of this discussion, however, I will need to present you with some information that may be a little confusing until we cover additional aspects of the cycle later in the chapter. Don't worry; we'll get there. It is much like building a puzzle. The first few pieces you put together do not give you much of an understanding of the whole picture, but the picture becomes clear as more pieces are in place. You may want to read through the chapter first to get an idea of what this cycle entails; then you might want to read the chapter a second time to absorb the details.

Let's start with oogenesis; the production of female gametes (Figure 15.6). The female gamete, the ovum, develops within structures called ovarian follicles. These follicles actually go through an interesting process of development as well. We will study their development once we understand the stages of development of the ova.

The first stages in the development of the ova begin very early in embryonic development with cells called primordial germ cells. They migrate into the developing ovary around the beginning of the fifth week of embryonic life. These cells differentiate into oogonia, the next stage in the pathway leading to the ovum. By the end of the third month of prenatal development, these have divided repeatedly and are in small clusters surrounded by cells that will later be part of the ovarian follicle. The oogonia differentiate into primary oocytes, the next developmental stage. By the fifth month of development, there are approximately 7×10^6 (7 million) such cells in the ovaries. Over the next couple of months, many of

these regress and die. As birth approaches, the surviving primary oocytes (perhaps 700,000 to 2 million in number) have all completed prophase of the first meiotic division (review Chapter 14 for details) and have arrested their meiotic division at that stage. These cells will remain in this stage until sometime after the young woman reaches puberty. By puberty, many of the primary oocytes will have regressed, leaving about 400,000. The rest have all died and been resorbed in a process that may involve apoptosis (programmed cell death); activation of genes that lead to death of the cell.

After puberty, each month, about 20 primary oocytes will become active and resume development. One of these 20 will successfully complete its development. The remaining 19 or so will be resorbed. The successful cell will proceed as follows.

It will complete its first meiotic division (as described in our previous chapter). One resulting daughter cell will receive almost all of the cytoplasm; it will become a secondary oocyte. The other daughter cell will receive very little cytoplasm and will become a first polar body. This will remain alongside of the secondary oocyte and ultimately will be reabsorbed.

The secondary oocyte will enter the second meiotic division. It will ultimately be released from the ovary (ovulated) as a secondary oocyte before this division has been completed. The second meiotic division will only be completed after a sperm enters the secondary oocyte (if that occurs). If a sperm enters the oocyte, it will complete its second meiotic division, only then becoming a mature ovum, ready to fuse nuclei with the sperm in the process of fertilization.

The details of this fascinating development are illustrated in Figure 15.6b. Please have a look at that figure before continuing. When you are ready, we will proceed with the development of ovarian follicles. These are the structures in which oogenesis occurs.

Ovarian Follicle Development

During the third month of prenatal life (in the developing female embryo), the embryonic ovaries begin to produce ovarian follicles. At this stage, they are primordial follicles and will all remain so for many years. Primordial follicles each contain a primary oocyte and are surrounded by a single layer of squamous follicular cells (Figure 15.6a).

As we just learned, after puberty (until menopause) about 20 primary oocytes reawaken each month. Each of these is in a primordial follicle, which similarly reawakens. The follicular cells of these primordial follicles increase in size and become cuboidal. Together with the primary oocyte, they produce a gelatinous membrane called the zona pellucida, separating the follicular cells from the oocyte. When the follicular cells become cuboidal and the zonal pellucida arises, the follicle becomes a primary follicle. Typically, only one primary follicle will successfully complete development through ovulation each month. The others will regress and be resorbed. We will follow the development of the successful follicle.

The primary follicle next becomes more complex. The follicular cells (also called granulosa cells) proliferate and become stratified (multilayered). Superficial to the granulosa cells, a basement membrane forms. Superficial to that, connective tissue is laid down. At this point, the follicle is a secondary follicle. As it continues to develop, a small, fluid-filled cyst called an antrum appears within the granulosa cells. Some physiologists now call this a tertiary follicle; others stick to the designation of secondary follicle.

The final stage before ovulation is that of a vesicular ovarian follicle, or Graafian follicle. Please examine the illustration and photomicrograph in Figure 15.6. Note that the antrum (the fluid-filled cyst) is now quite large. The follicle may actually measure up to 1 centimeter in diameter at this point. Also note that the follicular (granulosa) cells have now differentiated into several subtypes and have begun secreting estrogens. Immediately surrounding the zona pellucida is a layer of very tall cells called the corona radiata (meaning "spreading crown"). At the site of attachment of the corona radiata to the granulosa-lined wall of the antrum, we find a layer of modified granulosa cells called cumulus oophorus (*cumulus* means "a little mound"). While the vesicular ovarian follicle has been forming, the primary oocyte has become a secondary oocyte. Ovulation can now occur.

Under the influence of a sudden surge of LH, the vesicular ovarian follicle bursts, releasing the secondary oocyte and surrounding corona radiata. This is ovulation. Some women report that they actually can feel the bursting of the follicle during ovulation. The cells of the follicle that remain behind become a corpus luteum (meaning yellow body). This is an endocrinologically active structure, producing hormones such as estrogens and progesterone. Ultimately, this too recedes, becoming a corpus albicans (white body), which is nothing more than a small collection of scar tissue and does not produce hormones.

What Hormones Control All of This?

Meanwhile, back at the hormones. Starting at puberty, the hypothalamus begins to produce gonadotropin-releasing hormone (GnRH), which stimulates release of FSH and LH from the anterior pituitary (these were discussed in Chapter 13. Follicle-stimulating hormone is so named for stimulating the ovarian follicles described previously. Under its influence, the granulosa cells of these follicles produce estrogens and progesterone. LH is called luteinizing hormone because it causes development of the corpus luteum; in other words, it causes ovulation. Increasing levels of estrogens and progesterone have a negative feedback effect on GnRH, shutting off GnRH production; this leads, in turn, to decreasing FSH and LH levels, thus causing estrogens and progesterone levels to fall. The loss of estrogens and progesterone thereby release the negative feedback effect on GnRH; GnRH levels rise and the whole thing starts all over again. We will revisit this in a few moments.

One more fact to note is that the rising levels of estrogens have a transient positive feedback effect on the production of LH: hence, we see a spike of LH. It is this LH spike that causes ovulation.

A summary of the hormones of the female reproductive system is presented in **TABLE 15.1** and **FIGURE 15.7**. Please examine that table before proceeding.

Let's examine the other organs of the female reproductive system before putting all of this together in a synopsis of the female reproductive cycle.

■ Secondary Sex Organs of the Female
The Uterine (Fallopian) Tubes

Extending medially in an upward sweeping curve from the ovaries to the uterus are the uterine or Fallopian tubes (Figure 15.5). They begin with a wide, open area called the infundibulum (meaning funnel). It is fringed distally with fingerlike projections called fimbriae. The fimbriae graze the surface of the ovaries. During ovulation, the oocyte is expelled from the ovarian follicle, picked up by the fimbriae, and passed into the lumen of the uterine tube. As it moves medially along the uterine tube, it passes through the ampulla, a wide area, to the isthmus, a narrower area. Finally, it will reach the uterus itself.

The lumen of the uterine tube is somewhat star shaped to maximize surface area while limiting the volume of the lumen, and it is lined with simple columnar epithelium. Some of these epithelial cells possess cilia to propel the oocyte toward the uterus; others produce a secretion to maintain a moist nutritive environment for the oocyte and sperm. The wall also contains two spiral layers of smooth muscle that contract rhythmically to propel the oocyte along. Imagine the swimming capacity of the sperm that allows them to survive the trek upstream through the uterine tubes against the current created by the cilia and smooth muscle. If you have seen

Table 15.1   An Overview of the Major Hormones of the Female Reproductive System

Hormone	Source	Function
GnRH	Hypothalamus	Causes release of FSH and LH
FSH	Anterior pituitary	Stimulates follicle development and release of estrogen by follicle
LH	Anterior pituitary	Aids in follicle development, and stimulates release of estrogen and progesterone. A surge in LH causes ovulation
Estrogens (there are at least 6; B-estradiol is the major one)	Follicular (granulosa) cells	Stimulates development and maintenance of female reproductive structures and secondary sex characteristics. Causes proliferation of uterine lining (endometrium). High levels inhibit GnRH release (negative feedback)
Progesterone	Granulosa cells of corpus luteum	Causes maturation of endometrium in preparation for implantation
Prolactin	Anterior pituitary	Stimulates the production of milk by mammary glands that have been prepared by estrogens and progesterone
Oxytocin	Posterior pituitary	Causes contraction of uterine smooth muscle, facilitating the labor of childbirth. Also controls the milk letdown reflex, causing release of milk from mammary glands

GnRH = gonadotropin-releasing hormone; FSH = follicle-stimulating hormone; LH = luteinizing hormone.

films of salmon swimming upstream to spawn, you have some idea of the peril that the sperm face. Again we see a good reason for their vast numbers!

The distal one third of the uterine tubes is the site of fertilization. This allows enough time to pass between fertilization and entry of the early embryo into the body of the uterus so that it will be ready to implant on its arrival there.

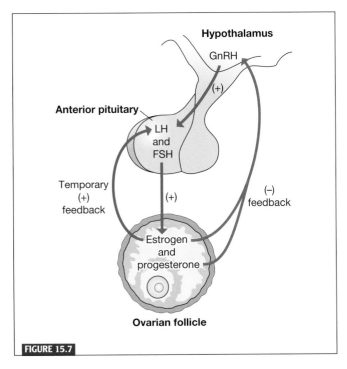

FIGURE 15.7

Control mechanisms for secretion of the hormones of the female reproductive system.

We learned that vasectomy is a procedure that blocks the passage of gametes (sperm) in men, as a permanent sterilization technique. A similar procedure, tubal ligation, can be performed in women. Tubal ligation involves interrupting the uterine tubes by cutting, cauterization, or the application of special clips. This too, is a permanent procedure that does not allow gametes to pass (in this case, the oocyte), thereby preventing pregnancy.

The Uterus

This pear-shaped organ has much smooth muscle and a very interesting mucosa, or lining. This arrangement enables it to support implantation and development of an embryo and then to deliver a full-term fetus. The uterine tubes join the uterus in its superior-lateral aspects. The uterus joins the vagina through the uterine cervix. **FIGURE 15.8** and Figure 15.5 show the anatomy of the uterus.

The uterine wall contains three layers: the perimetrium, which is simply visceral peritoneum; the myometrium, which consists of three thick layers of strong smooth muscle; and the endometrium, which lines the lumen. We will discuss the endometrium in detail.

The endometrium is the lush mucosal lining of the uterus and has three major components. The surface epithelium is composed of simple columnar epithelium with ciliated and secretory cells. This overlies the lamina propria or connective tissue layer. Extending from the surface epithelium into the lamina propria are tubular glands that produce mucus.

We can also divide the endometrium functionally into two layers: the stratum functionalis and the stratum

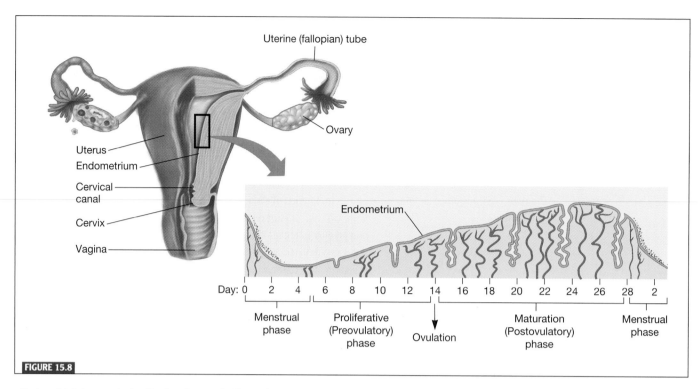

FIGURE 15.8

Endometrial changes during the female reproductive cycle.

basalis. The stratum functionalis is the upper (luminal) two thirds of the endometrium. During the menstrual cycle (later in this chapter), it grows and then matures to prepare for implantation of an embryo. If implantation does not occur, for instance, in months when fertilization does not occur, it dies and is sloughed off during menstruation.

The underlying layer, called the stratum basalis, does not meet this same fate. It serves as a stem cell layer, proliferating to replace the stratum functionalis after menstruation is complete.

The Vagina

This tubular organ allows entry of the penis during sexual intercourse for the reception of sperm by the female reproductive tract and, later on, for passage of the baby during delivery. It also serves as the passageway for menstrual secretions if pregnancy does not occur. Its highly distensible walls are lined with noncornified stratified columnar epithelium to withstand abrasion in this moist environment. Interestingly, the upper layers of this epithelium contain abundant glycogen. This glycogen feeds the bacterial inhabitants of the vagina that turn glucose (from the glycogen) into lactic acid, making the vaginal environment acidic for protection against pathogenic microorganisms. This is also a difficult environment for sperm to survive. They do so through the

neutralizing effects of the fluid component of semen. Lymph nodes are also present in the walls of the vagina for additional protection against infection.

The Vulva

The external genitalia of the female consist of the various components of the vulva: the labia majora and labia minora, and the clitoris (**FIGURE 15.9**). The labia majora are the most lateral portion of the vulva. They

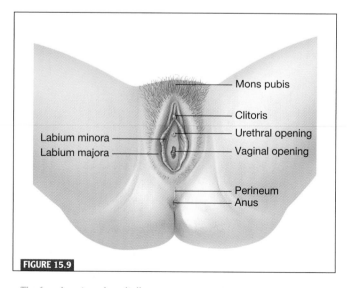

FIGURE 15.9

The female external genitalia.

consist of large skin folds containing pads of adipose tissue. Their outer surface is covered with coarse pubic hair. Their inner surface lacks hair. Both surfaces contain the glands common to skin in most locations (sweat glands and sebaceous glands, which will be discussed in Chapter 20).

The labia majora either completely (early in life) or partially (later on) enclose the labia minora. These two very thin skin folds (the labia minora) do not possess hair and are covered with stratified squamous epithelium possessing only a very thin cornified layer. They enclose a narrow, flattened area, the vestibule, which holds the vaginal and the urethral orifices. They meet anteriorly to enfold the clitoris. The clitoris is the female homolog of the penis (developmentally, they are the same structure). It contains two erectile structures similar to the corpus cavernosa, and a glans clitoris that is much like the glans penis. Aside from the size difference, the other major difference is the fact that the urethra does not travel through the clitoris. The clitoris is important in the female sexual response, arousal and orgasm.

There are also glands present in the vestibule. The paraurethral glands open into the floor of the vestibule, lateral to the urethral orifice. These are developmentally homologous to the male prostate and produce mucus. The greater vestibular glands are homologous to the bulbourethral glands in the male. Like those glands, the greater vestibular glands release a lubricating secretion during sexual arousal in preparation for intercourse. These secretions are released in the area of the vaginal orifice. The lesser vestibular glands, located throughout the vestibular floor, keep the vestibule moist. Their activity is not related to sexual arousal, but is for general vestibular maintenance.

The Female Reproductive Cycle: Putting It All Together

We have just covered a lot of material in a somewhat disjointed fashion. This was necessary to give you all of the pieces of the puzzle that is the female reproductive or menstrual cycle. The term *menstrual* refers to one part of the cycle: menstruation. The term *menstruation* is derived from the same root as the term *menses*, which refers to the bloody fluid that is expelled. *Menses* is from the Latin term for month, indicating the approximate (but variable) timing of this cycle.

As with all cycles, it is difficult to point to an actual beginning. Cycles, by their nature, have no easily definable beginning. We will assume certain conditions

for this cycle. We will consider it as lasting for 28 days, but it frequently lasts between 24 and 35 days. We will call the first day on which menses is discharged day one, and count all of the other days from that point. I will present this cycle in **TABLE 15.2**, for that is the most succinct way to examine and learn it. Note that for most phases, two names are given. One name pertains to the changes occurring in the ovary; the other name (the one in parentheses) refers to changes occurring in the endometrium. Examine this information carefully and compare it to what you have just read. It should firm up the information we have been covering.

Please also be aware that if pregnancy occurs, the early embryo and developing placenta produce the hormone human chorionic gonadotropin (HCG). This hormone maintains the corpus luteum, which is necessary for the production of progesterone, until the production of progesterone can be taken over by the placenta. Progesterone is necessary for the maintenance of the endometrium. The endometrium must be maintained to support the embryo. Even after the placenta develops and takes on this role, the corpus luteum persists, although its contribution becomes less significant. Home pregnancy-testing kits that change color to indicate pregnancy after urine has been added to them are based on the detection of HCG in the urine of the recently impregnated woman.

The Mammary Glands

The final organ we will consider in this section is the female breast (**FIGURE 15.10**). This is not to indicate that breast tissue is absent in the male; rather, it is underdeveloped. The effects of female hormones (estrogens and progesterone) include the development of the female secondary sex characteristics. One such characteristic is the development of the breasts.

The breasts are actually very important organs from the standpoint of the survival of the human species. They produce the proper nourishment for the developing baby, as well as providing substances needed for immunological defense in the newborn. Breastfeeding, therefore, gives babies a good start in life.

The mammary glands, or the glands of the breasts, are classified as branched tubuloalveolar glands. This means that they have a branching tubular structure (resembling a tree), and these branches end in small sacks, the alveoli. Here is where milk is produced. Notice the diagram of the mammary gland in Figure 15.10. One lobe of the 15 to 20 total lobes is shown in that diagram. These lobes are embedded in adipose tissue.

Table 15.2 Overview of the Menstrual Cycle*

Menstrual phase

Days 1–5

This phase is triggered by a sudden drop in estrogen and progesterone (due to loss of corpus luteum)

It is characterized by necrosis and sloughing of stratum functionalis, and discharge of this tissue, along with blood and mucus

The drop in estrogen and progesterone that triggered this phase results in an increase in (GnRH) and subsequent increase in (FSH) late in the phase

The increased FSH stimulates about 20 primary follicles to become secondary follicles

Preovulatory phase (proliferative phase)

Days 6–13

Estrogen is the primary hormone of this phase

GnRH levels are increasing, causing FSH and luteinizing (LH) levels to increase

This causes increased estrogen release from secondary follicles

Stratum functionalis is being replaced

One secondary follicle becomes a vesicular ovarian (Graafian) follicle

The vesicular ovarian follicle begins to produce progesterone during the last 1 or 2 days of this phase

Ovulation

Day 14

Luteinizing hormone (LH) is the primary hormone of this phase

Increasing levels of estrogens produce a transient positive feedback effect on LH levels; hence, LH levels spike

The spike in LH causes ovulation (rupture of the antrum and release of the secondary oocyte and surrounding cells from the vesicular ovarian follicle)

The vesicular ovarian follicle now becomes a corpus luteum and produces progesterone (and some estrogen) under the influence of LH

Postovulatory phase (maturation phase)

Days 15–28

Progesterone is the primary hormone of this phase

Corpus luteum secretes increasing levels of progesterone (and estrogen)

This causes maturation of the thickened stratum functionalis for implantation, if fertilization should occur

After about a week of rising progesterone and estrogen levels, GnRH levels fall (negative feedback), causing LH levels to fall

Decreased LH levels cause the corpus luteum to become a corpus albicans (scar tissue). This shuts off production of estrogen and progesterone

As estrogen and progesterone levels fall, the stratum functionalis begins to necrose (die) and menstruation begins

*This table presents a description of the cyclic changes that take place in the reproductive tract of a nonpregnant female. The role of this cycle is to prepare the female reproductive tract for the fertilization of an ovum and the implantation and gestation of the resulting embryo.

A typical cycle is described; however, be aware that much variation may exist among individuals, or between cycles in one individual. Also be aware that, as is true of many cycles in complicated systems, different ways of breaking up and describing this cycle are valid.

Estrogen and progesterone act permissively in preparing the mammary gland for the effects of prolactin. During gestation (pregnancy), the placenta produces the hormone human placental lactogen (HPL), which is also necessary for this process. At delivery, progesterone levels fall, allowing the increasing levels of prolactin to work: the mammary glands begin to produce milk. Some milk is stored in the lactiferous sinuses (Figure 15.10) and is released by contraction of smooth muscle and myoepithelial cells in the ducts. Myoepithelial cells are epithelial cells that have differentiated to include contraction as one of their abilities. Physical stimulation of the nipple by the suckling infant will stimulate release of oxytocin from the posterior pituitary. Oxytocin

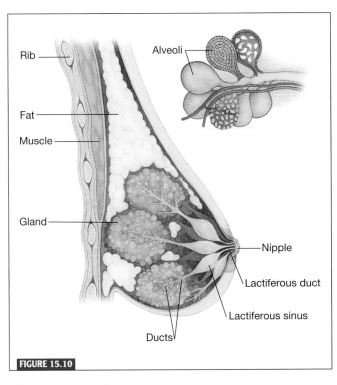

Rib

Fat

Muscle

Gland

Alveoli

Nipple

Lactiferous duct

Lactiferous sinus

Ducts

FIGURE 15.10

The mammary gland.

is involved in the milk letdown reflex, the release of milk from the mammary gland. Lactation (production of milk) may be continued over many months by the continuation of breastfeeding. Stimulation of the nipple causes release of prolactin releasing hormone (PRH) from the hypothalamus, resulting in sustained release of prolactin (necessary for milk production). If you are unclear on these hormonal interrelationships, please refer back to Chapter 13 for review.

This ends our discussions on the human reproductive system. This fascinating topic continues to be further elucidated as scientists and clinicians work to aid couples who have been unable to conceive children on their own. The foundation of knowledge you have just laid will help you to follow new developments with understanding. Please be sure to use the "What You Should Know" and "What Did You Learn?" sections that follow to assess your knowledge. This will help you to make certain that you really do understand what you have just read. Before proceeding to our next section, make sure you have re-examined any areas in which you find understanding deficient.

Breaching Homeostasis . . . When Things Go Wrong

Testicular Cancer

Testicular cancer, while overall relatively rare, is most often seen in young men between the age of puberty and midlife. Sometimes these young men have noticed the growth of these malignancies for months before bringing them to the attention of their physicians. This delay often has dire consequences: it allows these tumors to grow and spread beyond the confines of the testis, making a cure less likely. Just as society needed to overcome social mores to make women aware of the need for breast self-examination, the public now needs to be made aware of the need for testicular self-examination in men (**FIGURE 15.11**). Our society needs to overcome its squeamishness in discussing such matters, so young men will be encouraged to perform this needed examination and promptly report any irregularities to their physicians. In this way, treatment may begin promptly and we will reduce the needless deaths of the young men afflicted with testicular cancer.

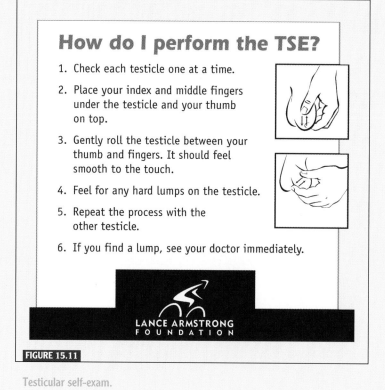

How do I perform the TSE?

1. Check each testicle one at a time.

2. Place your index and middle fingers under the testicle and your thumb on top.

3. Gently roll the testicle between your thumb and fingers. It should feel smooth to the touch.

4. Feel for any hard lumps on the testicle.

5. Repeat the process with the other testicle.

6. If you find a lump, see your doctor immediately.

LANCE ARMSTRONG
F O U N D A T I O N

FIGURE 15.11

Testicular self-exam.

What You Should Know

1. In either gender, the organ that produces the gametes is the primary sex organ.

2. The primary sex organ of the male is the testis.

3. The testes are located in the scrotum.

4. The scrotum is raised and lowered by the dartos and cremaster muscle to regulate the temperature of the testes.

5. Spermatogenesis occurs at a temperature approximately 3 degrees below that of the rest of the body.

What You Should Know (continued)

6. The seminiferous tubules of the testis are the site of spermatogenesis.

7. The testis is divided into many lobules by septae that are part of the tunica albuginea. Each lobule contains from one to three seminiferous tubules.

8. Spermatogenesis results in the production of approximately 300 million sperm per day.

9. Sustentacular (Sertoli) cells line the seminiferous tubules, and support and organize the developing germ cells.

10. Interstitial endocrinocytes (Leydig cells) are located between the seminiferous tubules and produce androgens such as testosterone.

11. The epididymis is the most proximal structure of the ducts leading from the testes to the exterior of the body. Sperm must mature in the epididymis to become fertile.

12. The ductus deferens is a long duct that conveys sperm from the epididymis to the ejaculatory duct. Smooth muscle in its walls contract during ejaculation to propel the sperm.

13. The ejaculatory duct is the site where sperm is mixed with the secretion of the seminal vesicle.

14. In males, the urethra conveys semen and urine from the body.

15. The fluid component of semen is produced mainly by the seminal vesicles and the prostate.

16. The bulbourethral glands provide a lubricating fluid before ejaculation.

17. The penis is the male copulatory organ. It contains two corpora cavernosa and one corpus spongiosum. These vascular structures provide the rigidity necessary for copulation.

18. The primary sex organ of the female is the ovary.

19. The ovary contains ovarian follicles in which oogenesis occurs.

20. Development of the ova begins in the early embryo and is completed as part of a monthly cycle in women during the years between puberty and menopause.

21. Several hormones control the development of ova and the endometrium. The cycle generated by these hormones is called the female reproductive cycle, or menstrual cycle.

22. The uterine (Fallopian) tubes convey the ova toward the uterus and are the site of fertilization.

23. The uterus is lined with endometrium and is the site of embryo development. Its walls contain much smooth muscle for delivery of the full-term fetus.

24. The vagina is the female copulatory organ, and the means by which the secretions of the female reproductive tract, and the fully developed fetus, exit the body.

25. The vulva encloses and protects the openings of the vagina and urethra.

26. You must know the stages of the female reproductive cycle, including what happens during each phase, which hormones are responsible, and how long each stage lasts.

27. The female breast, or mammary gland, is an important nutritive organ for human young. A complex interplay of hormones prepares the breast for this purpose, initiates and prolongs milk production, and ejects milk at the proper time.

What Did You Learn?

Multiple choice questions: choose the best answer.

1. The smooth muscle of the scrotum is called the:
   a. Cutaneous maximus
   b. Sternocleidomastoid
   c. Glans
   d. Dartos
   e. None of the above

2. At what temperature does spermatogenesis occur?
   a. Body temperature −6°
   b. Body temperature −3°
   c. Body temperature
   d. Body temperature +3°
   e. Body temperature +6°

3. Spermatogenesis occurs within the:
   a. Epididymis
   b. Seminiferous tubules
   c. Secondary follicles
   d. Ductus deferens
   e. None of the above

4. Which of the following cell types supports and nourishes the cells of the spermatogenic lineage (the cells that become sperm)?
   a. Germ cells
   b. Sertoli (sustentacular) cells
   c. Leydig cells (interstitial endocrinocytes)

5. The cell type that produces testosterone is known as:
   a. Spermatogonium
   b. Sertoli (sustentacular) cell
   c. Leydig cells (interstitial endocrinocytes)
   d. Germ cells

6. The life expectancy of spermatozoa after ejaculation (in the female reproductive tract) is:
   a. 6–12 hours
   b. 12–24 hours
   c. 48–72 hours
   d. 2 weeks

7. Sperm must mature for 10 days to 2 weeks in the:
   a. Testis
   b. Epididymis
   c. Ductus (vas) deferens
   d. Ejaculatory duct
   e. They do not mature until after ejaculation

8. Approximately how many sperm are produced per day:
   a. 50,000
   b. 100,000
   c. 850,000
   d. 300,000,000
   e. 2,500,000,000

9. Which gland secretes the coagulation protein fibrinogen:
   a. Seminal vesicle
   b. Prostate
   c. Bulbourethral (Cowper's) gland
   d. Testis
   e. None of the above secrete a coagulation protein

10. Which gland secretes enzymes that activate, and later degrade, coagulation proteins?
    a. Seminal vesicle
    b. Prostate
    c. Bulbourethral (Cowper's) gland
    d. Testis

11. Which of the following contains much smooth muscle to aid in ejaculatory propulsion?
    a. Prostate
    b. Bulbourethral (Cowper's) gland
    c. Both of the above
    d. Neither of the above

12. Which of the following contains much smooth muscle to aid in ejaculatory propulsion?
    a. Ductus deferens
    b. Ejaculatory duct
    c. Both of the above
    d. Neither of the above

13. Female secondary sex organs include all of the following except:
    a. Vagina
    b. Uterus
    c. Ovary
    d. Uterine (fallopian) tube
    e. All of the above are secondary sex organs

14. Identify the site of fertilization.
    a. Ovary
    b. Uterine (fallopian) tube
    c. Uterus
    d. Vagina

What Did You Learn? (continued)

15. Where is GnRH produced?

  a. Ovaries

  b. Testes

  c. Hypothalamus

  d. Anterior pituitary

16. The smooth muscle of the uterus is the:

  a. Myometrium

  b. Perimetrium

  c. Endometrium

  d. Periosteum

  e. Endomysium

17. The portion of the uterine lining that is sloughed off during menstruation is called:

  a. Theca interna

  b. Stratum basalis

  c. Adventitia

  d. Stratum functionalis

  e. Theca externa

18. The principal hormone of the postovulatory phase is:

  a. Estrogen

  b. Progesterone

  c. GnRH

  d. Prolactin

  e. HCG

19. The postovulatory phase ends as:

  a. A corpus albicans becomes a corpus luteum

  b. A vesicular ovarian follicle becomes a corpus albicans

  c. Twenty primary follicles become active

  d. A corpus luteum becomes a corpus albicans

  e. An antrum forms in a secondary follicle

20. The principal hormone of the preovulatory phase is:

  a. GnRH

  b. Progesterone

  c. Estrogen

  d. Inhibin

21. Ovulation is triggered by a sudden surge of:

  a. Estrogen

  b. GnRH

  c. FSH

  d. LH

  e. Emotion

22. In the typical menstrual cycle, the postovulatory phase begins on day:

  a. 5

  b. 12

  c. 15

  d. 28

23. Release of which of the following is influenced by a temporary positive feedback mechanism?

  a. FSH

  b. LH

  c. GnRH

  d. None of the above

24. Which of the following is hormonally active (releases hormones)?

  a. Corpus luteum

  b. Corpus albicans

  c. Both of the above

  d. Neither of the above

Short answer questions: answer briefly and in your own words.

1. Describe the pathway that sperm must follow as they travel from the testes to their exit from the male body. Name each structure through which they pass.

2. Indicate the function of each of the following glands:

  – Prostate

  – Seminiferous tubule

  – Bulbourethral gland

3. What is the purpose of the epididymis?

4. Draw a flowchart of the control mechanism for the release of estrogen and progesterone by the female reproductive organs. Indicate which organs secrete the hormones that regulate this release, and show, with arrows, any feedback loops that exist in this system.

5. If a woman ovulated today, her ovary released an oocyte that began its development many years ago. Please provide the life history of that cell, indicating the developmental changes it and the follicle that surrounded it went through.

6. List the stages of the female reproductive cycle and indicate what happens during each stage. Also list the hormones that regulate each stage and the days of a typical cycle that each stage covers.

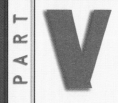

Moving Fluids and Gases

We are about to begin a very interesting section in our study of the human body. What makes this section so interesting? Several things; first, the organs and functions are dramatic, and visible to us in a variety of ways. As such, we all desire to know more about them. Second, diseases of these two systems play a major role in the health consciousness of our society, as well they should.

Cardiovascular disease is the cause of more than half of all deaths in developed societies. It accounts for more than twice the number of deaths attributed to cancers. The vast majority of cardiovascular pathologies are related to atherosclerosis. Advancements in our understanding of atherosclerosis have the potential to greatly reduce mortality rates from these illnesses, thereby increasing the lifespan of many individuals. The popular press is full of conflicting information on how we can improve our cardiovascular health. How can we decide whose advise is sound if we do not understand the tissues, organs, and systems they are talking about? Many people in our society are interested in the cardiovascular system for the insight knowledge of this system will provide into their own health-care decisions.

Respiratory illness, although not on the order of cardiovascular disease, is also a major source of mortality in our society. Even more so, it contributes to morbidity (the presence of illness) and related degradation in the quality of life for many people. Many among us want to understand this system so they will have a basis on which to interpret the information they receive from their health-care providers, and perhaps be better able to question their physicians about issues regarding their health. So, why do we study these two systems together?

Why Study the Cardiovascular and Respiratory Systems Together?

When we first discussed the generation of ATP as a source of energy in the body (Chapters 2 and 3), it became apparent that oxygen is very important in that process. Our discussions about metabolism also pointed to the need to remove the metabolic byproduct carbon dioxide from our bodies. These two substances can easily be exchanged with the external environment, but how can we get them there? The respiratory system provides a great place for that exchange to occur. But that is not where most of the oxygen is needed, nor where most of the carbon dioxide is generated. Ah, back to the concept of moving fluids as a mechanism for maintaining homeostasis. We need to move these gases in a fluid to get them to and from the respiratory system. The cardiovascular system provides the fluid (blood) and the motion (the pumping action of the heart).

Simply put, a respiratory system without a cardiovascular system would be useless, and moving substances to and from the respiratory system is a major concern of the cardiovascular system. These two systems must work hand in hand for homeostasis to be maintained. Hence, a discussion of one of these systems without a corresponding discussion of the other system would be pointless. We will discuss each of them in the next two chapters. First we will examine the cardiovascular system, then the respiratory system. I hope you will enjoy our discussions of these exciting topics.

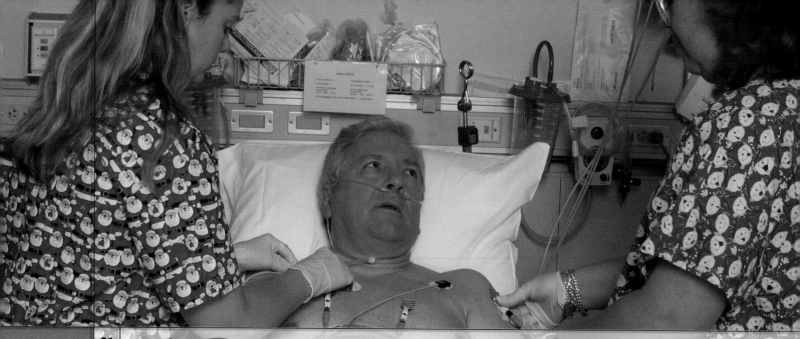

16 The River Within: Your Cardiovascular System

What You Will Learn

- The location and structure of your heart.
- The anatomy of the chambers of your heart.
- Which vessels convey blood to and from your heart.
- The names and locations of the valves of your heart.
- The anatomy and physiology of the electrical impulse generation and conduction system of your heart.
- The stages of the cardiac cycle and what happens in each stage.
- The factors that determine cardiac output and how cardiac output is regulated.
- The types of blood vessels and their structures.
- The gross anatomy of the cardiovascular system.
- The basic physics of blood as a moving fluid.
- The characteristics of your blood as a connective tissue.
- What cells are present in your blood, and what functions these cells perform.
- What actually determines your blood type.
- How plasma compares to other extracellular matrices.
- The mechanisms that allow your blood to clot.

Like a mighty river flowing within our bodies, moving fluids are essential for the maintenance of homeostasis. Just as a river carries life-sustaining water and nutrients to parched regions, so these moving fluids of the body nourish our tissues (**FIGURE 16.1**). Also like a river, the moving fluids within our bodies carry wastes away from our tissues.

16.1 Blood As a Moving Fluid

We have learned that the maintenance of homeostasis is crucial to our health and survival. We have also learned that moving fluids are an essential tool in the maintenance of homeostasis. When we think of fluids moving within the body, the first fluid that comes to mind is blood. In fact, as we think about the other moving fluids—interstitial fluid, lymphatic fluid, cerebrospinal fluid, and intracellular fluid—we realize that they are all related to plasma, the fluid component of blood. They all depend on plasma as the source for the substances from which they are made. In this chapter, we will consider the cardiovascular system. This is the system that contains the blood and conveys it throughout the body. The term *cardio* refers to the heart, while the term *vascular* refers to the blood vessels. The heart provides the force that moves the blood. We will begin our discussion with the anatomy and physiology of the heart and then move on to the blood vessels that provide the channels through which the blood flows. We will conclude with the blood itself, the fluid that flows in this inner river.

16.2 Your Heart

The heart is a truly amazing organ. Think about it. Your heart began its rhythmic contractions long before you were born and must continue them without interruption throughout your entire life. Each minute it beats approximately 70 times, for a total of over 100,000 beats per day. With each beat, it pumps approximately 70 ml of blood, for a total of approximately 7,000 liters per day. That translates to approximately 1,835 gallons, the equivalent of over 33 of the typical 55-gallon steel drums, each day of your entire life (**FIGURE 16.2**).

The heart is located in the mediastinum (**FIGURE 16.3a**). You may recall from Chapter 5 that the mediastinum is that mass of tissue in the thoracic cavity between the two pleural cavities. The pericardial cavity is a space within the mediastinum (Figure 16.3b). This is where we find the heart. Like the other body cavities, the pericardial space is lined with a serous membrane. This membrane is called the pericardium. Recall that these serous membranes are folded into two portions: one that lines the cavity, in this case the parietal pericardium, and one that lines the outer surface of the organ within the cavity, in this case the visceral pericardium. A potential space exists between the visceral and parietal pericardia called the pericardial space. The pericardial space contains a small quantity of serous fluid that lubricates the two membranes, allowing them to slide over each other easily as the heart beats.

The wall of the heart is composed of three layers (Figure 16.3c). The outer layer, the visceral pericardium, is also called the epicardium. The middle layer, composed of cardiac muscle, is by far the thickest layer. It is called the myocardium. The inner layer, the endocardium, is composed of simple squamous cells called endothelium. We will find endothelial cells lining any space through which blood flows (the chambers of the heart, arteries, capillaries, and veins).

The heart is about the size of a closed fist, and is roughly triangular in shape (not "heart-shaped," as you might expect). The tip of the triangle, the apex, is located inferiorly and to the left (**FIGURE 16.4**). The base of the heart, the "bottom" of the triangle, is superior and to the right. Four chambers make up the human heart. The two superior chambers are called atria. The larger, inferior chambers are called ventricles. The right and left atria are separated by the interatrial septum. The two ventricles are separated from one another by the interventricular septum. The atria and ventricles are separated from each other by atrioventricular valves, which will be described shortly. To understand the anatomy of the heart more fully, we must first consider how blood enters and exits the heart.

▪ The Great Vessels and the Path Your Blood Follows

The great vessels of the heart consist of those vessels that carry blood to and away from the heart (**FIGURE 16.5**). Blood leaves the heart through arteries and returns to the heart through veins. Throughout the body (referred to as the periphery), capillaries lie between the arteries and veins. It is in the capillaries that exchange of gases, nutrients, and wastes between blood and tissue and of gases between blood and the external environment occurs. Let's begin by thinking about blood leaving the left ventricle.

Blood leaves the left ventricle through the aorta. The aorta is a large artery. We will discuss the anatomy and physiology of arteries later in this chapter. As the aorta leaves the base of the heart, it ascends toward the head. This segment of the aorta is called the ascending aorta. The aorta next curves around to travel in an inferior

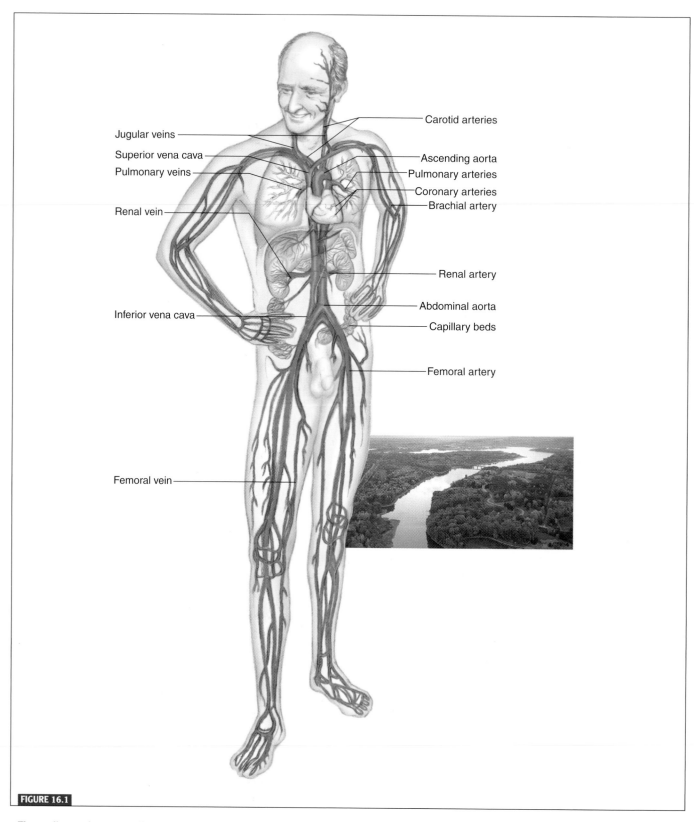

Jugular veins
Superior vena cava
Pulmonary veins
Renal vein
Inferior vena cava
Femoral vein

Carotid arteries
Ascending aorta
Pulmonary arteries
Coronary arteries
Brachial artery
Renal artery
Abdominal aorta
Capillary beds
Femoral artery

FIGURE 16.1

The cardiovascular system. Note its many similarities to a river.

direction. The curved portion is the arch of the aorta, while that which is traveling inferiorly is the descending aorta. Other vessels branch off of the aorta and distribute blood throughout the body. In other words, all of the blood distributed throughout the body, except the blood going to the lungs for gas exchange, begins in the aorta before entering other arteries.

After traveling through the body, blood must return to the heart's right atrium. It does this through several vessels. Blood returning from structures inferior to the heart, such as the legs and organs of the abdominopelvic cavity, returns through the inferior vena cava. Blood returning from structures superior to the heart, such as the brain, does so through the superior vena cava. Since the heart is an organ like any other, the walls of the heart must also have a vascular supply. **TABLE 16.1** lists the coronary arteries (the arteries that supply the heart wall with blood) and their major branches. Blood returns to the right atrium from the walls of the heart, through the coronary sinus.

Once blood has re-entered the heart in the right atrium, it passes into the right ventricle and then leaves the heart through the pulmonary trunk. The pulmonary trunk is a short length of artery that divides into the right and left pulmonary arteries. These convey the blood to the right and left lungs, respectively. The blood being brought to the lungs in this way is deoxygenated blood. It is being brought to the lungs for the exchange of gases between the blood and the external environment. Through this process, the blood will become reoxygenated. This oxygenated blood must next return to the left atrium of the heart. It does so through four pulmonary veins (two right and two left pulmonary veins). Blood entering the left atrium passes into the left ventricle and then leaves the ventricle through the aorta, as we discussed.

These are the two circuits through which the blood travels. Blood that is leaving the left ventricle to travel throughout the body, carrying oxygen and nutrients to the tissues of the body, and carrying wastes away from those tissues, is in the systemic circuit. Blood that is leaving the right ventricle to travel through the lungs, picking up oxygen and giving off carbon dioxide, is in the pulmonary circuit. What keeps the blood moving in only one direction? It makes sense that the blood must keep moving in one direction for circulation to be effective. How is that accomplished?

■ Heart Valves

When you have been in a crowd, entering a building, perhaps a movie theater, a concert hall, or a subway station, haven't you sometimes had to pass through some sort of

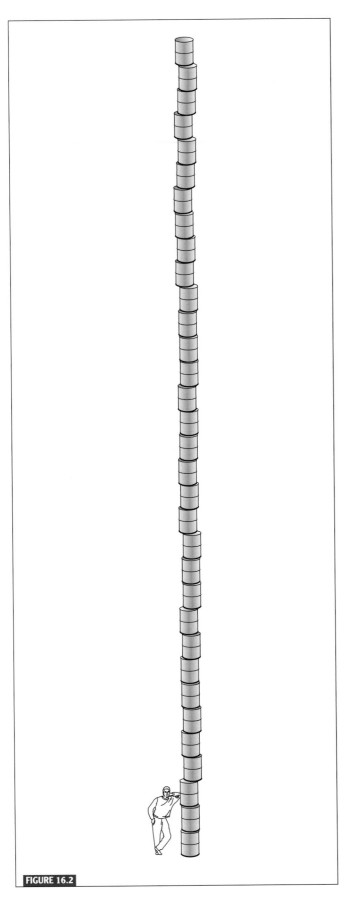

FIGURE 16.2

One day's cardiac output.

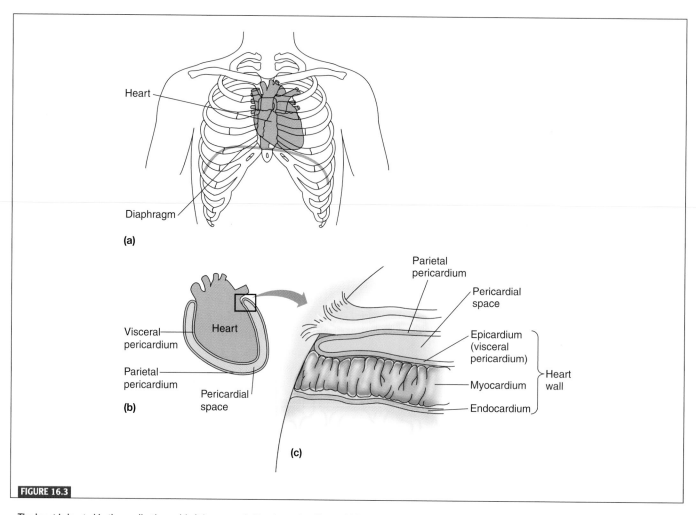

FIGURE 16.3

The heart is located in the mediastinum (a). It is surrounded by the pericardium, which contains the pericardial space (b). There are three layers to the heart wall (c).

a revolving gate or turnstyle? This is one means of ensuring order. People can only travel in one direction through the gate; it simply will not turn in the opposite direction (**FIGURE 16.6**). A similar mechanism is used to keep blood flowing in the proper direction. Valves are present in the heart between the atria and the ventricles (atrioventricular valves) and at the proximal end of the great arteries leaving the heart (semilunar valves). These valves are flaps, composed mainly of dense connective tissue. The right atrioventricular valve is called the tricuspid valve because it has three flaps, called cusps. The left atrioventricular valve is called the bicuspid valve (two cusps) and is also known as the mitral valve. A series of dense regular connective tissue cords attach the free edge of these cusps to the ventricle walls to keep the valves from moving beyond the closed position. The valves at the beginning of the pulmonary trunk and aorta are called semilunar valves because their cusps (flaps) are shaped like a half moon.

Let's try to picture for a moment how these valves work. We have not yet thought about how blood is moved through the heart. We will cover that in a few moments. Let's first consider the function of the heart valves. We will focus on the atrioventricular valves and begin by thinking about another situation entirely.

Imagine it is a hot summer night (**FIGURE 16.7a**). You are asleep in your bedroom. All of the windows in your house are open, as is your bedroom door. A storm begins to brew and the wind starts to blow. The wind is coming in your bedroom window, blowing through your bedroom door and your house, to exit through the windows on the opposite side (Figure 16.7b). As the wind increases, suddenly it blows your bedroom door shut, waking you with its slam. Haven't we all had this happen? What would have happened if, instead, the wind had come from the opposite direction? Instead of blowing in your bedroom window, it is entering the opposite side of the house and blowing out of your bedroom window (Figure 16.7c). Your bedroom door would be held open by the wind, not slammed shut. That is exactly how the valves in the heart function.

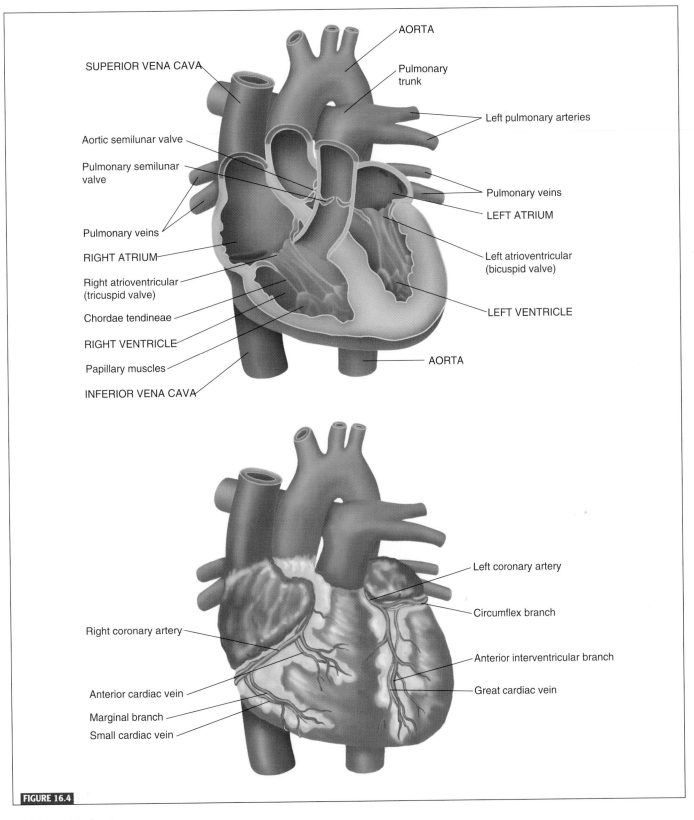

AORTA

SUPERIOR VENA CAVA

Pulmonary trunk

Left pulmonary arteries

Aortic semilunar valve

Pulmonary semilunar valve

Pulmonary veins

LEFT ATRIUM

Pulmonary veins

RIGHT ATRIUM

Left atrioventricular (bicuspid valve)

Right atrioventricular (tricuspid valve)

Chordae tendineae

LEFT VENTRICLE

RIGHT VENTRICLE

AORTA

Papillary muscles

INFERIOR VENA CAVA

Left coronary artery

Circumflex branch

Right coronary artery

Anterior interventricular branch

Anterior cardiac vein

Great cardiac vein

Marginal branch

Small cardiac vein

FIGURE 16.4

Anatomy of the heart.

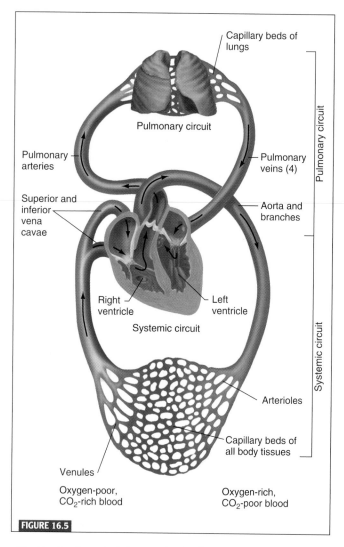

FIGURE 16.5

The blood pathway includes two circuits. The right ventricle supplies the pulmonary circuit, and the left ventricle supplies the systemic circuit.

When the pressure in the atria is greater than the pressure in the ventricles, blood flows from the atria into the ventricles (Figure 16.6). The ventricles are analogous to your bedroom, the atria are like the hallway outside of your bedroom, and the cusps of the atrioventricular valves are like your bedroom door. As long as blood is flowing from the atria into the ventricles, the

Table 16.1 The Coronary Arteries

Artery	Region Supplied*	Major Branches
Left	Left atrium and ventricle, interventricular septum	Anterior interventricular branch, circumflex branch, left anterior descending branch
Right	Right atrium and ventricle	Posterior interventricular branch, marginal branch

*Note that some overlap in regions supplied by each artery does occur.

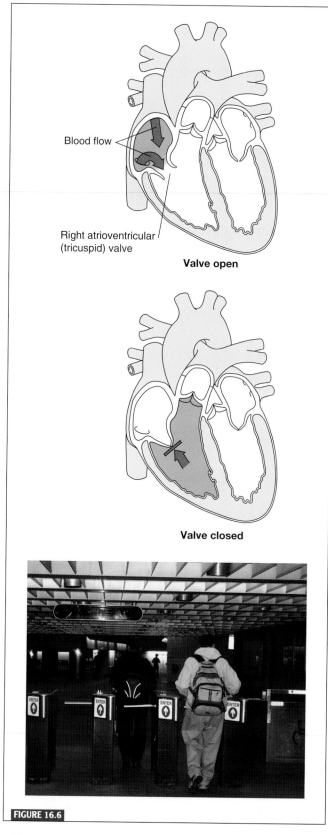

FIGURE 16.6

Like a turnstile used to keep crowds moving in one direction, the valves of the heart allow the blood to flow in only one direction.

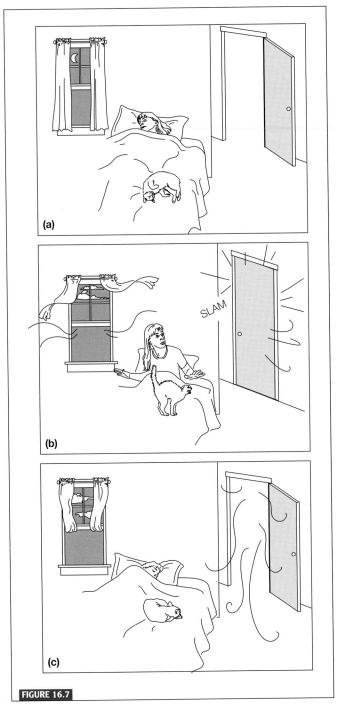

FIGURE 16.7

The valves of your heart work like a door in your home (a). They are closed by flow in one direction (b) and opened by the flow from the opposite direction (c).

valves will be held open. As the heart continues on its cycle (to be presented shortly), the pressure in the atria (atrial pressure) will decrease, and the pressure in the ventricles (ventricular pressure) will rise. When the ventricular pressure exceeds atrial pressure, blood will begin to flow backwards, from the ventricles into the atria. This is similar to the wind coming in your bedroom window. Just as the wind would blow your bed-

room door shut, the blood flowing in that direction forces the atrioventricular valves shut. This eliminates the possibility of blood flowing in the wrong direction.

What about the semilunar valves? When ventricular pressure is greater than arterial pressure (pressure in the pulmonary trunk and aorta), the semilunar valves are held open and blood flows from the ventricles into the arteries. When ventricular pressure falls below arterial pressure, the valves are pushed to the closed position by blood beginning to flow in the opposite direction. This keeps blood flowing in the proper direction.

■ Electrical Impulse Generation and Conduction

Recall from Chapter 8 that cells such as neurons and muscle cells generate electrical charges, called electrical potential, by pumping ions (charged particles) across their cell membranes. They produce a gradient of ions across their membrane and, in that way, become charged. Recall the cat and dog analogy and how it related to the generation of the electrical gradient (for review, see Figures 8.1 and 8.2). Also remember that this electrical potential can be quickly discharged as a wave of depolarization moving along the cell's surface. This wave of depolarization, and the repolarization that follows it, is called an action potential. If you do not remember this material, please review Chapter 8 before continuing in this chapter.

In Chapter 9, we learned how muscle cells contract and how this contraction was initiated by a muscle action potential. We also learned that there are three types of muscle, one of which is cardiac muscle. Let's briefly review the information on cardiac muscle at this time.

Cardiac muscle cells are generally rectangular in shape, although some are branched (**FIGURE 16.8**). They measure approximately 150 micrometers in length and are striated. One or sometimes two nuclei are centrally located, and special structures called intercalated disks make up the junctions between cells. These intercalated disks contain gap junctions, special pores that allow ions to flow from one cell to the next. Because of these structures, the cells of the myocardium function as one cell, rather than as many individual cells. They are, therefore, a functional syncytium, individual cells acting as if they were one large cell. Recall that skeletal muscle fibers are syncytia, or large cells with many nuclei. Cardiac muscle instead acts as if it were a syncytium, while being composed of individual cells.

Autorhythmicity is a special feature of cardiac muscle. Autorhythmicity means that these cells generate their own rhythm, the beat by which the heart contracts. So inherent is this self-generated beat that when embryonic heart cells grown in culture differentiate into cardiac

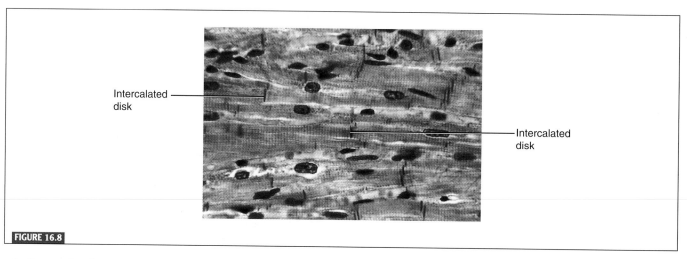

Cardiac muscle cells.

muscle, the single layer of cells in the culture flask will actually begin to beat! Autorhythmicity is caused by the cells having a slight permeability for sodium. As sodium ions leak in, the membrane reaches threshold and the action potential is triggered. This action potential causes the cardiac muscle cells to contract.

In some parts of the heart, the cardiac muscle cells have been modified to specifically generate or conduct action potentials, rather than to contract. These cells make up the impulse generation and conduction system (**FIGURE 16.9**). The components of this system are listed in **TABLE 16.2**.

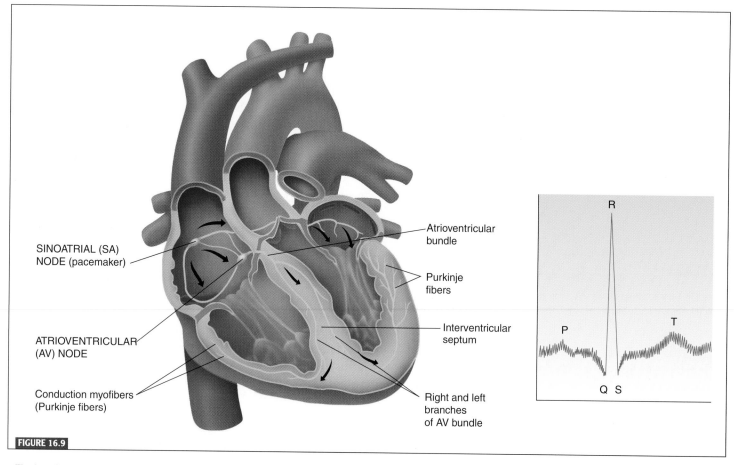

The impulse generation and conduction system of your heart. The fibrotendinous ring is shown in blue. Also shown is the tracing of an EKG. The p wave corresponds to atrial depolarization, the QRS complex to ventricular depolarization, and the T wave to ventricular repolarization.

Table 16.2	The Cardiac Impulse Generation and Conduction System	
Structure	**Location**	**Function**
Sinoatrial (SA) node	Right atrium, inferior to the opening of the inferior vena cava	Primary pacemaker
Atrioventricular (AV) node	Inferior portion of the interatrial septum	Secondary pacemaker
Atrioventricular (AV) bundle	Passes through the fibrotendinous ring	Conduction from the atria to the ventricles
Bundle branches (right and left)	Pass down either side of the interventricular septum	Distributes action potential through the ventricles
Conduction myofibers	Throughout ventricles	Distributes action potential through the ventricles

The primary pacemaker is the sinoatrial (SA) node, located in the wall of the right atrium. This is the heart's primary pacemaker simply because it is the heart's most rapid pacemaker. The cells of the SA node are more permeable to sodium than cells in other regions, allowing this node to reach threshold more quickly. The atrioventricular (AV) node acts as a secondary pacemaker. If the SA node fails to function, the AV node can take over, keeping the heart functioning, although at a slower pace and less efficiently. In normal functioning of the heart, the SA node generates an action potential that spreads across the atria and finally reaches the AV node. Here we have to think again about the structure of the heart.

The heart is separated into two electrical circuits by a disk of dense connective tissue called the fibrotendinous ring. The superior electrical circuit is composed of the atria and the two nodes we have already discussed. The fibrotendinous ring serves as an electrical insulator, separating this circuit from the inferior circuit. Each of the heart valves are also part of the fibrotendinous ring. All of the vessels of the heart enter and exit through the base of the heart so that the valves may all be part of this connective tissue structure.

The electrical activity of the atria must be coordinated with that of the ventricles to ensure proper heart function. To allow this coordination, the electrical activity that began in the SA node, spread across the atria, and finally reached the AV node, must have some way of passing through the fibrotendinous ring into the ventricles (the inferior electrical circuit). The atrioventricular bundle, also called the bundle of His (pronounced hiss), conducts the action potential through the fibrotendinous ring. It then splits into the right and left bundle branches, which travel down either side of the interventricular septum. From here, the action potential is carried rapidly throughout the ventricular myocardium by cells called conduction myofibers, or Purkinje cells. Like other cells throughout the conduction system, these are modified cardiac muscle cells that have differentiated into cells specialized in conduction rather than contraction.

The purpose of this entire system is to generate the beat or rhythm by which the heart contracts and to dis-

tribute that rhythm in a manner that allows for coordinated contractions of the atria and ventricles. It also must function in a way that causes cells throughout the ventricles to be depolarized at the same time so an effective contraction of the ventricles can occur. Electrocardiogram (EKG) is a method of monitoring the heart's electrical activity from the surface of the body (Figure 16.9).

The Cardiac Cycle

We are now ready to put together what we know about the anatomy of the heart, the heart valves, and the electrical activities of the heart. We will accomplish this by examining the cardiac cycle, the cyclic activity of the heart. Please understand that there are many ways to break down this cycle; this is but one way to do so. **TABLE 16.3** presents some definitions we will need. The actual cycle is presented in **FIGURE 16.10**. It is presented as an illustrated outline to aid your comprehension. Please keep in mind that this cycle is very rapid; with a cardiac rate of 60 beats per minute, the entire cycle takes 1 second.

Cardiac Output

Your body has mechanisms it can use to alter your cardiac output. Think about how your body uses moving fluids to maintain homeostasis. During periods of high metabolic activity, like when you are exercising, you need to move much more of these fluids to maintain homeostasis (**FIGURE 16.11**). Blood, being chief among these moving fluids, must be pumped at a much greater

Table 16.3	Terms Associated with the Cardiac Cycle
Term	**Definition**
Atrial pressure	Pressure in the atria
Ventricular pressure	Pressure in the ventricles
Arterial pressure	Pressure in the aorta and pulmonary trunk
Systole	Phase of contraction (high pressure)
Diastole	Phase of relaxation (low pressure)
Isovolumetric	No change in volume

I. Ventricular Filling

    A. This process begins when ventricular pressure falls below atrial pressure.

    B. The first phase is the period of *rapid ventricular filling* (a).

        1. This is the initial flow upon opening of the AV valves.

    C. The second phase is called *diastasis*.

        1. In this phase all contractions of the heart have stopped; the cardiac muscle is relaxed.

        2. The ventricles are still being filled with blood as it flows from the great veins through the atria into the ventricles.

        3. By the end of this phase, approximately 70% of the blood that enters the ventricles has done so.

    D. The third phase is the *period of atrial systole*.

        1. The sinoatrial (SA) node fires, sending an action potential across the atria.

        2. The atria are contracting in response to this action potential (atrial systole), ejecting more blood into the ventricles (b).

        3. Only about 30% of the blood that enters the ventricles does so during atrial systole.

II. Ventricular Systole

    A. The action potential now passes through the atrioventricular (AV) bundle into the bundle branches and spreads throughout the ventricles.

    B. In response to this, the myocardium of the ventricles begins to contract.

    C. This elevates the ventricular pressure.

    D. When ventricular pressure exceeds atrial pressure, the AV valves close, causing the first heart sound "lubb."

    E. This begins the *period of isovolumetric contraction,* the period in which the AV valves are closed, the semilunar valves are closed, the ventricles are continuing to contract, and no blood is being pumped (c).

    F. The *ejection period* begins when ventricular pressure exceeds arterial pressure. When this happens, the semilunar valves open and blood is ejected from the ventricles into the aorta and the pulmonary trunk. During the ejection period, slightly more than half of the volume of blood contained in the ventricles is ejected (d).

III. Ventricular Diastole

    A. The action potential has now passed through the ventricles, and they are starting to relax, entering *ventricular diastole*.

    B. As the ventricles relax, ventricular pressure begins to fall.

    C. When ventricular pressure falls below arterial pressure, the semilunar valves close, causing the second heart sound "dupp."

    D. The *period of isovolumetric relaxation* is the period in which the AV valves are closed, the semilunar valves are closed, the ventricles are continuing to relax, and no blood is being pumped (e).

    E. This period continues until the ventricular pressure falls below the atrial pressure, at which time the AV valves open and the ventricular filling stage begins.

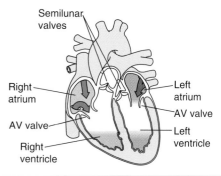

(a)

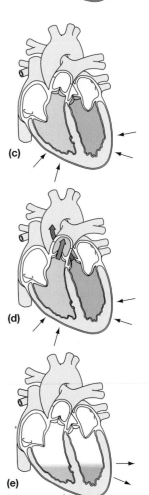

(b)

(c)

(d)

(e)

FIGURE 16.10

The cardiac cycle.

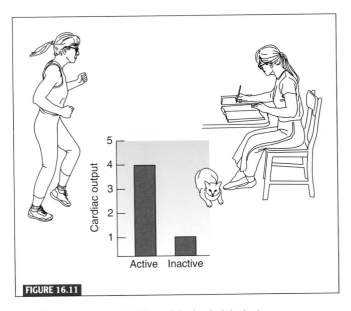

FIGURE 16.11

Cardiac output varies with the activity level of the body.

It is easy to imagine alterations in the heart rate. We have all noticed such alterations. Have you noticed how your heart races during and after heavy exercise, or when you watch a horror movie, or as you begin to take a difficult exam? We are most apt to notice increases in our heart rate, but obviously our body has the ability to increase or decrease heart rate as needed. As you are already aware, heart rate is regulated by the autonomic nervous system and the endocrine system (more on this in a moment).

How about the amount of blood pumped per cardiac cycle? You may also have noticed how your heart has at times felt as if it were really pounding: perhaps after exercising or when you had a fever. In doing so, you may have been observing your body's ability to increase the force of each ventricular contraction and, therefore, increase the amount of blood being expelled with each cardiac cycle.

We refer to the volume of blood pumped per ventricular contraction as the stroke volume. Stroke volume varies with the strength of ventricular contraction. A stronger (more forceful) contraction will start the ejection period sooner and continue that period longer, increasing the amount of blood pumped from the ventricle. Remember that the ejection period begins when ventricular pressure exceeds arterial pressure. The ejection period ends when ventricular pressure falls below arterial pressure. A more forceful contraction, therefore, will result in the ejection period beginning sooner and ending later. A longer ejection period achieves more complete emptying of the ventricles and a resulting increase in stroke volume.

So, which systems regulate the heart rate and force of ventricular contraction? The main regulators of homeostasis are the nervous and endocrine systems. They work together to control cardiac function. The autonomic nervous system directly innervates the myocardium. As part of this system, the cardiac center in the

rate during these peak demand periods than when you are at rest. It would not be efficient to have the heart circulating blood at such a high rate when it is not necessary to do so, like while you are reading this book.

So, how can we alter cardiac output? The two main ways of changing cardiac output are either to alter the number of cardiac cycles per minute (heart rate) or to alter the amount of blood pumped per cardiac cycle (per ventricular contraction). To picture this, think about bailing out a sinking rowboat (**FIGURE 16.12**). If the boat is sinking faster than you are bailing, you must alter your bailing to save yourself. You can bail faster (more buckets per minute). This is like increasing your heart rate. Alternatively, you could get a bigger bailing bucket (more water per scoop). This would be similar to increasing the strength of your heart's contraction and moving more blood per cycle.

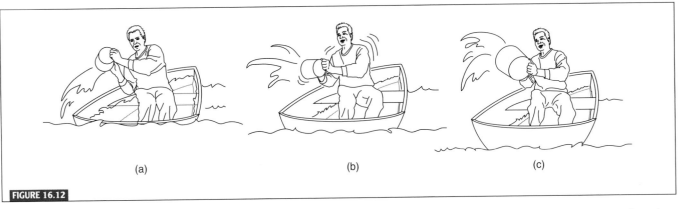

(a)   (b)   (c)

FIGURE 16.12

We can increase cardiac output much like we can increase the volume of water we are bailing out of a sinking boat (a). We can increase the number of cardiac cycles per minute, which is similar to bailing faster (b), or we can increase the amount of blood pumped per cardiac cycle, which is like using a larger bailing bucket (c).

medulla oblongata plays an important role in regulating heart rate. Through the activity of that center, the sympathetic nervous system increases heart rate and force of contraction, while the parasympathetic nervous system does the opposite. These two divisions of the autonomic nervous system work antagonistically to allow fine control of cardiac output. Information from blood pressure monitors in the carotid artery, the arch of the aorta, and the right atrium is used in this process.

The endocrine system produces hormones that affect cardiac output (detailed in Chapter 13). Epinephrine and norepinephrine (also called adrenalin and noradrenalin) from the adrenal medulla increase cardiac output. Recall how the adrenal medulla works in the interface between the sympathetic nervous system and the endocrine system to make the effects of the sympathetic nervous system global (systemic) and long lasting. Thyroid hormone also increases cardiac output, as one factor in its elevation of metabolic rate.

16.3 Your Blood Vessels

Blood vessels provide the channels through which the blood is distributed throughout the body and returned to the heart. Blood vessels come in a variety of types, based on their size, their form, and ultimately on the functions they are called on to perform. In this section, we will learn about the various types of blood vessels, and about how their structure contributes to their ability to perform their function. We will also learn the basic anatomy of the vasculature by learning the names of some major blood vessels.

■ The Types of Vessels

Let's start by thinking about taking a trip in a car (**FIGURE 16.13**). We may begin on a big interstate divided highway. After a while, as we approach our destination, we exit onto a smaller highway. It is still a major road, but perhaps it is not a divided highway. Later we exit onto a local road that takes us through a town. We pass through the business district where we can shop, get something to eat, or perhaps use the restrooms, if necessary. As we continue on our trip, we leave town and get on another local road, then on an intermediate highway, and again onto a big interstate divided highway. Blood vessels are arranged in a similar manner. Just as roadways of different types carry us to our destinations, blood vessels of different types transport blood around the body.

The blood vessels that carry blood away from the heart are called arteries. Like superhighways, the largest arteries do not go everywhere. The aorta is this type of

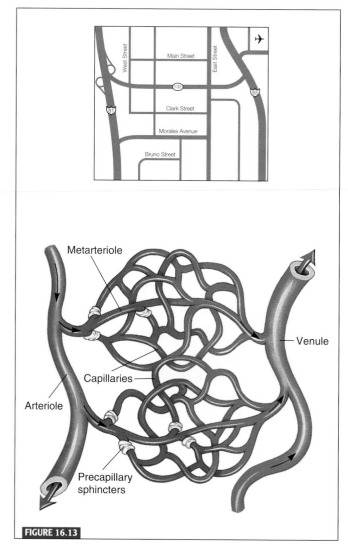

FIGURE 16.13

Just as we travel on different types of roads, our vasculature consists of several different types of vessels.

artery. It serves as a main distribution route, off of which branch medium-sized arteries. As these continue to branch to smaller arteries, we reach the smallest arteries, called arterioles. These are the equivalent of county roads that lead into a town. In towns we usually find small roads and numerous shops. Towns are the business districts where exchange takes place. In the vasculature, the capillary beds are similar to towns. Capillaries are the smallest blood vessels. Some are so fine that blood cells must pass through them single file. They are the business districts of the vasculature, the place where exchange occurs. Exchange in this case involves movement of gases, nutrients, and wastes between the blood and the surrounding tissues.

Once blood leaves the capillaries, it is heading back toward the heart. Veins are the vessels that carry blood toward the heart. The smallest veins, which begin at the end of the capillaries, are called venules. These join together and become medium and then large veins. The largest veins return blood to the right and left atria.

If we now consider the structure of these vessels, we can comprehend their function in more detail (**FIGURE 16.14**). The walls of blood vessels are generally composed of three layers. The luminal (innermost) layer is the tunica intima, the middle layer is the tunica media, and the external layer is the tunica externa, or adventitia.

The tunica intima is made up of the cells that actually line the lumen of the blood vessel and the underlying structures that support them. We learned about the cells that line the lumen earlier in this chapter (think, what are they called?). Every space that blood passes through must be lined with something that will not activate the clotting mechanism. This mechanism causes blood to clot at the site of an injury, protecting the body from excessive blood loss. If the blood were to clot within the blood vessels, as it does in a condition called disseminated intravascular coagulation (DIC), an extreme medical emergency would follow. Therefore, our blood vessels and the chambers of our heart are lined with endothelial cells, a cell type that shields the clotting mechanism from molecules deep to the endothelial cells that would trigger clotting.

Endothelial cells line blood vessels. As lining cells, endothelial cells must be epithelial. What type of epithelial cell would we find in this location? First, consider whether they are simple or stratified. Is this a site of abrasion? No, not really. The only substance that is in contact with these cells is blood, and that is a liquid. We know then that a simple epithelium would be found here. Endothelial cells must resist being lifted off their underlying basement membrane by the blood flowing by. In some locations, they must also allow diffusion to occur through them from the apical surface to the basal surface, or in the opposite direction. This is especially true in the capillaries, the "business district," where exchange occurs. What epithelial cell type offers a low profile to resist being lifted off of its basement membrane and also is flat enough to allow rapid diffusion through its thickness? Squamous cells meet those criteria. Endothelial cells are simple squamous epithelia.

Deep to the endothelial cells and their basement membrane, we find one more component of the tunica intima, an elastic membrane. This membrane, called the internal elastic lamina, underlies these structures to give some flexibility to the tunica intima, particularly in the largest arteries.

The tunica media is the thickest layer of most vessel walls. It is composed of different tissues in different types of vessels. Large arteries, such as the aorta, must expand as the ventricles contract to absorb some of the force of the surging blood. Through elastic recoil, as the ventricles relax, they must return to their original diameters. This propels the blood along the arteries even when the ejection period is over. To picture this, think about how a bagpipe player fills a bag with air as he exhales, allowing him to compress the bag to continue playing even when he inhales (**FIGURE 16.15**). This is similar to how these large arteries work. Their walls stretch during ventricular systole, absorbing some of the force of the ejected blood, and recoil during diastole to keep the blood flowing while it is not being ejected from the heart.

To accomplish this, the vessel wall must be able to stretch and recoil greatly. We know we must have a connective tissue here because this is not a lining. Which type of connective tissue allows for such stretching and relaxation? Elastic connective tissue with elastic fibers does.

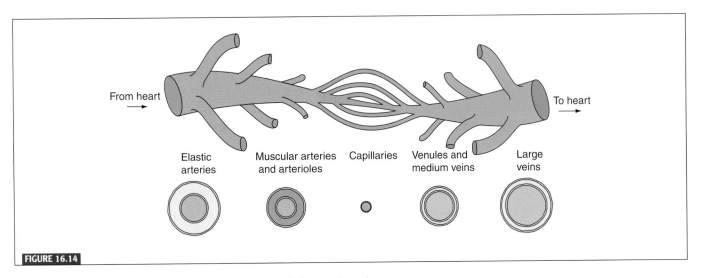

FIGURE 16.14

The composition and diameter of our blood vessel walls varies with the type of vessel.

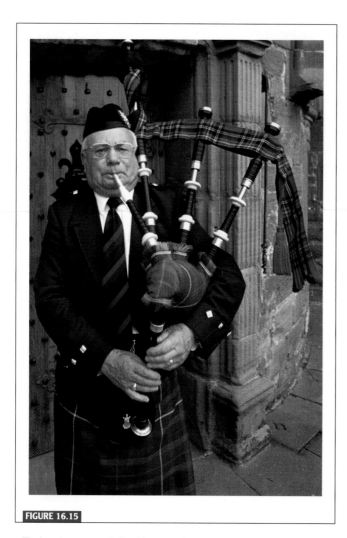

The bagpiper uses an inflated bag to maintain airflow through his instrument whether he is exhaling or inhaling. In much the same way, our aorta stretches as the heart pumps blood into it and recoils to keep the blood moving when the ventricle is no longer ejecting blood.

For that reason, large arteries that have elastic connective tissue in their tunica media are called elastic arteries.

Smaller arteries and arterioles have different characteristics and abilities than those of the large arteries. At any one time, blood is flowing through a very small percentage of your capillaries. This is very important. You do not have enough blood volume to fill all of your capillaries at one time. Even if you did, your heart does not have enough pumping capacity to maintain adequate blood pressure if blood were to flow through all of your capillaries at once. Imagine what would happen if you turned on every faucet in your house at one time, including the shower, the garden hose, and flushed the toilet. If you live in an apartment, picture all of your neighbors doing the same thing. What would happen to your water pressure?

For this reason, we must have a way to regulate flow through our capillary beds. The vessels that supply individual organs and individual capillary beds within those organs must have the ability to constrict, reduce, or shut off the flow through the capillaries. That sounds like the job of smooth muscle. In fact, the tunica media of the medium-sized arteries (such as the renal arteries) and the arterioles is composed of smooth muscle. Medium-sized arteries are, therefore, called muscular arteries.

Do we have any tunica media at all in our capillaries? Capillaries are the sites of exchange between the vasculature and the surrounding tissues. Substances such as oxygen and carbon dioxide must freely cross the vessel wall in these locations. Therefore, the tunica media (and tunica externa) are essentially absent from capillaries.

Since the capillary wall is so thin, the blood pressure in the capillaries must be very low to avoid rupture of the wall. For this reason, blood must be able to flow freely through the vessels following the capillaries. If these vessels, the venules and veins, restricted blood flow, pressure would build up in the capillaries and the capillary walls would be damaged. How do our veins avoid this pressure build-up? In addition to having diameters larger than the arteries and arterioles that supply the capillaries, the venules and veins have mainly elastic connective tissue in their tunica media, with little smooth muscle, compared to the arteries we have discussed. They have only a minimal ability to constrict and build pressure in the capillaries.

The tunica externa of arteries and veins is composed of loose connective tissue, containing collagenous and elastic fibers to support the vessel wall. This connective tissue is continuous with the connective tissue of surrounding structures, making it difficult at times to dissect individual vessels from those structures. In large veins, we also find some smooth muscle arranged longitudinally for strength.

There are now a couple of additional features of the vasculature that we must consider. Picture yourself relaxing on a bench and then suddenly standing up (**FIGURE 16.16**). In a more extreme case, picture yourself standing on your head and then suddenly standing upright (not so easy for some of us to picture). What would keep the blood that is in the veins in your legs from flowing backwards, away from your heart? Gravity would pull it in that direction, wouldn't it? That would be a bad thing, as it could result in a sudden drop in blood pressure. We are protected from that occurrence by the presence of valves in our large veins similar to the semilunar valves of the large arteries of our heart.

For the next feature we will consider, let's think again about our trip in the car. We are on our way to a

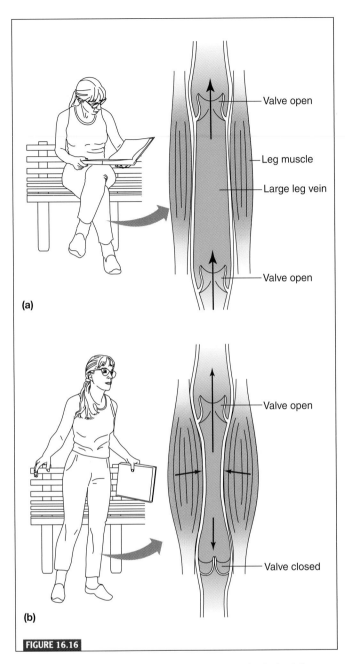

(a)

Valve open

Leg muscle

Large leg vein

Valve open

(b)

Valve open

Valve closed

FIGURE 16.16

Valves in our veins keep blood flowing toward the heart despite local changes in pressure.

popular seasonal destination, such as the beach or the mountains, and the road we travel passes through a town. Because of the narrow roads and traffic lights in the town, traffic backs up onto the highway, causing terrible congestion. Don't they sometimes build a by-pass around towns, allowing cars that do not need to go to the town to continue on their journey? This reduces such traffic congestion.

Arterioles have tunica media of smooth muscle. They also have a ring of smooth muscle called a pre-

capillary sphincter just before the capillary. These two features allow them to effectively shut off blood flow through a capillary bed. If many of the arterioles supplied by a single medium-sized artery were to be shut off, congestion similar to the traffic jam just described could occur. Toward the distal end of many arterioles we find a small vessel called a metarteriole. The metarteriole bypasses the capillary bed, connecting directly to the venule, in a manner similar to the highway bypass around a town. This eliminates vascular congestion just as the highway bypass eliminates traffic congestion.

16.4 The Gross Anatomy of Your Cardiovascular System: A Brief Atlas

The gross anatomy of the arteries and veins are presented as a miniatlas in **FIGURES 16.17–16.20**. Please study this anatomy before continuing on to our discussion of blood.

16.5 Fluids in Motion: Your Blood

Earlier in this chapter, the cardiovascular system was likened to a river, and we discussed that river in detail. We discussed its geography (our cardiovascular system's anatomy), the banks or shores that enclose it (the blood vessels), and the force that propels it (the action of the heart). We have not yet discussed what flows within it.

If you think that the fluid that flows in this internal "river," our blood, is mere river water, you are in for some surprises. This moving liquid is actually a connective tissue in liquid form. And just as our other mesenchymal derivatives are complex, so is our blood. It has a complex composition and an equally complex array of capabilities. Let's begin by continuing our "river" analogy and discuss the movement of this fluid, how it flows, and the pressures involved. Then let's think some more about blood as a connective tissue (mesenchymal derivative).

■ How Your Blood Moves: Axial Flow

Have you ever stood along a river bank, or perhaps on a small bridge, and watched sticks and other objects floating by? Perhaps you added a few small sticks to the flow and watched them disappear downstream. Was the flow of that river uniform across the surface, or did the middle and the edges of the stream move at different rates? You may have noticed that the flow was fastest in the middle of the river and slower along the bank. In fact, you may have noticed that the sticks and floating

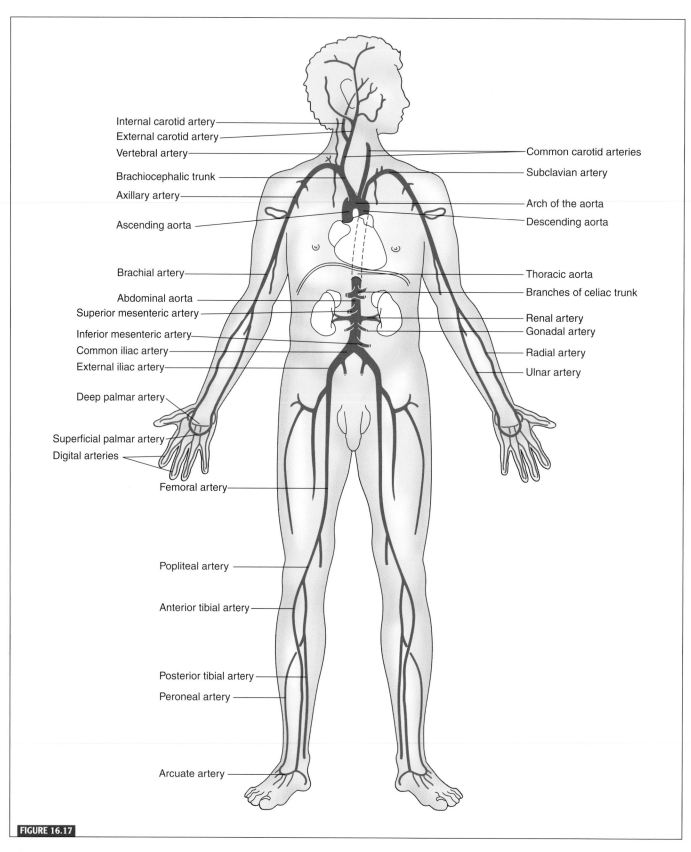

Internal carotid artery

External carotid artery

Vertebral artery

Brachiocephalic trunk

Axillary artery

Ascending aorta

Brachial artery

Abdominal aorta

Superior mesenteric artery

Inferior mesenteric artery

Common iliac artery

External iliac artery

Deep palmar artery

Superficial palmar artery

Digital arteries

Femoral artery

Popliteal artery

Anterior tibial artery

Posterior tibial artery

Peroneal artery

Arcuate artery

Common carotid arteries

Subclavian artery

Arch of the aorta

Descending aorta

Thoracic aorta

Branches of celiac trunk

Renal artery

Gonadal artery

Radial artery

Ulnar artery

FIGURE 16.17

Overview of the arteries.

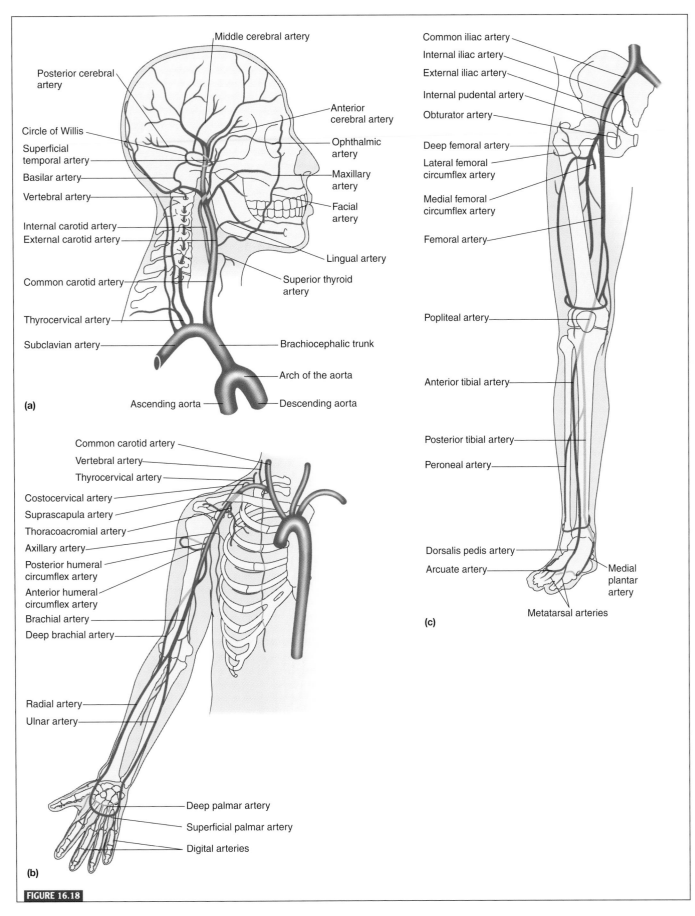

Middle cerebral artery

Posterior cerebral artery

Anterior cerebral artery

Circle of Willis

Ophthalmic artery

Superficial temporal artery

Maxillary artery

Basilar artery

Vertebral artery

Facial artery

Internal carotid artery

External carotid artery

Lingual artery

Common carotid artery

Superior thyroid artery

Thyrocervical artery

Subclavian artery

Brachiocephalic trunk

Arch of the aorta

Ascending aorta

Descending aorta

(a)

Common carotid artery

Vertebral artery

Thyrocervical artery

Costocervical artery

Suprascapula artery

Thoracoacromial artery

Axillary artery

Posterior humeral circumflex artery

Anterior humeral circumflex artery

Brachial artery

Deep brachial artery

Radial artery

Ulnar artery

Deep palmar artery

Superficial palmar artery

Digital arteries

(b)

Common iliac artery

Internal iliac artery

External iliac artery

Internal pudendal artery

Obturator artery

Deep femoral artery

Lateral femoral circumflex artery

Medial femoral circumflex artery

Femoral artery

Popliteal artery

Anterior tibial artery

Posterior tibial artery

Peroneal artery

Dorsalis pedis artery

Arcuate artery

Medial plantar artery

Metatarsal arteries

(c)

FIGURE 16.18

Detailed views of the arteries.

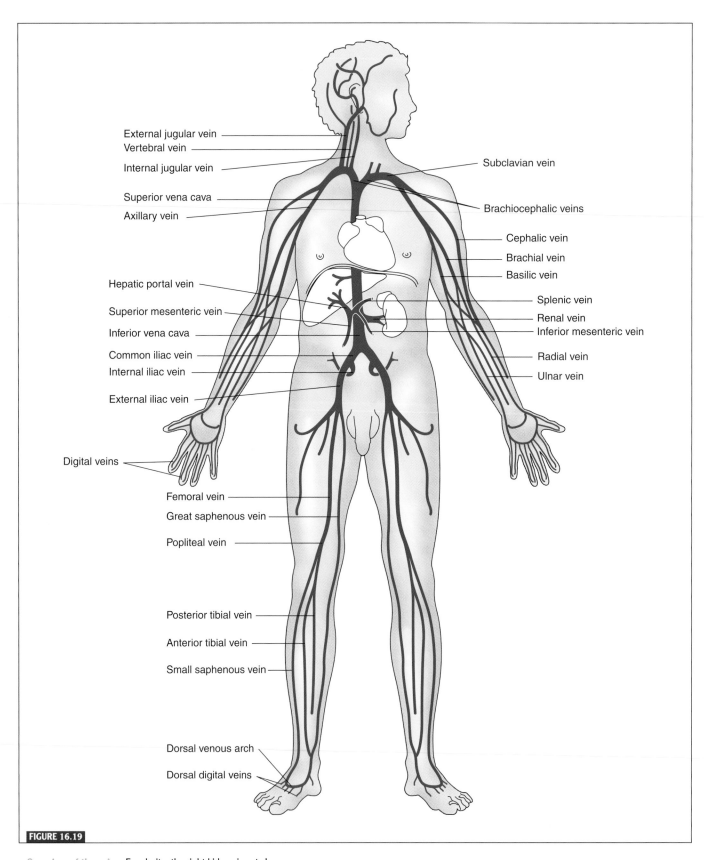

External jugular vein

Vertebral vein

Internal jugular vein

Superior vena cava

Axillary vein

Hepatic portal vein

Superior mesenteric vein

Inferior vena cava

Common iliac vein

Internal iliac vein

External iliac vein

Digital veins

Femoral vein

Great saphenous vein

Popliteal vein

Posterior tibial vein

Anterior tibial vein

Small saphenous vein

Dorsal venous arch

Dorsal digital veins

Subclavian vein

Brachiocephalic veins

Cephalic vein

Brachial vein

Basilic vein

Splenic vein

Renal vein

Inferior mesenteric vein

Radial vein

Ulnar vein

FIGURE 16.19

Overview of the veins. For clarity, the right kidney is not shown.

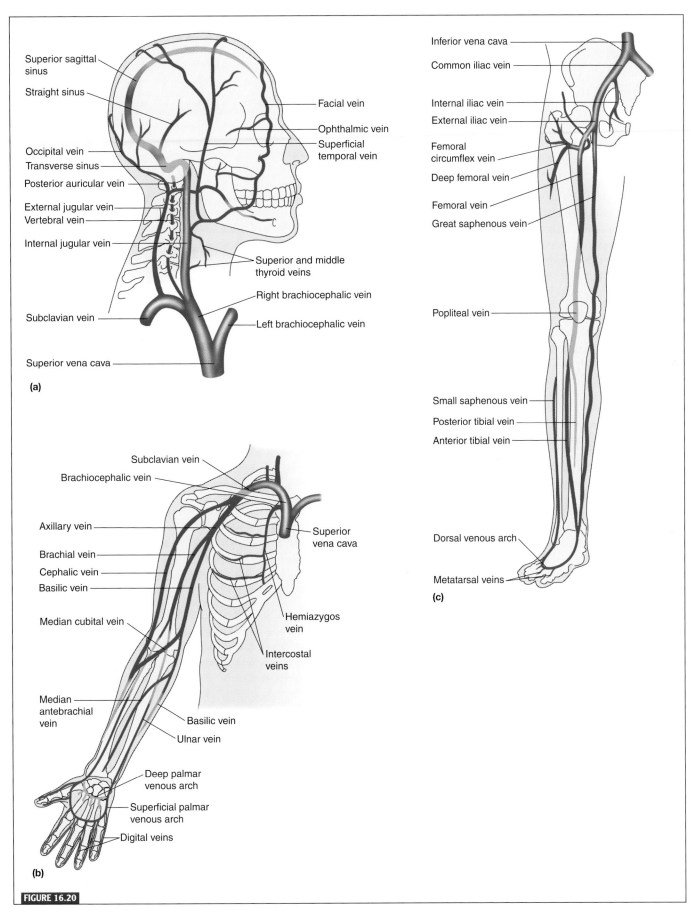

FIGURE 16.20

Detailed views of the veins.

debris tended to be pulled to the center of the stream into the fastest moving flow.

This illustrates the concept of axial flow. The term *axial* refers to the center line of some object, such as the axis of the earth (remember the axial skeleton). The axis of a river is its central region where the flow is fastest. The flow of blood in our vasculature exhibits axial flow, just like a river. The blood is moving fastest in the center of the vessel and slower along the edges (quick, think of the name of the cells that line all blood vessels). Just as floating objects were carried out into the fastest current in our river, objects moving in our blood are generally carried to its center. These objects are our blood cells. The largest cells (white blood cells) are carried in the center of the current. The smaller red blood cells, and even smaller platelets (cell fragments), are carried further out, but are still mainly in the fast-moving current. The slower-moving fluid, along the endothelial cell-lined walls of the vessel, actually carries relatively few cells.

I mention axial flow here so you can picture in your mind what actually occurs in a blood vessel. You will also need this information as we discuss inflammation in Chapter 21. Now, let's think a little about pressures.

■ A Balance of Pressures: Starling's Hypothesis

You already know something about blood pressure. If we were to measure the pressure in an artery as your heart was contracting, what would we call that pressure? O.K., systolic pressure. How about as your heart was relaxing? Good; diastolic pressure (isn't it amazing that I can tell in advance that you are answering these questions correctly?). These are mechanical pressures, and are what we generally think of when we think about blood pressure. But there is more to it than that. There are actually four types of pressure we need to think about as we consider the pressures in our blood vessels.

Look at the diagram in **FIGURE 16.21a** and notice that four types of pressure are listed, alongside arrows showing the direction of these pressures. Remember from our very early discussions in this text that, in addition to mechanical pressure (hydrostatic pressure), we also have osmotic pressure. Osmotic pressure is generated any time the concentrations of two solutions separated by a semipermiable membrane differ. In this case, the membrane is the wall of a blood vessel.

In examining Figure 16.21, you will notice that two different hydrostatic pressures oppose each other. Blood hydrostatic pressure is that pressure we normally think of as "blood pressure;" it is a force that pushes fluid out of the blood vessel. Interstitial hydrostatic pressure is

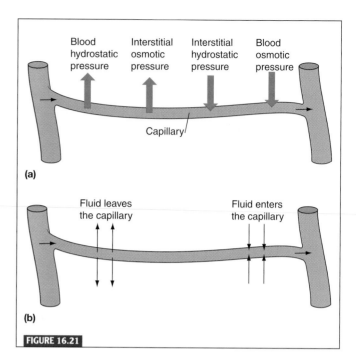

FIGURE 16.21

Starling's hypothesis explains that four pressures (a) balance to determine whether interstitial fluid is produced or removed from the tissues surrounding capillary beds. Fluid leaves capillaries in the proximal part of the capillary bed and reenters capillaries distally (b). Interstitial fluid also leaves tissues through lymphatic vessels.

the hydrostatic pressure of the fluid of the tissues. It pushes fluid into the vessel; if fluid is to leave a blood vessel, this is a force that must be overcome.

Interstitial osmotic pressure is another pressure that pulls fluid from the blood vessel. This pressure is prominent if the concentration of proteins and other substances is greater outside the vessel than inside the vessel. Blood osmotic pressure is the opposite of interstitial osmotic pressure. It is strongest when the concentration of proteins and other substances is greater within the vessel, when compared to the concentration outside the vessel.

What does all of this have to do with the movement of fluids? Simply this: when blood is traveling in our capillaries, it is traveling in a vessel with walls through which some components of blood can pass. The fluid component of blood, and many of the small molecules suspended in that fluid, can pass through the capillary wall in either direction. In the proximal region of any capillary (the beginning of a capillary bed), the sum of these four pressures favors the movement of fluid out of the capillaries, into the interstitial space. This is how interstitial fluid is formed. Interstitial fluid is very much like the fluid component of blood, except that it lacks the large proteins and clotting agents of blood. Also absent are the red blood cells, and white blood cells in large numbers.

In the distal portion of a capillary (at the far end of the capillary bed), these four pressures add up to a sum that favors the movement of fluid into the capillary from the interstitial space. This is how we get rid of some of the interstitial fluid. This is what occurs during homeostasis. These pressures, and hence their sum, change during certain pathological processes. You can imagine how interstitial fluid could build up in tissues if these pressures were to become unbalanced. This condition is called edema. That, however, is outside of homeostasis and not the topic of our current discussion (see inflammation, in Chapter 21). The concept of the balance of these pressures determining the movement of fluids across the capillary wall is described by Starling's Hypothesis.

■ Lymphatic Vessels

We also have a second set of vessels that carry interstitial fluid (the interstitial fluid that does not re-enter the capillaries) away from our tissues. Our lymphatic system is made up of a series of vessels and organs that pick up the remaining interstitial fluid and transport it as lymphatic fluid back into the vasculature (**FIGURE 16.22**). After certain injuries, or because of scarring after surgery, these vessels are sometimes blocked, leading to persistent edema. The smallest lymph vessels are similar to open-ended capillaries. They arise in the tissues and join together to form ever larger vessels until they become lymphatic trunks and, ultimately, either the thoracic duct or the right lymphatic duct. The thoracic duct empties its lymphatic fluid into the blood of the left subclavian vein. The right lymphatic duct empties its lymph into the blood of the right subclavian vein. Hence, in all cases the lymphatic fluid returns to the blood from which it originally came. These moving fluids (the fluid component of blood, interstitial fluid and lymphatic fluid) are all part of one great system, just as all water throughout the world is all part of one great system. The organs of the lymphatic system will be described in Chapter 21.

16.6 Your Blood As a Connective Tissue

Your blood has already been described as a connective tissue (mesenchymal derivative). If you recall the connective tissues, they all had three components: grapes, spaghetti, and Jell-O (whoops, I mean cells, fibers, and amorphous ground substance). Blood contains cells, the red and white blood cells. Blood also contains an extra-

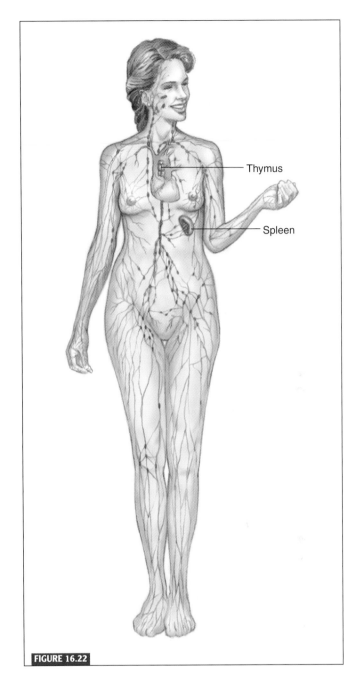

FIGURE 16.22

Lymphatic vessels.

cellular matrix (called plasma) of fibers and amorphous ground substance. We will examine each of these in turn.

■ The Cells of Your Blood

The cellular component of your blood makes up approximately 45 percent of its total volume. Within that population, we find a number of different cells types (**FIGURE 16.23**). But how did they arise; from where do these different cell types originate? During embryonic

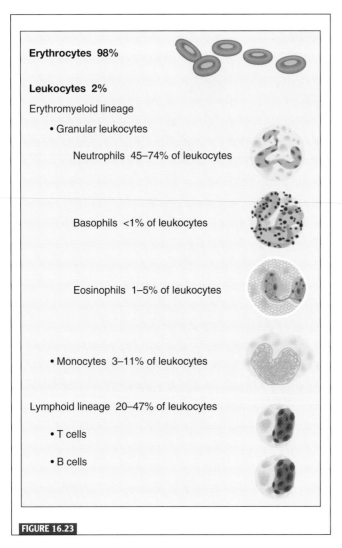

Erythrocytes 98%

Leukocytes 2%

Erythromyeloid lineage

• Granular leukocytes

Neutrophils 45–74% of leukocytes

Basophils <1% of leukocytes

Eosinophils 1–5% of leukocytes

• Monocytes 3–11% of leukocytes

Lymphoid lineage 20–47% of leukocytes

• T cells

• B cells

FIGURE 16.23

The cells of your blood.

development the primitive cells that would later give rise to your blood stem cells were formed in an extra-embryonic (not actually part of the embryo) membrane called the yolk sac. These cells migrated to various sites within the forming embryo, including the liver, bone marrow, spleen, thymus, and lymph nodes. These all became sites of hematopoeisis (formation of blood cells) in the embryo. During the perinatal period (around birth), this list was shortened: the liver and spleen ceased to participate. During childhood, the list is further shortened, and by adulthood, only the flat bones (coxal, ribs, sternum, and skull) and the vertebrae, plus the epiphyses of long bones, contain hematopoeitic red bone marrow. The lymph nodes also continue in one form of hematopoeisis, lymphopoeisis (production of lymphocytes). The thymus involutes by adolescence and no longer is capable of producing lymphocytes.

There are a couple of major lineages (families) of cells that are produced by hematopoeisis, and not all forms of hematopoeisis occur in all locations, even during childhood. The two major lineages are the lymphoid lineage and the erythromyeloid lineage. The lymphoid lineage produces the type of leukocytes (white blood cells) called lymphocytes. Lymphocyte stem cells are found in red bone marrow. Their daughter cells begin their differentiation in the bone marrow and then leave that location to mature in lymphoid organs (the thymus, lymph nodes, and spleen). Since they are not fully differentiated when they reach these organs, some cell division may also occur there. All of the cells in the other lineage are produced in bone marrow (hence the "myeloid" component of its name; *myeloid* means "marrow"). The "erythro" portion of the name refers to red blood cells, the erythrocytes. The erythromyeloid lineage produces red blood cells, the granular leukocytes, the cells of the monocyte-macrophage lineage, and megakaryocytes, which in turn produce platelets.

Although all of these different blood cell types ultimately developed from one embryonic precursor, in adults their stem cells are committed: they are restricted as to the differentiation pathways available to their daughter cells. Much of what we know about differentiation potential in stem cells comes from studies involving the effects of specific growth factors and related molecules, called colony-stimulating factors, on the hematopoeitic stem cells of bone marrow.

Interestingly, the blood contained in the umbilical cord contains stem cells capable of reconstituting the hematopoeitic tissues of an individual if his or her stem cell population is killed as part of the medical intervention for certain forms of cancer. So promising is this technology that an industry is developing around the collection and storage of these stem cells for use later in life, if needed. Some health insurance companies are even subsidizing the costs for individuals desiring to take advantage of these archiving opportunities as their infants are born; after all, if this stem cell–containing blood is not collected at birth, current technology does not enable it to be reconstituted later in life.

We will continue our discussion by examining each of the cell types present in blood. We will start with erythrocytes (red blood cells) and then consider leukocytes (white blood cells).

Erythrocytes

Let's start with the most abundant cells of your blood: the red blood cells. Red blood cells, or erythrocytes, are present in very large quantities. There are about $4.3–5.8 \times 10^6$ erythrocytes per milliliter of blood. Females tend to have slightly less than males. In tissue sections, they measure 5.5–6 micrometers, but they appear a little larger in blood smears because of the way they get compressed. About 98 percent of all the cells in our blood are erythrocytes. Their shape is that of a biconcave disk. That means they look like a disk, but one that someone held between their thumb and index finger (one each side) and pressed (see Figure 16.23).

Unlike almost all other cells in your body, mature erythrocytes lack nuclei. Their stem cells, located in red bone marrow, have nuclei, but these are lost in the differentiation process. Red blood cells in circulation are terminally differentiated and lack nuclei.

Red blood cells have the important task of carrying gases in your blood. In our next chapter, we will learn why this is necessary, but for now be aware that red blood cells contain a red pigment (giving them their color and their catchy name) called hemoglobin. Hemoglobin is a globular protein made up of four polypeptide chains and four iron molecules. Several types of hemoglobin exist, depending on which four polypeptide chains it contains. In the adult, most hemoglobin is the A type (HbA) and is composed of two alpha chains and two beta chains. The presence of two alpha chains and two gamma chains produces fetal hemoglobin (HbF). Other combinations also exist. Other than water, almost the entire weight of the red blood cell (about 90 percent) is hemoglobin.

Hemoglobin picks up (binds) oxygen when it is in an environment where oxygen is abundant. It gives up that oxygen when it is in an environment where oxygen is not abundant. If carbon dioxide is abundant, it binds carbon dioxide and releases it where it is not abundant. In effect, it works like a little delivery truck, carrying whichever of the two gases is present in large quantities to sites where they are lacking. As already stated, you will get more information on this in our next chapter.

Antigens on Erythrocytes: What's Your Blood Type?

This is a good time for us to examine the topic of blood typing. We are discussing erythrocytes, the cells that carry the blood group antigens, and we have already discussed the genetics that make this phenomenon possible. Some additional information will be presented in Chapter 21 that may aid your understanding of this topic.

You are probably aware that blood exists in different "types." You may even know your own blood type. When we discuss blood type, we are usually talking about the ABO blood group antigens, although other blood typing systems exist containing other antigens (Rh blood group, for example). Antigens are molecules that our immune system recognizes as foreign and mounts a reaction against. Our immune system produces molecules called antibodies that bind to specific antigens, initiating a response. This is a defense mechanism and is explained in detail in Chapter 21.

The ABO blood typing system is based on carbohydrate antigens that are found on red blood cells. If your cells have, for instance, the antigen that characterizes the A blood type on their surfaces, and you are transfused with B type red blood cells, your immune system will respond to the B antigen and a life-threatening event will ensue. The questions that concern us are: what are these blood group antigens, and what determines which blood group antigens are on our erythrocytes?

The blood group antigens in the ABO system are small carbohydrates that are added to the end of a glycolipid called the H antigen. The presence or absence of the H antigen is determined by a gene separate from that of the ABO system. If the H antigen is not present, no ABO antigens can be expressed. This is, however a relatively rare occurrence. So, let's assume we have the H antigen present.

The ABO gene is located on chromosome nine. At that one locus, we have three possible alleles (you remember that an allele is an alternate form of a gene, and a locus is the location of a gene). What do genes encode? Come on: you remember this from Chapter 14! Genes encode proteins. Since we are talking about a carbohydrate antigen, we know that this gene does not encode the actual carbohydrate. It must encode the enzyme that produces that carbohydrate. The type of enzyme that produces the ABO antigens (or more accurately, attaches them to the H antigen) is called a glycosyltransferase. Glycosyltransferases attach carbohydrates to other molecules in a highly specific manner.

The A allele (often written I^A) encodes a glycosyltransferase that attaches a specific monosaccharide to the H antigen, producing the A antigen. Your erythrocytes would carry the A marker. If you had the B allele (I^B), you would have a slightly different glycosyltransferase; one that would add a slightly different monosaccharide to the H antigen, producing the B marker. So what about the O allele (i)? It encodes a glycosyltransferase that does not work; it transfers no monosaccharide to the H antigen. Since you have two copies of this gene (one on each of your two analogous chromosomes nine), the combinations listed in **TABLE 16.4** are possible.

Notice that Table 16.4 lists the genotype (which alleles are present at this locus) and that two alleles are listed for each possible combination. The phenotype indicates the characteristic you express, based on the genes that are present. If a blood group antigen is present, whether you are homozygous for the trait (both alleles

Table 16.4 The Blood Types in the ABO system

Genotype	Phenotype	Accepts	Donates to
i/i	O	O	A, AB, B, O
I^A/I^A	A	O, A	A, AB
I^B/I^B	B	O, B	B, AB
I^A/i	A	O, A	A, AB
I^B/i	B	O, B	B, AB
I^B/I^A	AB	O, AB, A, B	AB

the same) or heterozygous for the trait (only one gene has that particular allele), you will express the trait. A person with one A allele will express the A antigen just as a person with two A alleles will. Note also that the presence of a particular antigen allows you to donate blood only to those who also have that antigen; donations to anyone else will result in a reaction by them, as they will recognize your blood as foreign. Only blood of the O type (i/i genotype) can be donated to anyone independent of their other antigens, as O is not recognized by anyone's immune system. Remember, the glycosyl-transferase encoded by the i allele is nonfunctional; it adds no monosaccharide to the H antigen. Since essentially all of us have the H antigen, none of us will recognize O type blood as foreign. There are rare people who do not express the H antigen, as mentioned. These people, with the so-called Bombay phenotype, are exceptions to the rules just explained.

Leukocytes

Our nonerythrocyte blood cells are all leukocytes, or white blood cells (Figure 16.23). When a sample of blood is spun in a centrifuge, the red blood cells will quickly settle to the bottom of the tube. A cream- to white-colored layer will rest on the settled erythrocytes. This layer is called the buffy coat and contains the leukocytes. Platelets, fragments of megakaryocytes, are also in the buffy coat. The number of leukocytes per milliliter of blood can vary widely in a normal healthy individual, depending on a wide array of factors. The leukocyte count is dependent on the time of day, temporal proximity to a meal, and even the site from which the blood was drawn. Obviously, the presence of a pathological process can push the leukocyte count well outside the normal range. The normal range for leukocytes is approximately 4,000–11,000 per milliliter.

We have a number of different types of leukocytes. We will continue here with the leukocytes in the erythromyeloid lineage. These include the granulocytes and the monocytes. There are three different types of granulocytes, and we will discuss each of them. We will also consider megakaryocytes at this time, although they exist in the bone marrow, not in circulation. Then we will continue on to the cells of the lymphoid lineage.

Leukocytes of the Erythromyeloid Lineage

Granular Leukocytes. There are three types of granular leukocytes: neutrophils, basophils, and eosinophils. All are named for the staining characteristics of granules present within their cytoplasm. Neutrophils are the most abundant, so we will consider them first.

Neutrophils account for about 45–74 percent of all leukocytes (bearing in mind that leukocytes account for only 2 percent of our blood cells). They have neutrophilic granules: granules that stain with dyes of neutral pH. These are the smallest granules seen in granulocytes. They also have distinctive nuclei. Their multilobed nuclei give them their other name: polymorphonuclear leukocytes or PMNs. They are about 12 micrometers in diameter.

The main function of neutrophils is phagocytosis. These short-lived cells leave the blood vessels and migrate through the tissues of the body in response to injury. In fact, they respond very quickly to injury as a main component in the early stages of inflammation. As very effective scavengers, they phagocytize bacteria, cellular debris, foreign matter, and anything else that does not belong in the tissues. They have, however, been implicated in contributing to the damage that occurs after heart attack, stroke, and other injuries because of their overexuberance.

Eosinophils make up 1–5 percent of the leukocyte pool and contain large granules that bind the stain eosin. Eosinophilic granules stain an orange-red color. Eosinophils measure between 9 and 12 micrometers in diameter, depending on the preparative technique used. The adherence of antibodies (to be considered later) target an object for attack by an eosinophil. In addition to phagocytosis, they also carry out their defense strategies by exuding substances capable of killing their targets: bacteria and parasites. They are involved in allergic reactions and inflammation.

Basophils contain granules that bind basic stains in specific preparations (do you see a pattern developing?). Basophils are our least common granulocyte, amounting to less than 1 percent of circulating leukocytes. Their activity is similar to that of the mast cells found in connective tissues. Through a process called degranulation, they release compounds such as heparin and histamine in response to various physical and chemical stimuli. The release of these compounds initiate inflammation at sites of injury.

Monocytes. Although they are leukocytes in the erythromyeloid lineage, monocytes are not granulocytes. They are instead in a differentiation pathway that we have often considered. You may recall that cells such as osteoclasts and microglia are in the monocyte-macrophage lineage. Monocytes are the leukocytes that differentiate into these other cell types when they enter the appropriate tissues. When activated, they become macrophages (which were discussed in Chapter 3) for their phagocytic abilities (macrophage means big eater). They constitute 3–11 percent of all leukocytes. They are difficult to distinguish from large lymphocytes in some preparations.

Megakaryocytes and Platelets. Megakaryocytes are being considered here as they are members of this lineage. They are not normally present in circulation, however, as they reside in red bone marrow. They have a very interesting life cycle. As they develop, they become larger and larger, producing and storing lots of cytoplasmic components. Then they begin to fragment off pieces of this cytoplasm, surrounded by plasmalemma, as small packets of themselves. These fragments are platelets. Platelets are released into circulation, where they participate in hemostasis (blood clotting) and mediation of inflammation.

The Lymphocytic Lineage

This is a much simpler lineage. There are only a couple of closely related cell types in this lineage. Lymphocytes account for 20–47 percent of leukocytes. Although some lymphocytes are relatively short lived, others live for decades. Lymphocytes arise in bone marrow but complete their maturation in lymphatic organs. There are two main categories of lymphocytes, designated by the letters B and T.

B lymphocytes (B cells to their friends) receive their "B" letter designation because they were originally described in the chicken, where they mature in the lymphatic organ called the Bursa of Fabricius (B for Bursa-dependent lymphocytes). Humans lack this organ; B cells mature in human lymph nodes. Mature B cells differentiate into plasma cells that produce antibodies. Antibodies are globular proteins that are important in the immune system and in immunologic defense of the body; resulting in their other name, immunoglobulins. We will learn about immunity in Chapter 21.

T lymphocytes look very similar to B cells, but have a different developmental pathway and perform different functions. T cells mature in the thymus (hence their "T" designation). T cells exist in several functional types, each of which plays a role in immunity. We will learn the details of T cell function in Chapter 21.

Figure 16.23 shows a diagram of each of the cells of blood and indicates their relative abundance. Familiarize yourself with this information before proceeding.

■ Plasma As an Extracellular Matrix

We have already decided that blood is a connective tissue. That being the case, there are two more components (after cells) we need to discuss. Together they are called extracellular matrix. Extracellular matrix consists of amorphous ground substance and fibers. If this does not seem familiar to you, perhaps you had better review Chapter 4.

In blood, the extracellular matrix is in liquid form. This is so for two reasons. Like Jell-O that has not set, the amorphous ground substance is liquid. Also, the fibers are present only in a nonpolymerized form; instead of having actual fibers, usually blood only contains the parts necessary to make fibers. The fibers are only assembled as part of the clotting process.

So, what is this extracellular matrix? Well, if we remove only the cells from blood, we are left with plasma. Plasma is the extracellular matrix of blood. It contains both the amorphous ground substance and the fibers. If we allow the plasma to clot, the clot that forms contains fibrin, along with some other components. The "fiber" component of this connective tissue is the fibrin. The fluid that remains once we remove the clot from the plasma is serum. In other words, serum is blood minus the cells and fibrin (along with a few other components of the clot). Serum is the amorphous ground substance of this connective tissue.

Now all that is left to discuss is hemostasis (blood clotting).

16.7 Hemostasis

Look at this word carefully. *Hemostasis* is easily confused with the word *homeostasis*, but their meanings are completely different. You already know what homeostasis means, so I won't bore you with that. Hemostasis means blood clotting (although it can also mean lack of blood flow). The blood clotting system is very important to the maintenance of homeostasis and life itself. Without the ability to clot our blood, we would have a difficult time surviving the minor bumps and traumas of everyday life. This becomes very apparent when we examine the lives of those who suffer from hemophilia, a group of disorders of the blood-clotting system.

Please examine **FIGURE 16.24**. It describes the blood-clotting system. Note that we have a number of clotting factors that are in circulation at all times. These are

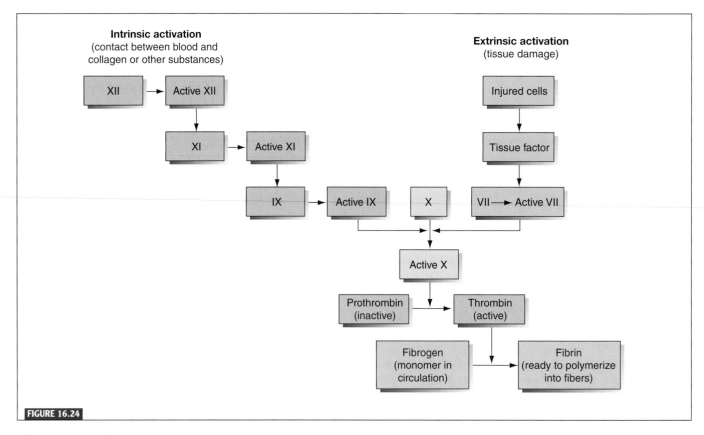

FIGURE 16.24

The clotting cascade.

produced by the liver. There are two pathways to the activation of the clotting system. The intrinsic pathway is triggered by the exposure of blood to negatively charged surfaces. The relevant surface in the body is collagen. The blood is sequestered from contact with collagen by the endothelial cells. When a vessel is injured, the endothelial cells are damaged and the blood comes in contact with collagen.

The extrinsic pathway is triggered by substances liberated from injured cells, such as the smooth muscle cells of the blood vessel wall. Both pathways lead to activation of the circulating thrombin (from prothrombin), which cleaves the circulating protein fibrinogen. This liberates active fibrin, which polymerizes into the fibers

we discussed previously. These are an integral component of a clot. Platelets also play a major role in clotting. When activated, they become "sticky" and form a plug that acts to temporarily stop the leaking blood. After a while, they contract to tighten up the clot, making the plug more secure.

This ends our discussion of blood. I hope you have found this topic interesting and can now see blood as an important tissue, rather that just a red liquid that lets you know when you have been cut. Be sure to look over the "What You Should Know" and "What Did You Learn?" features of this chapter. You will need this information to understand topics presented in our next chapter and in Chapter 21.

Atherosclerosis

Atherosclerosis is a term with which we are all familiar. We see it in the popular press, we hear about it on television programs, in health food ads, and in information about diets (whether scientifically based or fad diets based on quackery). What actually is atherosclerosis? Is it merely fat smeared along the walls of our arteries, or is it a complex pathophysiologic process? If you guessed that it is a complex process, you are correct. It is also the topic of this "Breaching Homeostasis" section.

Atherosclerosis is one form of arteriosclerosis. Arteriosclerosis is a category of disease that involves hardening of the arteries (*arterio* indicates arteries; *sclerosis* indicates a loss of elasticity or flexibility). There are several types of arteriosclerosis. Atherosclerosis is one type.

The initial changes in the pathway leading to atherosclerosis are found in all people. Developing during infancy and childhood; these lesions are called "fatty streaks." They are characterized by the transportation of lipids into the tunica intima of arteries, the oxidation of these lipids, and ultimately their phagocytosis by macrophages called *foam cells* (because of their foamy appearance after ingesting the lipids). Smooth muscle cells also phagocytize some lipids (very uncharacteristic smooth muscle behavior) and become *myointimal cells.* Extracellular collagen and lipids also accumulate. These changes occur in all people independent of genetics, diet, or environment, and are observable in the aorta by 1 year of age and in the coronary arteries by 10 years of age. In many people, they progress no further. In some people, however, these lesions progress after years of dormancy. This progression is dependent on the risk factors we will discuss at the end of this section.

This next step is termed *plaque formation* and is the start of atherogenesis, as it ultimately leads to an *atheroma* (a term I will explain momentarily). These changes occur focally within fatty streaks. More macrophages enter the lesion and produce substances that cause smooth muscle cells of the tunica media to proliferate. These smooth muscle cells then migrate into the lesion (into the tunica intima). There they lay down collagen (again uncharacteristic behavior for smooth muscle). This results in a "fibromuscular cap" immediately deep to the endothelium. The lesion is now called a plaque.

The next step is the actual development of an atheroma. The term *atheroma* is from the term *athero,* Greek for gruel (boiled grain or cereal, the slurry fed to orphans in Charles Dickens' stories). This term describes the consistency of the center of the lesion that is developing at this time. This step may follow plaque formation or plaques may lie dormant for years. They may even regress. Nevertheless, this process may ensue. Macrophages within the lesion die. As they die, they release enzymes that degrade (digest) the center of the lesion. Small blood vessels, called vasa vasorum, that normally supply the tissue of the walls of the artery begin to proliferate. As they do so, their newly developed branches are slightly leaky and bring in platelets. The platelets release factors that cause more smooth muscle proliferation and migration into the lesion (positive feedback). Scar formation begins within the lesion and calcium deposits form within the necrotic (dead) tissue. Expansion of the lesion causes the fibromuscular cap to become stretched and thin. The center of the lesion is now lumpy and gruel-like, hence the name atheroma.

The next step involves progression of the atheroma to a complicated atheroma. The arterial wall has been weakened by this lesion. Endothelial cells may be torn off by the passing blood, like shingles off a roof in a storm. The necrotic debris in the center of the lesion may then begin to leak out into the blood. Exposure of these substances to the blood causes the blood to clot (thrombus formation). If this occurs in the coronary arteries, a myocardial infarction may ensue. If the location is one of the cerebral arteries, a stroke may be the result (see Chapter 12's "Breaching Homeostasis"). It can also lead to an aneurysm (bulging of the artery like a weakened garden hose), or to damage in downstream organs caused when fragments of the thrombus (intravascular clot) break off and travel in the blood (as an embolus) until they block a smaller artery. Needless to say, many of the outcomes of atherosclerosis are quite bad. Atherosclerosis contributes to one half of all deaths in North America and is the number one killer world-wide.

So, what can we do to reduce our risk of developing atherosclerosis? Some risks are beyond our control (we can't change our genetics), but we can diminish their impact by altering those things we can affect. For instance, controlling hypertension and diabetes mellitus, and never beginning to smoke (or quitting if you have already made the wrong decision in that regard) will greatly reduce risk. Regularly monitoring your blood lipid profile and taking steps to improve any aberrant readings involves your health-care provider, and will ultimately be extremely beneficial. Proper diet and exercise may be all that is required. Your health-care provider may also prescribe medication. If so, sticking to the regimen prescribed may greatly improve your chances of a long and healthy life.

What You Should Know

1. Blood is a moving fluid and is important in the maintenance of homeostasis.

2. Your heart is located within the pericardial cavity, in the mediastinum.

3. The walls of your heart are made up of three layers: the epicardium, the myocardium, and the endocardium.

4. Your heart has four chambers, two atria and two ventricles.

5. Blood enters your left atrium from the four pulmonary veins, and leaves your left ventricle through the aorta. Blood leaving the left ventricle is entering the systemic circuit.

6. Blood enters your right atrium through the superior vena cava, the inferior vena cava, and the coronary sinus. Blood leaves your right ventricle through the pulmonary trunk. Blood leaving the right ventricle is entering the pulmonary circuit.

7. Valves control the direction of blood flow through your heart. The atrioventricular valves lie between the atria and ventricles. The right atrioventricular valve is the tricuspid. The left atrioventricular valve is the mitral or bicuspid.

8. The electrical impulses that set your heart rate are generated by specialized cells within your heart. The primary pacemaker is the sinoatrial node.

9. You must know the sites of impulse generation and the path of conduction through your heart.

10. The cardiac cycle is the cycle of activity your heart follows as it pumps blood. It is a combination of electrical and mechanical activities. You must know the stages of the cardiac cycle and what happens during each stage.

11. Cardiac output is determined by the number of contractions per minute and the volume of blood pumped per contraction. Alterations in heart rate or the strength of contraction will alter cardiac output.

12. Arteries are the high-pressure vessels that carry blood away from your heart, toward your capillaries.

13. The largest of your arteries are elastic arteries, named for the elastic connective tissue that is so prominent in their walls. Your smaller arteries are muscular arteries. They contain smooth muscle in their walls to regulate blood flow.

14. Capillaries are the site of exchange between your blood and the cells and tissues of your body.

15. Veins carry blood from your capillaries back to your heart. The pressure in your veins must remain relatively low, so their diameters must be greater than that of your arteries.

16. Fluid moves between your blood and your tissues through the walls of your capillaries. The direction and rate of this movement is determined by the pressures defined in Starling's Hypothesis.

17. Your blood is a connective tissue and as such contains cells, amorphous ground substance, and fibers.

18. Numerous cell types can be found in your blood. You must know the names, descriptions, and functions of each of these cell types.

19. The amorphous ground substance of your blood is the fluid component of blood, called serum.

20. Serum plus fibrin and other clotting proteins is plasma. Fibrin is the fiber component of this connective tissue.

21. A blood clot is made up of fibrin and platelets. The fibrin component of a clot is generated by a complex system of clotting factors, most of which are produced by your liver.

What Did You Learn?

Multiple choice questions: choose the best answer.

1. As it lies within the mediastinum, the base of the heart is located in the _____ position.

   a. Superior

   b. Inferior

   c. It depends on whether you are standing or lying down

   d. The heart does not have a base

2. The pericardial space contains which of the following?

   a. Serous fluid

   b. Mucus

   c. Blood

   d. Lipid

   e. Air

What Did You Learn? (continued)

3. Which of the following is also known as visceral pericardium?

   a. Epicardium

   b. Myocardium

   c. Endocardium

   d. None of the above

4. Which of the following does not return blood to the right atrium?

   a. Superior vena cava

   b. Inferior vena cava

   c. Pulmonary veins

   d. Coronary sinus

   e. All of the above return blood to the right atrium

5. Blood entering the aorta is actually entering the:

   a. Systemic circuit

   b. Pulmonary circuit

   c. Both of the above

   d. Neither of the above

6. Blood entering the aorta is leaving the:

   a. Left atrium

   b. Left ventricle

   c. Right atrium

   d. Right ventricle

7. The left atrioventricular valve is called the:

   a. Tricuspid valve

   b. Mitral valve

   c. Both of the above

   d. Neither of the above

8. The atrioventricular valves close when:

   a. The atria contract

   b. The papillary muscles contract

   c. The pressure in the atria exceeds the pressure in the ventricles

   d. The pressure in the ventricles exceeds the pressure in the atria

9. The second heart sound is created when:

   a. The atrioventricular valves open

   b. The atrioventricular valves close

   c. The semilunar valves open

   d. The semilunar valves close

10. During isovolumetric contraction, which valves are closed?

   a. Atrioventricular valves

   b. Semilunar valves

   c. Both of the above

   d. Neither of the above

11. Which portion of the cardiac conduction system is the heart's primary pacemaker?

   a. AV node

   b. SA node

   c. AV bundle

   d. Bundle branches

   e. Conduction (Purkinje) myofibers

12. The correct sequence of the path of cardiac impulses is:

   1. Atrioventricular (AV) node

   2. Sinoatrial (SA) node

   3. Conduction myofibers (Purkinje fibers)

   4. Atrioventricular bundle (bundle of His)

   5. Right and left bundle branches

   a. 1,2,3,4,5

   b. 2,4,5,3,1

   c. 3,2,1,5,4

   d. 2,1,4,5,3

   e. None of the above

13. Which of the following is not true of the fibrotendinous ring?

   a. It electrically insulates the right atrium from the left atrium

   b. It contains the atrioventricular valves

   c. It contains the semilunar valves

   d. It electrically insulates the atria from the ventricles

   e. All of the above are true

14. During the periods of rapid ventricular filling and diastasis, the ventricles become _____ filled with blood.

   a. 30 percent

   b. 50 percent

   c. 70 percent

   d. 100 percent

15. Cardiac output can be increased by:

   a. Increasing the heart rate

   b. Increasing the amount of blood pumped per contraction

   c. Both of the above

   d. Neither of the above

16. Heart rate will be reduced by increased _____ nervous system activity.

   a. Sympathetic

   b. Parasympathetic

   c. Either of the above

   d. Neither of the above

What Did You Learn? (continued)

17. _____ carry blood away from the heart.
    a. Arteries
    b. Veins
    c. Both of the above
    d. Neither of the above

18. _____ are high-pressure vessels.
    a. Capillaries
    b. Arteries
    c. Veins
    d. None of the above
    e. All of the above

19. The tunica media of a small artery is mainly composed of:
    a. Smooth muscle
    b. Elastic connective tissue
    c. Cardiac muscle
    d. Collagenous fibers

20. Endothelial cells line the walls of _____.
    a. Arteries
    b. Veins
    c. Capillaries
    d. The chambers of the heart
    e. All of the above

21. Axial flow, as seen in blood vessels, indicates that the _____ objects are carried toward the middle of the moving stream.
    a. Largest
    b. Smallest
    c. Neither of the above; it has nothing to do with size

22. Based on Starling's law, fluid _____ capillaries through the capillary wall at the proximal portion of the capillary bed.
    a. Leaves
    b. Enters
    c. Neither of the above; fluid never crosses the capillary wall

23. In adult humans, hematopoeisis occurs in:
    a. The marrow of flat bones, such as the sternum
    b. The marrow of the diaphysis of long bones, such as the femur
    c. Both of the above
    d. Neither of the above

24. In infants, hematopoeisis occurs in:
    a. The marrow of flat bones, such as the sternum
    b. The marrow of long bones, such as the femur
    c. Both of the above
    d. Neither of the above

25. Which of these granular leukocytes are most numerous?
    a. Eosinophils
    b. Basophils
    c. Neutrophils
    d. They are equally numerous

26. A person with B blood can accept transfusions from:
    a. A type donors
    b. AB type donors
    c. Both of the above
    d. Neither of the above

27. A person with B type blood can give transfusions to:
    a. A type recipients
    b. AB type recipients
    c. Both of the above
    d. Neither of the above

Short answer questions: answer briefly and in your own words.

1. List the three layers of the heart wall and indicate the tissue that comprises each layer.

2. List the coronary arteries and the regions of the heart that they supply with blood.

3. Explain the two circuits within the circulatory system and indicate the pathway the blood follows through the heart to enter each circuit. You may choose to draw a diagram to enhance your explanation.

4. List the stages of the cardiac cycle and indicate what happens during each stage. A good exercise to aid your learning is to explain this cycle to a friend or relative who has not studied anatomy and physiology. If you can explain it so that they understand it, you will aid your own comprehension and retention.

5. Please explain what is meant by "blood types." How do the alleles of the ABO blood type gene determine the markers that appear on our erythrocytes? Who can donate blood to whom? Who can accept blood from whom?

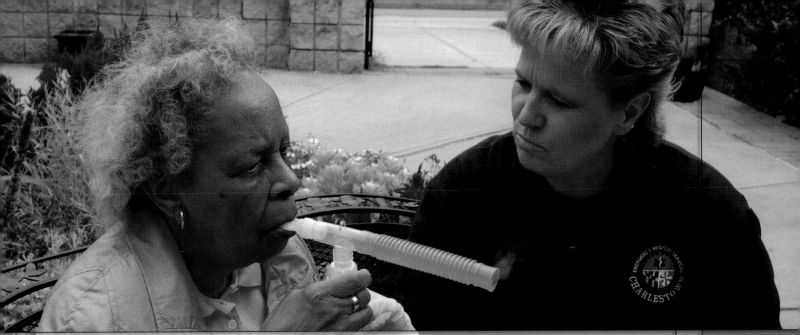

Every Breath You Take: Your Respiratory System

17 CHAPTER

What You Will Learn

- The interaction between the respiratory and cardiovascular system.
- The internal structure of your nose.
- The functions of your nose.
- The regions of your pharynx and the type of epithelium that is present in each region.
- The structure of your larynx and the way your larynx protects your respiratory tract from materials intended for your digestive tract.
- The structure and function of your trachea.
- The anatomy of your bronchi.
- How your alveoli serve as the site of gas exchange between your blood and the external environment.
- How pulmonary ventilation works when you are at rest and during times of forced breathing.
- The role of surfactant in reducing elastic recoil in your alveoli.
- The manner in which oxygen and carbon dioxide are exchanged with the atmosphere and transported in the blood.
- How the activity of your respiratory rate is regulated.

17.1 A Partnership

This fascinating system works hand-in-hand with the cardiovascular system. While the cardiovascular system provides the transportation mechanism for moving gases around within the body, your respiratory system provides a site for exchange of gases between the internal and external environments. As mentioned in the introduction to this section, an understanding of either system requires some knowledge of the other system. We are now ready to learn about the respiratory system.

First, we must learn the anatomy of this system. It is actually quite simple and will allow us to exercise our understanding of what tissues and, particularly, what epithelial cell types we would expect to find in a location based on the needs of that structure. If you understand the material we learned in Chapter 4, this will be easy. If you need a little brush up on that material, now is your opportunity. Next, we need to think about some basic physics of gases. Again, this is an interesting topic and one you can easily understand with a little effort. Let's get started.

17.2 The Anatomy of Your Respiratory System

We are studying another pathway, a set of ducts through which a substance is conveyed (**FIGURE 17.1**). Unlike the previous systems we have studied, however, this one is open to the external environment and carries air. We will start at the very opening of this system on the outside of your body and work our way in.

■ Your Nose

The nose is actually more than it appears to be (**FIGURE 17.2**). Sure it is a very obvious structure, sitting prominently on your anterior midline, but we may fail at first to grasp its functional significance and internal structure.

The nose has an external component, made up of a hyaline cartilage core, overlaid with skin externally and

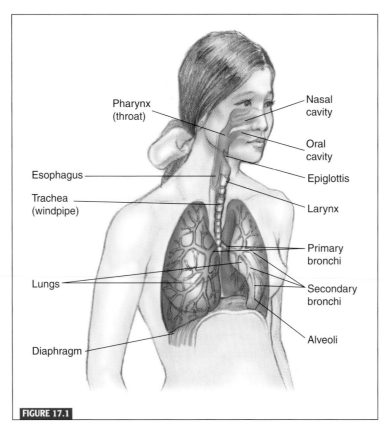

FIGURE 17.1

The respiratory system.

stratified squamous epithelium containing hair follicles internally. The hair is present as the first portion of the nose's filter mechanism. The cavity within the external nose is called the vestibule, as it lies outside of the more significant internal nasal cavity.

The internal nasal cavity, like the vestibule, is divided into two spaces by the nasal septum. The internal nasal cavity is mainly lined by pseudostratified ciliated columnar epithelium containing goblet cells for mucous production. A well developed vasculature lies deep to this epithelium, resembling the erectile tissue we discussed in the reproductive system. Engorgement of these vessels with blood and the associated tissue swelling are main components of a "stuffed nose."

On the lateral walls of the internal nasal cavity are the nasal conchae, or turbinates, that we learned about during our discussion of the skeletal system (**FIGURE 17.3**). These three bony plates are responsible for swirling the air that passes through the nose. This swirling is important for the effective functioning of the nose. The nose, you see, has important functions other than just holding your eyeglasses in place.

Think about what happens when you clean out a dusty attic or basement. Afterward, when you blow your nose, the discharge is quite muddy. Would you like all of that particulate matter in your lungs? Certainly not, and the nose is there to filter it out for you.

Think about what the turbulence caused by air passing over the conchae accomplishes. As you inhale through your nose, the air column spins. This spinning forces dust and other particulate matter to the outside of the column, where the velocity is slower. In this reduced velocity, the dust particles settle out of the moving air. When the dust contacts the mucus that covers the epithelium of your nasal cavity, it sticks and is trapped. This is a very effective filter.

Now, what about other nasal functions? Have you ever gone outside on a cold, dry winter morning and breathed in deeply? I'm talking about air that is very cold and very dry. If you breathe in deeply through your mouth, it will choke you and make you gasp. If you breathe in through your nose, it's fine. That's because the air is conditioned by your nose before it reaches the delicate structures deeper in your respiratory tract. The blood passing deep to the epithelium imparts warmth to that lining and, hence, warms the air. Moisture evaporates from the mucus and enters the air, moistening it so it will not dry out the delicate epithelia of your lower respiratory tract. The nose, you see, is quite important. In fact, we have not even discussed its role in olfaction here. As mentioned in Chapter 12, the internal nose is the site of the olfactory receptors that help maintain

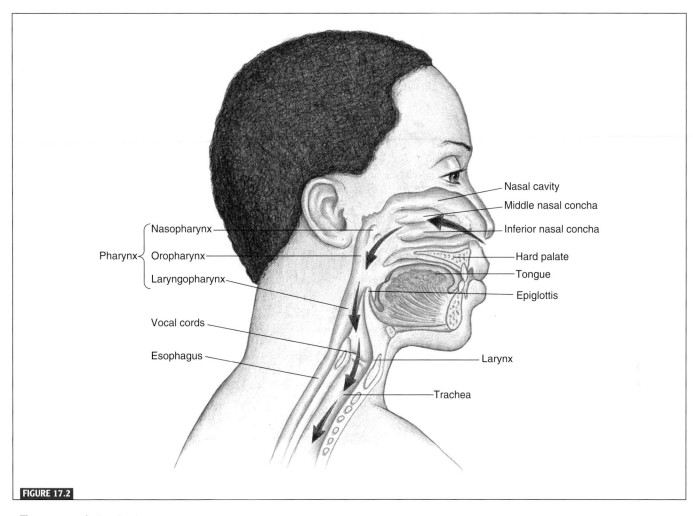

FIGURE 17.2

The upper respiratory tract.

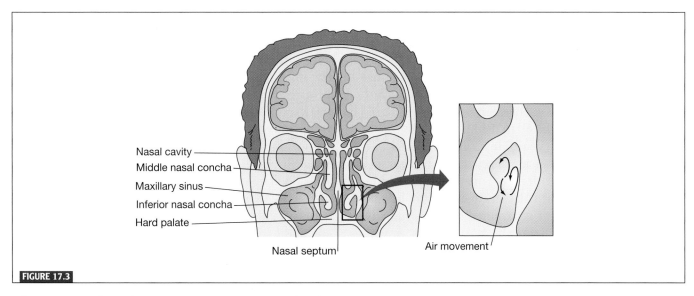

FIGURE 17.3

The nasal cavity. The nasal concha causes air to swirl as it passes through this cavity.

your homeostasis by letting you know what is and is not safe to eat, drink, and inhale.

Your Pharynx

The next portion of the respiratory tract is the pharynx (Figure 17.2). The pharynx actually has three component regions. The first region is part of the respiratory tract only, as only air is meant to pass through it. It is the nasopharynx and extends from the internal nares at the posterior aspect of the internal nose to the level of the oral cavity. The next portion of the pharynx is the oropharynx, which lies posterior to the oral cavity. Both air and ingested matter pass through the oropharynx, making it part of both the respiratory and digestive tracts. The laryngopharynx is the third region. It begins inferior to the oropharynx and ends at the larynx. Food and air also pass through this region.

So, in what way must these three regions differ from one another? Well, you might think of a few answers to that question, but please focus on their epithelia for a moment. Based on what you know of the characteristics of different epithelia and the tasks required in these three regions, can you predict what epithelium would be present in each region? Sure you can. Only air passes through the nasopharynx, so does it need a lot of abrasion resistance? No, air is not that abrasive. It does, however, need to be able to produce mucus. What would be the appropriate cell shape for that purpose (look back at Figure 4.3 in Chapter 4, if you need to)? O.K., columnar epithelium is called for here. Since we want to be able to move this mucus, perhaps we had better include cilia. Now, how important is it that we keep this basement membrane covered, and how likely are cells to be killed by substances we inhale? For defense purposes it is very important that we keep the basement membrane covered, yet we are likely to lose cells to viruses, chemical fumes, and other things in the air. We had better use pseudostratified ciliated columnar epithelium in the nasopharynx.

Is this a good choice for the oropharynx? Well, think about it. Do you ever eat hard foods (pretzels, potato chips, crackers, nuts, or cookies; I must stop as I'm getting hungry, and you'll be off to the kitchen)? Are these foods abrasive? Sure they are. How can we protect our oropharynx from this abrasion? Pseudostratified columnar epithelium won't work here. Squamous epithelium is a better choice, in particular stratified squamous epithelium. But do we want it cornified or noncornified? This is a moist environment, isn't it? It must be, or you would not be able to swallow those crackers (they need lubrication). A cornified layer does not do too well in a moist environment (notice your fingers after spending too long in dishwater). So, we must have a noncornified

stratified squamous epithelium in the oropharynx. Since the laryngopharynx has similar requirements, the same epithelium is found there.

Your Larynx

Here is a very interesting structure (Figures 17.2 and 17.4). The larynx is inferior to the pharynx and is the site where the respiratory and digestive systems branch apart. The trachea (respiratory system) and the esophagus (digestive system) depart from the inferior aspect of the pharynx. The larynx is involved in keeping the appropriate substances in the right channels.

The larynx is composed of nine pieces of cartilage, the hyoid bone, and the true and false vocal cords. You can easily identify your thyroid cartilage; it is your "Adam's apple." The others are not so easy to identify. **FIGURE 17.4** illustrates their locations.

When you swallow, the larynx must close the opening of your trachea to keep food or drink from entering. We all know what it feels like if it is not successful. How does it perform this task? Often people describe the epiglottis as a "trap door" that closes off the proximal end of the trachea. Think about it, though; of what is the epiglottis composed? Being elastic cartilage, it lacks the ability to move on its own. As you swallow, the muscles of your tongue move the epiglottis somewhat downward as the larynx moves up to meet it. Hold your finger on your "Adam's apple" and swallow. Did you feel your Adam's apple rise? You felt the larynx elevate as part of the process of swallowing. That elevation raises the opening of your trachea into contact with the epiglottis, which has been pushed down by your tongue, thus closing the opening and forcing the ingested material into the esophagus where it belongs.

The larynx does have another function, however. It is the site of voice production. Two paired folds of mucosa exist within the larynx. The superior pair are the false vocal cords, which do not play a role in voice production. The inferior pair are the true vocal cords. As air passes through them, these vibrate at different frequencies to make sounds at different pitches. Have you ever grasped the opening of a balloon as the air was passing out through the opening? You may have noticed that, if you pulled it into a slit, a screeching sound was produced. If you pulled the balloon tighter, the pitch rose. It fell if you relaxed the latex a bit. That is exactly how your voice produces sounds of different pitches; it is done by adjusting the tension of the true vocal cords as air passes between them.

Your Trachea

Feel the tube that extends downward from your larynx. Do you feel the ridges running around this tube? This

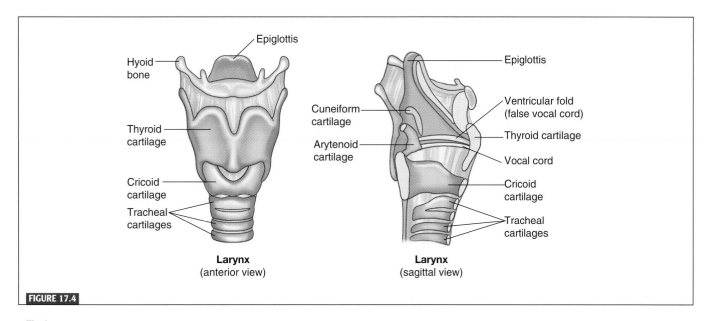

Hyoid bone

Epiglottis

Thyroid cartilage

Cricoid cartilage

Tracheal cartilages

Larynx
(anterior view)

Cuneiform cartilage

Arytenoid cartilage

Epiglottis

Ventricular fold (false vocal cord)

Thyroid cartilage

Vocal cord

Cricoid cartilage

Tracheal cartilages

Larynx
(sagittal view)

FIGURE 17.4

The larynx.

tube is your trachea. The trachea is the next portion of your respiratory tree. It extends from your larynx to your primary bronchi. It lies just anterior to your esophagus (**FIGURE 17.5a**).

The trachea is composed of connective tissue lined with pseudostratified ciliated columnar epithelium that includes goblet cells. Mucous glands are present in the walls. Rings of hyaline cartilage add rigidity to the walls. We'll discuss the cartilage further in a moment. First, let's think about the epithelium. Why would we find these types of epithelial cells and mucous glands at this location? Again, to filter out debris. Debris that makes it past your nose (perhaps you inhaled through your mouth) may be in the air traveling through the trachea. We do not want this material to reach the lungs. The mucus of the trachea gives us an additional filter. Dust becomes trapped in this mucus. The cilia move the mucus superiorly toward the larynx. As mucus reaches the larynx, it is coughed up slightly and swallowed; this is not exactly an attractive thought, but what an effective way for disposing of the debris that would otherwise clog our lungs. Incidentally, there are substances in cigarette smoke that disable the beating of these cilia, leading to the coughing heard even in the beginning smoker (long-term smokers have other problems); so at the risk of sounding like a public service announcement, don't smoke!

Now, what about the cartilage? Did you ever eat chicken noodle soup through a straw (maybe as a youngster, when you were home sick and were bored)? What happened when a piece of chicken (or noodle) got stuck on the end of the straw? The straw collapsed. That is

what would happen if you did not have cartilage rings in your trachea and you breathed in forcefully. The trachea would collapse and air would not travel through it. You may have noticed that vacuum cleaners have stiff hoses, or a springlike coil to stiffen their hose walls. The same principle applies there; they work just like your trachea.

There are 16 to 20 cartilage rings in your trachea, and they are "C"-shaped. The open region of the "C" points in the posterior direction. This allows your esophagus to expand as food passes through it and to bulge toward the trachea, which it could not do if the rings formed complete circles. This allows you to swallow boluses of food that otherwise might get stuck.

■ Your Bronchi

At its most inferior limit, the trachea branches, becoming the right and left primary bronchi, which go to the right and left lungs, respectively (Figure 17.5a). The right primary bronchus is more vertical and wider in diameter than the left; therefore, deeply aspirated objects tend to be found there. Where the bifurcation of the trachea into the primary bronchi takes place, we find the *carina tracheae,* a small ridge. Carina tracheae are extremely sensitive and will cause reflex coughing when touched. This is another mechanism for keeping foreign objects out of the lungs.

The primary bronchi branch into secondary, or lobar, bronchi. There are five lobes to the human lungs (Figure 17.5a). The right lung has three lobes; the left lung, two. Think about the anatomical arrangement of the heart and you will see why more lung tissue is to the right of the midline. There is one secondary bronchus

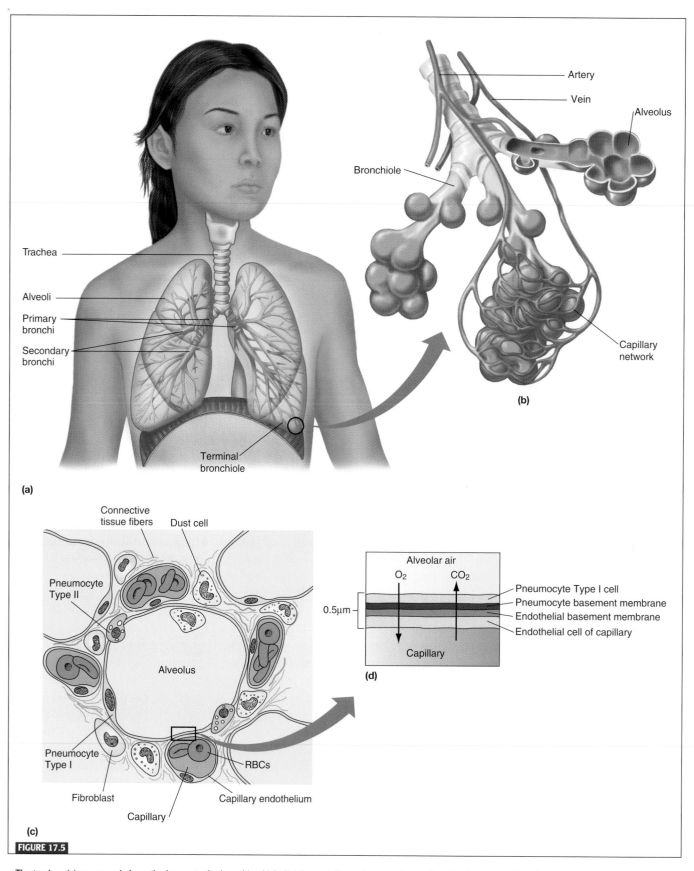

(a)

(b)

(c)

(d)

FIGURE 17.5

The trachea (a) conveys air from the larynx to the bronchi, which distribute air throughout the lungs. The alveolar wall (b) includes pneumocyte type I and II cells (c), dust cells and the endothelial cells of the alveolar capillaries. Gases must cross a thin membrane (d), composed of pneumocyte type I cells and their basement membrane, and endothelial cells and their basement membrane to diffuse between the blood and the alveolar air.

per lung lobe. These secondary bronchi branch into tertiary bronchi, which branch into bronchioles.

As we have been moving through the branches of bronchi, the walls of these airways have been changing. We noted that in the trachea there are "C"-shaped rings of hyaline cartilage. As we have moved through successive branches of bronchi, gradually these rings have given way to successively smaller plates of cartilage. In our next airways, the bronchioles, the cartilage is completely absent, replaced instead by smooth muscle. The epithelium has also been changing. By the time we reach the bronchioles, the pseudostratified, ciliated columnar epithelium has been replaced by a simple, low columnar epithelium. The smaller branches of the bronchioles have a simple cuboidal epithelium.

These changes, most notable in the bronchioles, result from the need for less mucus further down the respiratory tree. In fact, excess mucus production in the bronchioles, together with excessive contraction of bronchiole smooth muscle, is characteristic of asthma. Why then does this smooth muscle even exist in this location? It is here as a final safety net to keep toxic gases out of the alveoli. Alveoli are the final stop in this pathway and the site of gas exchange between the internal and external environments.

■ Your Alveoli

This is the actual location of gas exchange, the reason for the existence of your lungs. Alveoli have an amazing structure, well designed for their purpose (Figure 17.5c). The term *alveolus* means little cavity or space. It is given to the functional unit in the lungs: the alveolar sacs and the alveolar ducts that connect them to the bronchioles. The lung is a large network of alveoli. Often when students first encounter actual lung tissue, they are surprised at its apparently solid nature. They have expected it to be more like a balloon or series of small balloons. In fact, the alveoli of the lungs are microscopic to barely macroscopic. This is necessary to provide enough surface area for sufficient gas exchange to occur. The alveolar surface area in the average adult is approximately 750 square feet. That is an area slightly larger than the floor of a three-car garage!

Your Alveolar Membrane

The membrane across which gas exchange occurs has a large surface area, as already pointed out, but it also must be very thin. If it were not very thin, the diffusion of gases would be impeded. This membrane is diagrammed in Figure 17.5d. Note that it is composed of four layers: the epithelial cells that line the alveolar lumen; the basement membrane of those cells; the basement membrane

of the endothelial cells that line the capillaries; and the endothelial cells themselves. The order in which they are listed here is the order in which oxygen encounters them as it diffuses from air to blood. Carbon dioxide (CO_2) traveling in the opposite direction, encounters these layers in the reverse order. The entire thickness of this membrane is only 0.5 micrometer.

The epithelial cells of the alveolar membrane include very flat squamous cells called pneumocytes type I, and pneumocytes type II, which are cuboidal cells and are scattered among the more numerous pneumocytes type I. The type II cells produce surfactant, which we will discuss shortly.

An additional cell, the dust cell, is also present. These cells are in the monocyte-macrophage lineage, and from that you should be able to surmise their role. They phagocytize any debris that makes it past all of the filters we have already discussed. They also phagocytize any cellular debris that may be present in the alveoli.

Circulation in the Alveolar Walls

As you already have learned, the lungs receive all of the blood pumped by the right side of the heart (**FIGURE 17.6**). It comes to the lungs through the pulmonary trunk and right and left pulmonary arteries. It leaves through the four pulmonary veins. The lungs also have a second blood supply, giving them a dual blood supply. They receive blood from the left side of the heart, like any other organ. This is necessary for supplying the tissues of the lungs with oxygen; the blood supplied by the right side of the heart is deoxygenated. This is not necessary for the alveolar membrane per se, but for the tissues of the airways and other structures.

The blood from the right side of the heart flows through fine capillaries within the alveolar wall. These capillaries are so small in diameter that the erythrocytes pass through them single file. This ensures ready diffusion of gases into and out of these cells as they pass through the lungs. This makes for extremely efficient gas exchange. We will discuss this gas exchange in a few moments and the transportation of respiratory gases as well. We must first think about how we move air into and out of the lungs.

17.3 Pulmonary Ventilation: It's As Easy As Breathing In and Out

Let's start with the anatomic location of the lungs (**FIGURE 17.7**). You know that they are in your thoracic cavity; in fact, they are in two subdivisions of your thoracic cavity called the pleural cavities. These cavities are

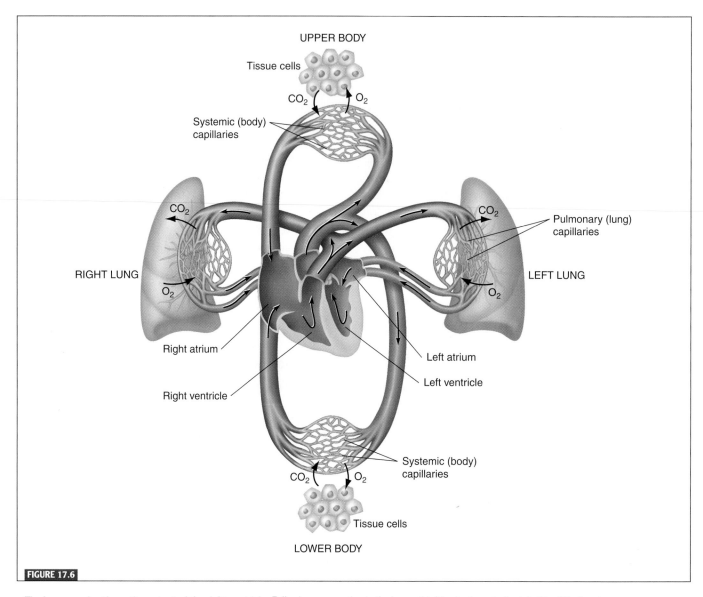

FIGURE 17.6

The lungs receive the entire output of the right ventricle. Following oxygenation in the lungs, this blood returns to the left side of the heart.

lined with parietal pleura, and the lungs themselves are covered with visceral pleura (both linings are a type of serous membrane, or mesothelium). You will recall from Chapter 5 that these pleural membranes are actually part of the same membrane; their location marks them as parietal or visceral. The space between the two is called the intrapleural space.

Now, let's think about something else. Imagine that you have a cylinder that has a plunger in it (**FIGURE 17.8a**). If I were to pull on the plunger, what would happen to the pressure in the cylinder? Pulling on the plunger would cause a negative pressure to develop in the cylinder. Pushing on the plunger would develop positive pressure. If this cylinder had a hole in it, pushing on the plunger would cause air to leave the cylinder through

the hole. Pulling on the plunger would cause air to enter the cylinder through the hole.

If we were to put a balloon in the cylinder and connect its opening to the hole, pulling on the plunger (making the space within the cylinder larger) would inflate the balloon. Pushing on the plunger (making the space within the cylinder smaller) would cause the balloon to deflate. You can make just such a device using a 20-cc syringe, a small cork that has a hole in it, and the finger of a rubber glove (in place of a small balloon). This is illustrated in Figures 17.8a–c.

So, other that a little balloon trick, what have we accomplished? Picture the balloon as your lungs. The hole that connects the balloon to the outside of the cylinder is your trachea and bronchi. The cylinder and

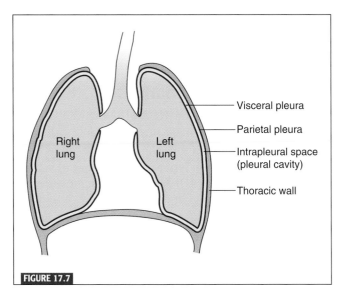

FIGURE 17.7

The lungs reside in the pleural cavities, subdivisions of the thoracic cavity. They are lined with a serous membrane called the pleura. The intrapleural space is located between the visceral and parietal pleura.

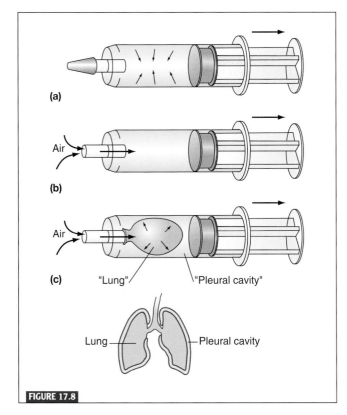

FIGURE 17.8

Changing the volume of a closed cylinder alters the pressure in the cylinder (a). Changing the volume of an open cylinder causes air to enter or exit the cylinder (b). Changing the volume of a cylinder containing a balloon that is open to the outside of the cylinder (c) inflates or deflates the balloon. This is how we inflate and deflate the lungs as we inhale and exhale. This model mimics the anatomical arrangement of the respiratory system.

plunger are the walls of your thoracic cavity. The space between the balloon and the cylinder is your intrapleural space (again note Figure 17.8c).

When you make your thoracic cavity larger, you make the intrapleural pressure (the pressure in the intrapleural space) more negative. This "pulls" on the tissues of your lungs and causes air to rush into your lungs through your airways. When you make your thoracic cavity smaller, you make the intrapleural pressure greater (more positive), forcing air out of your lungs through your airways and out of your body. It's really that simple. You do not have the direct ability to make your lungs larger and smaller; instead, you make the cavities in which they reside larger and smaller, raising and lowering the pressure around your lungs, and thereby causing them to inflate or deflate.

So, how do you make your thoracic cavity larger and smaller? The answer to this question involves the various ways in which we breathe. You are well aware that you do not always breathe the same way. You need various levels of pulmonary ventilation, depending on what you are doing. When you are sitting reading this text, you need only quiet breathing, or *eupnea*. I know that you find this subject stimulating, but the simple truth is, to maintain homeostasis while reading this book, you do not need to move that much air into and out of your lungs. Now, as soon as you finish studying, you will run to your friends' house to teach them the exciting things you have learned. You will need a higher level of pulmonary ventilation for that exercise; this will require forced (labored) breathing. We will consider eupnea (quiet breathing) and forced breathing separately.

■ The Muscles of Respiration: Eupnea and Forced Breathing

Pulmonary ventilation (breathing) involves two steps, inhaling and exhaling. We will consider these two steps first in eupnea and then in forced (labored) breathing.

During eupnea, there are two types of inhalation (breathing in) that you may use: shallow (costal) breathing and deep (diaphragmatic) breathing. Keep in mind that we are talking only about inhalation here; we will cover exhaling during eupnea in a moment. The inhalation of shallow breathing requires contraction of the external intercostal muscles. The external intercostals pull the ribs upward and outward, increasing the volume of the thoracic cavity and causing inhalation. Inhalation during deep breathing of eupnea involves the diaphragm. The diaphragm is normally dome shaped. As the muscle of the diaphragm contracts, the diaphragmatic dome becomes flattened. This increases the volume of the thoracic cavity and causes inhalation to occur. Often during eupnea, inhalation involves some combination of shallow and deep breathing. Singers have long understood the value of the types of inhalation in varying their singing timbre. Talk to some well-trained singer that you know, and you will find that they are well acquainted with this concept.

Exhalation during eupnea is completely passive. No muscle contraction causes exhalation during eupnea; it occurs when the muscles of inhalation are relaxed. The elastic recoil of the tissues of the thoracic wall and the lungs themselves will cause exhalation to occur (more on this elastic recoil in a moment).

During the inhalation of forced breathing, we use the muscles already mentioned (external intercostals and diaphragm) plus additional muscles. Think of how you breathe after running hard; you apply great force when moving air into your lungs. The additional muscles of forced inhalation are the scalenes, which elevate the two most superior ribs: the pectoralis minor, which elevates ribs three through five; and the sternocleidomastoids, which elevate the sternum.

Exhalation during forced breathing is also an active process; it requires the contraction of a couple of muscles. This may be necessary during vigorous exercise, when talking, shouting, singing, or when playing your bassoon. During any of those activities, you must be able to forcefully move air from your lungs. You do this by contracting the internal intercostals and the abdominal muscles. The internal intercostals pull the ribs inward and downward; the abdominal muscles push on the organs of the abdominopelvic cavity, which, in turn, push upward on the diaphragm.

Now, let's return to the concept of elastic recoil. This is the force that allows passive exhalation and that must be overcome to allow inhalation.

■ Elastic Recoil and Surfactant

Have you ever overfilled a glass of water and had the water sort of pile up instead of spilling over, adhering to itself and extending above the top of the glass?

This ability is dependent on the presence of surface tension. Water, you recall from Chapter 2, is a polar molecule (polar solvent). Each molecule of water has a positive pole (end) and a negative pole. This causes water molecules to stick together like little magnets. Across the surface of the water, this cohesiveness pulls inward, trying to make the surface as small as possible. This causes water to generate elastic recoil. Elastic recoil is the inward pulling we see in rubber bands, balloons, and water after they have been stretched. The elastic recoil of elastic fibers in the walls of the lungs, muscle fibers in the thoracic cavity wall, and in the moisture covering the alveoli (all 750 square feet of them) must be overcome to allow inflation to occur.

Let's think about a little balloon trick (**FIGURE 17.9**). If we connect two balloons together through a rubber hose, blow one up almost completely and the other up only partially, and then allow air to flow between them, in which direction do you think the air will flow? Will it flow from the more inflated balloon into the less inflated balloon, equalizing their sizes? Will there be no net flow of air, with the two balloons staying their original size? Will the small balloon deflate further into the larger balloon? You can answer this question experimentally by making this device, or you can think about what you already know about how balloons behave. Is

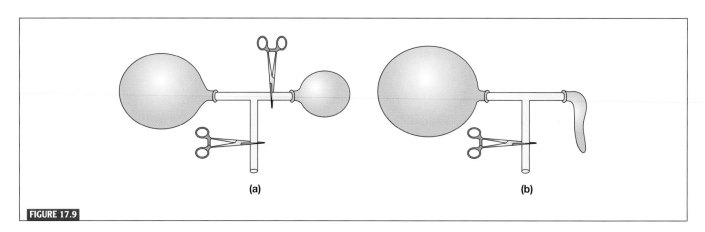

(a)　　　　　　　　　　　　　　　　　(b)

FIGURE 17.9

If we interconnect two balloons that are inflated unequally (a), the less-inflated balloon will completely deflate into the more-inflated balloon (b). This is due to differences in their elastic recoil. Moisture in our alveolar membranes provides elastic recoil that must be reduced to keep a similar phenomenon from occurring in our lungs.

it easier to blow a puff of air into a completely deflated balloon or a partially inflated balloon? When blowing up a balloon, isn't the first puff or two the hardest? Once some air is in the balloon, it gets easier. That is because elastic recoil is greatest in the least-filled balloon. The latex walls of the balloon are thickest when the balloon is the least filled, and, therefore, it has the most elastic recoil. For this reason, in our device described previously, the less inflated balloon will further deflate, adding its air to the more inflated balloon.

What is the point of all this? After all, we are studying physiology, not balloon tricks. The point is this: your alveoli act in the same way as these balloons do. The surface tension of the moisture in your alveoli will generate elastic recoil to the greatest degree in the least inflated alveoli. This potentially could cause your least inflated alveoli to completely collapse, pushing their air into your more fully inflated alveoli. This would not be good for your lungs or your overall homeostasis. We need a mechanism that will equalize the surface tension (elastic recoil) across all of your alveoli, and we, in fact, have such a mechanism.

Detergents reduce the surface tension of water. You know this to be true: water without detergent will bead-up on a smooth surface due to the surface tension of the water (**FIGURE 17.10**). Add detergent (dishwashing liquid) and it smoothly sheets across the smooth surface: the detergent reduces the surface tension. Our lungs possess a substance that acts like a detergent. The pneumocyte type II cells that we learned about earlier produce surfactant. Surfactant is a phospholipid that acts as a detergent and reduces elastic recoil in our lungs. As an

alveolus deflates, its surface area diminishes, leaving more surfactant per unit area of surface. This causes surfactant to have a greater effect in more deflated alveoli and less of an effect in more inflated alveoli. This equalizes the elastic recoil from one alveolus to the next, protecting our delicate alveolar membranes.

One last fact about surfactant. Without this substance, the elastic recoil of our lungs would be so powerful that they would completely deflate at the end of every exhalation. This would make inhalation very difficult; every inhalation would be like filling a completely empty balloon. We all know what that is like from having fallen hard on our anterior or posterior surface at some time, and "knocked the wind out of our sails" (overdeflated our lungs). Our lungs, in fact, normally do not completely deflate from the time we draw our first breath onward. We have reflexes that do not allow us to overdeflate (or overinflate) them. Without surfactant, we would be unable to keep them from fully deflating; the elastic recoil would be too great.

Infants born prematurely often suffer from respiratory distress. The major cause of this is that pneumocyte type II cells do not start to make surfactant until very late in fetal development. Premature birth (before sufficient surfactant production, which begins at 28 weeks and increases through 36 weeks) causes many infants to experience difficulty in inflating their lungs. Increased surface tension causes their alveoli to completely deflate during each exhalation, instead of remaining partially inflated. Fortunately, effective therapies for this condition have been (and continue to be) developed.

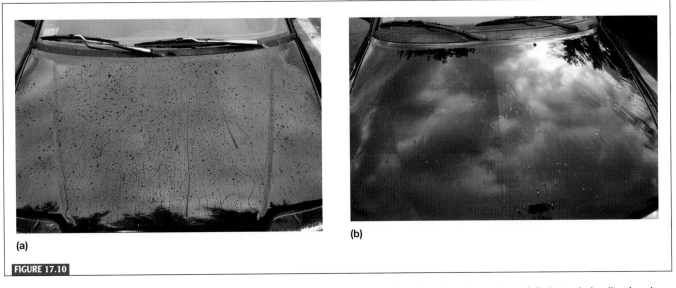

(a)

(b)

FIGURE 17.10

Surface tension causes water to bead up on a waxed surface (a). Detergent added to the water (b) reduces the surface tension and eliminates the beading. In a similar manner, surfactant reduces surface tension and elastic recoil in our alveoli.

17.4 Behavior of Respiratory Gases: Exchange and Transport

Individual gases in the air act like goats, not like sheep. Have you ever tried to herd sheep or goats? When you try to get a herd of sheep to do something, they either all do it, or none of them do it. There is no individual initiative among sheep. They act as one unit. Goats, on the other hand, are strict individualists, even when in a herd. They all do their own thing; go their own way, independent of each other (this makes herding them very frustrating). That is how gases in a mixture act. They each exert their own pressure as if the other gases were not present. There is no interaction in their individual behaviors. This is the basic message of Dalton's Law. This law is one of the invariable laws of physics (of which Scotty in the original "Star Trek" often spoke) that help us to make sense out of our universe. Dalton's Law tells us that each gas in a mixture of gases exerts its own pressure as if the other gases were not present. This is important to us since the air we breathe is not one gas, but a mixture of several gases (**FIGURE 17.11**).

Individual gases diffuse based only on their individual pressures. We refer to the pressure exerted by one gas in a mixture as the partial pressure of that gas. A gas will diffuse from the location where its partial pressure is higher to the location where its partial pressure is lower, independent of the other gases in the mixture. This is an important concept that we will use momentarily.

Now that we know a little bit about how gases act in a mixture, let's think about how they act in a liquid, like water. Henry's law tells us that the concentration of a gas in a liquid is proportional to the concentration of that gas in the atmosphere above the liquid, but is dependent on a solubility coefficient. This law explains the carbonation of beverages.

Before you open a bottle of ginger ale, the concentration of gases in the ginger ale is proportional to the concentration of those gases in the atmosphere above that liquid (the ginger ale), as much as is allowed by the solubility of those gases in ginger ale. In other words, if there is a lot of a particular gas (CO_2, for instance) in that little bit of atmosphere that exists between the ginger ale and the cap of the bottle, there will be a lot of that particular gas (CO_2) in the ginger ale, assuming that the gas is readily soluble in ginger ale.

When you open the bottle, the atmosphere of the bottle escapes and is replaced by the atmosphere that we all know and love. The gases dissolved in the ginger ale must now equilibrate with those of the new atmosphere. If there is more of a particular gas in the new atmosphere than there was in the old atmosphere, that gas will diffuse into the ginger ale. In the case of CO_2, there is far less in the new atmosphere than there was in the old atmosphere: it must diffuse out of the ginger ale. In fact, this change in circumstances causes it to come out rather abruptly, and we see the bubbles of CO_2 emerging until equilibrium is reached (and the soda therefore becomes "flat"). How could we make it bubble again? We could again incubate it below an atmosphere high in CO_2 before returning it to our own atmosphere; we could take it to a planet with an atmosphere that has less CO_2 than the atmosphere of earth; or, for that matter, we could take it to a planet with an atmosphere that has less of some other gas (i.e., nitrogen) than the atmosphere here and watch the nitrogen bubble out. In any event, it is cheaper just to buy a new bottle of ginger ale!

So, what's with all this ginger ale talk? What does it have to do with anatomy and physiology? Well, the same principles that cause CO_2 to move between the atmosphere and the ginger ale also cause gases to move between the external environment and your blood. External respiration, the movement of gases between the external environment (the atmosphere) and your blood, is regulated by Dalton's law and Henry's law. We will also need Henry's law when we consider how gases are transported in blood. Let's examine how external respiration works.

■ External Respiration

We must begin by examining the concentrations of gases in the blood and atmosphere within the lungs. The partial pressures of CO_2 and oxygen in atmospheric air are 0.3 and 159.5 mm Hg, respectively. This is not the par-

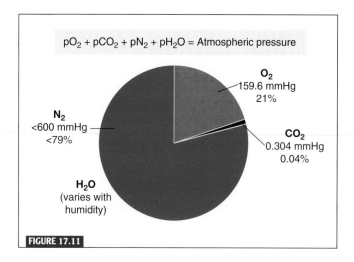

$$pO_2 + pCO_2 + pN_2 + pH_2O = \text{Atmospheric pressure}$$

O₂
159.6 mmHg
21%

N₂
<600 mmHg
<79%

CO₂
0.304 mmHg
0.04%

H₂O
(varies with humidity)

FIGURE 17.11

Several gases are present in our atmosphere. Atmospheric pressure is the sum of their partial pressures. Partial pressure is indicated by p. Note that mmHg is a unit for measuring pressure.

Table 17.1   Partial Pressures in External Respiration

	Alveolar Air	Deoxygenated Blood	Oxygenated Blood
pCO_2	40	45	40
pO_2	105	40	105

tial pressure of these gases in the air in the lungs, however. Since you do not completely empty your lungs of air at any exhalation, air remains in the airways and in the alveoli as they do not completely deflate. Alveolar air has the following partial pressures: $pCO_2 = 40$ mm Hg, $pO_2 = 105$ mm Hg. Deoxygenated blood (that which is coming to the lungs from the right side of the heart) has the following partial pressures: $pCO_2 = 45$ mm Hg, $pO_2 = 40$ mm Hg. These partial pressures are listed in **TABLE 17.1**.

Oxygen moves from alveolar air into the blood because the partial pressure of oxygen is greater in alveolar air than it is in the blood. According to Dalton's law, it must move from where its pressure is greater to where it is less. Carbon dioxide moves from deoxygenated blood into the alveolar air; again, it is moving according to its two relative partial pressures. Quite simply, both gases are diffusing as if no other gases were present. The concentration of these gases in oxygenated blood matches that of alveolar air because gas exchange in the lungs is so efficient. This is true because of the great area available for gas exchange, the small diameter of pulmonary capillaries, and the thinness of the alveolar membrane. So, what happens in the tissues? There (in internal respiration) we are dealing with the same principles.

■ Internal Respiration

Internal respiration describes the movement of gases between the blood and the tissues of our bodies (including interstitial fluid). We begin with oxygenated blood and end up with deoxygenated blood. The partial pressure of oxygen and CO_2 in each of these locations is listed in **TABLE 17.2**.

Table 17.2   Partial Pressures in Internal Respiration

	Oxygenated Blood	Tissues	Deoxygenated Blood
pCO_2	40	45	45
pO_2	105	40	40

Again, Dalton's law dictates that CO_2 moves from the tissues into the blood and that oxygen moves from the blood into the tissues. In this way, deoxygenated blood is generated. If you are unsure of this concept, reread the "External Respiration" and "Internal Respiration" sections of this chapter and look again at Tables 17.1 and 17.2. Pay attention to the numbers (partial pressures) associated with each gas in each location. Remember that whenever we have two locations with different pressures for the same gas, if that gas can move, it will move from where the pressure is higher to where the pressure is lower. That is how oxygen moves from the air into the blood and from the blood into the tissues. That is also how CO_2 moves in the opposite direction. So, if that is all there is to it, let's quit now and go have some fun. Oh, wait a minute; that can't be all there is to it. How do we actually transport these gases in our blood? We'd better examine that now.

■ Transportation of Gases in Your Blood

Can you jump into a pond and swim around underwater all day, breathing the water in and out as you go? (Don't actually go try this; take a wild guess.) You probably said that no, you could not do that. Why can't you do that? You could probably physically move water into and out of your lungs. (Actually, some people can. In others, the laryngospasm that occurs to keep foreign objects out of the respiratory tree is so great that they wouldn't actually drown, they would suffocate.) So, if you can physically move water into and out of your lungs, why won't that keep you alive? For that answer, we need to think back to Henry's law. Remember the solubility coefficient in his law? The amount of a gas that can dissolve in a liquid is dependent on how soluble it is in that liquid. The solubility coefficient of oxygen in water is too low; water can't hold enough oxygen for us to use it as our atmosphere.

So, if water is not good at holding oxygen (low solubility coefficient) and if our blood is mostly water, how can it hold enough oxygen to keep us alive? Hemoglobin is the answer (**FIGURE 17.12**). The hemoglobin in our red blood cells enables our blood to carry great amounts of oxygen. Hemoglobin acts as a carrier for oxygen, picking up oxygen where it is abundant (in our lungs) and releasing it where it is not abundant (in our tissues). It really is amazing how this works (**FIGURE 17.13**). The amount of oxygen bound to hemoglobin in our blood is dependent on the partial pressure of oxygen in our blood. In oxygenated blood, the partial pressure of oxygen is 105 mm Hg. At this partial pressure, our hemoglobin is essentially completely filled with oxygen. We

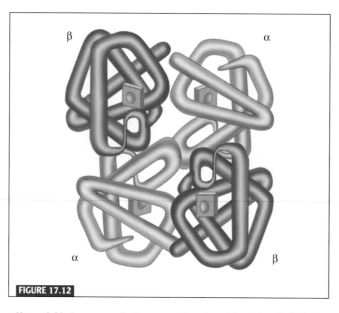

FIGURE 17.12

Hemoglobin is composed of two α and two β protein chains. Each chain includes an iron-containing heme group (shown in red).

would say that it is about 100 percent saturated with oxygen.

In our tissues, the partial pressure of oxygen is 40 mm Hg. At this partial pressure, our hemoglobin gives up about 25 percent of its oxygen so that oxygen can diffuse into the tissues. The result is a lot more oxygen delivered to the tissues than would be accomplished merely by dissolved oxygen diffusing out of our blood. That also gives us a reserve supply of oxygen still bound to hemoglobin. That reserve supply is important when our tissues are using greater quantities of oxygen, such as the oxygen needed by muscles during exercise.

As the partial pressure of oxygen drops below 40 mm Hg, our hemoglobin gives up its oxygen at a greatly increased rate. This keeps our tissues within the range of homeostasis, even when they are consuming great quantities of oxygen. Other factors that lead to increased delivery of oxygen from hemoglobin include decreased pH (more acidic conditions) and increased tempera-

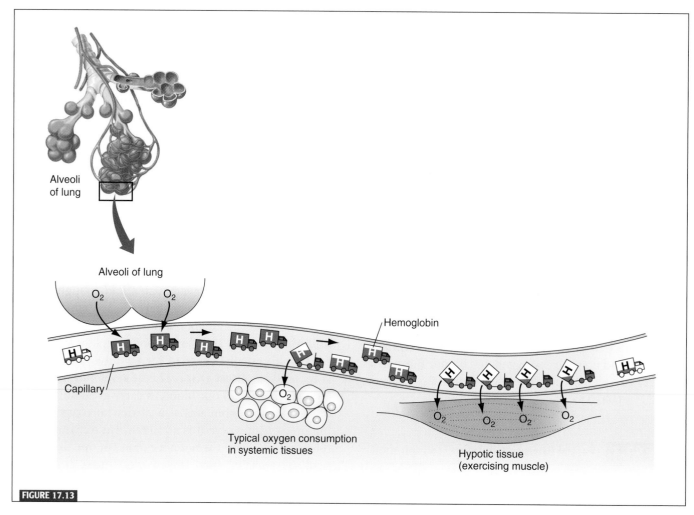

FIGURE 17.13

At the partial pressure of oxygen in alveolar air (105 mm Hg), hemoglobin becomes approximately 100% saturated with oxygen. At the partial pressure of oxygen we generally see in tissues (40 mm Hg), hemoglobin gives up about 25 percent of that oxygen (becoming 75% saturated with oxygen). As the partial pressure of oxygen in tissue drops further (as in exercising muscle), hemoglobin releases oxygen more readily. This maintains tissue pO_2 as close to 40 mm Hg as possible.

ture. Both of these conditions exist when tissues are highly metabolically active (such as muscle when exercising). What a system! The most oxygen is delivered where we need oxygen the most.

Now, what about CO_2? Can we move a lot of CO_2 simply dissolved in the fluid of our blood? No, Henry's law again plays a role here. Only about 7 percent of the CO_2 we move in our blood can travel dissolved in the plasma (**FIGURE 17.14**). How about bound to hemoglobin? We learned in Chapter 16 that hemoglobin binds CO_2 when it is in great supply and oxygen is in low supply. But again, we do not move that much of our CO_2 in that manner. Only about 23 percent of the CO_2 that we move can be transported bound to hemoglobin. That leaves us with 70 percent of our CO_2 needing a transport mechanism. This is where the enzyme carbonic anhydrase comes to the rescue.

Carbonic Anhydrase and the Transport of CO_2

Carbonic anhydrase is an enzyme that catalyzes the following reaction:

$$H_2O + CO_2 \rightarrow H_2CO_3 \rightarrow H^+ + HCO_3^-$$

Put into words, this means that carbonic anhydrase combines water and CO_2 to form carbonic acid (H_2CO_3). Carbonic acid can then ionize to a hydrogen cation (as part of the definition of an acid) and a bicarbonate anion (HCO_3^-). Since carbonic anhydrase is in erythrocytes, and since they are in the blood in which we need to transport CO_2, we can convert CO_2 to car-

bonic acid, and ultimately bicarbonate, for transport. Seventy percent of the CO_2 we transport is in this form.

Given that we transport so much CO_2 as bicarbonate, we can look for other ways in which this affects our delivery of blood gases. The bicarbonate diffuses out as the chloride ion diffuses into our red blood cells. This exchange is important for osmotic balance, and is called the *chloride shift*. By delivering bicarbonate into our plasma, we have had an additional effect on the plasma. Bicarbonate is part of the *carbonic acid-bicarbonate buffer system*.

Transportation of CO_2: Role in pH Regulation

Buffer systems are combinations of chemicals that replace strong acids with weak acids and strong bases with weak bases (review in Chapter 2). This helps to maintain homeostasis from the standpoint of acid-base balance whenever it is threatened by a strong acid or base. Most buffer systems are composed of a weak acid and either a weak base or the salt of the acid. As you recall from Chapter 2, an acid is a molecule that ionizes to the cation hydrogen and some anion other than a hydroxyl group. A base is a molecule that ionizes to the hydroxyl anion and some cation other than hydrogen. A molecule that binds hydrogen ions will also make an aqueous solution basic (in effect, it takes H^+ away, leaving more OH^- behind). A salt is a molecule that ionizes to any cation other than hydrogen and any anion other than a hydroxyl group. If a molecule ionizes to the cation hydrogen and the hydroxyl anion, it is water. A strong acid or base is merely one that ionizes more completely. A weak acid or base ionizes less completely (a greater percentage remain in the un-ionized form).

The most common buffer system in our extracellular fluids is the *carbonic acid-bicarbonate buffer system*. In this system, we have a weak acid (carbonic acid) and the salt of that acid (sodium bicarbonate), which acts like a weak base (even though we are well aware that it is not a base). When a strong base is introduced into the system, it reacts with the weak acid (carbonic acid) to make more of the salt (sodium bicarbonate). It works with the strong base sodium hydroxide, as shown in the following:

$$NaOH + H_2CO_3 \rightarrow H_2O + NaHCO_3$$

Sodium hydroxide	Carbonic acid	Water	Sodium bicarbonate
Strong base	Weak acid		Salt of the acid

When the system is challenged by a strong acid, the salt (acting as a weak base) is consumed, and more of the

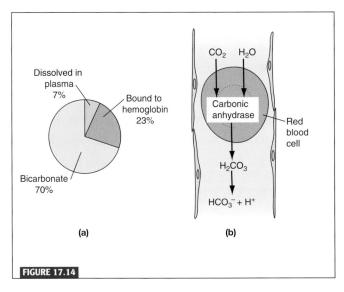

FIGURE 17.14

Most of the carbon dioxide that is transported in the blood travels as bicarbonate (a). Bicarbonate is generated by carbonic anhydrase, which is present in red blood cells.

weak acid (carbonic acid) is produced. This is shown in the following using hydrochloric acid as the strong acid:

$$HCL + NaHCO_3 \rightarrow NaCL + H_2CO_3$$

Hydro-chloric acid	Sodium bicarbonate	Sodium chloride	Carbonic acid
Strong acid	Salt of the acid (acting as a weak base)	Salt	Weak acid

When a large amount of CO_2 is being produced, carbonic acid is being produced. This tends to acidify the blood, but since this is a weak acid and is part of this buffer system, the effects of this potential decrease in pH are minimized. This reduced pH also results in oxygen being released more readily from hemoglobin, so more oxygen is delivered to the site of CO_2 production (where oxygen is being consumed).

O.K., so we know how gases are exchanged and how they are transported. Do we know what regulates our pulmonary ventilation? That is our next topic.

17.5 Regulation of Breathing

We learned in a previous chapter that the heartbeat is generated intrinsically within the heart. Although the CNS may modify that rate, the rate is generated independently of the CNS. Such is not the situation for respiration. If you were to disconnect my CNS from my muscles of respiration, I would stop breathing immediately. (I will leave it to you to consider how that disconnection could be achieved.) Centers within our brainstem regulate our breathing. We learned about those centers in Chapter 12. At that time, I told you that I would tell you more about those mechanisms later on. Now is later on; it's time to learn how the CNS controls respiration.

Remember the medullary rhythmicity area (Chapter 12)? It contains an inspiratory area on its dorsal aspect and an expiratory area on its ventral aspect (**FIGURE 17.15**). The inspiratory area causes the muscles of inspiration to contract. It rhythmically sends stimulatory impulses to those muscles. The expiratory area is only active during forced (labored) breathing. It too sends rhythmic stimulatory impulses when active, but its impulses go to the muscles of expiration.

But that's not all there is to it. We need to consider how those rhythmic impulses are generated. That involves the two respiratory areas we learned about in the pons. The apneustic area continually sends stimulatory impulses to the inspiratory area of the medullary rhythmicity area to prolong inspiration. The pneumotaxic area stops inspiration, thereby allowing expiration by

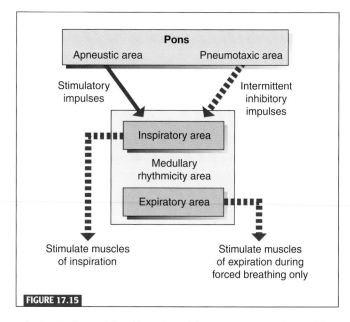

FIGURE 17.15

Centers in the medulla oblongata and the pons cooperate to regulate respiration.

overriding the stimulatory impulses from the apneustic area with rhythmic inhibitory impulses. If the pneumotaxic area is destroyed, the subject will inhale maximally, hold it for 10–20 seconds, then give a brief, ineffective exhale before maximally inhaling again. This does not result in effective pulmonary ventilation and is not consistent with life.

Other influences also regulate pulmonary ventilation. These include stretch reflexes that do not allow us to overinflate or overdeflate our lungs, and cortical influences that allow us to hold our breath. Can we voluntarily hold our breath "to death?" One is reminded here of the young child who, on not being allowed to leave the table until he or she eats all of their peas, threatens to hold his or her breath to death. Can this be done? The answer is no. Here is the reason.

Chemical stimuli are also involved in regulating our respiratory rate. Our nervous system monitors the blood in a typical negative feedback arrangement to regulate the rate of our pulmonary ventilation. These chemical monitoring systems will override the voluntary mechanisms and not allow you to hold your breath too long. While it is true to say that oxygen and CO_2 are both monitored, it is also misleading to say that. The monitoring of oxygen is generally not that effective. By the time blood oxygen levels drop enough to trigger increased respiration, damage due to low oxygen levels may already have been done. Carbon dioxide levels are the real indicators used to regulate pulmonary ventilation.

Actually, that is not quite true either. It is not CO_2 levels that are directly monitored, but blood pH as an indirect indicator of CO_2 levels. Think about it; if most of our CO_2 is transported as bicarbonate, which is generated by the ionization of carbonic acid, doesn't an increase in CO_2 lead to an increase in blood hydrogen ion levels (a decrease in pH)? Want to go through that again? Carbon dioxide is converted to carbonic acid, which ionizes to bicarbonate and a hydrogen cation. If we monitor the hydrogen cation levels, we will have an indication of how much CO_2 is being transported. If the pH of the blood gets too low, it means there is too much CO_2 (as bicarbonate) in the blood, and we need to increase the respiration rate to bring the pH back up. Look at **FIGURE 17.16** to help clarify that point.

■ A Cautionary Tale

One last thing before we leave the respiratory system. Here is a practical application for the concepts of blood gas transport and the regulation of respiration. When young kids are at the local swimming hole, don't they eventually have a contest to see who can stay under the longest? So, there they are, lined up at the edge of the water, and some of them hyperventilate before going under. They probably believe they are putting more oxygen into their blood so that they can stay under longer. You now know that they can not add more oxygen to their blood. At the partial pressure of oxygen that we see in oxygenated blood, hemoglobin is 100 percent saturated with oxygen. It simply can't hold any more.

But they can drive down the CO_2 levels in their blood. Since CO_2 (monitored indirectly as pH) is used to determine when the voluntary regulation of respiration (holding your breath) must be overridden (when respiration must be resumed), the system can be "tricked" by driving down the CO_2 levels. When the breath is held longer, because the voluntary system is not overridden, the oxygen level of the blood may be brought dangerously low. This can cause one to pass into unconsciousness, which is a very dangerous state when under water.

So, when you see kids doing that stunt, stop them and explain why it's unsafe. It will give you a chance

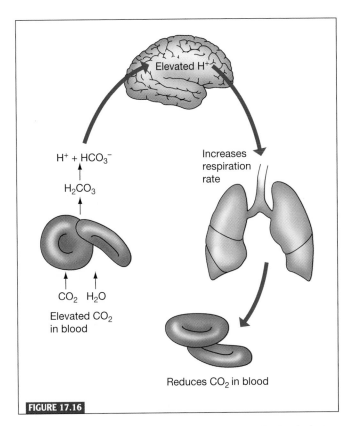

FIGURE 17.16

Because carbon dioxide is converted to carbonic acid by carbonic anhydrase, elevated blood CO_2 concentrations cause a decrease in blood pH (elevated levels of hydrogen ions). The nervous system monitors blood pH as an indirect measure of blood CO_2 levels. In response to a decreased pH, the nervous system increases the respiration rate, thereby reducing blood CO_2 levels.

to practice your knowledge of what you have learned, it will expose them to the exciting world of anatomy and physiology, and it may help save one of them from drowning.

That's it for the respiratory system. What did you think? Interesting, but complex, huh? Make sure you understand it by using the "What You Should Know" and "What Did You Learn?" features of this chapter before moving on. We will again revisit the regulation of blood pH in Chapter 20. You might have to come back and review this information then if you do not take the time to make certain you know it now.

Breaching Homeostasis . . . When Things Go Wrong

Chronic Bronchitis and Emphysema: COPD

Respiratory diseases are quite common in developed societies. Often the air we breathe is contaminated to the point that it challenges our respiratory systems' ability to cope: homeostasis is breached and disease ensues. Sometimes our personal behavior (smoking) or the work we do (workplace exposures to pollutants) contribute greatly to the problem. In this "Breaching Homeostasis" section, we will discuss two chronic obstructive diseases of the lung. The term *chronic* tells us that these diseases are of long duration. The term *obstructive* tells us that they involve an increased resistance to air flow.

Chronic bronchitis is the most common of the chronic obstructive diseases. The term *bronchitis* points to inflammation of the bronchi. A major characteristic of this illness is hypersecretion of mucus in the bronchi. Its diagnosis is based on patient history, as opposed to laboratory findings or pulmonary measurements. It is diagnosed in patients who have a history of a productive cough for a significant number of days during at least three consecutive months in at least two consecutive years. These criteria distinguish chronic bronchitis from recurrent bouts of acute bronchitis. Long-term inhalation of irritants can result in chronic bronchitis. Smoking increases risk by as much as one order of magnitude. In some cities, the incidence of chronic bronchitis may approach 25 percent of the population. Infectious agents also play a role in its etiology. Chronic bronchitis can lead to cor pulmonale, right-sided cardiac failure caused by pulmonary pathology. It also frequently leads to recurrent pulmonary infections and, ultimately, pulmonary failure. These, in turn, can result in death.

Emphysema is characterized by destruction of alveolar and alveolar duct walls, resulting in permanent enlargement of these airways. Through random examination of lungs at autopsy, emphysema has been determined to be quite common. Obviously, many of these cases are subclinical and played no role in the deaths of these people. Unfortunately, it is not always this inconsequential. The major contributor to risk of emphysema is smoking, although breathing polluted air also contributes to the development of this disease even in nonsmokers.

Smoking and other pollutants may cause an increase in inflammatory cells in the alveoli and small airways. This, in turn, may lead to increased levels of proteolytic enzymes (released by these cells) within the lungs. These enzymes destroy the elastic fibers in the alveolar walls, thereby weakening the walls. Destruction of the alveolar walls results in enlarged airways (if you knocked down the internal walls in your home, you would ultimately have larger but fewer rooms). This reduces the area available for gas exchange and destroys the internal structure of the lungs. This structure had helped to hold the airways open; its destruction leads to collapsed airways and increased resistance to air flow. Ultimately, emphysema may become debilitating and life threatening.

When seen together, chronic bronchitis and emphysema result in a condition called chronic obstructive pulmonary disease (COPD for short). Chronic obstructive pulmonary disease is quite common, as chronic bronchitis and emphysema are rarely seen individually and usually will ultimately coexist in the same patient, even if at presentation only one of them was diagnosed.

What can we do to avoid these illnesses? First, do not begin smoking, and if you already smoke, quit right now. Second, try to live in as clean an environment as possible, avoid heavy exercise when the air is highly polluted (high smog days), and wear the proper respirator whenever you are working in an unclean environment. Why not discuss any specific air pollution exposures you might encounter with your health-care provider? He or she will help you determine how best to minimize your risk.

What You Should Know

1. A functional partnership exists between the respiratory and cardiovascular systems: the respiratory system provides the site for gas exchange between the air and the blood, and the cardiovascular system transports gases in the blood, to and from the respiratory system.

2. The core of your external nose is made of hyaline cartilage.

3. The internal nasal cavity is lined with pseudostratified ciliated columnar epithelium.

4. Nasal conchae, or turbinates, swirl the column of air passing through your internal nose to condition (filter, warm, and moisten) the air. This protects the delicate alveoli within your lungs.

5. Your pharynx is composed of three regions: the nasopharynx, the oropharynx, and the laryngopharynx. The first of these is lined with pseudostratified ciliated columnar epithelium, while the later two are lined with noncornified stratified squamous epithelium.

6. Your larynx is composed of nine pieces of cartilage, the hyoid bone, and the true and false vocal cords.

7. Your trachea leads from your larynx to your bronchi. It is lined with pseudostratified ciliated columnar epithelium. It is supported by "C"-shaped rings of hyaline cartilage.

8. Your primary bronchi bifurcate off of your trachea. In each successive branch of bronchi, the amount of supporting cartilage becomes more diminished and the epithelium is ultimately reduced to simple low columnar.

9. In the bronchioles, the cartilage is replaced by smooth muscle and the epithelium has been reduced in height to simple cuboidal.

10. The alveoli are the site of gas exchange in your lungs. The alveolar membrane consists of the alveolar epithelium and their basement membrane, and the endothelial cells and their basement membrane.

11. Pneumocyte type I cells are the simple squamous epithelium of the alveoli. Pneumocyte type II cells are also found in the alveolar epithelium. These cuboidal cells produce surfactant. Dust cells are the resident macrophages of the alveoli.

12. The capillaries of the alveolar wall are so fine that erythrocytes must pass through them single file.

13. A slightly negative intrapleural pressure keeps the lungs partially inflated. Increasing this negative pressure causes the lungs to inflate; decreasing this negative pressure, or causing it to become positive, causes the lungs to deflate.

14. During eupnea we use the external intercostals and the diaphragm to inhale. Exhalation is passive; no muscles are contracted to cause deflation of the lungs.

15. During forced inhalation, we use the same muscles as during eupnea, plus the scalenes, the pectoralis minor, and the sternocleidomastoid.

16. During forced exhalation, we use the internal intercostals and the abdominal muscles.

17. Surfactant reduces the elastic recoil in our lungs that is produced by the surface tension of the moisture that coats the alveoli. Surfactant is important in that it allows us to inflate our lungs easily, keeps them from overdeflating when we exhale, and allows all of the alveoli to inflate evenly.

18. The gases in our atmosphere interact according to specific physical laws. You must know Dalton's law and Henry's law.

19. The net movement of gases by diffusion is from a region where their partial pressure is greater to a region where their partial pressure is lower.

20. Most of the oxygen transported in your blood is carried on hemoglobin in your erythrocytes.

21. Hemoglobin gives up (releases) oxygen more readily when the partial pressure of oxygen is low (especially below a partial pressure of 40 mm Hg), or when the pH is low.

22. Although some CO_2 is transported in solution and on hemoglobin, most is transported as bicarbonate.

23. Carbonic anhydrase (present in erythrocytes) combines CO_2 and water to form carbonic acid, which ionizes to bicarbonate plus the hydrogen ion.

24. The production of carbonic acid from CO_2 causes the blood to become more acidic. Carbonic acid acts as the weak acid in our carbonic acid-bicarbonate buffer system.

25. Chemical stimuli overrule the voluntary cessation of pulmonary ventilation. The concentration of CO_2 in our blood is monitored indirectly as blood pH. Low blood pH stimulates pulmonary ventilation.

What Did You Learn?

Multiple choice questions: choose the best answer.

1. The external nose is supported by a core of:
   a. Bone
   b. Fibrocartilage
   c. Hyaline cartilage
   d. Elastic cartilage

2. What does the nose do to the air that passes through it?
   a. It warms it
   b. It moistens it
   c. It filters it
   d. It does all of the above
   e. It does none of the above

3. The oropharynx is lined with:
   a. Pseudostratified ciliated columnar epithelium
   b. Cornified stratified squamous epithelium
   c. Noncornified stratified squamous epithelium
   d. Simple cuboidal epithelium

4. The epiglottis contains:
   a. Smooth muscle
   b. Skeletal muscle
   c. Hyaline cartilage
   d. Elastic cartilage
   e. None of the above

5. The trachea is supported by "C"-shaped cartilage rings. Which way does the open portion of the "C" face?
   a. Anteriorly
   b. Laterally
   c. Posteriorly
   d. Randomly in any direction

6. Place the following components of the alveolar membrane in order as they would be crossed by carbon dioxide:
   1. Pneumocytes
   2. Endothelial cells
   3. Endothelial basement membrane
   4. Pneumocyte basement membrane
   a. 1,4,3,2
   b. 1,4,2,3,
   c. 2,3,4,1
   d. 2,3,1,4

7. Which of the following is true of the cells that phagocytize debris within the lungs?
   a. They are called dust cells
   b. They are in the monocyte-macrophage lineage
   c. Both of the above
   d. Neither of the above

8. Which of the following are simple squamous epithelial cells?
   a. Pneumocytes type I
   b. Pneumocytes type II
   c. Both of the above
   d. Neither of the above

9. _____ contract(s) to cause inspiration during eupnea.
   a. External intercostals
   b. Diaphragm
   c. Either of the above
   d. Neither of the above

10. _____ contract to cause expiration during eupnea.
    a. Internal intercostals
    b. External intercostals
    c. Either of the above
    d. Neither of the above

11. The force for elastic recoil in the lungs is produced by:
    a. Elastic fibers distributed throughout the lungs
    b. The surface tension of water as moisture in the lungs
    c. Both of the above
    d. Neither of the above

12. What is the effect of surfactant on surface tension?
    a. It increases surface tension
    b. It decreases surface tension
    c. It has no effect on surface tension
    d. Surfactant, what's that?

13. Surfactant is produced by:
    a. Dust cells
    b. Pneumocytes type I
    c. Pneumocytes type II
    d. Pneumocytes type III

14. Henry's law tells us that:
    a. Each gas in a mixture exerts its own pressure as if the other gases were not present
    b. The concentration of a gas in a liquid is proportional to the concentration of that gas in the atmosphere above the liquid and dependent on a solubility coefficient
    c. Gases in a mixture do not act independently; their pressures interact to produce unpredictable phenomena
    d. The concentration of a gas in a liquid is independent of the concentration of that gas in the atmosphere above the liquid

What Did You Learn? (continued)

15. Alveolar air contains _____ oxygen than atmospheric air.

  a. More

  b. The same amount

  c. Less

16. With oxygen at a partial pressure of 105 mm Hg (as in oxygenated blood), hemoglobin is approximately _____ percent saturated with oxygen.

  a. 20

  b. 40

  c. 50

  d. 75

  e. 100

17. With oxygen at a partial pressure of 40 mm Hg (as is usually the case in our tissues), hemoglobin is approximately ___ percent saturated with oxygen.

  a. 20

  b. 40

  c. 50

  d. 75

  e. 100

18. Most of the CO_2 in our blood is transported as:

  a. Carbon dioxide bound to hemoglobin

  b. Carbonic anhydrase

  c. Carbon dioxide dissolved in the plasma

  d. Bicarbonate

19. As the amount of CO_2 in the blood increases, the pH of the blood:

  a. Increases

  b. Decreases

  c. Does not change

  d. The effect of CO_2 content on blood pH is determined by the oxygen content of the blood

20. The pneumotaxic area is in the:

  a. Medulla oblongata

  b. Midbrain

  c. Pons

  d. Cerebellum

Short answer questions: answer briefly and in your own words.

  1. What is the role of the nasal conchae in the function of the nose?

  2. How is food kept from entering your trachea as you swallow?

  3. How is dust kept from injuring your lungs? Please explain each of the safety mechanisms that protect your lungs from dust.

  4. Draw and label the anatomy of your respiratory system. Be sure to show the proper number of lobes for each lung, the structures that carry air to and from these lobes, and the position of the lungs within the body.

  5. Please explain why your lungs receive blood from both sides of your heart.

  6. Explain how the lungs are inflated and deflated during eupnea and forced breathing.

  7. What is the role of surfactant?

  8. How is your respiratory rate regulated?

Management of Nutrients and Wastes

PART VI

Why Study the Gastrointestinal and Urinary Systems Together?

You may wonder what the next two systems that we are about to study have to do with each other. At the outset, you may think that the gastrointestinal (digestive) and urinary systems have little in common. Both of these systems are, however, materials-handling systems. In the case of the gastrointestinal system, the materials being managed are the substances ingested (food and drink) and the wastes generated in the process. In the case of the urinary system, we are dealing with a number of metabolic wastes, most notably the nitrogenous wastes, although it has several other important functions as well. These are two very interesting and important systems, so I hope you will take your time and study them carefully. You will find that both of these systems give you an opportunity to exercise many of the concepts that you have learned while studying anatomy and physiology. This will enable you to firm up what you are not sure of and to derive satisfaction from what you know well. So, let's begin.

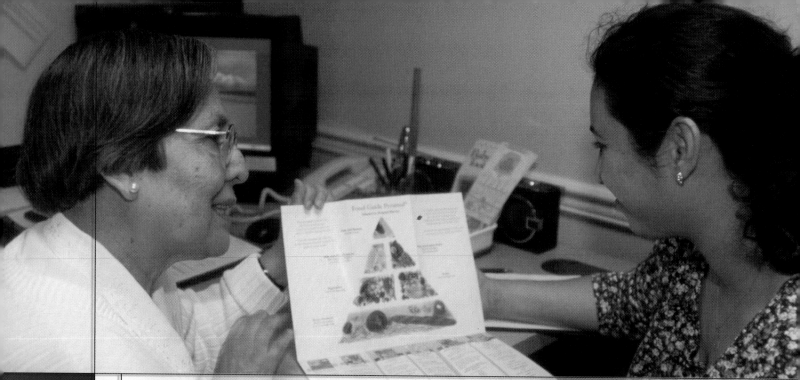

18 Your Gastrointestinal System

What You Will Learn

- That there are two major components in the gastrointestinal system.
- The names of the membranes that support your alimentary canal.
- The functions of your gastrointestinal system.
- The anatomical features of each region of your alimentary canal, including your mouth, pharynx, esophagus, stomach, small intestine, and large intestine.
- The internal structure of your teeth.
- The various forms of digestion that occur in each region of your alimentary canal.
- How the activity of your stomach is regulated.
- How the various substances that you eat are absorbed in your small intestine.
- The effects of vitamins.
- How the activities of your small intestine are regulated.
- How feces are formed in your colon.
- The location, structure, and activities of your accessory organs of digestion.
- How your pancreas, liver, and gallbladder are connected to your duodenum.
- Why bile is important.
- How the liver processes proteins, carbohydrates, and lipids.
- The details of lipid metabolism.

18.1 One System: Two Basic Components

This important system has two basic components: the alimentary canal (digestive tract) and the accessory organs of digestion (**FIGURE 18.1**). There are several ways to approach the study of this system. In one method of study, the alimentary canal and the accessory organs are integrated in such a way that you study the alimentary canal until you reach the point where one of the acces-

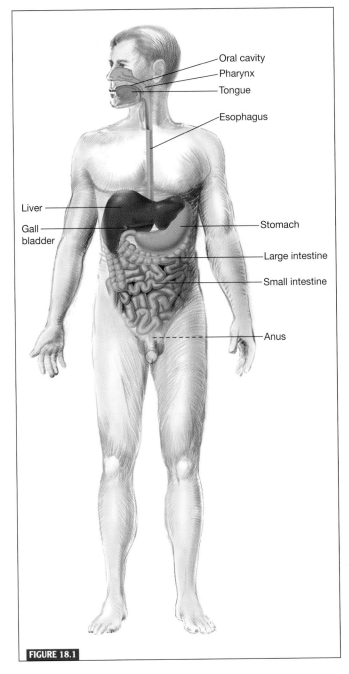

Oral cavity
Pharynx
Tongue
Esophagus
Liver
Gall bladder
Stomach
Large intestine
Small intestine
Anus

FIGURE 18.1

The digestive system.

sory organs plays a role. At that point, you switch to that organ before again continuing down the alimentary canal.

The other approach to this system involves studying the entire alimentary canal before studying any of the accessory organs. This is the approach we will take. The reason for this is simple. The alimentary canal is one continuous structure, a tube running from your mouth to your anus. The accessory organs are associated with this tract, but are not a part of it. When the two are integrated into one discussion, students are sometimes mislead into thinking, even if only subconsciously, that the materials moving through the alimentary canal take detours to these other organs before returning to the canal to continue their journey. Although these students understand the concept correctly when asked about it, their confusion is more subtle in nature and is there nonetheless. I would really like to help you avoid this possible source of confusion. The best way I know of to do this is to study the alimentary canal in its entirety before examining the accessory organs.

The one drawback to this approach is that at times I must ask you to hold a thought until later in the chapter. I may introduce a subject and then tell you that we must revisit it after we have studied the accessory organs. This will not impede your learning, but will actually help it in the long run. So, with that introduction, let's begin.

18.2 Your Alimentary Canal

Your alimentary canal is one continuous tube running from your mouth to your anus. You will recall from Chapter 5 that we have a tube-in-a-tube body plan. We are roughly tube shaped, and there is a tube that runs through our bodies. The alimentary canal is that tube. The lumen of the tube, while apparently within your body, is actually an exterior space: the environment within the alimentary canal is an external environment. To bring substances into the body itself, these substances must cross the walls of this tube.

This tubular structure is almost 30 feet long. Think about your garden hose; it may be of similar length. Has it ever become tangled up? Most likely, it has. Our alimentary canal could do the same if it were not well supported along much of its length. We have double folds of peritoneal membrane that extend from the body wall to the alimentary canal to physically support and provide vascular and nervous access to this canal. This structure also provides for storage of energy as adipose tissue, immune protection of the alimentary

Table 18.1 The Supporting Membranes of the Alimentary Canal and Associated Structures

Membrane	Location
Falciform ligament	Suspends liver to anterior abdominal wall and diaphragm
Lesser omentum	Suspends stomach and proximal small intestine to liver
Greater omentum	A four-layered structure overlying much of the intestine
Mesentery	Holds the small intestine in folds
Mesocolon	Holds the large intestine in position

canal through the presence of lymphatic nodules, and lubrication of this structure through the secretion of a serous (thin, watery) fluid. The names of these membranes in different locations are listed in **TABLE 18.1** and illustrated in **FIGURE 18.2**.

Although it is one long tube, the alimentary canal has a number of distinct regions. These regions differ in

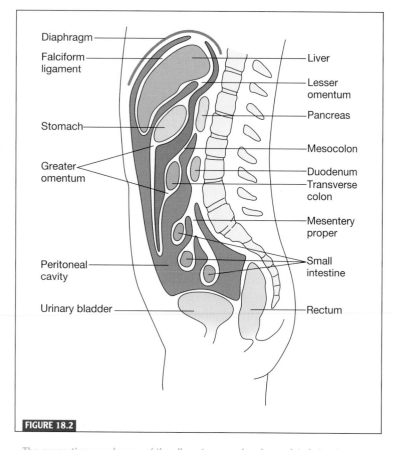

FIGURE 18.2

The supporting membranes of the alimentary canal and associated structures.

structure and function, and we must consider each separately. They include the following: the mouth, the pharynx, the esophagus, the stomach, the small intestine, and the large intestine. The large intestine includes the cecum, colon, rectum, and anus. In fact, several digestive tract structures have distinct regions within them. We will name and consider each of these as we come to them.

■ Some Definitions

To discuss the functions that occur in the alimentary canal, we need to know some terminology. First of all, *digestion* is a term associated with one name for this system. Digestion is merely the breakdown of ingested substances. Two types of digestion occur in the digestive system: mechanical digestion and chemical digestion. Mechanical digestion is the process we use to break food into particles that can be transported in the alimentary canal and worked on by chemical means. All of the muscular activities of the alimentary canal, including chewing, swallowing, churning, and propelling substances along, are mechanical digestion.

Chemical digestion is the process we use to break down molecules in our food into smaller molecules that can be absorbed through the wall of this canal into our bodies. In most locations, this is an enzymatic process. In the colon, it is the work of a resident population of bacteria.

Absorption is the mechanism used to move substances across the wall of the digestive tract. Once substances are absorbed, they can be transported either in blood vessels or lymphatic vessels. Many of the nutrients absorbed by the alimentary canal are transported to the liver through the hepatic portal system. You will recall portal systems from our discussion of the anterior pituitary gland in Chapter 13. A portal system is a vascular arrangement where a capillary bed in one organ drains into veins that subsequently feed capillaries in another organ (remember the interoffice mail analogy?). In the case of the hepatic portal system, the first capillary bed is in the walls of the alimentary canal. These drain into the hepatic portal vein, which supplies sinusoids (capillarylike structures) in the liver. We will learn more about this later in this chapter.

■ An Architectural Plan

One additional piece of necessary introductory information is how the walls to this tubular structure are

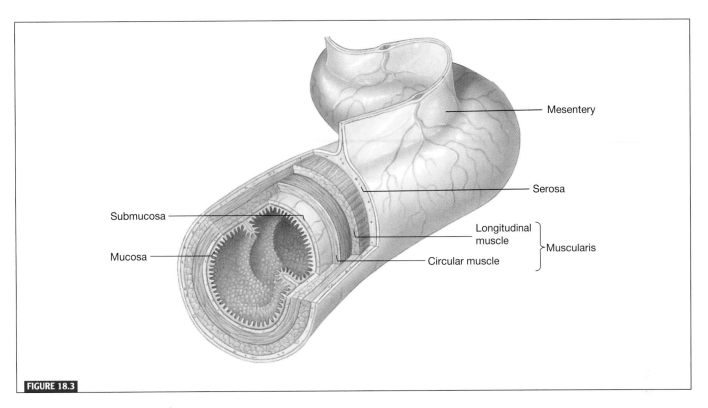

FIGURE 18.3

The layers of the alimentary canal.

arranged. There are distinct layers to this wall (as shown in **FIGURE 18.3**): a mucosa, a submucosa, a muscularis, and a serosa.

The mucosa is the innermost layer. It consists of an epithelial layer; a lamina propria, or layer of connective tissue, blood and lymph vessels; and a muscularis mucosa, or thin layer of smooth muscle. The muscularis mucosa causes the mucosa to rise into folds. The next layer is the submucosa, which is highly vascular connective tissue, containing nerve plexuses. Next, we have the muscularis, which in most places consists of two layers of smooth muscle. The inner layer is arranged in a circular pattern, while the fibers of the outer layer run longitudinally. In the stomach, the muscularis has three layers: circular inner and outer layers with a longitudinal middle layer. Here we also find nerve plexuses. Finally, for the parts inferior to the diaphragm, we have the serosa, composed of visceral peritoneum. We have already discussed how this serous layer connects the alimentary canal to the body wall. If this tube is directly attached to the body wall (parts of it are retroperitoneal, meaning "behind the peritoneum"), the surface exposed to the body cavity is covered with serosa, while the posterior aspect is covered with adventitia, connective tissue.

We are ready to begin; so on to the mouth.

■ Your Mouth

Your alimentary canal begins at your mouth. While we will not spend much time discussing your mouth, there are a few interesting facts that we must consider. First of all, can you predict what type of epithelium is present in your mouth? Think of the roles the mouth performs and what epithelium would be best suited for the task. If you named noncornified stratified squamous epithelium, you are correct. Remember that this epithelium provides abrasion resistance, yet can withstand the moist environment dictated by the need for lubrication in the mouth.

The teeth are also present in the mouth. They are diagrammed in **FIGURE 18.4**. An individual tooth is also shown in Figure 18.4. Notice the layers of a tooth, which are composed of both hard and soft tissue. In the center of each tooth is the soft pulp cavity. This contains connective tissue, blood vessels, and nerves. The parenchymal cells of the pulp are odontoblasts, specialized columnar epithelial cells. You may recall from Chapter 4 that the columnar form is often used for cells that have secretory functions. Here is no exception. The odontoblasts produce dentin, which makes up the majority of the tooth, and is a hard tissue of the tooth. Dentin, which is 75 percent inorganic salts and 25 percent

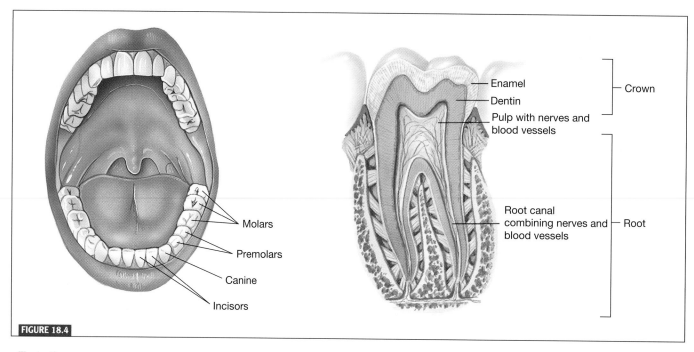

FIGURE 18.4

The teeth.

protein, differs greatly from our other main hard tissue, bone, in that it is acellular.

Superficial to the dentin, in the part of the tooth that is exposed, we find enamel. This part of the tooth, called the crown, is covered in enamel as the tooth is being produced. That enamel is made by ameloblasts, which are then lost to erosion as the tooth is used. Therefore, enamel is permanent. The cells that produced it are no longer present. Enamel is 98 percent inorganic salts and only 2 percent protein.

The unexposed portion of the tooth (the part covered by the gingiva or gums and the part within the bony socket) is called the root. Roots are covered in cementum rather than enamel. The socket is lined with modified periosteum, called the periodontal membrane or ligament. This joint was introduced in Chapter 7 as a gomphosis, an example of a fibrous joint that is synarthrotic (described in Chapter 7). At the apex or bottom of the tooth is the apical foramen, which is an opening for the access of nerves and blood vessels.

Your tongue is also present in your mouth. This structure holds many of your taste buds (Chapter 12) and is necessary for moving food around the mouth during chewing and swallowing. Interestingly, your tongue is the only structure in which skeletal muscle contains branched fibers. If someone accuses you of speaking with a "forked-tongue," you can assure that person that your tongue is not forked, but some of the muscle fibers in it may be!

Obviously, mechanical digestion in the mouth includes chewing and, as such, is very important. Chemical digestion also begins in the mouth with the digestion of some carbohydrates. The process of breaking complex carbohydrates into disaccharides begins here. The enzyme involved is salivary amylase. A lipid-digesting enzyme, lingual lipase, is produced by the submucosal glands of the mouth. It is, however, largely ineffective. For the most part lipid digestion waits until later in the alimentary canal.

■ Your Pharynx

During our discussions of the respiratory system, we learned that the pharynx is composed of three regions: the nasopharynx, the oropharynx, and the laryngopharynx. We also learned that the oropharynx and laryngopharynx serves as a passageway for food (and drink), as well as air. The pharynx participates in the initiation of swallowing by moving the food being swallowed toward the esophagus, elevating the soft palate to close off the opening to the internal nose, and elevating the larynx to close off the entrance to the trachea. You may want to review the structure of the pharynx now, described in Chapter 17.

■ Your Esophagus

The next segment of your alimentary canal is your esophagus. This muscular tube is located posterior to your trachea. You will recall from Chapter 17 that the respiratory tract and alimentary canal diverge at the larynx, with the trachea being in the anterior position. The "C"-shaped cartilage rings of the trachea open toward the esophagus so that meatball sandwich you wolf down while running to your anatomy and physiology lecture can make it down. It would be a shame to choke to death right before an exciting anatomy and physiology lecture!

The esophagus begins at the upper esophageal sphincter and ends at the lower esophageal sphincter. These sphincters regulate the movement of substances through the esophagus. The upper esophageal sphincter prohibits the inadvertent entry of air into the alimentary canal. The lower esophageal sphincter prohibits the movement of substances from the stomach into the esophagus. The low pH of the gastric secretions would damage the esophagus if the lower esophageal sphincter did not prevent this reflux. In fact, many people experience "heartburn" and even esophageal ulcers when the lower esophageal sphincter does not function adequately.

The esophagus is lined with noncornified stratified squamous epithelium and has a muscular wall. The muscle tissue of the esophagus is interesting. In the proximal one third of this tube, the muscle is of the skeletal type. In the distal one third, it is smooth muscle. In the middle, the muscle is a mixture of these two types. For this reason, swallowing (also called deglutition) begins with a voluntary effort and ends as an involuntary reflex. Swallowing involves peristalsis. To picture peristalsis, take a very long toothpaste tube. Put your fingers around its distal end (opposite end from the cap) and press to constrict the tube slightly. With the cap off, slide your fingers toward the cap end. This should cause lots of toothpaste to come out. (By the way, I don't actually mean for you to do this; just imagine it. Toothpaste costs money!) This is a fair representation of peristalsis. It takes about 1 second to swallow liquids. It generally takes 4–8 seconds to swallow solids and semisolids; however, some solids (like peanut butter) may take a little longer.

The chemical digestion that began in the mouth by the action of salivary amylase continues here as there is nothing present to stop the activity of this enzyme. The lipid-digesting activity of lingual lipase continues here but really does not accomplish a great deal because of the short time available and the hydrophobic nature of lipids. No additional enzymatic digestion begins here.

■ Your Stomach

Here is an interesting organ. Your stomach (**FIGURE 18.5**) is a "J"-shaped enlargement of your alimentary canal,

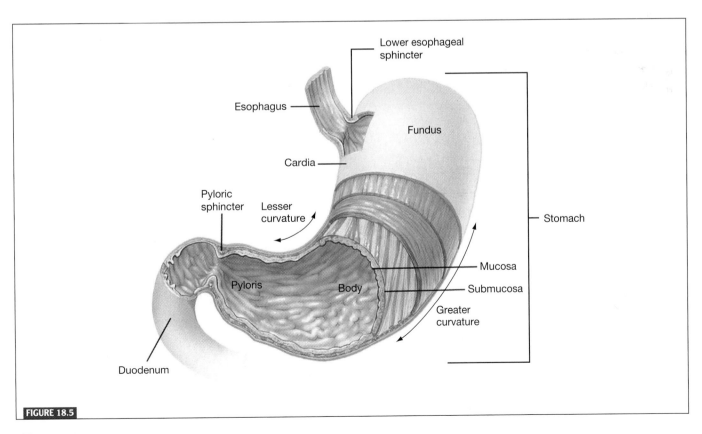

Lower esophageal sphincter

Esophagus

Fundus

Cardia

Pyloric sphincter

Lesser curvature

Stomach

Mucosa

Pyloris   Body

Submucosa

Greater curvature

Duodenum

FIGURE 18.5

The stomach.

designed for mechanical and chemical digestion and, to some degree, the storage of food. The location of the stomach is largely to the left of your midline. This puts the union of the esophagus and the stomach (at the lower esophageal sphincter) in the midline. To the left of the esophagus is the fundus, and to the right of it is the cardia. Unlike the rest of the stomach, the fundus is not primarily for digestion. When you eat a big meal, you are introducing more food than the stomach can process at one time. The fundus serves as a storage area, a sort of warehouse in which the excess food can be stored. Food is released slowly from the fundus for processing in the body of the stomach.

The body of the stomach is inferior to the fundus and the cardia. As we move through the stomach's body, we reach the pylorus. The pylorus is the most distal portion of the stomach and ends where the small intestine begins. At this junction, we find the pyloric sphincter. Just as the lower esophageal sphincter guards the entrance to the stomach, the pyloric sphincter regulates the exit from the stomach. During gastric activity, the pyloric sphincter never completely relaxes; it only opens slightly. This allows only liquid to be squirted from the pylorus (stomach) into the duodenum (small intestine), and this only happens slowly. Otherwise, the low pH of the gastric secretions and the solid material that might also get through would damage the lining of the small intestine.

The stomach is a highly muscular organ with three layers of smooth muscle in its muscularis (two circular layers sandwiching a longitudinal layer). The mucosa (lining) of the stomach is thrown into longitudinal folds called rugae. These allow expansion of the stomach as it fills with food.

Microscopic examination of the mucosa also reveals an interesting architecture. Deep pits, called gastric pits, open from the surface, carrying epithelium into the lamina propria. You can picture this arrangement in the following way. Take a bowl of Jell-O and cover it with plastic wrap. Plunge your fingers into the Jell-O so that the plastic wrap lines the indentations that your fingers make. Now imagine that the Jell-O is the lamina propria and the plastic wrap is the epithelium. The surface of the bowl of Jell-O is the lining at the lumen of the stomach. The holes left by your fingers are the gastric pits.

Now picture these pits actually going a little deeper, because the bases of the pits open into gastric glands. What would be the reason for this arrangement? What purpose do these gastric pits and glands serve? Think about the great increase in surface area afforded by this design. Then think about how, by increasing the surface area in this manner, you would increase the secretory capacity of the epithelium. With that, we must consider what types of epithelial cells are present.

Epithelial Cells of Your Stomach

The epithelium of the stomach is of the simple columnar variety. There are several distinct cell types present. Chief cells produce pepsinogen, the precursor of the main gastric enzyme, pepsin. Pepsin is a protein-digesting enzyme. Some digestive enzymes are produced in an inactive form and are only activated after delivery into the lumen. If the cell were to work with active digestive enzyme, it would be like a munitions factory working with live bombs, very dangerous indeed. These cells also produce the lipid-digesting enzyme lipase, but as we will soon learn, its activity is insignificant.

Parietal cells produce hydrochloric acid (HCl), a strong acid that is responsible for the low pH of the stomach (around pH 2). Production of this acid is an interesting process, beginning with the production of carbonic acid from carbon dioxide and water by the enzyme carbonic anhydrase. Dissociation of the anion bicarbonate and the cation hydrogen gives us one of the two ions needed for HCl production. This hydrogen is combined with a chloride anion to produce HCl. The bicarbonate is returned to the blood and actually causes an increase in blood pH during digestion. Parietal cells also produce intrinsic factor, which works as a carrier for vitamin B_{12} absorption. In the absence of intrinsic factor, this vitamin cannot be absorbed.

Mucous cells produce mucus, as one would expect. It is important to point out, however, that these cells are not goblet cells. Normally no goblet cells are present in the stomach. The difference between mucous cells and goblet cells is the way in which the mucus is stored. In goblet cells, it is stored as a large droplet to be released all at once. In mucous cells, it is stored in numerous small vacuoles to be released as an ongoing dribble. The harsh environment of the stomach makes a constant coating of mucus necessary. Although this protects the epithelium, the life span of a mucous cell on the luminal surface is only about 3 days.

Deep in the gastric pits, the stomach epithelium also contains endocrine cells. These cells produce the peptide hormone gastrin, which is important in the regulation of gastric activity.

The Regulation of Gastric Activity

So, we know which pieces are present; now let's think about how they work. We may assume that gastric secretion of enzymes and acid, as well as muscle activity (churning), must increase after a meal to achieve digestion. But how is that increase regulated?

Think about a pizza. Sure, you can picture a pizza, can't you? What would you like on it? Pepperoni, perhaps, maybe extra cheese, or some mushrooms. Can't you see the steam rising off of it? Can't you see the strings of cheese stretching as you pull a piece away? If you can imagine these things, you have probably just increased gastric activity through a reflex action. Simply imagining food, hearing it being prepared, or smelling it will start the process. The process is further activated by the entry of food into the stomach. It is under the control of both the nervous and endocrine systems.

Parasympathetic stimulation increases these activities. The hormone gastrin also has these effects. Gastrin is released in response to parasympathetic stimulation and the presence of proteins in the stomach. The food that was ingested is now being digested. Digestion, and the mixing of food with gastric secretions, changes the food into a liquid or semiliquid state. It has a consistency similar to very loose oatmeal. This liquid is called chyme and is the state that food must come into before it can be processed by the small intestine. Little by little, chyme is squirted through the pyloric sphincter into the small intestine. As food enters the small intestine, the enterogastric reflex reduces gastric secretion and muscular activity. This reduces the possibility of damaging the small intestine by overwhelming it with stomach acid.

So, the mechanical digestion that occurs in the stomach involves the churning activity of mixing waves. The chemical digestion that occurs in the stomach involves the digestion almost purely of proteins by pepsin. Pepsinogen is activated to pepsin by the low pH of the gastric secretions. Pepsin digests polypeptide chains (proteins) into di- and tripeptides. The other gastric enzyme, gastric lipase, is for all intents and purposes inactive. Think about what fats do when they are placed in water (i.e., greasy pots and pans in a sink of water without detergent). Since lipids are hydrophobic and no detergent is present in the stomach, these fats clump together into a form that the lipase simply can not physically reach. We will have to wait until later in the alimentary canal to digest lipids.

The carbohydrate digestion that began in the mouth with salivary amylase, and continued in the esophagus because there was nothing there to stop it, is stopped here. The pH of the stomach is simply too low to allow that enzyme to work. The carbohydrates are not all reduced to disaccharides at this point, but further digestion must wait until further down the alimentary canal.

Very little absorption occurs in the stomach. The thick mucous coat that keeps the harsh digestive agents away from the epithelium also imposes a barrier to absorption. Some electrolytes (ions) and water (by osmosis), as well as some drugs, are absorbed here. Among drugs absorbed in the stomach, alcohol is most notable. Since its solubility is equal in water and in lipids, it is difficult for the body to keep alcohol from diffusing everywhere. This accounts for its rapid absorption and resulting CNS effects.

Gastric emptying takes from 2 to 6 hours, with high carbohydrate meals emptying the fastest. You know this to be true, as you may have noticed that rice-based meals leave you hungry very quickly. High-fat meals take the longest to empty from the stomach. You also are most likely aware of that phenomenon. Think about how you feel "stuffed" for hours after eating some greasy meal.

With that, we will move further down this canal. Keep in mind that chyme is now being squirted through the pyloric sphincter into the small intestine. This chyme is a mixture of liquefied food and gastric secretions, and contains partially digested proteins and carbohydrates. The lipids present have not yet been digested to any degree.

◼ Your Small Intestine

Your small intestine makes up the largest portion of your alimentary canal. It is composed of three regions that are best distinguished histologically (**FIGURE 18.6**). The first region, the duodenum, is only about 10 inches long. In fact, the term *duodenum* comes from the Latin term for the number 12: the duodenum measures about the width of 12 fingers. It wraps around the head of the pancreas.

The next region of the small intestine is the *jejunum*, meaning "empty." It is about 8 feet in length. The final region of the small intestine is the ileum. *Ileum* is from the Latin term meaning "groin"; however, it is also related to the Latin term for "twisted." This is the longest portion of the small intestine, measuring about 12 feet and ending at the ileocecal valve. The ileocecal valve does not allow substances that have left the small intestine to re-enter it.

Now, you may be wondering how an organ that is approximately 21 feet in length (about the depth of the average garage) can be called the "small" intestine. This designation has to do with its diameter, not its length. The small intestine is about 1 inch in diameter, whereas the large intestine is about 2.5 inches in diameter.

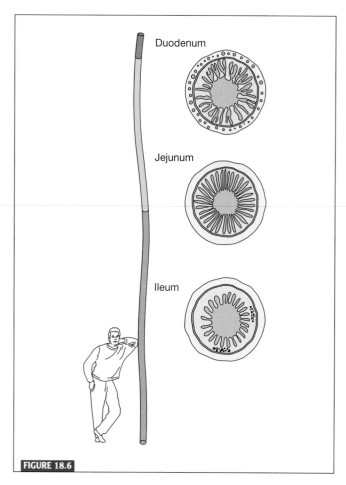

The small intestine. This diagram shows the relative lengths of the regions of the small intestine. The shape and abundance of villi vary throughout the small intestine. The duodenum is characterized by the presence of glands in the submucosa. Lymphatic nodules are present in the lamina propria of the ileum.

The mucosal arrangement of the small intestine is that of crypts and villi (**FIGURE 18.7**). Crypts are invaginations like the gastric pits we saw in the stomach. Villi are fingerlike projections extending out into the lumen. Both are present to increase surface area for secretion, digestion, and absorption. The duodenum also has glands in the submucosa for production of a protective alkaline mucus.

The simple columnar epithelium of the small intestine has three major cell types. The majority of the cells in the small intestine are enterocytes (meaning intestinal cells). These cells have microvilli on their apical surface to increase their surface area. The second most common cells in the small intestine are goblet cells for mucus production. Finally, we have enteroendocrine cells found deep in the crypts. Enteroendocrine cells produce the intestinal hormones we will learn about in a moment.

The epithelial cells of the small intestine are very short lived and are constantly being replaced. Stem cells found in the base of the crypts are continuously dividing. Their daughter cells differentiate as they move up the crypts in a migration reminiscent of moving up an escalator. They are ultimately shed from the villi.

The secretion of the small intestine, intestinal juice, is produced in abundance. It is slightly basic, again to counteract the acidity of the chyme coming from the stomach. The small intestine produces a number of digestive enzymes, which make their way from the enterocytes into the intestinal juice. These enzymes are collectively called brush-border hydrolases because they are found on the brush border (microvilli) of the enterocytes. We will return to these enzymes when we discuss chemical digestion in the small intestine.

Mechanical Digestion in Your Small Intestine

Two general types of mechanical digestion occur in the small intestine. Segmentation is the major movement of the small intestine. It simply involves a localized back and forth "sloshing" motion to mix the chyme with intestinal juice and keep it moving across the enterocytes. Have you ever put Jell-O into your mouth and "sloshed" it back and forth from one cheek to the other? This liquefies it very quickly. If you have done this, you have a good idea of how segmentation works in the small intestine. If you have not done this, at the risk of upsetting your dining companions (who will accuse you of playing with your food), you should try it and explain that it is an experiment for your anatomy and physiology class. The other major motion of the small intestine is peristalsis. Peristalsis in the small intestine is a weak wave of contraction that moves from the proximal end to the distal end, propelling the contents along.

One additional type of small intestinal movement should be considered here. The entry of food into the stomach triggers a reflex in the ileum called the gastroileal reflex. The gastroileal reflex causes peristaltic waves to occur in the ileum and also causes relaxation of the ileocecal sphincter. This moves the contents of the ileum into the first segment of the large intestine to make way for the meal that is just being consumed.

Chemical Digestion in Your Small Intestine

O.K., what is the chemical composition of the consumed substances entering the small intestine? Carbohydrates: partially broken down into disaccharides. Proteins: partially broken down into di- and tripeptides. Lipids: relatively unchanged to this point. Let's think about how we will complete their digestion.

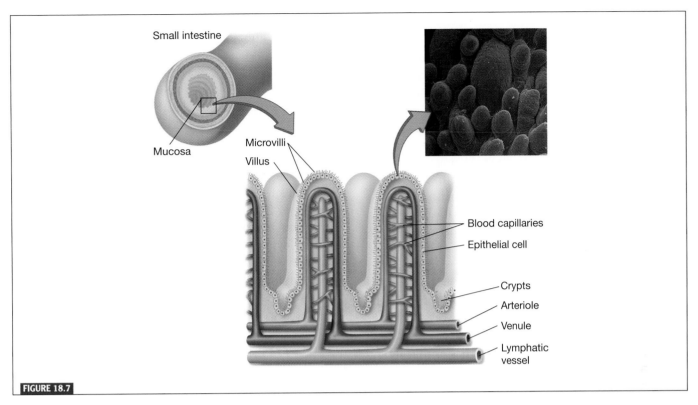

Small intestine

Mucosa

Microvilli

Villus

Blood capillaries

Epithelial cell

Crypts

Arteriole

Venule

Lymphatic vessel

FIGURE 18.7

The small intestinal mucosa is folded into villi and crypts. The epithelium covers the lamina propria, connective tissue containing abundant blood vessels and lymphatic vessels.

Pancreatic enzymes play a major role in small intestinal chemical digestion. We will consider those in greater detail after we make it through the alimentary canal (figuratively speaking, of course). For now, I will mention them and their activities.

Carbohydrate digestion resumes in the small intestine through the activity of pancreatic amylase, an enzyme very much like salivary amylase. It too breaks carbohydrates down into disaccharides. Disaccharides are broken down into monosaccharides by brush-border hydrolases that are produced in the enterocytes. There are many such enzymes, and to attempt to name them would be beyond the scope of our current work. Suffice it to say, they have names that are descriptive of their activity or substrate. They have their effects both while bound to microvilli and after being released into the chyme.

Protein digestion began in the stomach by the action of pepsin. This activity is continued in the small intestine by three enzymes from the pancreas: trypsin, chymotrypsin, and carboxypeptidase. These enzymes break polypeptides into di- and tripeptides. These must be broken down further into individual amino acids. That is done by brush-border hydrolases. Again, there are many different brush-border proteases, and to name them would not achieve our aim.

Chemical digestion of lipids is a fascinating process that really can only be understood after a discussion of the pancreas and, especially, the liver. We will go into detail on the digestion and absorption of lipids toward the end of this chapter.

Nucleic acids are broken down in the small intestine by nucleases. These too are from the pancreas.

Absorption in Your Small Intestine

Ninety percent of the absorption that takes place in our alimentary canal occurs in the small intestine. This accounts for the great length of this structure. The surfaces of the villi are the primary sites of absorption. This is easily understandable, as they wave about in the chyme like fronds of seaweed pushed about by the ocean currents. All of the types of cellular transport we discussed in Chapter 4 are used in this process. If you do not remember the details of diffusion, facilitated diffusion, osmosis, and the forms of active transport, now would be a good time to look back at them. Here, we will briefly discuss absorption of each chemical class. We will skip absorption of lipids until the end of the chapter, when we are better prepared to discuss it. Let's begin with electrolytes and water.

Electrolytes and Water

Absorption of electrolytes (acids, bases, salts, and the ions of which they consist) is best considered together with absorption of water. The two are tightly linked. The small intestine has a lot of water to deal with each day. Approximately 9 liters (think of 4.5 of the 2-liter soda bottles full of water) enter the small intestine each day. What, you ask? How can we possibly drink that much water? The answer is that we don't. That is the point of all this absorption. Through food or drink, we ingest about 1.5 liters of water per day. The remaining approximately 7.5 liters of water comes from salivary, gastric, and intestinal secretions. Regardless of the source, however, most of it must be absorbed. It is difficult for people in the developed world to take diarrhea very seriously; we see advertisements making fun of it all the time; and at most, to us, it is a discomfort and inconvenience. In the developing world, however, this is not the case. Diarrhea is a major killer in much of the world. As you think of the 9 liters of water that enter the small intestine and all of the electrolytes contained in that water, you get some sense of how that can be so. If we could not reabsorb a great deal of that water, we would dehydrate very quickly, indeed.

So, how do we absorb that water, and how much of it actually is absorbed? Of the 9 liters entering the small intestine, somewhere between 8 and 8.5 liters are absorbed in the small intestine. All of this absorption occurs through osmosis. You remember osmosis: diffusion of water across a semipermeable membrane. The electrolytes that are absorbed set up a concentration gradient that favors absorption of water. In particular, much sodium is absorbed by active transport, often in a coupled mechanism. Anions, such as chloride, follow the sodium. This sets up the osmotic balance that water follows. Always think about water following sodium, and you won't be far wrong. We will see that again in the kidneys. Calcium ions are also absorbed by active transport via a parathyroid hormone- and vitamin D-dependent mechanism.

Carbohydrates

All carbohydrates are absorbed as monosaccharides. Glucose and galactose are absorbed in a coupled transport system that requires the presence of sodium. Fructose is absorbed via facilitated diffusion.

Proteins

For the most part, for proteins to be absorbed, they must be broken down into individual amino acids. Certain specific di- and tripeptides can be absorbed into the intestinal epithelium, but this is the exception, not the rule. Further, these peptides must be broken down into individual amino acids before their transport in the blood. These facts should make you incredibly skeptical of any dietary supplement in the form of a protein that promises amazing health results. Remember that since the body does not, as a rule, absorb proteins in any form other than individual amino acids, the body never actually sees the protein that is being touted by its supplier.

Sodium-coupled active transport mechanisms are used to absorb amino acids. There are about four such mechanisms, one for each category of amino acid. We can break our 20 amino acids into four categories, based on the characteristics of their side chains. The categories are the following: acidic, neutral nonpolar, neutral polar, and basic. It is important to note that, although the body can either manufacture or transform other amino acids into many of the 20, some are available only in our diet. These are the essential amino acids and must be present in our diet for protein synthesis to occur. In the absence of an amino acid that is specified in the messenger RNA for a particular protein, that protein can not be synthesized. Substitutions are not allowed. Therefore, a well-balanced diet is necessary for the maintenance of homeostasis.

Vitamins

Vitamins are organic substances that are not proteins, carbohydrates, fats, or minerals, yet are absolutely necessary for the maintenance of homeostasis and usually can not be produced by our bodies. That really is the point; we must ingest them to remain healthy and, ultimately, to avoid death. Usually only very small quantities are required. They are not used as a source of energy or as building blocks for structural molecules in our bodies. Most often, they act as coenzymes (something necessary for an enzyme to function) in energy-transfer systems or as regulators of metabolism. The small intestine is where most vitamins are absorbed (see **TABLE 18.2** for the names and activities of the vitamins).

There are two major categories of vitamins: fat soluble and water soluble. The fat-soluble vitamins (A, D, E, and K) are absorbed by diffusion along with fats (to be considered later in this chapter). The water-soluble vitamins (the B vitamins and C) are absorbed by diffusion. The one exception to this is vitamin B_{12}, which requires the presence of intrinsic factor for its absorption by active transport.

Regulation by and of Your Small Intestine

Endocrine and neural control mechanisms regulate the activity of the alimentary canal. Again, in the small intestine, we see that the parasympathetic nervous system acts for energy restoration by increasing the activity of

Table 18.2 The Vitamins

Water-soluble Vitamins	Effect
B$_1$, thiamine	Coenzyme in catalytic reactions. Necessary for carbohydrate metabolism
B$_2$, riboflavin	Coenzyme role in carbohydrate and protein metabolism. Important for epithelium, eyes, and blood
Niacin	Coenzyme in glycolysis and cellular respiration. Inhibits cholesterol synthesis and assists in triglyceride degradation
B$_6$, pyridoxine	Essential for amino acid (especially tryptophan) metabolism. Important in immunoglobulin synthesis
Pantothenic acid	Necessary for the citric acid cycle in mitochondrial production of ATP. Necessary for gluconeogenesis and lipid synthesis
Biotin	Necessary for pyruvic acid breakdown in ATP synthesis. Important in lipid and nucleic acid synthesis
Folate	Important in hematopoiesis and nucleic acid synthesis
B$_{12}$, cyanocobalamin	Important in erythropoiesis (formation of red blood cells), methionine synthesis, choline synthesis, and the citric acid cycle in mitochondrial production of ATP
C	Important in protein metabolism, especially in the synthesis of extracellular matrix proteins and for the maintenance of mucous membranes. Antioxidant with immune system functions
Fat-soluble Vitamins	**Effect**
A	Necessary for rhodopsin production. Involved in osteoclast/osteoblast activity regulation. Necessary for epithelial health
D	Role in calcium and phosphate absorption in the alimentary canal, and resorption in the kidneys
E	Important antioxidant, necessary for erythropoiesis and nucleic acid synthesis
K	Necessary for synthesis of clotting factors

ATP = adenosine triphosphate.

this structure. The enteroendocrine cells produce hormones that play a regulatory role elsewhere in the digestive system. These hormones are presented in **TABLE 18.3**. With this, we are ready to move into the large intestine (don't take that literally).

■ Your Large Intestine

Here we are at the large intestine. There are numerous differences between the small intestine and the large in-

testine. We will discuss them in a moment, but first we need to consider some gross anatomy. The entire large intestine is about 5 feet long and 2.5 inches in diameter. There are three main regions to the large intestine: the cecum, the colon, and the rectum. We will discuss each of these three regions in turn.

The large intestine begins at the ileocecal valve, a sphincter we have already discussed. This is the doorway between the ileum and the cecum, the first portion

Table 18.3 Hormones of the Small Intestine

Name	Effects on Stomach	Effects on Accessory Organs
Gastrin*	Increased secretion and motility	None
Secretin	Reduced secretion and motility	Increased pancreatic exocrine secretion (particularly bicarbonate ions); increased bile secretion from the liver
CCK	Reduced secretion and motility	Increased pancreatic exocrine secretion (particularly enzymes); increased bile secretion from the gallbladder
GIP	Reduced secretion and motility	Increased release of insulin from the pancreatic islets

CCK = cholecystokinin; GIP = gastric-inhibiting peptide.
*Gastrin is produced in the stomach and small intestine.

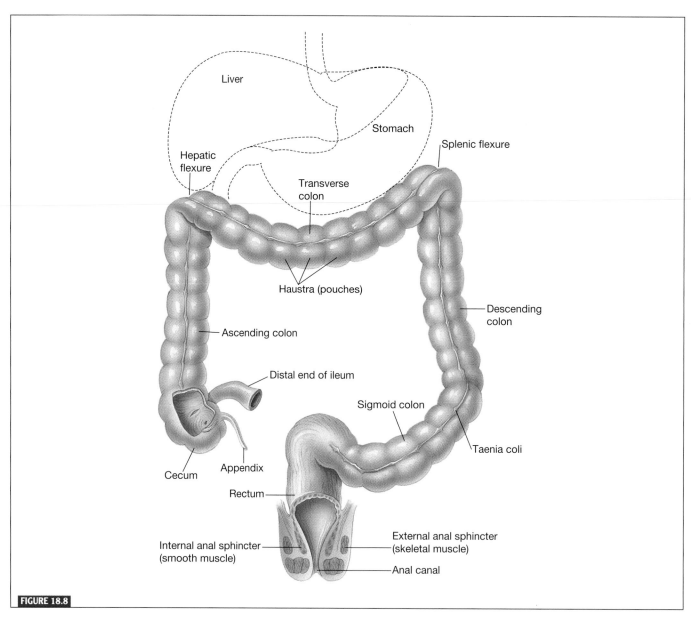

Liver

Stomach

Splenic flexure

Hepatic flexure

Transverse colon

Haustra (pouches)

Descending colon

Ascending colon

Distal end of ileum

Sigmoid colon

Cecum

Appendix

Taenia coli

Rectum

Internal anal sphincter (smooth muscle)

External anal sphincter (skeletal muscle)

Anal canal

FIGURE 18.8

The large intestine.

of the large intestine (**FIGURE 18.8**). The term *cecum* comes from the Latin term meaning "blind," for this is a blind pouch or cul-de-sac. It is small in humans (6 × 7.5 cm), but it can be quite large in some grass-eating nonruminants (like the horse, in which it is big enough for you to crawl inside). In humans, it has a small (up to 10 cm) fingerlike appendage extending from its inferior and posterior surface: the vermiform appendix. The appendix is a layered structure, like other portions of the alimentary canal; however, it is mainly composed of lymphatic tissue and, as such, has an immune system function. As you may have experienced, it often becomes inflamed (appendicitis) and must be removed.

We leave the cecum and enter the colon. The colon has several anatomical regions with which we must be-

come familiar. The first region is the ascending colon, running superiorly along the right lateral aspect of our abdominal cavity. It turns 90 degrees to the left, as the hepatic flexure. It then becomes the transverse colon, running from right to left across the anterior aspect of the abdominal cavity, just inferior to the stomach and liver. When it reaches the left side, it again turns 90 degrees to run in an inferior direction as the descending colon. This turn is called the splenic flexure (that is, the turn between the transverse colon and the descending colon). How can you keep the order of the two flexures straight? Remember that they are in alphabetical order (hepatic before splenic). If you also remember that the splenic flexure is on the left side, you will always remember where the spleen is.

The descending colon travels down the left side of the abdominopelvic cavity, and the anus is in the midline; if these two structures are to connect, we must have more "bends in the road." We do; the sigmoid colon (*sigmoid* meaning "S"-shaped) extends from the descending colon on the left to the rectum in the midline. It is the last region of the colon.

The colon is easily recognized grossly by its pouched appearance (Figure 18.8). These pouches, or haustra, are produced by three distinct bands of smooth muscle that run longitudinally along the colon. These muscular bands, the taenia coli, remain slightly contracted and produce these pouches. To imagine this, picture the sleeve of your shirt pushed up partway. Notice that the tubular sleeve gains a number of pouches from being shortened in this way. That is what the haustra are like.

The rectum is the final 8 inches of your large intestine. It is for the storage of fecal matter before its removal by the reflex action called defecation. It extends from the sigmoid colon to the anus, the distal orifice leading from your alimentary canal. The anus is held closed by two muscular sphincters. The internal anal sphincter is of smooth muscle; its action is, therefore, involuntary. The external anal sphincter is skeletal muscle and is under voluntary control.

We will spend our time discussing the colon, although you can assume that the activities of the cecum are very similar. The rectum, on the other hand, is simply for storage before evacuation at the proper time.

What would you expect of the histology of the colon? Well, to answer that, you might need to know a little about its function. The colon is responsible for less than 10 percent of the absorption performed in the alimentary canal (we will discuss this absorption in a moment). Its main job is feces formation: removing water from the matter that reaches it, and turning that matter into feces. Given that, you can assume that we will find a different structure here than we saw in the small intestine.

Picture for a moment a large river in the far north. In fact, a river that meets the sea and has boats coming in and out in the warm months. This river freezes in the winter, and large masses of ice travel down it toward the sea. Would it be a good idea to have long docks extending out from the shoreline into the current during the winter months? No, and you can picture why not, if you think about what the moving ice would do to the docks.

Now picture your colon. They may not be large blocks of ice, as in the river, but as well-formed masses of feces move along, could you picture what they would do to villi if they were present? The villi, like the docks, would not withstand that punishment. The colon contains crypts, but no villi (**FIGURE 18.9**).

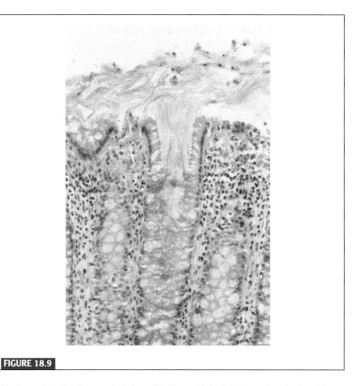

The large intestine has crypts but no villi. The goblet cell is the main colonic epithelial cell type. Goblet cells produce mucus, which flows from the crypts (shown here) into the colonic lumen.

What type of epithelium would you expect to find here? Before we answer that, let's think about the differences between the colon and small intestine. Do we need vast numbers of enterocytes here, as we had in the small intestine? Remember, they had microvilli on their apical surfaces to give lots of surface area for absorption. Since little absorption is going on here, they are probably not that necessary. How about the second most common cell type from the small intestine: the goblet cell. Since we need to keep the feces moving (we all know what happens if they don't), we had better keep them well lubricated. The goblet cell, therefore, is the main cell type in the colon, and these cells are present in a simple columnar epithelium (Figure 18.9).

Again, we have stem cells and endocrine cells in the bases of the crypts. The daughter cells differentiate into mainly goblet cells and some enterocytes, as they migrate up the crypt toward the lumen. Once they reach the luminal surface, they are sloughed off.

Mechanical Digestion in Your Large Intestine

Large intestinal movements begin as substances to be processed enter the cecum. Movement from the cecum is slow: it takes time to remove enough water to turn this material into a paste, which will be further thickened in the colon itself. We already learned that the gastroileal reflex causes the contents of the ileum to enter the cecum as the stomach is being filled with the next meal. The ileocecal valve constricts as the cecum becomes filled in a negative feedback arrangement: as the cecum becomes full, this sphincter restricts flow to keep it from becoming overfilled.

Colonic movements begin as substances enter the haustra (the pouches of the colon). Each haustrum contracts as it becomes filled up, pushing its contents to the next haustrum. This is called haustral churning.

Peristalsis also plays a role here. These waves of contraction, running distally, occur more slowly here than elsewhere in the alimentary canal.

Mass peristalsis is a distinct colonic movement. It is stronger than peristalsis and begins in the middle of the transverse colon. Mass peristalsis moves the contents of the lower half of the colon into the rectum. The presence of food in the stomach triggers this reflex action, thereby making room for the material arriving from the ileum. This is called the gastrocolic reflex. For this reason, you may notice that the urge to defecate usually occurs shortly after mealtime. Those who work in the geriatric health-care system (nursing homes) are often quick to make this association.

Chemical Digestion in Your Large Intestine

Now here's something different from what we've seen before. Chemical digestion in the large intestine is not based on the activity of enzymes from the alimentary canal or accessory organs. Chemical digestion in the large intestine is the work of bacteria that reside there. Remember, mucus is secreted in great quantity into the colon, but enzymes are not.

Bacteria ferment the remaining nutrients into simple compounds. Carbohydrates are broken down into carbon dioxide, hydrogen, and methane gas. This is the source of colonic flatus. So, next time, blame it on the bacteria!

Proteins or amino acids that reach this point are converted into simple chemical substances such as indole and skatole (which give feces their characteristic odor), hydrogen sulfide, and fatty acids.

The liver, which we have not yet studied, converts hemoglobin recycled from erythrocytes into bilirubin. Bilirubin is delivered to the small intestine in bile from the liver. The bilirubin that makes it to the colon is converted to urobilinogen by bacterial action. Urobilinogen gives feces their characteristic color.

Some vitamins are produced by the bacteria of the colon. These include some B vitamins and vitamin K.

Absorption in Your Large Intestine

As mentioned, the main responsibility of the colon is feces formation. That is important because we can not afford to lose the water that enters the colon each day, or we would dehydrate. Of the nearly 1 liter that enters the colon daily, only about 100 milliliters leaves the colon in the feces. This is accomplished by osmosis; as electrolytes and other solutes are absorbed, water follows by osmosis, making the feces more compact. There is a limit to the benefit here, however.

The average daily fecal mass in parts of the world where people eat a diet low in animal fat but high in grain (a high fiber diet) is nearly three times that of people eating the high-fat, low-fiber diet typical in the United States. Now, you may ask, why would we want those bigger stools? Well, the transit time through the colon is greatly reduced by producing bulkier, more fluid stools. Simply put, because there is more of it, it can't be kept around as long. The amount of water that is removed is directly related to how long the feces take to make it through the colon. The longer it takes to move materials through the colon, the harder the resulting stools become. The colon has an easier time moving larger, looser stools. It is also exposed to toxic byproducts of fermentation for a shorter period. Certain colonic diseases that plague western society (i.e., colon cancer and diverticulitis) are virtually unknown by people in cultures that eat this low-fat, high-fiber diet. Doesn't this give you one more reason to watch what you eat?

With this, we exit the alimentary canal. We will now consider the accessory organs of digestion before returning to the digestion, absorption, and metabolism of fats.

18.3 Accessory Organs of Digestion

■ Your Salivary Glands

Saliva is an important fluid. It keeps the mouth, oropharynx, and laryngopharynx moist; lubricates food for ease in swallowing; dissolves substances in our food, thereby enabling our sense of taste; and begins the process of chemical digestion. Saliva is produced by two types of glands (**FIGURE 18.10**). Buccal glands, which lay within the mucosa and submucosa of the mouth, contribute a small amount of saliva. Their secretion is the source of lingual lipase. The larger amount is produced by the glands we typically think of as "salivary glands." Although saliva is secreted continuously, its secretion increases in response to the presence of food and decreases in response to stress. The parasympathetic nervous system increases saliva production; the sympathetic nervous system decreases saliva production.

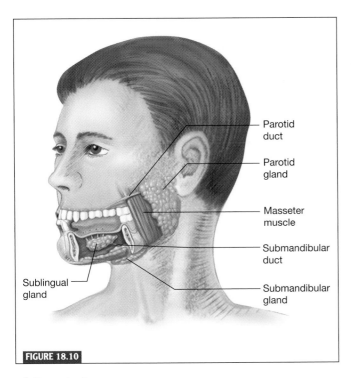

FIGURE 18.10

Salivary glands.

This accounts for the dry mouth you experience when frightened. There are three pairs of salivary glands: the parotids, the submandibulars, and the sublinguals.

Saliva is actually a combination of several types of secretions produced by these glands. Of the nearly 1.5 liters produced daily, our saliva is 99.5 percent water. It also contains salts and ions; bicarbonate, which serves as a buffer; dissolved gasses; nitrogenous wastes; several serum proteins; the enzyme lysozyme, which kills bacteria; salivary amylase for digestion of carbohydrates; and mucin. Mucin is a glycoprotein that swells greatly in water and serves as an effective lubricant, that is, it forms mucus.

The parotid glands are inferior and anterior to the ears. They deliver their secretion to the vicinity of the second upper molars. They produce a serous (watery) secretion containing salivary amylase. The submandibular glands are inferior to the tongue and medial to the mandibles. They deliver their secretion to the floor of the mouth at the anterior aspect of the base of the tongue. In fact, you can observe these ducts if you look in the mirror, lift your tongue, and look either side of the lingual frenulum. The lingual frenulum is that ridge you will observe running medially on the inferior surface of the anterior part of your tongue. The submandibular glands produce a serous secretion, mucus, and salivary amylase.

The sublingual glands are anterior, medial, and superior to the submandibular glands. Their secretion is delivered through several ducts, lateral to the tongue, in the floor of the mouth. These ducts can also be observed in the mirror, posterior to those of the submandibular glands; however, they are not as easy to see. They produce mainly mucus.

■ Your Pancreas

This organ has already been discussed as an endocrine gland. Here we must draw attention to its exocrine component. The exocrine component makes up 99 percent of the pancreas and is composed of secretory units called acini. An acinus is merely a group of secretory cells arranged in a saclike manner. The word *acinus* comes from the Latin word for grape, as the structure resembles grapes arranged on a stem of secretory ducts. This structure is shown in **FIGURE 18.11**. The location of the pancreas and its ducts are shown in **FIGURE 18.12**.

The liquid secreted by the excretory pancreas is called pancreatic juice. Nearly 1.5 liters of pancreatic juice are produced per day. It is composed of water, plus electrolytes; sodium bicarbonate, which acts as a buffer; and a variety of enzymes. The protein-digesting enzymes trypsin, chymotrypsin, and carboxypeptidase are all secreted in an inactive form to protect the pancreas from accidental digestion. The inactive forms are called trypsinogen, chymotrypsinogen, and procarboxypeptidase, respectively. They are activated by enterokinase, a phosphorylating enzyme produced by the small intestinal epithelium.

Pancreatic lipase for lipid digestion, ribonuclease and deoxyribonuclease for nucleic acid digestion, and pancreatic amylase for carbohydrate digestion are also produced here. All of these enzymes are delivered to the duodenum through one or two ducts. I say "one or two" because this is one of those places in which there is some variability in the anatomy of different individuals. All people have the duct called the pancreatic duct (of Wirsung). Some people also have a second duct, the accessory duct (of Santorini). In some individuals, this duct is present but incomplete. Whether or not this second duct is present does not matter at all to the functioning of this gland. Notice that I am putting part of the names of each of these structures in parentheses. The names of these structures are currently used without this portion (the name of the person who described the structure). I include that portion of the name because you may find it in your supplemental reading. Also, I find that including this portion of the name makes these ducts easier to remember. Use them or ignore them as you choose.

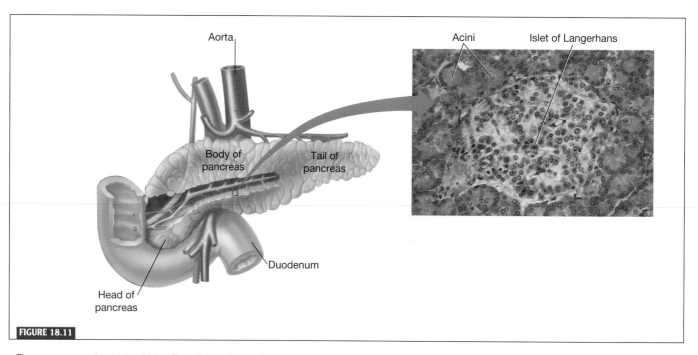

FIGURE 18.11

The pancreas contains acini and islets. The acini are the exocrine component of the pancreas and produce digestive enzymes for delivery to the duodenum. The islets are endocrine structures and were discussed in Chapter 13.

Notice the simplified drawing in Figure 18.12. This is a "roadmap" view of the anatomy of the ducts of the pancreas, liver, and gallbladder. The relationships of these structures are more easily understood when drawn this way than in a more "anatomically correct" drawing.

Please familiarize yourself with this anatomy before proceeding to the liver. Note that the secretions of the liver, gallbladder, and pancreas are all delivered to the duodenum through the hepatopancreatic ampulla (of Vater) at the duodenal papilla. Note also that the opening of

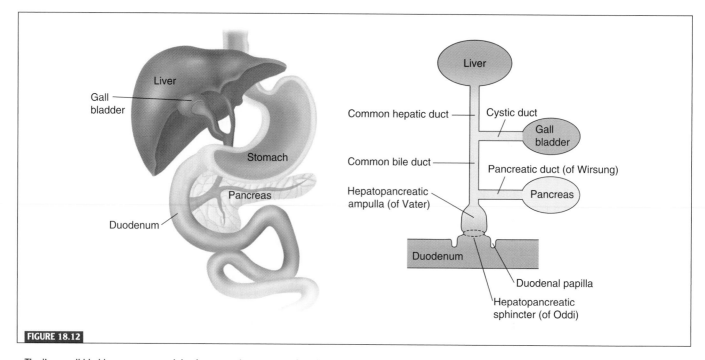

FIGURE 18.12

The liver, gall bladder, pancreas, and duodenum are interconnected as shown. The schematic diagram makes this anatomy easier to comprehend.

this papilla can be constricted by the hepatopancreatic sphincter (of Oddi).

Your Liver

Your liver is one of the most amazing organs in the human body. The range of its activities is truly mind boggling. As you study this organ, you will see why proper functioning of the liver is so crucial to the maintenance of homeostasis. So important is its functioning that, even if as much as 75 percent of your liver were removed, you would still be able to survive. Your liver has that much excess functional capacity, barring extenuating circumstances, of course. In fact, your liver has the ability to regenerate after such tissue loss; its cells would increase their rate of division and in a short time would replace the lost tissue.

Your liver is located inferior to your diaphragm and weighs a little more than 3 pounds. It is divided up into different numbers of lobes by different anatomists.

Based on the circulatory arrangement, there are two major lobes: the right and left lobes. The left lobe is associated with small caudate and quadrate lobes.

The liver is composed of many functional units called lobules (**FIGURE 18.13**). Each lobule consists of a central vein from which radiate plates of hepatocytes, the parenchymal cells of the liver. The arrangement of these plates is reminiscent of the spokes of a wheel, radiating out from a central hub. Between the plates of hepatocytes, we find sinusoids lined with endothelial cells. Blood flows through these sinusoids on its way to the central vein. Kupffer cells, the resident cells of the monocyte-macrophage lineage, roam through the sinusoids and among the hepatocytes phagocytizing debris. This makes the liver an effective blood filter.

If you have seen liver (i.e., calves liver with bacon and onions), it may surprise you to learn that this is an epithelial structure: hepatocytes are epithelial cells. This is surprising because of the dense arrangement of these

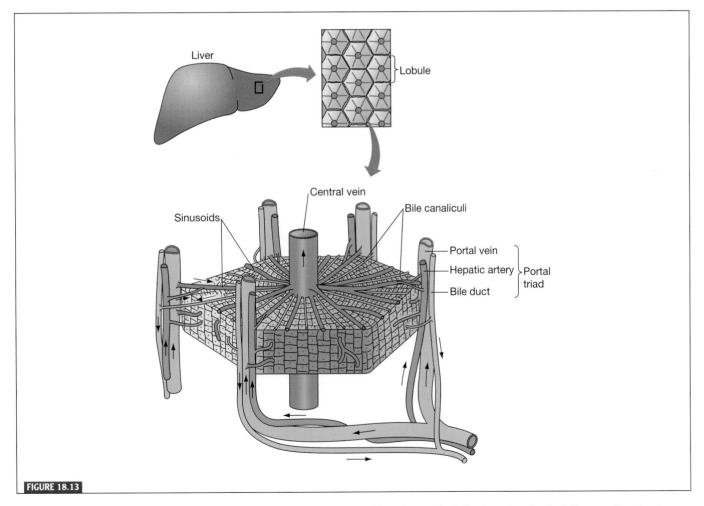

FIGURE 18.13

Liver lobules. Hepatocytes are arranged in rows within the lobule, extending outward from the central vein like the spokes of a wheel. The rows of hepatocytes are separated by sinusoids. Hepatocytes line bile canaliculi.

cells; epithelial cells must line something. What do the hepatocytes line?

Between the hepatocytes, we find small canals called bile canaliculi (Figure 18.13). This is what the hepatocytes line. The canaliculi carry bile, the liver's main product, to bile ducts, which join to form the right and left hepatic ducts. The right and left hepatic ducts join to form the common hepatic duct that exits from the liver. Notice the common hepatic duct in Figure 18.12.

The liver has a dual blood supply. Do you remember what a portal system is? We discussed portal systems in Chapter 13 while describing the anterior pituitary.

The liver receives blood that has already passed through capillary beds in the alimentary canal, through the hepatic portal vein. The hepatic portal vein delivers newly absorbed nutrients directly to the liver for processing. The liver also receives blood through the hepatic artery. This artery delivers oxygenated blood to the liver. Blood from both of these supplies flows together in the sinusoids and exits the liver through hepatic central veins leading to the inferior vena cava.

Bile Synthesis and Secretion

In a moment, we will learn of the many functions that the liver fulfills. First, it is important to understand that the liver produces bile. Bile is the secretion of the liver. It has both secretory (as a useful product) and excretory (as a waste) roles. You may know what bile is like from vomiting it up during some illness. It is a yellow-brownish-green liquid. Your liver produces about 1 liter of bile per day. It consists of water, bile salts and pigments, cholesterol, lecithin, and ions. Bile salts are polar derivatives of cholesterol, the major one being glycholate (**FIGURE 18.14**). Together with the bile phospholipid lecithin, they act as detergents to emulsify fats (more

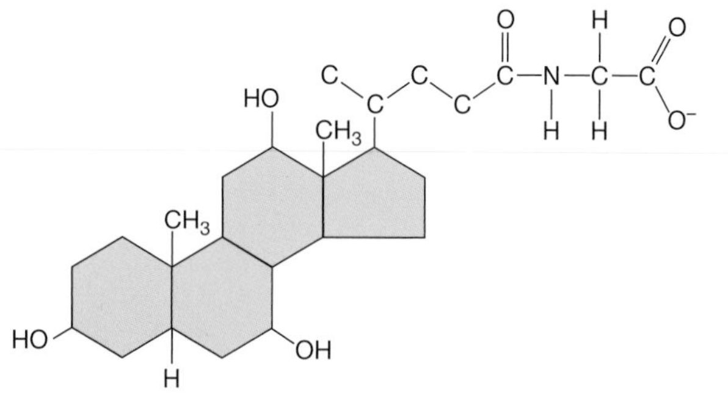

FIGURE 18.14

Glycholate, a bile salt derived from cholesterol.

on that in the "Lipid Metabolism" section at the end of this chapter).

The main bile pigment is bilirubin. About 70 percent of bilirubin is the product of erythrocyte degradation, which occurs mainly in the spleen. When old erythrocytes (the life span of an erythrocyte is only about 4 months) are degraded, something must be done with the hemoglobin contained in them. While much of this large protein can be broken down into amino acids for recycling, the iron-containing heme group would become toxic if allowed to accumulate. After removing much of the iron for recycling, heme groups are converted to bilirubin, mainly by macrophages, and then delivered to hepatocytes for excretion. Bilirubin is processed by the hepatocytes and added to the bile. It is then transported to the duodenum for excretion in the feces. Bilirubin gives bile its rather unappealing color. Bilirubin is converted to urobilinogen in the colon, giving feces their color.

Parasympathetic stimulation and the hormone secretin cause increased bile release from the liver. It is also stimulated by high rates of blood flow to the liver and increased rates of bile synthesis, which can be influenced by diet.

During times when bile is being synthesized but is not needed in the small intestine (no meal is being digested), it is stored in the gallbladder. The gallbladder is a pear-shaped pouch, 3–4 inches long, attached to the right lobe of the liver. It is lined with simple columnar epithelium. Its functions are the storage and concentration of bile. While being stored, bile may be concentrated up to tenfold by the removal of water. As we have seen elsewhere, the epithelial cells of the gallbladder transport ions out of the bile, and water follows by osmosis. This is the mechanism of bile concentration.

The gallbladder contracts in response to cholecystokinin (CCK) from the enteroendocrine cells of the small intestine. Remember that secretin stimulates bile secretion from the liver, while CCK causes bile release from the gallbladder.

Functions of Your Liver

So, in addition to producing bile, what does the liver do, anyway? At more than 3 pounds, there is enough of it that it better do something important! It certainly does do a number of important things. Let's look at some of them.

The liver serves as a reservoir for the storage of energy (glycogen), minerals, and vitamins. It is also an important filter of the blood; the Kupffer cells (macrophages) found here phagocytize bacteria and worn-out blood cells, thereby eliminating them from circulation.

Imagine all of the molecules that circulate in our blood that have biological effects. Many of them (hormones, for example) are produced within our bodies. Others are contained within the food we eat as either naturally occurring substances or man-made products. Drugs taken to restore homeostasis during an illness, or for other legitimate or illicit reasons, also fall into this category. We also absorb molecules through our skin and respiratory tracts that have potential effects on our bodies. All of these molecules must be inactivated or we would soon be overwhelmed. The liver is the main site of inactivation of bioactive and potentially toxic substances. The smooth endoplasmic reticulum of the hepatocytes contains enzyme systems capable of breaking down many substances. The main enzyme system for this purpose is called the mixed-function oxidase system. In almost all cases, the activities of this system are to our benefit. In some cases, however, the resulting products turn out to be more toxic than the substance with which the liver started. Furthermore, when some drugs are administered for a long period of time to treat chronic conditions, the dosage must be repeatedly increased, and ultimately the drug may completely lose efficacy because of the increased ability of the liver to degrade the drug. All in all, it is amazing how this organ can adapt to deal with the innumerable substances that are delivered to it.

What about other forms of metabolism? We know that the alimentary canal delivers much of the nutrients it absorbs directly to the liver through a portal system (**FIGURE 18.15**). This system is made up of capillaries in the walls of the alimentary canal that drain into the hepatic portal vein. This vein directly supplies the hepatic sinusoids, delivering the absorbed nutrients to the hepatocytes. Ultimately, this blood leaves the liver through the hepatic veins, which connect to the inferior vena

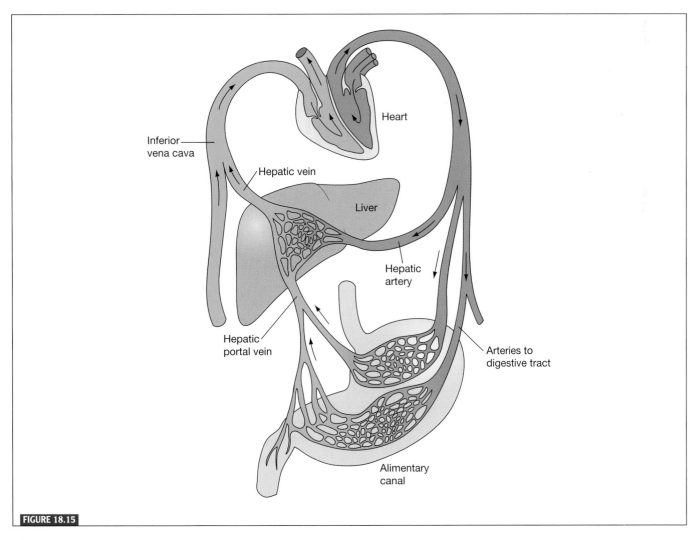

FIGURE 18.15

The hepatic portal system.

cava. The liver must, therefore, be able to process large quantities of nutrients. It is able to do this; we will briefly discuss its role in each of the categories of molecules about which we have learned.

Protein metabolism in the liver takes many forms. Your blood contains many proteins that are produced in your liver. These include albumin, the main molecule responsible for the blood's osmotic balance, and the proteins of the blood-clotting system. To produce these proteins (or any proteins, for that matter), all of the amino acids required must be present. In some cases, that means all 20 amino acids must be available. If some are not present, synthesis of that protein cannot occur.

The liver is the main site where amino acids may be either synthesized or converted: an abundant amino acid into a less-abundant one. Obviously, not all amino acids are interchangeable in this way; some transformations are possible, while others are not. About half of our 20 amino acids are essential amino acids; they must be present in our diet as we can neither synthesize them nor convert other amino acids into them. For some, however, this conversion can be important. Our liver, therefore, is important in maintaining appropriate levels of availability of amino acids.

If we are producing proteins and synthesizing or converting amino acids here, what about protein and amino acid degradation? This is also the main site of protein and amino acid degradation in the body. We may degrade proteins as part of a recycling effort to rid the body of unneeded, worn-out proteins. We may also degrade proteins (and their amino acids) to release the energy and atoms they contain for other uses (more in a moment). In either case, this is the main place to do it.

So, what actually happens to amino acids that come out of the proteins we are degrading? A major step in their breakdown is deamination: removal of the amino group (NH_2) from the amino acid. The amino group becomes ammonia (NH_3), which is a toxic nitrogenous waste. The liver again comes to the rescue by converting ammonia into the less toxic nitrogenous waste urea (see **FIGURE 18.16**) for excretion by the kidneys. So, if the liver can produce and degrade proteins, and synthesize,

convert, and degrade amino acids, what can it do with carbohydrates?

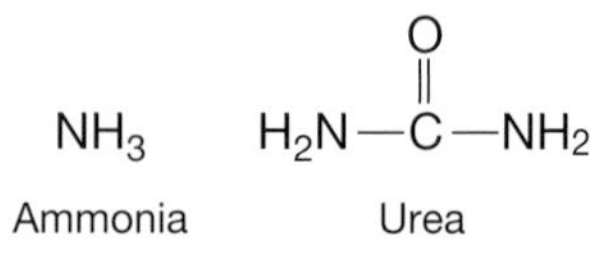

The liver has a long list of abilities when it comes to carbohydrates (**FIGURE 18.17**). It has an important role in our carbohydrate homeostasis: in response to insulin and glucagon, it maintains blood glucose levels within the necessary range. It is a major site of glucose storage in the form of glycogen. Therefore, it is capable of glycogenesis, production of glycogen, and glycogenolysis, breakdown of glycogen to free glucose for use as energy. Gluconeogenesis also occurs here. Gluconeogenesis is the de novo production of glucose using proteins and lipids, but not carbohydrates, as the source of material. It is used when glucose is in short supply and is another reason that protein and amino acid breakdown occur in the liver. Obviously, glycolysis (breakdown of glucose to generate ATP) also occurs here.

18.4 Lipid Metabolism: We Saved the Best for Last

This is where the liver really gets interesting. We will cover all of lipid metabolism (digestion, absorption, processing, and excretion) here. This is the last topic we will cover in this chapter, and we needed all of the other "pieces of the puzzle" before we could discuss these processes. It is sometimes good to "save the best for last."

■ Lipid Digestion and Absorption

Most of the lipids we consume are triglycerides that, as you recall from way back in Chapter 2, are composed of one glycerol molecule with three fatty-acid side chains. We need to follow fats, composed mainly of this molecule, through the alimentary canal (**FIGURE 18.18**).

We start with the fats in the mouth. Although mechanical digestion is occurring, very little chemical digestion of fats can occur in the mouth: lingual lipase (fat-digesting enzyme) is present but not especially effective. We follow these fats through the esophagus where, again, little chemical digestion of fats will occur. Next, in the stomach, gastric lipase is present; however, it too is ineffective. Why are these two lipases ineffective?

What happens when you place greasy dishes in a sink of water without detergent? The molecules of grease (lipids) aggregate or stick together. This is because they are hydrophobic (nonpolar) molecules in an aqueous environment. Remember that the water molecules are polar; water is a polar solvent. The situation is similar for the lipids in your saliva or stomach.

That still may leave you wondering why the lipase doesn't work. Picture a picnic for you and everyone else

$$NH_3 \qquad H_2N-\overset{\overset{\displaystyle O}{\|}}{C}-NH_2$$

Ammonia   Urea

FIGURE 18.16

The nitrogenous wastes ammonia and urea.

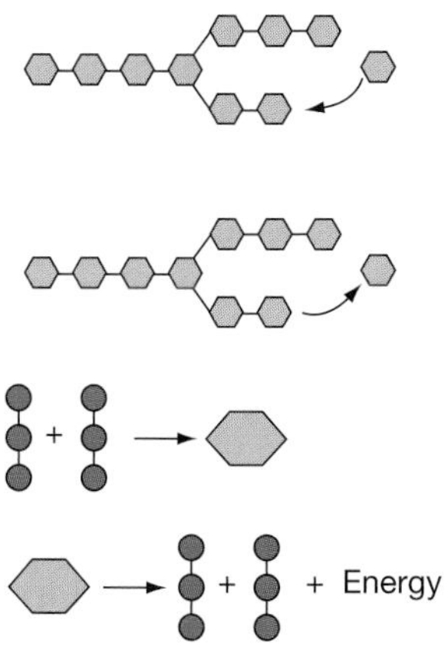

	Term	Definition
	Glycogenesis	Production of glycogen: storage of glucose in the form of glycogen
	Glycogenolysis	Breakdown of glycogen: release of glucose from glycogen storage
	Gluconeogenesis	De novo synthesis of glucose: production of glucose from protein or lipid precursors
	Glycolysis	Breakdown of glucose to two pyruvic acids, resulting in the production of two molecules of ATP

FIGURE 18.17

Forms of carbohydrate metabolism.

in your school. The caterer at this picnic decided to make meatballs for everyone to eat, but instead of making lots of small meatballs, he made one giant one. This meatball is huge, large enough to feed your entire school. There is one problem, however. Your schoolmates simply do not have access to it in an efficient manner. They have no way to distribute portions of this giant meatball, so everyone must gnaw away from the outside of it. This really would not work; it would take far too long to eat it that way. It is a similar situation with the fats in the stomach. Because they are in the form of large globules (because of their hydrophobic nature), the lipase molecules simply can't get to the fat molecules to digest them. So again, essentially no fat digestion occurs here.

Next, our essentially undigested fats enter the small intestine. Here is where things begin to happen. Bile is delivered to the duodenum from the liver and gallbladder through the duodenal papilla. The bile salts and lecithin present in the bile act as detergents. Much the way dishwashing detergent breaks up droplets of fat in your dishwater, these molecules break up (emulsify) fats in the chyme into droplets about 1 micrometer in diameter. Lipase can work on these small droplets of fat.

Lipase breaks each molecule of the triglycerides into one monoglyceride (a glycerol with one fatty acid side chain) and two fatty acids. Now we're making progress with the fats. Short-chain fatty acids (those with perhaps 12 carbons or less) can be directly absorbed into the intestinal epithelium at this point. The problem is that most of the side chains are long-chain fatty acids, and we also have the monoglycerides to think about.

Fatty acids of more than about 12 carbons and monoglycerides are still hydrophobic molecules in an aqueous medium; they still want to clump together. They need a carrier to travel within the chyme. Again, bile comes to the rescue. Bile salts, which are polar, form small (2.5 nanometer) spheres around groups of monoglycerides and fatty acids. These spheres, called micelles, can diffuse around in the chyme until they reach the epithelium. There the contents of the micelles are released and diffuse through the phospholipid bilayer of these cells (they are absorbed). The bile salts remain behind to carry more lipids within the chyme.

If you are having trouble picturing this, think of it this way. If you wanted to drive across a river in your car and there was no bridge, you would have a problem. In essence, your car is "hydrophobic;" it can not move about in a watery environment. A ferryboat could carry your car about in the water until it reached the place where your car could be "absorbed" onto the land. The car is like the lipids; the ferryboat is like the bile salts (Figure 18.18).

Once the lipids are absorbed by the intestinal epithelium, they are processed into triglycerides in preparation for export from the epithelium. We must get them to the liver for further processing. We have a problem, however; the lipids that have been absorbed must again travel in an aqueous medium. Triglycerides, phospholipids, and cholesterol molecules that have been absorbed into the intestinal epithelium are packaged with carrier proteins and leave the intestinal epithelium as structures called chylomicrons. As for the bile salts, most are ultimately reabsorbed, but a percentage is lost each day in the feces.

Chylomicrons travel first in the interstitial fluid, then in lymphatic vessels, and later in the blood. They do not directly diffuse into capillaries because of their large size; they have easier access to the open-ended lymphatic vessels. They travel into the blood of the left subclavian vein with the lymphatic fluid and then into general circulation.

Most of the fatty acids contained in the circulating chylomicrons are removed for use in adipose and muscle tissue before ever reaching the liver. The triglycerides that reach the liver (in the chylomicrons) are broken down into glycerol and fatty acids. Hepatocytes then reassemble them into triglycerides and package them with carrier proteins called apoproteins for transport in the blood stream as lipoproteins. We are about to learn about a few classes of lipoproteins. They differ from each other in their relative content of various lipids and in the actual apoproteins of which they are composed. Keep in mind that the apoproteins are produced by the liver and are the portion of the lipoprotein that determines where the lipids will be delivered. It is as if they are different types of envelopes, carrying different addresses. The "address" on the apoprotein envelope determines which cells will receive the lipid contained within that apoprotein envelope.

The liver produces very low-density lipoproteins (VLDLs), mainly for the delivery of fatty acids to adipose tissue for storage. Once the adipose cells remove triglycerides from the VLDLs, they are transported back to the liver. The lipids they contain are then repackaged by hepatocytes, converting them into low-density lipoproteins (LDLs). Low-density lipoproteins travel through the blood delivering their contents, mainly cholesterol, to tissues throughout the body. Their ability to deliver cholesterol to cells in arterial walls makes elevated LDL levels a risk factor in people with a genetic predisposition for atherosclerotic disease.

As the cells that receive LDLs degrade them and use the cholesterol they contain for cell membrane syntheses, steroid syntheses, and other purposes, excess cholesterol diffuses out of these cells into the blood. This cholesterol must be packaged for transport back to the liver (remember, lipids can not travel in the bloodstream without a carrier). The liver produces apoproteins for this purpose.

The liver produces the apoproteins of high-density lipoproteins (HDLs) and releases them into the blood. They act like small lipid "sponges," traveling through the blood absorbing the lipids that were delivered to cells throughout the body by the LDLs, but not needed by these cells. Their lipid "scavenging" removes lipids that could be used by the cells of arterial walls in the development of atherosclerotic lesions; hence, increasing levels of HDLs in people with a genetic predisposition for atherosclerotic disease has a protective value against the development of these lesions (see the "Breaching Homeostasis" section in Chapter 16). High-density lipoproteins transport lipids back to the liver so they can be processed into bile salts for delivery to the duodenum. In this way, the lipids in your diet are used for energy by your cells (either through their own breakdown or through their use in gluconeogenesis), for the production of lipids needed by your cells (i.e., plasmalemma, prostaglandins, and steroids), and in the digestion and absorption of more dietary lipids. Figure 18.18 depicts fat absorption and metabolism in detail.

This ends our discussion of the digestive system. This has been a lot of material, and there is a lot to remember about what happens where in the alimentary canal. Be sure to use the "What You Should Know" and "What Did You Learn?" features of this chapter before moving on.

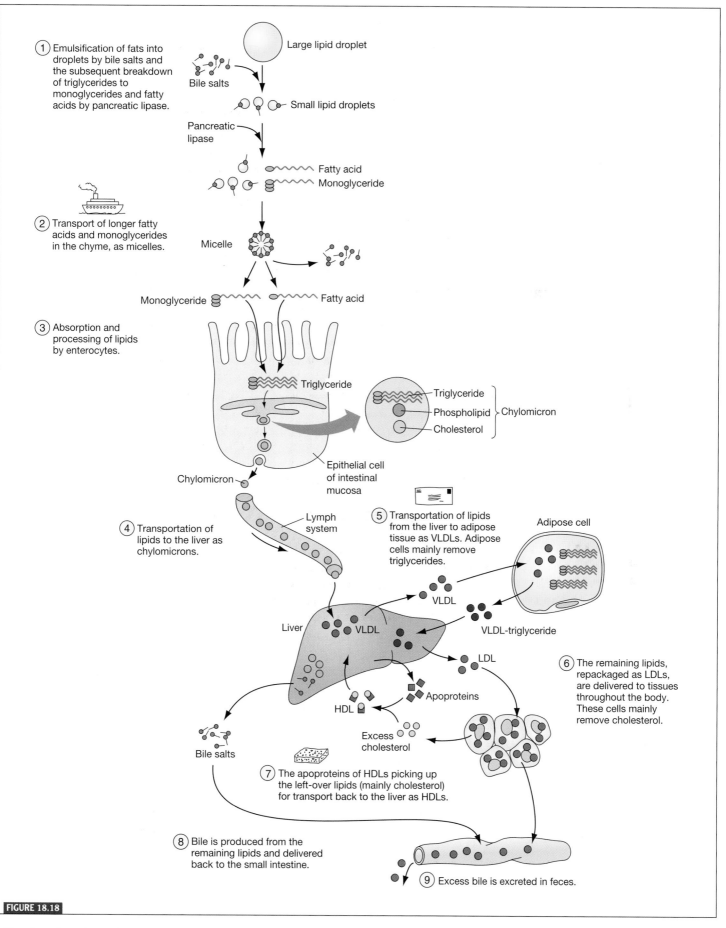

1. Emulsification of fats into droplets by bile salts and the subsequent breakdown of triglycerides to monoglycerides and fatty acids by pancreatic lipase.

Large lipid droplet

Bile salts

Small lipid droplets

Pancreatic lipase

Fatty acid
Monoglyceride

2. Transport of longer fatty acids and monoglycerides in the chyme, as micelles.

Micelle

Monoglyceride   Fatty acid

3. Absorption and processing of lipids by enterocytes.

Triglyceride

Triglyceride
Phospholipid   } Chylomicron
Cholesterol

Epithelial cell of intestinal mucosa

Chylomicron

4. Transportation of lipids to the liver as chylomicrons.

Lymph system

5. Transportation of lipids from the liver to adipose tissue as VLDLs. Adipose cells mainly remove triglycerides.

Adipose cell

VLDL

VLDL-triglyceride

Liver   VLDL

LDL

6. The remaining lipids, repackaged as LDLs, are delivered to tissues throughout the body. These cells mainly remove cholesterol.

Apoproteins

HDL

Excess cholesterol

Bile salts

7. The apoproteins of HDLs picking up the left-over lipids (mainly cholesterol) for transport back to the liver as HDLs.

8. Bile is produced from the remaining lipids and delivered back to the small intestine.

9. Excess bile is excreted in feces.

FIGURE 18.18

Digestion, absorption, and transportation of lipids.

Breaching Homeostasis . . . When Things Go Wrong

How Laxatives Work

You know those television advertisements in which a lady starts talking about her husband's diarrhea in various inappropriate places? Well, we're not going to talk about diarrhea here; rather, the opposite. Did you ever wonder how laxatives work? That's what we're about to discuss.

We have just learned that feces are formed in the colon by removing water from the remaining waste. We also learned that the longer the transit time through the colon, the less water will be left in the feces. You can well imagine that a very hard, dry stool is difficult for the colon to move along. It sounds like positive feedback, doesn't it: the longer it takes to move the feces along, the smaller and harder it gets. The smaller and harder it gets, the longer it takes to pass it through. Well, I'm sure you get the idea.

So, what can be done to keep it moving? Laxatives can help. Let's see how they work. Laxatives can increase peristalsis, increase the liquid content of feces, or perform some combination of these functions.

You know that a high fiber diet works as a natural laxative. Some prepared laxatives work in a similar manner. They add mass to or "bulk-up" the feces. Methycellulose is a common active ingredient in these laxatives (incidentally, it is also used in many prepared foods and in wallpaper paste). We cannot digest or absorb it, so it makes it to our colon in a form that can bind water, resulting in a bulky, soft bowel movement. The increased fecal mass promotes peristalsis. The increased water content aids movement as well.

To increase water content, thereby lubricating and aiding movement, some laxatives alter the osmostic balance to keep water in the colon lumen. Ingestion of an ion or salt that is not readily absorbed has this effect. Magnesium ions are not readily absorbed. Salts of magnesium, therefore, work well for this purpose.

Some products increase peristalsis and water content at the same time. Think about the effect of hot pepper sauce accidentally introduced into your eyes. In fact, some "tear gas" products are hot pepper extracts. Similarly, some plant products irritate the colon, causing increased secretion of mucus and peristalsis. These "irritant" laxatives tend to be effective but harsh.

Sometimes classified as laxatives, stool softeners are actually emulsifying agents. Detergent-like preparations, like surfactants, they work to reduce surface tension. This promotes the mixing of fecal fat and water, producing a looser, more easily propelled stool.

If you think you are in need of a laxative, it is best to discuss the situation with your health-care provider. Pharmacists can also provide helpful suggestions. If you find you need these agents on more than rare occasions, you really need to seek professional advice; they can be habit forming and lead to other, more serious conditions. Furthermore, the underlying cause for your need should be addressed.

A diet that is high in fiber and low in fat can reduce your need for laxatives by performing the same function naturally. Diets of this type can help you to reduce your risk of a number of serious illnesses. Be sure to include lots of fruit and vegetables, as well as whole grains, in your diet daily.

What You Should Know

1. Your gastrointestinal system is composed of an alimentary canal and several accessory organs of digestion.
2. Your alimentary canal is a continuous tube running from your mouth to your anus.
3. Your alimentary canal is supported by a number of membranes, including the lesser omentum, mesentery, and mesocolon.
4. Digestion is the breakdown of ingested substances and it is carried out by mechanical and chemical means.
5. Absorption is the way in which we move ingested substances that have been broken down from the lumen of the alimentary canal into our bodies.
6. Your alimentary canal is a layered structure composed of a mucosa, submucosa, muscularis, and serosa.
7. Carbohydrate digestion begins in your mouth through the activity of salivary amylase.
8. Teeth have a complex structure of hard and soft tissue.

What You Should Know (continued)

9. The hard tissue, or dentin, of your teeth is produced by odontoblasts, and is covered with enamel.

10. Access to your esophagus is regulated by upper and lower esophageal sphincters.

11. Noncornified stratified squamous epithelium lines the muscular walls of your esophagus.

12. The carbohydrate digestion begun in your mouth continues as food passes through your esophagus.

13. Your stomach is an enlarged area of your alimentary canal with several distinct regions.

14. Your stomach's fundus is a storage area used during large meals.

15. The mucosa of your stomach is arranged into gastric pits, which greatly increase its surface area.

16. The simple columnar epithelium of your stomach contains a variety of cell types modified for specific purposes.

17. Gastric activity is regulated by neural and hormonal means.

18. Carbohydrate digestion is suspended in your stomach, but protein digestion begins here.

19. Your small intestine consists of your duodenum (proximal 10 inches), your jejunum (the next 8 feet), and the ileum (the distal 12 feet).

20. The mucosa of your small intestine is folded into villi and crypts.

21. The simple columnar epithelium of your small intestine is mainly composed of enterocytes with absorptive and secretory functions.

22. Pancreatic enzymes, bile from your liver, and enzymes produced by your small intestinal epithelium all play a role in chemical digestion in your small intestine.

23. You must know the names and activities of the digestive enzymes used in your small intestine.

24. The small intestine is the major site of absorption in your alimentary canal.

25. You must know in which form the various classes of compounds are absorbed.

26. Vitamins are necessary for the maintenance of homeostasis, yet generally cannot be produced by our bodies. These can be broken into two groups based on their solubility.

27. A few hormones are produced by cells in your small intestine. These regulate specific activities of your gastrointestinal system.

28. Your large intestine is composed of your cecum, colon, and rectum. Your colon has several anatomical regions. You must be familiar with these regions.

29. Crypts are present in your colonic mucosa, but villi are not.

30. The major cell type in the simple columnar epithelium of your large intestine is the goblet cell.

31. The major function of your large intestine is feces formation.

32. Digestion in your large intestine is by bacterial action, not the effect of enzymes.

33. Water, electrolytes, and some vitamins are absorbed in your large intestine.

34. Buccal glands, the parotid glands, and the sublingual glands produce saliva. You must know the locations of these glands.

35. Your pancreas has exocrine as well as endocrine functions. Its exocrine functions involve the production of a number of digestive enzymes.

36. Your liver, gallbladder, and pancreas are connected to your duodenum by several ducts that connect together and ultimately open into the duodenal papilla. You must be familiar with this anatomical arrangement.

37. Your liver is the site of bile synthesis. Bile is necessary for digestion and absorption of lipids. It is also an excretory product allowing us to eliminate hemoglobin breakdown products and excess lipids.

39. The gallbladder stores and concentrates bile.

40. The liver plays important roles in the metabolism of proteins, carbohydrates, and lipids. You must be familiar with these roles.

41. Dietary lipids must be emulsified by bile salts and lecithin to be digested by pancreatic lipase.

42. Digested components of dietary lipids are transported in chyme by bile salts as structures called micelles.

43. Absorbed lipids are transported from the small intestine as lipoproteins called chylomicrons.

44. Adipose and muscle tissue use fatty acids contained in chylomicrons.

45. After processing the remaining contents of the chylomicrons, the liver sends lipids to adipose tissue as VLDLs. The adipose tissue removes mainly fatty acids.

46. Upon their return to the liver, the remaining lipids are processed into LDLs for transport to tissues throughout the body. Mainly cholesterol is removed by these tissues.

47. The apoproteins of HDLs remove lipids from the blood and transport them to the liver (as HDLs) for processing into bile.

What Did You Learn?

Multiple choice questions: choose the best answer.

1. Your esophagus is:
   a. A component of your alimentary canal
   b. An accessory organ of digestion
   c. Both of the above
   d. Neither of the above

2. The greater omentum:
   a. Suspends the liver
   b. Suspends the stomach and proximal small intestine
   c. Holds the small intestine in folds
   d. Holds the large intestine in position
   e. None of the above is correct

3. Chewing is an example of:
   a. Chemical digestion
   b. Mechanical digestion
   c. Both of the above
   d. Neither of the above

4. The epithelium of the mouth is:
   a. Simple squamous
   b. Cornified stratified squamous
   c. Noncornified stratified squamous
   d. Simple columnar

5. Which of the following is untrue regarding the enamel of your teeth.
   a. It is made by ameloblasts
   b. It is almost completely made of inorganic salts
   c. It is replaced throughout life, as it is lost to erosion
   d. All of the above are true

6. Chemical digestion of which of the following starts in your mouth?
   a. Proteins
   b. Carbohydrates
   c. Lipids
   d. All of the above
   e. None of the above

7. Which type of epithelium is found in the esophagus?
   a. Simple squamous
   b. Cornified stratified squamous
   c. Noncornified stratified squamous
   d. None of the above

8. Which portion of your stomach is most distal?
   a. Body
   b. Fundus
   c. Pylorus
   d. Cardia

9. Chemical digestion of which of the following starts in your stomach?
   a. Proteins
   b. Carbohydrates
   c. Lipids
   d. All of the above
   e. None of the above

10. Chief cells produce:
    a. Pepsinogen
    b. Hydrochloric acid
    c. Mucus
    d. Gastrin
    e. All of the above

11. Why is pepsin produced in its inactive form (pepsinogen) and later activated?
    a. It's not
    b. So it won't damage the cells that produce it
    c. Because it is not very potent and must be saved up
    d. Actually, pepsinogen is the active form and pepsin the inactive

12. The duodenum:
    a. Is the most distal portion of the small intestine
    b. Is about 8 feet long
    c. Both of the above are correct
    d. Neither of the above is correct

13. The small intestinal mucosa contains:
    a. Villi
    b. Crypts
    c. Both of the above
    d. Neither of the above

14. Pancreatic amylase digests:
    a. Proteins
    b. Carbohydrates
    c. Lipids
    d. All of the above

15. Carbohydrates are mainly absorbed as:
    a. Complex carbohydrates
    b. Trisaccharides
    c. Disaccharides
    d. Monosaccharides

What Did You Learn? (continued)

16. Which of the following is a fat-soluble vitamin that is important in rhodopsin production?
    a. Pantothenic acid
    b. Niacin
    c. A
    d. E
    e. B_1

17. Cholecystokinin:
    a. Reduces stomach motility and secretion
    b. Increases bile secretion from the liver
    c. Both of the above
    d. Neither of the above

18. The mucosa of the large intestine contains:
    a. Villi
    b. Crypts
    c. Both of the above
    d. Neither of the above

19. The main epithelial cell type of the colon is the:
    a. Mucous cell
    b. Chief cell
    c. Enterocyte
    d. Goblet cell
    e. Parietal cell

20. Chemical digestion in the large intestine is mainly by:
    a. Enzymatic action
    b. Bacterial action
    c. Fungal action
    d. There is no chemical digestion in the large intestine

21. The presence of food in the stomach triggers a muscle contraction that begins in the middle of the transverse colon and moves the contents of the distal colon into the rectum. This contraction is called:
    a. Haustral churning
    b. Peristalsis
    c. Mass peristalsis
    d. Making-room contraction

22. The longer the transit time through the large intestine, the:
    a. More water is removed from the feces
    b. The more water is added to the feces
    c. Transit time has nothing to do with the amount of water that is in the feces

23. The _____ glands are inferior and anterior to the ears.
    a. Parotid
    b. Sublingual
    c. Buccal
    d. None of the above

24. The exocrine portion of your pancreas is composed of units called:
    a. Pancreatic islets
    b. Acini
    c. Ziti
    d. Linguini

25. _____ is a major step in the degradation of amino acids.
    a. Desalination
    b. Deamination
    c. Deanimation
    d. Deglutition
    e. Desquamation

26. Glycogenesis is:
    a. The de novo synthesis of glucose: production of glucose from protein or lipid
    b. Production of glycogen
    c. Breakdown of glycogen, releasing glucose
    d. Breakdown of glucose to lactic acid

27. Which of the following is the major site for inactivation of hormones, drugs, and toxins?
    a. Pancreas
    b. Gallbladder
    c. Liver
    d. Stomach
    e. None of the above

28. Why are lingual lipase and gastric lipase ineffective at breaking down fats?
    a. Because lipases digest carbohydrates
    b. Who says they're ineffective? They work great
    c. Because of the hydrophobic nature of fats
    d. Because fats are protected by bile until they reach the small intestine
    e. None of the above

29. Digested fats are transported in chyme by bile salts as:
    a. Chylomicrons
    b. Micelles
    c. VLDLs
    d. LDLs
    e. HDLs

What Did You Learn? (continued)

30. The lipoproteins that carry lipids back to the liver for processing into bile are called:

a. Chylomicrons

b. Micelles

c. VLDLs

d. LDLs

e. HDLs

Short answer questions: answer briefly and in your own words.

1. List the structures of the alimentary canal in order starting at the mouth and ending at the anus. Be sure to include the specific regions of the small intestine and the colon (including flexures).

2. Please explain two mechanisms that protect the stomach from being digested?

3. Describe the differences in mucosal structure between the small intestine and the large intestine. What are the reasons for these differences?

4. For each of the following, list what enzymes are responsible for their digestion, where their digestion begins, and in what form they are absorbed.

   – Proteins

   – Carbohydrates

   – Lipids

5. Draw and label a diagram showing the ducts that connect the liver, gallbladder, pancreas, and duodenum. Is there any duct that can be included that is not necessarily present in all people?

6. Briefly explain the functions of the liver.

7. Draw a diagram that shows the various ways in which lipids are transported in the chyme and in the blood. Be sure to indicate the names of the lipoproteins at each step.

Your Urinary System

What You Will Learn

- The functions of your urinary system.
- The anatomy of your urinary system.
- The structure of the functional units of your kidneys.
- How nephrons are arranged within your kidneys.
- The steps involved in urine production.
- How filtrate is produced.
- How filtrate is modified in the production of urine.
- The role of your kidneys in the maintenance of blood pH.
- The role of your kidneys in fluid and electrolyte balance.
- The role of your kidneys in blood pressure regulation.

19.1 Functions of Your Urinary System

Of all our organ systems, this is perhaps one of the most underrated by those not familiar with its functions (it sometimes has an image problem). The fluid that gives this system its name just does not seem all that interesting to some (although it really is). This system plays a number of fascinating and critical roles in the maintenance of homeostasis. It is important in the elimination of metabolic wastes and excess ions, such as nitrogenous wastes and excess hydrogen ions. We will revisit

the nitrogenous waste situation in a moment; first, let's think about ions. If we could not eliminate excess hydrogen ions, what would that do to the pH of our bodies' fluids? It would make them overly acidic. Since this system is important in hydrogen ion elimination (and for other reasons that we will discuss), we must therefore consider that it is important in acid-base homeostasis. How about other ions? We have repeatedly mentioned sodium ions during our discussions. That's because of their abundance and importance: they are the most abundant cation in our extracellular fluids, and our extracellular fluid volume is highly dependent on the abundance of sodium. Since the urinary system regulates the amount of such ions in our bodies, it must play a major role in fluid and electrolyte balance. By regulating the fluid and electrolyte balance of our bodies, and through the production of renin, the urinary system also plays a major role in the regulation of blood pressure.

As we begin our discussion of the urinary system, we should mention the fluid that provides the name for this system. Why is this fluid important? Urine is the fluid that is produced by our kidneys. Its main constituent is water, but it also contains excess ions and nitrogenous wastes. While it is important to have the ability to eliminate ions and water that are not required by the body, the nitrogenous wastes are also of interest to us; their buildup could lead to a life-threatening breach of homeostasis. Let's think about nitrogenous wastes now.

■ Nitrogenous Wastes: Where Do They Originate?

The existence of nitrogenous wastes has already been introduced. In Chapter 18, we learned that proteins can be broken down into their constituent amino acids, and amino acids can be broken down into the atoms of which they are composed. This may be necessary, for example, during gluconeogenesis. During gluconeogenesis, we need the energy stored in the amino acids; we also need the carbon, hydrogen, and oxygen that the amino acids contain. We must remove the amino groups from the amino acids that are being broken down, regardless of the reason for this degradation. The amino group becomes ammonia (NH_3) when it is removed from the amino acid. We produce quite a bit of ammonia because we deaminate lots of amino acid molecules every day. Think about how much protein we ingest. Amino acids that are contained in those proteins and are not needed for protein synthesis will be deaminated. Obviously, we have to deal with a lot of ammonia.

Ammonia is a nitrogenous (nitrogen-containing) waste. It is also toxic. It is produced mainly in the liver, but the liver is also the place that converts it into the less toxic nitrogenous waste, urea. Urea represents a final product of protein degradation and is the chief nitrogenous waste found in urine. Eighty to 90 percent of the total nitrogen content of urine is in the form of urea. Elimination of urea is an important urinary system function. Let's now learn about the structure of this system so we can understand its physiology.

19.2 Anatomy of Your Urinary System

The anatomy of this system is perhaps the simplest of any system we have studied (**FIGURE 19.1**). There are two kidneys, each of which is connected by a muscular tube, called a ureter, to the single urinary bladder. A single duct, the urethra, leaves the urinary bladder and exits the body at the tip of the penis in males and in the vulva in females. Note the similarity between the terms *ureter*, of which you have two, and *urethra*, of which you have one. Be sure that you look carefully if you see these terms on an exam. It is easy to be tricked into thinking you see one when the other is actually written.

The urinary bladder is a muscular sack that stores urine and provides the force for its expulsion from the body. This expulsion of urine (urination, or micturition) is largely a reflex action over which we learn limited voluntarily control. One interesting feature of this organ is that it is lined with an epithelium found in no other system. Transitional epithelium is composed of irregularly shaped cells that are specially adapted to

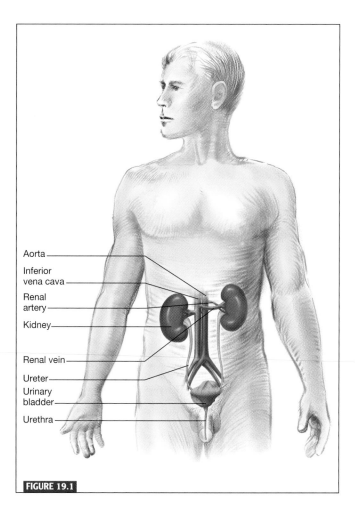

Aorta
Inferior vena cava
Renal artery
Kidney
Renal vein
Ureter
Urinary bladder
Urethra

FIGURE 19.1

The urinary system.

stretch as the bladder fills and recoil back as it empties. We learned of this epithelium in Chapter 4.

The kidneys are, oddly enough, shaped like kidney beans (**FIGURE 19.2**). They are about 4.5 inches long, 2.5 inches wide, and 1 inch thick. They are embedded in the posterior wall of the abdominal cavity, but only the surface, which is exposed to the cavity, is covered with the peritoneal lining. For this reason, they are really not within the abdominopelvic cavity, but are actually posterior to it. This position is called retroperitoneal. They are directly covered by a heavy capsule of dense irregular connective tissue. This capsule does not allow the kidneys to swell as urine is produced. This forces the urine to flow out of the kidneys, rather than pooling within them.

The notched side of the kidney, which is medial as they sit in the body, is called the hilus. The hilus is the

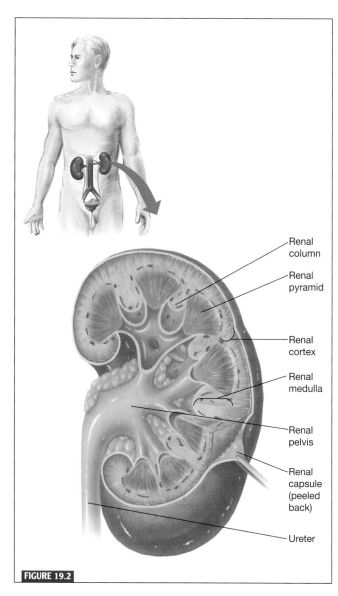

FIGURE 19.2

Gross anatomy of the kidney.

kidneys' connection point for blood vessels, nerves, and the ureters. The kidneys receive blood through the renal arteries (*renal* means "pertaining to the kidneys"), which branch directly from the aorta. Blood exits the kidneys through the renal veins that lead directly to the inferior vena cava. The reason that the kidneys are so directly connected to the body's great blood vessels is that they receive approximately 25 percent of the cardiac output. The reason for this major supply of blood will be readily apparent when we look at how the kidneys work.

◼ The Nephron: Functional Unit of Your Kidneys

Each kidney is composed of approximately 1 million nephrons (**FIGURE 19.3**). Nephrons are the functional units of the kidney; in other words, these 1 million functional units are each one unit of the actual machinery that makes urine. Let's look at their structure in the following paragraphs. Be sure to refer to the diagram (Figure 19.3) as you read this description.

The Renal Corpuscle

Each nephron begins at a renal corpuscle. A renal corpuscle consists of a capsule (the glomerular capsule, or Bowman's capsule) surrounding a tuft of capillaries called the *glomerulus* (meaning "little ball"). The glomerular wall is composed of special endothelial cells that are surrounded by cells called podocytes. *Podocytes* (meaning "foot cells") have small extensions called *pedicels* ("little feet"). The pedicels of the podocytes wrap around the capillaries of the glomerulus just like your fingers could wrap around the cardboard tube from a roll of paper towels (see **FIGURE 19.4**). Just as you could have a small space between your fingers as they wrap around the tube, small spaces called filtration slits are present between the pedicels. Filtration slits contain a slit membrane. Another very thin (0.1 micrometer) membrane is present between the endothelial cells and the pedicels. It is similar to a basement membrane, but lacks the fine structure we would see in a basement membrane. For this reason, it is called a basal lamina. Lying between the capillary tufts of the glomerulus are mesangial cells. Mesangial cells organize the tuft, assure a clean lamina at all times, and produce numerous regulatory agents. Although their specific functions are beyond the scope of this text, it is worth being aware of mesangial cells, as they play an important role in numerous kidney diseases.

The space between the glomerulus and the glomerular membrane is called the glomerular space, or Bowman's space. This space is drained by the tubules of

Renal column

Renal pyramid

Renal cortex

Renal medulla

Renal pelvis

Renal capsule (peeled back)

Ureter

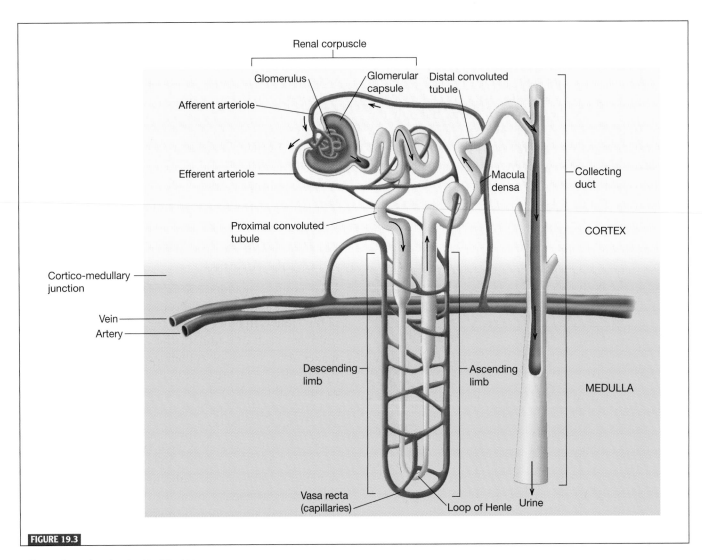

FIGURE 19.3

The nephron, functional unit of the kidney.

the nephron that we will discuss in a moment. There is an interesting feature of the vascular supply to the glomerulus that we must discuss first.

Think about a typical capillary bed. Capillaries usually receive their blood from arterioles that have smooth muscle in their walls to regulate blood flow into the capillary bed. Capillaries are usually drained by venules, which are larger in diameter than arterioles and have walls mainly composed of elastic fibers. This is so they will not restrict flow out of the capillary, for to do that would build pressure in the capillary, possibly damaging this fine-walled vessel.

The vascular arrangement of the glomerulus is different from this (**FIGURE 19.5**). While an arteriole supplies these capillary tufts, another arteriole also leads away from them. The arteriole that supplies blood to the glomerulus is called the *afferent arteriole*. The one that drains the glomerulus is called the *efferent arteriole*. We

learned these terms in conjunction with nerve fibers leading to and from the CNS. If you remember that, you will have no problems understanding the meaning of these terms here.

Why would we have arterioles leading away from capillaries in the renal corpuscle? Recall the difference between the arteriole wall and the venule wall, and you will see that the arteriole has the ability to restrict flow. This structure would indicate that we need to develop pressure in the glomerulus. In fact, we do need to develop hydrostatic pressure there. We will get back to this topic in a little while.

The Tubules of Your Nephron

The rest of the nephron is made up of tubules or ducts. Bowman's space is drained by the proximal convoluted tubule. Note that structure in Figure 19.3. You will see that its name is fitting: it is proximal (near the begin-

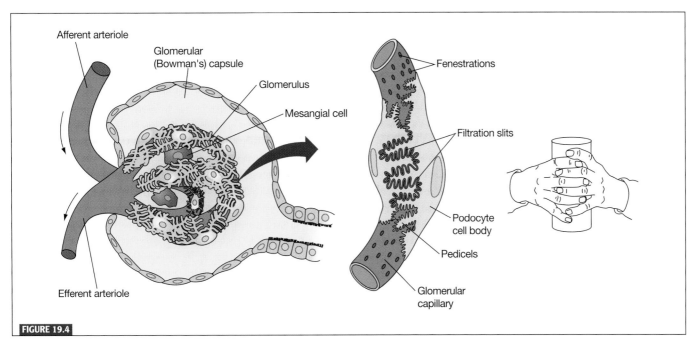

Structure of the renal corpuscle.

ning of this tubular structure) and convoluted (twisted). It leads to a long looping tubule, the loop of the nephron or the Loop of Henle. There are two regions in this loop. We begin with the descending limb, then turn 180 degrees and travel back toward the renal corpuscle in the ascending limb.

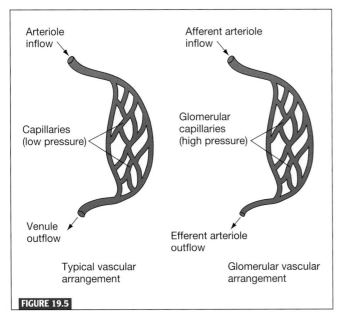

FIGURE 19.5

The vascular arrangement of the glomerulus differs from the typical vascular arrangement. In place of a venule, the glomerular capillary is drained by an efferent arteriole. This results in increased pressure in the glomerular capillary.

The next segment of the nephron is the distal convoluted tubule, again aptly named. This empties its contents into a collecting duct. Many nephrons dump their contents into each collecting duct.

The Juxtaglomerular Apparatus

One additional feature of the nephron we need to think about here is the juxtaglomerular apparatus (big name, little structure). Where the distal convoluted tubule lies adjacent to the afferent arteriole, both have special cells in their walls. The complex of these two structures is the juxtaglomerular apparatus. The distal convoluted tubule contains cells called macula densa because of their dense-appearing nuclei. The afferent arteriole contains juxtaglomerular cells. This structure has special functions we will discuss shortly.

O.K., let's recap the structures of the nephron. It begins with a renal corpuscle containing a glomerulus, which is contained within the glomerular space surrounded by the glomerular, or Bowman's capsule. The glomerulus is a tuft of special capillary that is supplied with blood by an afferent arteriole and drained by an efferent arteriole. Bowman's space is followed sequentially by the proximal convoluted tubule, the descending limb and ascending limb of the loop of the nephron, the distal convoluted tubule, and the collecting duct.

■ Gross Anatomy of Your Kidneys

Let's look at a longitudinal section through the kidney (Figure 19.2). Notice that two regions are apparent: an outer cortex and an inner medulla. The medulla is made up of two types of tissue: pyramids and columns. Deep within the kidney, we see a number of spaces: the calyces and the pelvis.

The cortex is primarily composed of renal corpuscles and the convoluted tubules that are located near them. The columns of the medulla are composed of the same structures. The pyramids of the medulla have a striped appearance. This is because they contain the loop of the nephron, with its ascending and descending limbs, and the collecting tubules. These ducts all run parallel to each other, descending and ascending from the most superficial part of the medulla to the deepest part alongside the pelvis.

The purpose of the nephron is to produce urine. That urine needs to get from the nephron to the ureters. This is where the collecting tubules, the calyces and the pelvis, are involved. This anatomy can be compared to a tributary system in which small streams flow into rivers, rivers flow into bays, and bays flow into oceans. The collecting ducts (small streams) empty their contents into the minor calyces (rivers) that flow into major calyces (bays), and ultimately into the renal pelvis (ocean). The pelvis is drained by a ureter.

So, we now know where the kidneys are, and what their internal structure is like, both histologically and grossly. We also know that urine is made here. Let's examine how that process works.

19.3 How to Make Urine in Three Easy Steps

There are three processes involved in urine production. We will study each of the three sequentially. Understand, however, that only the first step (glomerular filtration) is really "sequentially" the first; the other two (tubular resorption and secretion) occur simultaneously, although differently in different regions of the nephron.

■ Glomerular Filtration

Do you own a coffee maker, the kind in which the ground coffee beans sit in a filter while water drips through it? That's right, a filter-type coffee maker. Even if you don't own one, you can imagine how they work. This process is called filtration. So, what actually is filtration? It is the process whereby a fluid is forced through a membrane by pressure. It can be used to separate suspended substances out of the fluid. Water and dissolved "coffee" make it through the paper membrane filter in your coffee maker, but the ground coffee beans

stay behind (or if yours is like mine, most of them do, anyway).

Filtration is the job of the renal corpuscle and, in particular, the glomerulus. Let's look at each part of our definition of filtration as regards our glomerulus. Let's start with the fluid.

O.K., what fluid are we filtering? Right, we are filtering the fluid component of blood.

In fact, the entire volume of your blood is filtered about 60 times per day. That's astounding when you think about it. Your blood volume is somewhere around 5 liters (1.35 gallons), slightly more if you are male, slightly less if you are female. Filtered 60 times per day, that makes 300 liters (81 gallons) of fluid being passed through the filter each day. (If you are having trouble picturing that volume, imagine 150 of the large 2-liter soda bottles.)

So, what is the filter of our definition in our glomerulus? As we have already learned, the walls of the glomerulus are made up of three layers: the endothelial cells; the basal lamina; and the pedicels of the podocytes, with their slit membranes in filtration slits. This entire structure is called the endothelial-capsular membrane, or the glomerular filtration membrane (**FIGURE 19.6**). The total surface area of this membrane in all glomeruli in both of your kidneys is approximately equal to the surface area of your skin! It is through this membrane that filtration occurs. The endothelial cells contain porelike openings called fenestra.

Fluid is pushed through this membrane, but just as in your coffee maker, suspended substances are left be-

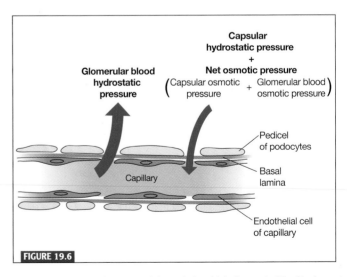

FIGURE 19.6

The presence of an efferent arteriole results in a high glomerular blood hydrostatic pressure. This pressure exceeds the sum of the pressures that oppose the movement of fluid through the glomerular filtration membrane. Filtration is the outcome of this balance of pressures.

hind. In the case of our blood, the fluid that makes it through the filter is called filtrate. Filtrate contains everything blood contains except cells and large proteins (i.e., albumin and immunoglobulins). Water, amino acids, small proteins, vitamins, glucose, nitrogenous wastes, and lots of other compounds make it into filtrate.

We now know what the fluid is and what the membrane is, so how about the pressure? In the case of your coffee maker, the pressure is generated by gravity. In the case of your glomeruli, we must add four pressures together to come up with the actual pressure promoting filtration. Recall Starling's hypothesis from Chapter 16 which told us that in a capillary bed we could add four pressures together (blood hydrostatic pressure, blood osmotic pressure, interstitial hydrostatic pressure, and interstitial osmotic pressure) and come up with a net pressure that would promote the movement of fluid either out of the capillaries (making interstitial fluid) or into the capillaries (removing interstitial fluid). The same pressures apply here, although we usually apply different names to them (see Figures 16.24 and 19.6). The only difference is that the blood (capillary) hydrostatic pressure (blood pressure as we think of it) is much greater here than in any other capillary. It is higher because we have an efferent arteriole restricting flow out of the capillary. It is like putting your fingers over the end of your garden hose. If your hose has some very small holes in it, won't water squirt out of those holes when you restrict the flow with your fingers? In fact, the hydrostatic pressure in our glomerular capillaries is about 60 mm Hg, roughly twice that of other capillaries. When these pressures are added together, we end up with a total pressure of only 10 mm Hg in favor of filtration. It's not much, but it is enough. You can see why the efferent arterioles are important; without them no filtration would occur. Simply put, filtration occurs because blood hydrostatic pressure is sufficient to overcome the forces opposing filtration.

This net pressure does, of course, vary. It is under the control of your autonomic nervous system. Parasympathetic stimulation increases glomerular hydrostatic pressure; hence, there is increased filtration. Sympathetic stimulation reduces glomerular hydrostatic pressure, leading to deceased filtration. This makes great sense; do you want to have to stop and find a bathroom when you are running from danger?

That's it for filtration. But is filtrate the same as urine? Could it possibly be that simple; you make filtrate and urinate it out? Think it through. You filter your entire blood volume 60 times per day and glucose, sodium, and other important substances make it into the filtrate.

If you were to urinate out filtrate, you would dehydrate and lose these important substances so rapidly that you could not keep up with the demand to replace them. You would rapidly die. We had better modify this filtrate before releasing it as urine.

■ Tubular Resorption

Tubular resorption is the movement of substances from the filtrate back into the blood. It is extremely important for the reasons just mentioned. We must reduce the volume of filtrate from 300 liters per day to the 1.5 liters or so that we actually urinate. We must also remove many substances from the filtrate that we can not afford to lose, as it would be too costly (in biological terms) to replace them. Resorbed substances include small proteins, amino acids, glucose, and ions such as sodium, chloride, calcium, potassium, and phosphorous. Bicarbonate is also resorbed, and acts as a buffer for the blood (more on this in a moment). Urea, although a nitrogenous waste that must be eliminated, is also resorbed to some degree.

Since water will follow ions and other substances through osmosis, resorption of these components of filtrate results in absorption of water wherever it can be resorbed. Note in **FIGURE 19.7** that some cells in the nephron are shaded, others are not. Where the cells are not shaded, the tubule is permeable to water, and water will be resorbed along with these other substances. Where the cells are shaded, the tubule is impermeable to water, and water cannot be resorbed. Where the cells are partially shaded (dashed line), the permeability of the tubule to water is variable. We will discuss how this works in the section titled "Renal Control of Fluid Volume."

Active and passive mechanisms are used to resorb various substances. In fact, the single most "expensive" use of energy by the kidneys is that of sodium resorption. Sodium is resorbed by active transport with other ions and water following (where water can follow, that is). We are unable to resorb all of the sodium that is present in filtrate, however, so some remains in our urine. This is the reason we have a daily dietary need for sodium. Tubular resorption is also why some people have to restrict the sodium in their diet.

Some people are better at resorbing sodium than others. This is a genetic characteristic; historically, these genes developed and were selected for in regions of the world where salt (and, therefore, sodium) was in short supply. The ability to resorb sodium more effectively (reducing the amount of sodium lost in the urine) was a good thing. When people have that genetic characteristic in our society, however, with its all-too-abundant

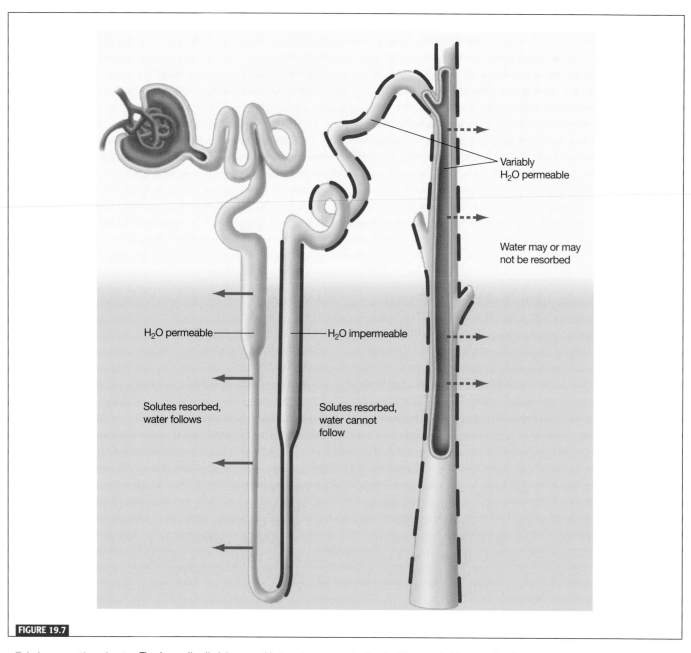

FIGURE 19.7

Tubular resorption of water. The descending limb is permeable to water, so water is absorbed by osmosis. The ascending limb is impermeable to water, so osmosis cannot occur there. The distal convoluted tubule and collecting duct are variably permeable to water, so osmosis in those locations can be regulated.

sodium, problems arise. Since these people are now consuming more sodium than they are excreting, the sodium level in their bodies increases. Since water follows sodium, this leads to a higher than desirable fluid (blood) volume and high blood pressure. See, the resorption of sodium has everything to do with genetic hypertension.

This also allows our kidneys to regulate blood volume through tubular resorption. We will look at renal regulation of blood volume later in this chapter.

What about glucose? How much of that do we excrete in our urine? The answer, normally, is none. We should not be excreting glucose in our urine; it should be completely resorbed. Let's think about how that works.

Picture a hallway in your school that has classrooms opening onto it and a doorway at each end (**FIGURE 19.8**). At one end of the hallway, someone is releasing cats. These cats are running down the hallway toward an open door at the other end. We do not want them to escape out of that door. In the entryway of each classroom, we

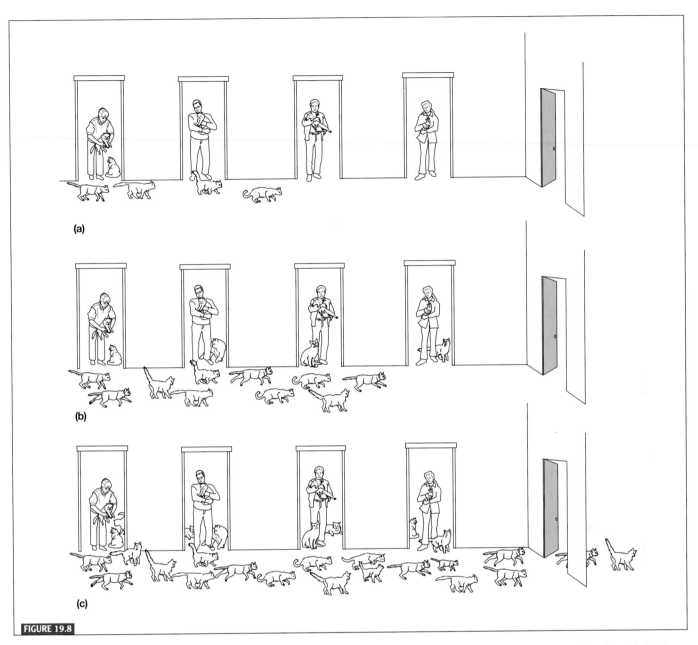

FIGURE 19.8

Resorption of sodium is like gathering cats from a hallway. When the number of cats running down the hallway is low, all of the cats are easily collected before they reach the open door at the end of the hall (a). As the number of cats increases (b), the job becomes more difficult. When the number of cats exceeds the ability of the people in the doorways to collect them, some of the cats escape from the hallway (c). Under the conditions of homeostasis, glucose is completely resorbed from filtrate (like panels a and b). In diabetes mellitus, the blood (and, therefore, filtrate) concentration of glucose exceeds the resorption ability of glucose carriers in the tubules and glucose "escapes" in the urine.

have positioned one student to grab cats as they pass and place them in the classroom, where they will be safe. They can't escape out the open door at the end of the hallway if they are in the classrooms.

If one cat per minute is running down the hallway, they will all be "resorbed" into the classrooms; none will make it the length of the hallway and out the door. This may also be true at 10 or 20 cats per minute: your

classmates should easily be able to grab and "resorb" that many cats. But if we reach 100 cats per minute, there will be too many for your classmates to catch. Some will make it through and out the door at the end of the hallway.

This is exactly how the resorption of glucose works. Glucose is resorbed through active transport. Under normal circumstances, there are sufficient glucose carriers to resorb all of the glucose that enters the tubules in the filtrate. If, however, more glucose enters the tubules than that number of glucose carriers can handle, just like the cats running out the door at the end of the hall, glucose will make it through the entire length of the tubule and be eliminated in the urine. The maximum amount of glucose that the tubule can resorb is called the tubular transport maximum, or Tmax. The plasma concentration of glucose at which we will exceed Tmax is called the renal threshold. People with diabetes mellitus often have elevated blood glucose levels. When their glucose level exceeds the renal threshold, the "cats make it to the end of the hallway," or glucose is not completely resorbed and appears in their urine. This is why a urine analysis to detect glucose is part of the diagnosis for diabetes mellitus.

■ Tubular Secretion

Tubular secretion is the next process of urine formation that we need to discuss. This is the process of taking additional substances out of the blood and adding them to the urine. It is a special way of dumping things we don't need or want, or taking out the trash, in a way. Potassium, hydrogen, and some other ions are secreted. Ammonia and urea are secreted (wait a minute, that must mean that urea is filtered, resorbed, and secreted; something interesting is going on there).

We will revisit the secretion of urea and potassium as part of our discussion of renal control of fluid volume and the secretion of hydrogen when we discuss renal influence on blood pH. Let's get into those topics now.

19.4 Acid-Base Balance and Renal Influence on Blood pH

As one factor of homeostasis, the maintenance of the acid-base balance of our blood and other fluids is extremely important. Low blood pH (acidosis) can be generated in a number of ways, including respiratory and renal failure, disturbances in fat metabolism, and excessive lactic acid production. High blood pH (alkalosis) can be generated through severe vomiting (excessive loss of gastric acid), diarrhea and hypersecretion of aldosterone (disturbance of other ion levels leading to hydrogen ion loss), and excessive antacid consumption.

In Chapter 17, we learned that carbon dioxide is converted to carbonic acid by carbonic anhydrase, and that the respiratory rate is determined by blood pH. Note how, by increasing or decreasing respiratory rate, we will alter the amount of carbonic acid present in the blood and therefore alter blood pH. This is one mechanism in the maintenance of acid-base balance. We also know (Chapters 2 and 17) that buffer systems are important in the maintenance of acid-base balance. The carbonic acid-bicarbonate buffer system is one such mechanism. Now let's examine the important role that the kidneys play in this aspect of homeostasis.

Just like our erythrocytes, the cells of the proximal convoluted tubule, distal convoluted tubule, and collecting duct contain carbonic anhydrase, which combines carbon dioxide with water to form carbonic acid. The carbonic acid then dissociates into its cation (hydrogen) and anion (bicarbonate). The hydrogen is secreted into the developing urine (**FIGURE 19.9**). This step acidifies the urine; in turn, this aids in retarding bacterial growth and in keeping solutes from precipitating. Rather than making the urine overly acidic, however, the hydrogen ions can reassociate with filtered bicarbonate, forming the weak acid, carbonic acid. Secreted hydrogen ions also can combine with nitrogenous wastes. NH_2 or NH_3, the amino group from amino acids, can accept an additional hydrogen ion, producing NH_3 (ammonia) or NH_4^+ (the ammonium ion). This keeps hydrogen ions from diffusing back into the blood. The primary role of this secretion of hydrogen is to raise the pH of the blood, protecting against the development of acidosis. The importance of this lies in the fact that so much of our metabolism and diet tends to acidify blood. In eliminating excess hydrogen ions from the blood, the urinary system is protecting us against acidosis.

This is not the only way in which the kidneys fight acidosis, however. The bicarbonate that is produced, as carbonic acid dissociates within the tubule epithelium, is ultimately resorbed. By adding bicarbonate to the

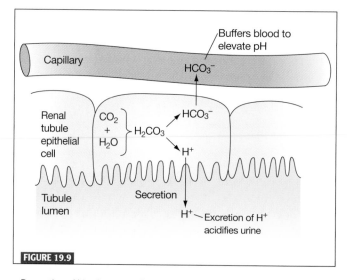

FIGURE 19.9

Resorption of bicarbonate and secretion of hydrogen ions serves to increase the pH of the blood and decrease the pH of the urine.

blood, the kidneys are further buffering the blood. These bicarbonate anions bind hydrogen cations to form carbonic acid in the blood. By accepting the hydrogen ions that dissociate from stronger acids, this weak acid protects our blood against becoming excessively acidic. Alternatively, the bicarbonate may bind sodium to form sodium bicarbonate, the salt that acts as a weak base in the carbonic acid-bicarbonate buffer system.

But what about alkalosis? How do our kidneys help us to avoid that homeostatic imbalance? Our bodies are actually not particularly good at counteracting a pH shift in this direction. Our ability to reduce our respiration rate, thereby acidifying the blood by a buildup of CO_2 (again, producing carbonic acid), is limited by our need for oxygen. Our kidneys compensate by decreasing the secretion of hydrogen ions and decreasing the resorption of bicarbonate.

19.5 Renal Control of Fluid and Electrolyte Balance

The role of the urinary system in controlling the fluid volume and the concentration of electrolytes in the body (for our purposes, ions such as sodium, potassium, and calcium) is manifold. It makes perfect sense, however, for the kidneys to play a major role in these important aspects of homeostasis. What other system is so well suited for either eliminating or conserving large quantities of water? Likewise, what system can so readily adjust the fluid concentration of specific ions? Let's start now by considering how the kidneys alter the fluid volume of the body to maintain homeostasis.

■ Renal Control of Fluid Volume

Wherever sodium is transported across the epithelium of the nephrons, if water can follow, it will follow. As already indicated diagrammatically (Figure 19.7), various regions of the nephron differ in their permeability to water. The proximal convoluted tubule and the descending limb are permeable to water: resorption of sodium and other substances here will result in the resorption of water. The ascending limb is impermeable to water: resorption of solutes here (i.e., sodium and urea) will not result in the resorption of water; instead, it will result in a decrease in the concentration of filtrate. The distal convoluted tubule and collecting ducts are variably permeable to water and will be discussed separately.

Eighty percent of the water that the kidneys are able to resorb will always be resorbed. The kidneys can not alter their resorption of that quantity of water. This is called obligatory water resorption. Facultative water resorption accounts for the additional 20 percent of the water that the kidneys are able to resorb. That percentage of water resorption is optional, so if the body is underhydrated (needs water), there is additional water available to resorb. If the body has excess water, it will not be resorbed; instead, it will be allowed to pass in the urine. This resorption depends on a concentration gradient in the interstitial fluid of the medulla as the "force" for moving water. We will first consider what happens if the body has too much water (needs to get rid of some), and then what happens if the body is dehydrated and needs to conserve water.

Too Much Water in Your Body? Urine-Dilution Mechanisms

When you have been drinking plenty of water, you may have noticed that your urine becomes clear. It is obviously not as concentrated as when you are somewhat dehydrated. How do the kidneys make this dilute urine? That is the question we must first answer.

Filtrate has a concentration slightly less than that of the plasma from which it is made (we will consider it equal to that of serum or interstitial fluid, about 300 milliosmoles). Milliosmoles simply represents a unit of concentration, related to molarity, discussed in Chapter 2. As resorption removes solute from the filtrate in the proximal convoluted tubule and the descending limb, water follows. However, since the ascending limb is impermeable to water, as substances are resorbed there, water can not follow. Therefore, the concentration of the filtrate will decrease. It is not that we are adding water (solvent), it is that we are removing solute (urea, sodium, and other electrolytes). By the time the filtrate reaches the distal convoluted tubule, the concentration of the filtrate (now nearly urine) has dropped to about 65 milliosmoles, really quite dilute. Since the permeability of the distal convoluted tubule and the collecting duct to water is variable, if we do not make it permeable (FIGURE 19.10a), no water will be resorbed from this point on, and our urine will be very dilute (concentration of 65 milliosmoles). That is quite simply how dilute urine is formed. Solutes are resorbed and water is not allowed to follow. Now let's think about what happens when we are dehydrated and must resorb that water.

Too Little Water in Your Body? Urine Concentration Mechanisms

Let's start by thinking about a concentration gradient that exists in the renal medulla. You know that the pyramids within the renal medulla are composed of the descending and ascending limbs of the loops of the

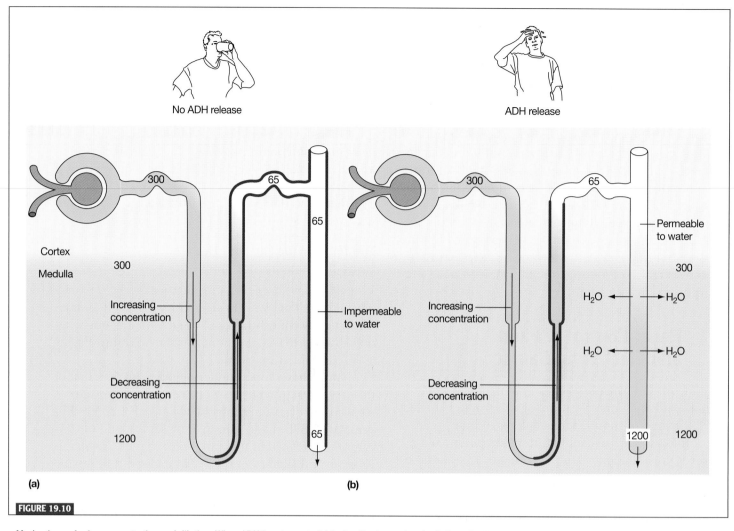

No ADH release

ADH release

Cortex

Medulla

Increasing concentration

Decreasing concentration

Impermeable to water

Increasing concentration

Decreasing concentration

Permeable to water

$H_2O \leftarrow \rightarrow H_2O$

$H_2O \leftarrow \rightarrow H_2O$

(a)

(b)

FIGURE 19.10

Mechanisms of urine concentration and dilution. When ADH is not secreted (a), the distal convoluted tubule and collecting duct are impermeable to water, resulting in dilute urine. When ADH is secreted (b), these structures are permeable to water, allowing water to leave by osmosis, resulting in concentrated urine.

nephrons and the collecting tubules running parallel to each other. Running alongside these tubules are loops of capillaries called vasa recta. Vasa recta carry away (in the blood) the substances that are resorbed by the nephron. As substances (i.e., urea, sodium, and other electrolytes) are reabsorbed into the descending loop of the vasa recta, they are carried deeper into the medulla, allowing less additional substances to be picked up. A similar situation exists in the ascending limb of the vasa recta, which is picking up water from the descending limb of the loop of the nephron. It's all by diffusion after all; so a delicate balance is set up between the amount of solutes resorbed into the interstitial fluid and the amount of solute carried away by the vasa recta.

Because of this balance, the concentration of the interstitial fluid varies between the corticomedullary junction (where the cortex and medulla meet) and the deep medulla. The interstitial fluid at the cortico-medullary junction has a concentration similar to that of the rest of the body, about 300 milliosmoles. As we travel deeper into the medulla, the concentration of the interstitial fluid increases, until we reach a maximum concentration deep in the medulla of 1,200 milliosmoles. Now think about the filtrate/urine that is traveling through the nephron. It begins with a concentration of about 300 mOsm. At first, both solute and solvent is being removed, but as it travels into the ascending limb and water can no longer follow the solutes that are resorbed, its concentration drops to 65 milliosmoles. When it next travels into the distal convoluted tubule and collecting duct, it is traveling through tubules where water permeability can be altered. If additional water needs to be removed from the urine, the walls will be made water permeable (Figure 19.10b). When the walls of the collecting duct are water permeable and the collecting duct descends down through an interstitial fluid with an osmolarity (concentration) of 1,200 milliosmoles (highly concentrated), water will move out of the collecting duct into the interstitial fluid by osmosis. This will increase the concentration of the urine (by removing solvent, water) to 1,200 milliosmoles. The urine will be much more concentrated because the water it held has been resorbed back into the interstitial fluid to then be taken away in the blood within the vasa recta. What an elegant means of controlling the fluid levels in the body!

But wait a minute! How did we alter the permeability of the distal convoluted tubule and collecting tubule (where it really matters)? That permeability is altered by a mechanism you already know. Cells in the hypothalamus monitor the osmolarity of the blood. When you are dehydrated, they stimulate release of antidiuretic hormone (ADH) from the posterior pituitary (In Chapter 13, I told you we would get back to this!). Antidiuretic hormone causes water resorption in the kidneys by causing the distal convoluted tubules and collecting ducts to become water permeable. Then the concentration gradient of the renal medulla can do its thing, and the water is resorbed.

Hence, we've seen the role of the kidneys in regulating the body's fluid (water) content, and we know that fluid content is related to blood pressure (Chapter 16). Do you think that is all there is to it? No, of course not! We have only been altering the amount of water that we are resorbing; can't we also alter the amount of certain solutes that we resorb?

■ Control of Ion Concentrations: Mechanisms You Already Understand

As we have been discussing tubular secretion and resorption of various electrolytes, it should have brought back memories of our endocrine system discussions. Didn't we learn about the endocrine system's regulation of various ion concentrations? Recall from Chapter 13 that, in some cases, the target cells of these hormones were in the kidney, specifically the tubule epithelia. In addition to altering osteoclast behavior, parathyroid hormone increases calcium resorption and phosphate secretion in the kidneys. Aldosterone increases resorption of sodium, and indirectly bicarbonate and the chloride ion. It also increases secretion of potassium and hydrogen. Sodium is the most abundant cation in our extracellular fluids and it plays a direct role in deter-

mining the volume of those fluids. For those reasons alone it is worth considering its regulation in detail. Let's do that now.

Sodium Resorption: Influence and Dependence on Blood Pressure

The amount of sodium in your body plays a major role in determining your blood pressure, as we have already discussed earlier in this chapter. Since water follows sodium, when you resorb sodium, water follows if it can. And if it does, your blood volume goes up. If your blood volume goes up, your blood pressure goes up. So in a typical negative feedback situation, if your blood pressure drops, you resorb more sodium to compensate. But how do you regulate the amount of sodium you resorb? That is what we will now discuss.

Remember the juxtaglomerular apparatus? Sure you do; it is composed of the juxtaglomerular cells of the afferent arteriole and the macula densa of the distal convoluted tubule. We need to think about this structure for a moment.

When the juxtaglomerular cells of the afferent arteriole detect low blood pressure, they secrete renin into the blood (**FIGURE 19.11**). Renin, you will recall from Chapter 13, is the enzyme that activates the renin-angiotensin system. We will review how it works.

Angiotensinogen is produced by the liver and is in circulation at all times. It is in an inactive form. When renin comes in contact with angiotensinogen, it cleaves off a piece, making angiotensin I, which is also inactive. As angiotensin I circulates in the blood (mainly, when it passes through the lungs) angiotensin-converting enzyme (ACE) cleaves it to angiotensin II. Angiotensin II is the active molecule.

Angiotensin II has several effects. One effect is that it stimulates release of aldosterone. (Remember the mineralocorticoids? Where do they originate?) Aldosterone increases sodium resorption (and, hence, water resorption) mainly in the distal convoluted tubule and collecting duct.

Angiotensin II is also a potent vasoconstrictor, having its strongest effect on the efferent arterioles. The general vasoconstriction it causes raises blood pressure throughout the body. The increased constriction on the efferent arterioles specifically raises the hydrostatic pressure in the glomeruli, assuring filtration even if blood pressure is low. Remember, we need to remove nitrogenous and other wastes from the blood even if we have low blood pressure.

The macula densa cells of the distal convoluted tubules also play a regulatory role. They monitor sodium

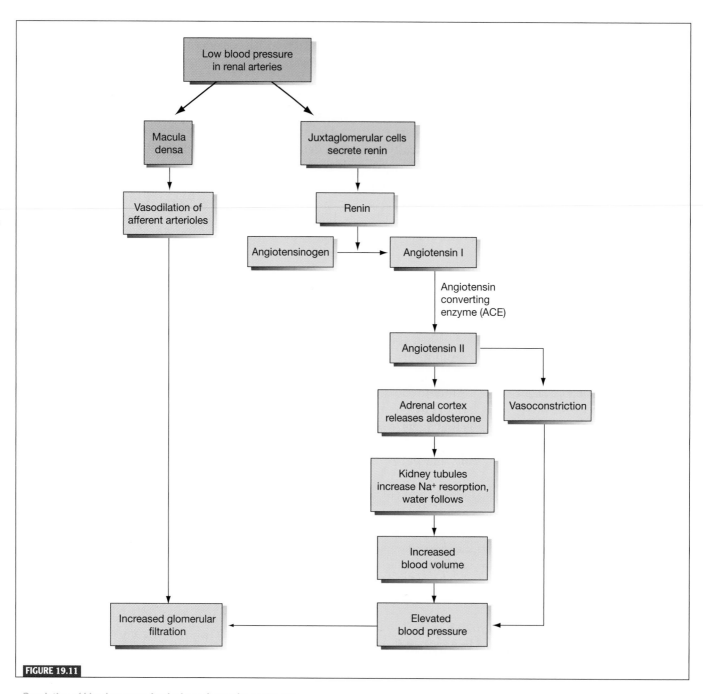

FIGURE 19.11

Regulation of blood pressure by the juxtaglomerular apparatus.

ions passing in the filtrate much the way you could count cars passing on the highway. Perhaps you only were counting red cars. This would give you an indirect measure of the overall amount of traffic. By "counting" sodium ions, the macula densa gets an indirect measure of the amount of filtrate being produced. If, in this way, it detects low filtrate production, it takes steps to increase it. Macula densa cells cause the afferent arterioles to dilate, thereby increasing glomerular hydrostatic pressure and filtration. They also trigger release of renin by the juxtaglomerular cells, producing the effects just described.

Well, there you have it. That is what the urinary system does. Understanding the process through which urine is produced kind of increases your respect for urine, doesn't it? Before we get too carried away, why not look over the "What You Should Know" section and try the questions in "What Did You Learn?" to make sure you really get it. Then, let's proceed to the final section of this text.

Breaching Homeostasis . . . When Things Go Wrong

Urolithiasis: Urinary Stones

You may be familiar with urinary stones. Since about 5 percent of all adults (males more often than females) experience them at some point, you are likely to know people who have experienced them, if you have not yet had any yourself. So, what are urinary stones (also called urolithiasis), what are they made of, and why do people get them? These are the questions to be addressed in this "Breaching Homeostasis."

Urinary stones are hardened chemical deposits that can form anywhere in the urinary tract, making the common term *kidney stones* potentially misleading. Most often (80 percent of the time) they are unilateral, even though many may exist on the one side. Usually they are very small (2–3 millimeters), although one type can be very large. Although they can be quite painful, even very large stones are often incidental findings at autopsy, having never come to clinical attention and having had no notable impact on the person's life.

They come in four types, based on their chemical composition. Calcium stones, made of precipitated calcium salts, make up about 75 percent of all urinary stones. Excessive calcium absorption in the digestive tract, leading to high concentrations of calcium in the urine (hypercalciuria) is the usual cause. These excessive calcium levels can be triggered by hyperparathyroidism, vitamin D intoxication, or a variety of other causes. Bacterial infections in the urinary tract can also contribute to precipitation of calcium salts, producing these stones.

Struvite stones make up 15 percent of cases. These are composed of magnesium salts and are the stones most likely to become quite large. A single struvite stone may fill the entire renal pelvis. These most commonly develop as complications of renal tract infections.

Approximately 5 percent of urolithiases are composed of uric acid. Gout, a metabolic disorder leading to abnormally high levels of uric acid in the urine, is a common cause, but 50 percent of cases have no history of gout. These are generally idiopathic (the cause is unknown).

Finally, we have the relatively rare cystine stones, composed primarily of the amino acid cystine. These develop in people with a heritable (genetic) disorder of amino acid metabolism.

Urinary stones may be passed spontaneously or may require medical intervention. Fortunately, a variety of ultrasound techniques are available to break up troublesome stones, easing their passage.

What You Should Know

1. Your urinary system has many important functions, including elimination of metabolic wastes and excess ions; maintenance of the pH, ion concentrations, and volume of our extracellular fluids; and a role in the regulation of blood pressure.

2. Nitrogenous wastes, one form of metabolic waste eliminated by the urinary system, are generated by the deamination of amino acids.

3. Your liver converts ammonia into urea, the main form of nitrogenous waste eliminated by your kidneys.

4. You have two kidneys, each of which is drained by one ureter. The ureters convey urine to your urinary bladder (one only). One urethra carries your urine from your bladder to the exterior of your body.

5. The nephron is the functional unit of your kidneys. Each kidney contains approximately 1 million nephrons.

6. Nephrons consist of a renal corpuscle and associated tubules. These tubules include the proximal convoluted tubule, the descending limb and ascending limb of the loop of the nephron (loop of Henle), the distal convoluted tubule, and a collecting duct.

7. The renal corpuscle consists of the glomerulus, which is a tuft of modified capillaries, and the glomerular capsule.

8. Unlike other capillaries, glomeruli are drained by arterioles called efferent arterioles.

9. The juxtaglomerular apparatus consists of the macula densa of the distal convoluted tubules and the juxtaglomerular cells of the afferent arteriole.

10. Urine production involves glomerular filtration, tubular resorption, and tubular secretion.

What You Should Know (continued)

11. Glomerular filtration is the process whereby fluid from your blood, minus large proteins and cells, is pushed through the endothelial-capsular membrane by the force of the sum of the four pressures present in your glomeruli.

12. Your entire blood volume is filtered 60 times per day.

13. Tubular resorption is the process of removing needed substances from the filtrate and returning them to the blood.

14. Some substances, glucose for example, are completely resorbed unless their concentration in the blood exceeds the maximum amount that the renal tubules are capable of resorbing.

15. Some substances, sodium for example, are incompletely resorbed, leading to a daily loss that must be replaced by dietary intake.

16. Tubular secretion is the process of taking additional substances from the blood and adding them to the urine as it is being produced.

17. Carbonic acid is produced in the kidneys; as it ionizes, the bicarbonate is resorbed and the hydrogen ion is secreted. This elevates the pH of the blood.

18. Your kidneys can alter their resorption of bicarbonate and secretion of hydrogen ions to compensate for acidosis and alkalosis.

19. Most of the water that can be resorbed by your kidneys is always resorbed. This is called obligatory water resorption.

20. Under the influence of ADH from the posterior pituitary, the kidneys can alter the concentration of the urine. Concentrated urine is excreted when we must conserve water in the body. Dilute urine is excreted when we have excess water that we must eliminate.

21. The endocrine system regulates the renal resorption of some ions.

22. The juxtaglomerular apparatus is involved in the regulation of sodium resorption. Low blood pressure in the afferent arteriole causes the juxtaglomerular cells to secrete renin. Renin activates the renin-angiotensin system. Activated angiotensin (angiotensin II) constricts muscular arteries, including efferent arterioles, and triggers release of aldosterone from the adrenal cortex. Aldosterone stimulates sodium resorption.

23. The kidneys influence blood pressure by controlling the blood volume through urine dilution and concentration mechanisms, and through the renin-angiotensin system.

What Did You Learn?

Multiple choice questions: choose the best answer.

1. The kidneys are located within which body cavity?
   a. Thoracic
   b. Abdominal
   c. Pelvic
   d. Pleural
   e. None of the above

2. Which of the following is not a function of your urinary system?
   a. Eliminating metabolic wastes
   b. Maintaining fluid-electrolyte balance and pH
   c. Maintaining blood pressure
   d. Maintaining extracellular fluid volume and ion concentration
   e. All of the above are functions of your urinary system

3. The duct that conveys urine from the bladder to the exterior is known as:
   a. Urethra
   b. Nephron
   c. Ureter
   d. Collecting tubules

4. Ammonia and urea are nitrogen-containing wastes, and result mainly from:
   a. Carbohydrate catabolism
   b. Protein anabolism
   c. Carbohydrate anabolism
   d. Protein catabolism
   e. None of the above

5. You have two of which of the following?
   a. Ureter
   b. Urethra
   c. Both of the above
   d. Neither of the above

6. Which of the following is larger in diameter?
   a. Afferent arteriole
   b. Efferent arteriole
   c. They have equal diameters

What Did You Learn? (continued)

7. Place the structures below in the correct sequence, as developing urine would pass through them.

    1. Loop of the nephron (of Henle)

    2. Distal convoluted tubule

    3. Proximal convoluted tubule

    4. Renal corpuscle

    5. Collecting tubules and ducts

    a. 3,2,1,4,5

    b. 3,4,1,2,5

    c. 4,3,1,2,5

    d. 4,3,2,1,5

    e. 2,3,1,4,5

8. Juxtaglomerular cells are found in the:

    a. Afferent arteriole

    b. Efferent arteriole

    c. Proximal convoluted tubule

    d. Distal convoluted tubule

9. Pyramids and columns are parts of the renal:

    a. Medulla

    b. Cortex

    c. Both of the above

    d. Neither of the above

10. The entire blood volume is filtered:

    a. Ten times per day

    b. Ten times per hour

    c. Sixty times per hour

    d. Sixty times per day

    e. One hundred times per day

11. Which of the following is/are found in normal filtrate?

    a. Large proteins

    b. Glucose

    c. Both are found within filtrate

    d. Neither is found within filtrate

12. The movement of substances from filtrate back into the blood is called:

    a. Filtration

    b. Tubular resorption

    c. Tubular secretion

    d. None of the above

13. Which of the following is not resorbed?

    a. Urea

    b. Small proteins and amino acids

    c. Glucose

    d. Calcium

    e. All of the above are resorbed

14. Which of the following is normally <u>completely</u> resorbed?

    a. Glucose

    b. Calcium

    c. Urea

    d. All of the above

    e. None of the above

15. Which of the following is secreted?

    a. Urea

    b. Ammonia

    c. Both of the above

    d. Neither of the above

16. What is the effect of tubular secretion of H^+ ions on the blood?

    a. Elevation of blood pH

    b. Decrease of blood pH

    c. No change in blood pH

    d. H^+ ions are not secreted

17. Which structure is permanently permeable to water?

    a. Distal convoluted tubule

    b. Descending limb

    c. Ascending limb

    d. Collecting tubule

18. A person is suffering from a pulmonary condition that causes an elevated blood CO_2 level. The kidneys will compensate by _____ secretion of H^+ and _____ resorption of bicarbonate.

    a. Increased, increased

    b. Decreased, decreased

    c. Increased, decreased

    d. Decreased, increased

19. Long loops of capillaries that travel deep into the medulla along with the loop of the nephron are called:

    a. Vasa vasora

    b. Vasa recta

    c. Vasa sinusoida

    d. Vasa whoknowsa

20. An elderly person has accidentally ingested an entire box of antacid in a very short time. This person is likely to develop:

    a. Acidosis

    b. Alkalosis

    c. Neither of the above

What Did You Learn? (continued)

21. After a severe bout of vomiting, one would expect the kidneys to:

    a. Secrete more H^+

    b. Secrete less H^+

    c. Not alter the secretion of H^+ in any way.

22. Antidiuretic hormone affects urine concentration by altering permeability of which of the following structures?

    a. Proximal convoluted tubule

    b. Descending limb

    c. Ascending limb

    d. Collecting tubules

    e. None of the above

23. You are adrift in a life raft and ran out of water a day ago. How concentrated should your urine be?

    a. 3,000 mOsm

    b. 1,200 mOsm

    c. 600 mOsm

    d. 60 mOsm

24. You have just come from your job as a taste tester in a bottled water factory, and it was a very long day. Which of the following will currently be impermeable to water?

    a. Distal convoluted tubule

    b. Collecting duct

    c. Both of the above

    d. Neither of the above

25. In response to low blood pressure, the juxtaglomerular apparatus secretes:

    a. Renin

    b. Angiotensinogen

    c. Both of the above

    d. Neither of the above

26. A diuretic prescribed by your health-care provider causes you to increase your urine output. This will _____ your blood pressure.

    a. Increase

    b. Decrease

    c. Have no effect on

Short answer questions: answer briefly and in your own words.

1. What is a nephron? Briefly describe its structure and function.

2. Please describe the steps involved in urine production.

3. What is a juxtaglomerular apparatus and what does it do?

4. Describe the mechanism the kidneys use to influence blood pressure. If you have a genetic condition that causes you to resorb sodium more efficiently than others, what will this do to your blood pressure? What can you do about it?

5. Describe the mechanisms used by the kidneys to influence the pH of the blood. If a nonathlete ran a marathon, how would the kidneys compensate for the resulting changes in blood pH?

6. Describe the unique vascular arrangement of the glomerulus. Why is this unusual arrangement necessary?

7. Why does diabetes mellitus cause excessive urine volume?

Defending Your Body

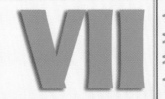

The Integumentary and Immune Systems: Why Study Them Together?

Your body is like a mighty fortress. Why a fortress, you ask, instead of some other structure? Well, just as a fortress is designed to withstand attacks from hostile forces, your body needs to be able to defend itself from a wide variety of attacking agents. A fortress has a wall capable of repelling many of its enemies. Your body has a similar wall, the main organ of the integumentary system: your skin. A fortress has an internal defense force, dedicated to vanquishing enemies that breach the wall and enter its inner spaces. Likewise, your body has an immune system capable of recognizing invading microorganisms, cells behaving aberrantly, and many other potential enemies.

For these reasons, we will study these two systems together. Our last two chapters will allow you to further use many of the facts and concepts you have learned while reading this text. It is a good idea to look back over any concepts of which you feel unsure as you encounter them in this, the final section in your first study of the human body.

20 The Great Wall and More: Your Integumentary System

What You Will Learn

- The many functions of your integumentary system.
- The anatomy of your skin.
- How and why melanocytes provide pigmentation for your skin.
- The role of the integumentary appendages.
- The structure and functions of your hair and nails.
- The names, locations, and secretions of the glands associated with your skin.

20.1 Like the Wall of a Mighty Fortress: The Functions of Your Integumentary System

As we consider your skin, the main component of your integumentary system, we may begin by noting its similarity to a great wall, such as we would find around a fortress. It certainly performs many of the same functions as such a wall. It defines the outer boundaries of our bodies, it serves as a somewhat impenetrable barrier to ward off invading injurious agents, and it protects us against the harsh effects of the environment.

As we come to know more about skin, however, we may begin to appreciate it as a living, self-repairing organ with attributes that the walls of a fortress could never replicate. Let's list some of these important functions now.

It controls entry into and exit from the body; in part by the fact that it is relatively impermeable to water (it is somewhat waterproof). Unfortunately, many organic solvents can pass directly through this barrier. It blocks ultraviolet light, protecting our internal organs from the effects of these rays. In fact, exposure to sunlight causes our bodies to increase the pigmentation that blocks the entry of this form of energy. With that in mind, another function is the synthesis of vitamin D (**FIGURE 20.1**). Our skin uses ultraviolet light to perform this synthesis. Our integumentary system is important in the thermoregulation of our bodies. Even the vascular arrangement of our skin is modified to aid in this important function. Sensory receptors are present in our skin, allowing us to sense our external environment. Special cells of our immune system are also present here, to mount a defense when invading microbes are present. Our skin protects us

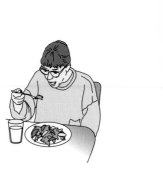
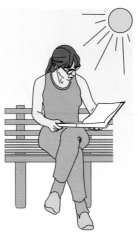
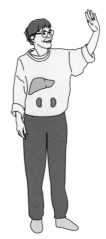
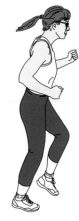

1. Provitamin D is ingested.

2. Provitamin D is converted into previtamin D by sunlight.

3. Previtamin D converts spontaneously to Vitamin D₃, which is activated by the liver and kidneys.

4. Active Vitamin D is necessary for calcium and phosphate homeostasis and for healthy bones.

FIGURE 20.1

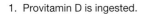

Synthesis of active vitamin D.

from damage by abrasion and physical impact. It also plays a minor role in excretion, through the production of sweat. Let's take a brief look at a few of the more specialized functions before turning to the anatomy of skin.

■ Specialized Functions of Your Skin

Vitamin D Synthesis: The Skin's Role

Rickets (in children) and osteomalacia (in adults) are bone diseases that can be caused by vitamin D insufficiency. Rickets was once very common in northern countries where there is a seasonal lack of daylight. Rickets has been largely eliminated in the developed world because of the supplementation of vitamin D in the diet. Osteomalacia is still prevalent in some cultures that require women to be completely covered (except for their eyes) when in public. With this talk of bone diseases, you may be asking yourself whether we are still discussing the skin, or have we turned to some other topic. Let's look at the skin's role in the avoidance of these diseases.

Vitamin D, a cholesterol derivative, is necessary for normal bone physiology. It is readily absorbed in the alimentary canal, and as such, dietary sources can supply our needs. What happens, however, if we don't have a sufficient intake of this vitamin? We produce our own in the following way.

The vitamin D synthetic pathway begins with pro-vitamin D (dehydrocholesterol), a cholesterol-related compound. When the skin is exposed to ultraviolet light, pro-vitamin D in the skin is converted to pre-vitamin D, which spontaneously converts to vitamin D₃ (chole-

calciferol). Vitamin D₃ is then activated in a pathway involving the liver and the kidneys. Active vitamin D (calcitrol) is necessary for calcium and phosphate absorption in the small intestine and resorption in the kidneys. As you know, calcium is very important for the production and maintenance of bone.

So, how can we be assured of adequate vitamin D intake? We can take steps to be sure that it is adequately supplied in our diets (vitamin D-supplemented milk is much more pleasant than the cod liver oil of days gone by). We can also try to spend some time in the sunlight, enabling our skin to fulfill this important function, as long as we take precautions to avoid overexposure (see this chapter's "Breaching Homeostasis").

Thermoregulation: Your Skin's Role in Temperature Homeostasis

You are well aware of the cooling effects of sweating; we discussed these effects in Chapter 5 when thinking about homeostasis and negative feedback. When your temperature rises, as during hot weather or when you are exercising, your integumentary system wets the surface of your skin with sweat. As the water present in sweat evaporates, it absorbs heat, drawing it away from the body's surface. Our goal, however, is not just to cool the surface of the body, but to maintain temperature homeostasis throughout the body. Again, our moving fluids play an important role. Special arterial-venous anastomoses (shunts that bypass capillaries) are present within the deeper layers of the skin. These arteries dilate while we sweat, allowing a great rate of blood flow, cooling the blood, which then circulates through our internal organs, cooling them in turn. This lowers the temperature of the whole body, not just the surface.

How about when we are not too hot, but too cold? Here again, the integumentary system has a role to play. Adipose tissue in the deep region of the skin serves as insulation, just as fiberglass or a similar material insulates your home against heat loss. Vascular changes opposite to those that occurred when your body was too hot now take place. The vascular supply to your skin constricts, reducing flow, thereby keeping the warm blood away from the body's surface where it would be cooled.

Sensory Reception: What's Out There?

Your integumentary system is important in allowing you to sense your environment and gain the information you need to protect yourself. Isn't this also like the wall of a fortress? Don't fortress walls contain some form of openings or windows to allow for identification of approaching friends or foes (see Figure 20.2)? Your skin has a number of such sensory devices. They sense such qualities as touch, pressure, temperature, and pain. These receptors are described in **TABLE 20.1**.

Security Force at the Wall: Immune Defense of Your Skin

A good fortress has a security force at the ready, prepared for defense should the wall be breached. This is also true of our skin; immune surveillance is one of its roles. Langerhans cells are members of the monocyte-macrophage lineage that are specialized not for phagocy-

tosis, like most of the cells in this lineage, but to watch for invading enemies (microorganisms) and to inform other immune cells of their presence. These cells are present in our skin. Their function will be described in Chapter 21.

Excretion: Elimination of Wastes at the Wall

Note that when we discuss sweat in the sweat gland section of this chapter, the chemical composition of sweat resembles that of urine. While not of great importance as an excretory organ, the skin does eliminate a small quantity of wastes through sweat.

Now, on to the anatomy of skin.

20.2 The Anatomy of Your Skin

Your skin is your largest organ. Its mass is about 16 percent that of your entire body (impressive). It has a surface area of 1.5–2 square meters. We will first look at the skin itself and then consider other structures associated with it.

Your skin has three layers: the epidermis is the most superficial; then the dermis; and last, the hypodermis. We will examine each of the three layers separately. Look at the diagram in **FIGURE 20.2** for clarity.

■ Your Epidermis

Your epidermis is the most superficial (outermost) portion of your skin. It overlies the dermis, and their line of contact is thrown into folds to increase surface area. This arrangement keeps the epidermis well adhered to the dermis.

The epidermis is the epithelial component of this organ and is a cornified stratified squamous epithelium. These epithelial cells are called keratinocytes because of the large amount of keratin they accumulate as they differentiate. The epidermis is composed of four to five layers, depending on location: the stratum basale, the stratum spinosum, the stratum granulosum, the stratum lucidum (only on fingertips, palms, and soles), and the stratum corneum. Let's look at each layer individually.

The stratum basale is, as the name implies, the basal layer. It is well anchored to a thin basement membrane and is made up of a single layer of low columnar cells. These cells are the stem cells of the epidermis; they proliferate, providing daughter cells that migrate up through the other layers, differentiating as they go. The importance of these stem cells is that your epidermis is replaced continually, individual cells lasting only about 30 days, more or less depending on the specific location. It is important to note that the mitotic rate of the epidermis increases while you sleep. Sleep is, therefore,

Table 20.1 Skin-Associated Sensory Receptors

Receptor	Sensations	Structure
Tactile (Meissner) corpuscle	Touch, pressure, and vibration	Elongated connective tissue capsule surrounding dendrites
Merkel disk	Touch and pressure	Merkel sensory cell surrounded by dendrites
Lamellated (Vater-Pacini) corpuscle	Pressure and vibration	Onionlike layered connective tissue surrounding dendrites
Hair root plexuses	Touch	Free nerve endings (dendrites) wrapped around hair follicles
Free nerve endings	Temperature and pain	Free nerve endings (dendrites)

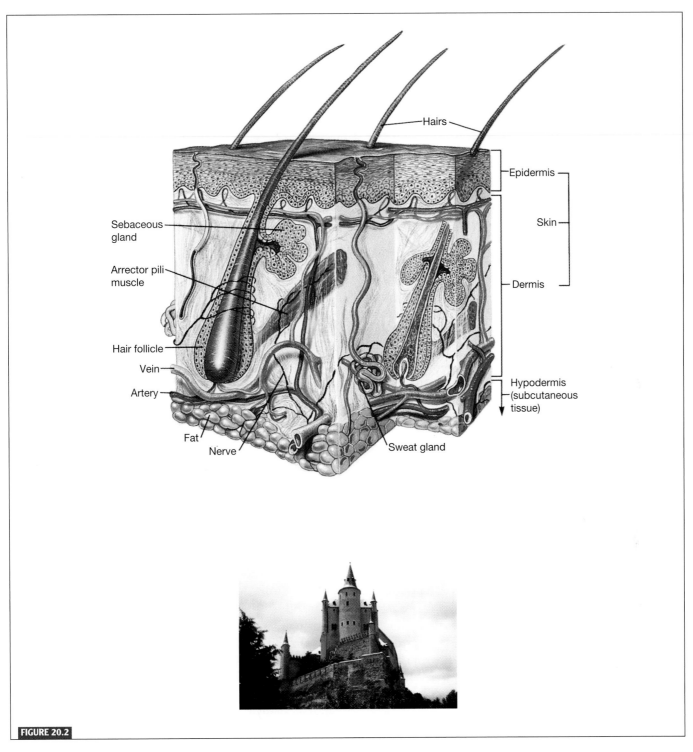

FIGURE 20.2

Anatomy of the skin.

important in promoting healthy skin. From the stratum basale, cells move into the stratum spinosum.

The stratum spinosum is made up of cuboidal cells to low-cuboidal cells. As the keratinocytes move up through the layers, they differentiate. Gaining a flattened morphology is one part of this differentiation process. This layer is thicker in areas of high abrasion, thinner in more protected areas. There may be as many as 10 layers of cells in the stratum spinosum. Despite the differentiation that is occurring here, these cells divide at an even faster rate than those of the basal layer. From here, cells move into the stratum granulosum.

The stratum granulosum comprises three to five layers of flattened cells. These well-differentiated cells are not mitotically active and have, in fact, begun to degenerate. As the keratinocytes move up through the layers, as noted, they are differentiating. This involves accumulation of large amounts of the keratin intermediate filament proteins and other proteins that link the keratin together. They also accumulate (and in the stratum granulosum, exude) phospholipids and other substances that repel water and "glue" the cells together. This produces a water-resistant barrier. Organic solvents can dissolve these substances and pass through this barrier, however, so be careful with paint thinner, gasoline, and similar materials.

The stratum lucidum, the next layer, is most apparent in exposed, abraded areas of skin, such as the fingertips, palms, and soles. It may be altogether absent in other areas. Again, the keratinocytes are moving upward. Here they are flattened, filled with keratin and related proteins, lack nuclei, and are tightly packed together. Next they enter the stratum corneum.

The cells of the stratum corneum, or cornified layer, are filled with tightly packed keratin and keratin-related proteins. Apoptosis has occurred, killing the keratinocytes. Enzymes from lysosomes have digested all of their organelles; they are, in fact, dead cells. Cells are constantly shed from the stratum corneum, and just as constantly replaced from below. Much of the dust we see in the places where we live and work is actually cells of the stratum corneum that have been shed (desquamated). An interesting laboratory anecdote is that, when scientists began studying the keratin proteins, the keratin polypeptides of the epidermis were frequently encountered as contaminants in samples of cells that don't contain keratin. It turned out that epidermal proteins made it into these samples from the ubiquitous desquamated epidermal cells in our environment! The thick calluses you may develop on your hands after performing hard work are actually a thickened stratum corneum. In areas of your skin exposed to very little abrasion, the stratum corneum may be quite thin.

In addition to keratinocytes, there is an additional cell type present in the epidermis that we will consider here. It is the melanocyte, the cell responsible for skin pigmentation.

Melanocytes and Skin Pigmentation

Melanocytes are the cells responsible for skin pigmentation. They are associated with the epithelium of the epidermis, but are not actually a part of that epithelium. They are interspersed among the cells of the stratum basale at a rate of one melanocyte per four to 12 associated keratinocytes. This number varies based on the location on the body, not based on gender or skin color. In fact, people of different skin color have similar numbers of melanocytes.

Melanocytes sit among the epithelial cells looking much like spiders sitting on their backs with their legs pointed upward (**FIGURE 20.3**). The "legs" of these "spiders," the cytoplasmic extensions of the melanocytes, reach out to epidermal cells (keratinocytes) of the basale and spinosum strata. Where the melanocytes contact these cells, the membrane of each epithelial cell has an indentation that accepts the melanocyte extension. This allows the transfer of the pigment produced by melanocytes to the keratinocytes.

Melanocytes produce melanin, a pigment that is derived from the amino acid tyrosine. They package this brown-black pigment in small (0.7×0.3 micrometer) football-shaped packets called melanosomes. Melanosomes are delivered up the cytoplasmic extensions to the keratinocytes. The keratinocytes, in turn, store and degrade the melanosomes. The rate of formation of melanin granules and the storage of melanosomes in the keratinocytes determine the degree of pigmentation present in the skin.

The "tanning" effect of the sun, darkening of the skin after sun exposure, is caused by a few interrelated phenomena. The melanin already present in melanosomes darkens by a photochemical reaction. This preexisting melanin is also released into the epidermal cells from the melanocytes more rapidly. The melanocytes also increase their rate of melanin synthesis.

The importance of this pigmentation lies not in any aesthetic benefit, but in the ability of melanin to block the harmful ultraviolet irradiation present in sunlight. As you sit in the sun, keep in mind that the very rays that induce the increased pigmentation you seek also causing damage. Perhaps a good sun screen is actually an improvement in protection from these rays.

Dermatoglyphics: Fingerprints

Doesn't *dermatoglyphics* sound like the term for some strange type of writing, or even a body decoration? In a way it is. We are all aware of the ridges that are present on the palms of our hands and fingers, and the soles of our feet and toes. These fingerprints, handprints, and footprints are called dermatoglyphics. Their function is to provide traction, just like the tread on your car's tires. The individuality of these ridges has been the basis for identification by the police and other legal entities for many years (**FIGURE 20.4**). The high points are called ridges; the grooves between them are sulci. Their pattern seems to be determined by multiple alleles on numerous genes, so incredible numbers of patterns are possible. They actually appear very early in life; about the 13th week in utero.

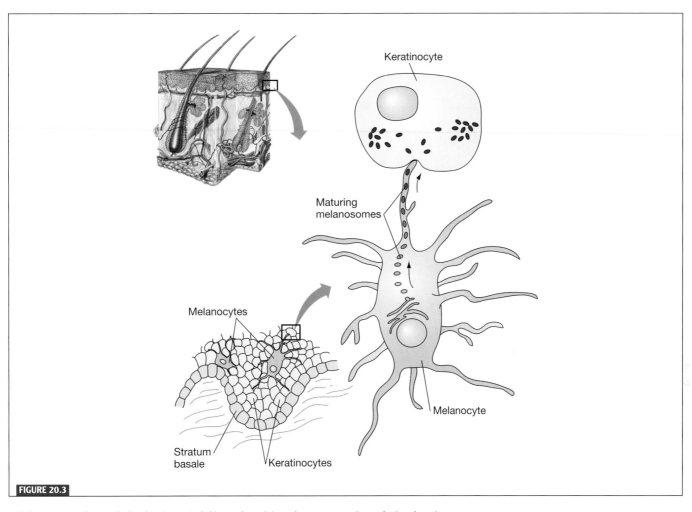

Melanocytes produce melanin, the pigment of skin, package it in melanosomes, and transfer it to keratinocytes.

■ Your Dermis

Deep to your epidermis is your dermis. The thickness of the dermis varies with location. It is at its thickest (3 mm) on the soles of your feet. It has a two-layered structure. The superficial layer (just deep to the epidermis) is called the papillary layer (Figure 20.2). It is composed of loose connective tissue with abundant mast cells, macrophages, and leukocytes. These immune and inflammatory cells are present to protect against any invaders that might make it through the epidermis. This is like having a security force patrolling the perimeter of our fortress just inside the wall.

The next layer of the dermis is the reticular layer. It is composed of dense irregular connective tissue and is the thicker of the two layers. It imparts much strength to the dermis and, hence, to your skin.

Common to both layers are abundant collagenous fibers for strength, and elastic fibers to allow your skin to stretch and recoil back to shape as you move. There are also many nerves present, including sensory nerves terminating as free nerve endings, tactile (Meissner)

corpuscles, and lamellated (Vater-Pacini) corpuscles, described in Table 20.1. These receptors allow you to continually sense your external environment.

The epidermal appendages, which we will discuss in a few moments, extend into the dermis. These include epidermal glands and hair follicles. First, let's consider the next layer.

■ Your Hypodermis: The Subcutaneous Tissues

Deep to the dermis, we find a layer of loose connective tissue called the hypodermis. Depending on the location, these tissues may allow the skin some freedom of movement or may hold it more rigidly. Where the skin is allowed freedom of movement, increased amounts of adipose tissue are present, and in some locations this fat may be quite thick. As we learned earlier in this text, this adipose tissue can be important. It is, in fact, stored energy. It also provides thermal insulation and an absorbent cushion against impact. The adipose cells are distributed as lobules with septae (walls) of dense connective tissue.

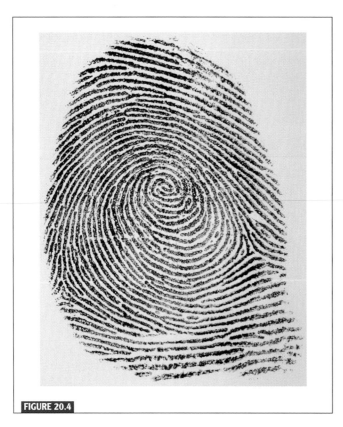

FIGURE 20.4

A fingerprint.

It is this connective tissue that keeps the skin from sliding around over the underlying tissues. In locations where the skin has freedom of movement, loose connective tissue with less adipose tissue is present. These locations are the sites used for subcutaneous injections, into this very connective tissue, in fact.

20.3 Integumentary Appendages: The Structures Associated with Your Skin

Included in the appendages associated with our skin (also called adnexa) are hair, nails, and several types of glands. We will discuss each appendage separately.

■ Your Hair

Hair is an amazing appendage of our skin. We may think of hair as purely decorative, and in fact the cosmetics industry would probably be happy if we did think of it that way. Hair actually has a number of important functions. While we most often think of hair in conjunction with the top of our heads; much of our hair is not there. Hair is spread across almost the entire body and is present with different textures in different locations.

It serves as a filtering mechanism to keep foreign objects out of our noses, ears, and eyes. On our heads, it provides thermal insulation, cushions us from minor bumps, and blocks ultraviolet rays (well, it provides these functions for some of us, anyway). On the surface of our bodies, it protects against abrasion, allowing our clothing and other surfaces to slide across our surface with less loss of cornified epithelial cells. Through the associated plexus of sensory nerves, hair acts as an "early warning system" for certain dangers. The movement of our hair by an angry wasp may help us to avert a dangerous sting. Even air currents moving our hairs as we grope about in the dark may give us subtle information about our environment. Hair even plays a role in human courtship and reproduction.

So, what actually is hair? The actual hair shaft (that which we think of as hair) is an organized structure constructed from dead, cornified epithelial cells. The cosmetic and shampoo industries might want us to believe that our hair shafts are living appendages on which their potions can have magical health effects. We must keep in mind when viewing their advertisements that they are talking about dead cells.

The hair follicle is, however, a different matter. Hair follicles are mainly epidermal structures that extend downward into the underlying dermis. They have a complex structure, as shown in **FIGURE 20.5**. Follow along with that figure as we examine the hair follicle.

The hair follicle is an ingrowth of epidermis into the underlying dermis, called the root sheath. It is surrounded by the glassy membrane (a thickened basement membrane), and by a dense sheath of dermal connective tissue. Near the epidermis, the root sheath has a single layer, but nearer the base of the follicle, two layers are present, an internal root sheath and an external root sheath. The base of the follicle has an onionlike layered structure, the hair bulb. The epithelial cells of this structure are differentiated for specific purposes.

In the center of the bulb, we find large vacuolated cells that form the medulla, or middle of the hair shaft. These cells are surrounded by others that form the cortex of the hair shaft. These cells contain large amounts of keratin. Moving outward to the next layer, we find cells that form the hair cuticle, its outermost layer. These cells become a shinglelike layer on the outside of the hair shaft. The individual cells of this layer (the "shingles") are called epicuticles. They are the equivalent of extremely flattened cornified keratinocytes.

The epicuticle arrangement is one of the differences between the different types of hair we find in different locations on the body. For example, scalp hair has epicuticles with smooth borders, arranged in a regular

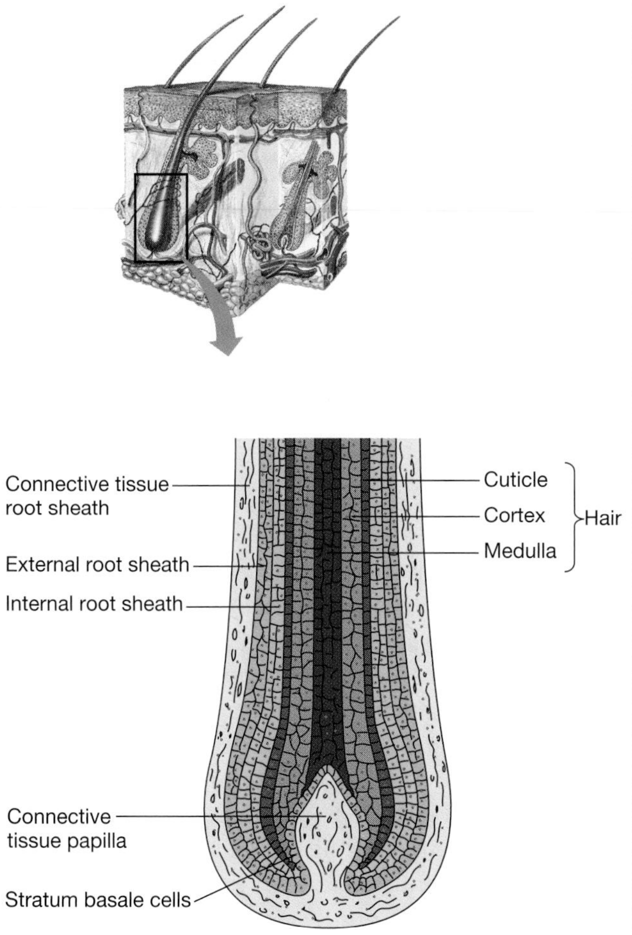
Connective tissue root sheath
External root sheath
Internal root sheath
Connective tissue papilla
Stratum basale cells
Cuticle
Cortex
Medulla
Hair

FIGURE 20.5

A hair follicle.

transverse order. Pubic hair has an irregular epicuticle arrangement with uneven borders. The epicuticle borders of eyebrow hair are smooth, but the epicuticles are arranged irregularly.

The outermost cells in the bulb are the cells of the internal root sheath that, as already pointed out, do not reach the surface of the skin.

Both the medullary and cortical hair cells contain melanin pigment. This pigment, produced by melanocytes, is passed to the cells of the bulb much like it is passed to other epidermal cells. Different forms of melanin are responsible for the differences we see in hair color. While the genes do not specify the hair color per se, they provide the plan for the enzymes that produce the melanin and arrange the melanin in the melanosomes, thereby indirectly determining the hair color. Differences between the amino acid sequences in these enzymes result in differences in the pigments they produce. Refer to Chapter 14 if you are unclear on this.

Arrector pili muscles attached to the follicle can elevate the hair shaft from the surface of the skin. We are all familiar with the feeling of the hair "standing up" on the backs of our necks in response to cold temperatures or a sudden fright. This is for heat conservation (in the cold) and to make us look larger and more imposing (as part of the fight-or-flight response). Seems rather ineffective with the small amount of hair humans possess! Sympathetic stimulation causes contraction of the arrector pili muscles. Interestingly, unlike almost all other sympathetic neuroeffector junctions that use norepinephrine as their neurotransmitter; the arrector pili (and some skin-associated glands) neuroeffector junctions use acetylcholine. Before discussing the skin-associated glands, let's consider the nails.

Your Nails: Finger and Toe

Of course, we all know where to find our nails: on the dorsal surfaces of the distal portions of our fingers and toes. Other than when to cut them, how much do we think about them? Well, they are actually very useful accessories on these appendages (O.K., on the fingers more so than the toes). They help us to grip objects; try opening a soda can without them. They are also useful defensively (again, the fortress theme).

The nail body (that which we think of as the nail) is a cornified plate largely composed of keratin (**FIGURE 20.6**). Nail bodies are as dead as our hair shafts (again, beware overzealous cosmetics ads). They adhere to the nail bed, a thickened epithelial layer. The proximal, deep portion of the nail bed is the nail root, the site of production of the nail body.

At the base of the exposed portion of the nail body is the pale, half-round lunula. It is an area of reduced vascularity, although its function is not known. The stratum corneum is modified along the proximal and distal edges of the nail body to seal the nail to the skin.

Now, onto the skin-associated glands.

Skin-Associated Glands

Several types of glands are associated with the skin. Different types of secretions are produced by these glands for different purposes. Some secretions specifically protect the skin and hair; others are important in thermoregulation of the body. Let's consider each type of skin-associated gland separately.

Sebaceous Glands

Sebaceous glands are made up of large, fat-filled cells that appear clear in standard histological preparations. The reason for this intracellular lipid is that their secretion is largely lipid. They produce an oily secretion that

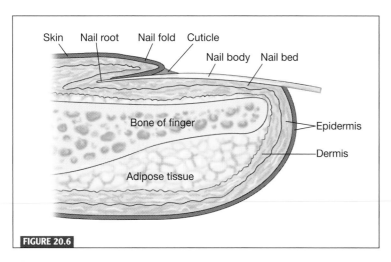

FIGURE 20.6

Fingernail anatomy.

is released into the hair follicles. Arrector pili contraction forces this secretion to the surface of the epidermis. This secretion, called sebum, is composed of triglycerides, cholesterol and related compounds, free fatty acids, electrolytes, and proteins. It serves as a lubricant and keeps hair and cornified epithelial cells from drying out (excessive removal by shampooing causes dandruff). It also discourages bacterial growth.

Some sebaceous glands are grouped into sebaceous follicles, independent of hair follicles. They release their secretions directly on the surface through their own ducts. They are concentrated on the face, trunk, nipple area, and male genitalia. Androgens increase their activity in both sexes. Derangements in sebaceous follicle activity are largely responsible for the development of acne.

Sweat Glands: Merocrine and Apocrine

Sweat glands (sudoriferous glands) are present in two types: *apocrine glands* and *merocrine glands*. Although this terminology, which refers to mechanisms of secretion, is not entirely accurate, it persists as a useful way to distinguish between these two different glands. We will discuss each separately.

Merocrine glands are small tubular structures present in the superficial dermis. They release their secretion directly onto the body's surface through their own ducts. While they are widely distributed across the surfaces of our bodies, they are especially abundant on the palms of our hands and soles of our feet (hence, sweaty palms when nervous). Their secretion is mainly water, but also contains nitrogenous and other metabolic wastes and electrolytes (mainly sodium chloride). Sounds kind of like urine, doesn't it? In fact, it does have an excretory function, and its volume is reduced by ADH, just like that of urine. Athletes generally produce this secretion in a higher volume and at a lower concentration as part of their adaptive response to regular exercise; this

is the secretion used for cooling the body. Its low pH also protects the skin through antibacterial action.

Apocrine glands are not widely distributed across the surface of the body; they are localized to the axilla, pubis, circumanal region, and areola (**FIGURE 20.7**). Like sebaceous glands, they release their secretion into hair follicles. These are relatively large glands, 3–5 millimeters in diameter, and are embedded in the subcutaneous tissues. Their cloudy, sticky secretion has its own odor, but also promotes bacterial growth, producing further odor. Their activity increases greatly at puberty, and they also undergo histological changes in women as they go through their menstrual cycle.

Ceruminous Glands: Earwax

Cerumin (earwax) was discussed in Chapter 12. It is a fatty substance produced by modified sweat glands along the external auditory meatus of the external ear. Although it may become troublesome when overproduced, it is useful in trapping unwanted foreign material heading toward your tympanic membrane. It also repels some insects (and we all know how annoying an insect in the ear can be).

That's it for the skin-associated glands. While it is tempting to rush at this point in our text, spend some time with the "What You Should Know" and "What Did You Learn?" features of this chapter, making sure you know what you think you know. Then proceed into our final chapter: The Immune System.

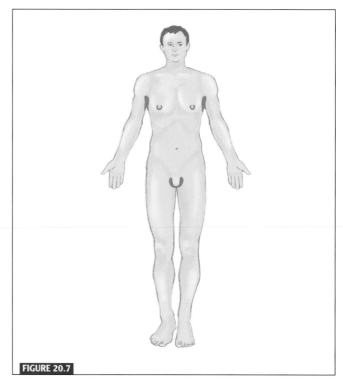

FIGURE 20.7

The locations of the apocrine sweat glands are shown in red. They include the axilla, areola, pubis, and circumanal region (not shown).

Skin Cancer

Skin cancer: how serious could that be? After all, it's only skin deep, right? Actually, skin cancer can be very dangerous, disfiguring, and even life threatening. Let's think about this common form of cancer for a few moments. Several distinctly different forms of skin cancer exist. We will discuss basal cell carcinoma, squamous cell carcinoma and its premalignant precursor actinic keratosis, and malignant melanoma.

Basal cell carcinoma is not actually a true carcinoma, but an epithelioma. We have already learned that a carcinoma is a malignancy of epithelial cells. The term *malignant* implies a number of things about a neoplasm, including that it has the ability to metastasize or migrate to distant parts of the body. Basal cell carcinoma almost always lacks that ability. Epithelioma implies a nonmalignant tumor of epithelial origin. Basal cell epithelioma (carcinoma) is an epithelial tumor since it arises from the basal cells of the integumentary adnexa. The term *carcinoma* is generally applied to this lesion regardless of this inaccuracy.

Does this lack of metastatic capacity indicate that basal cell carcinomas are to be taken lightly? No, indeed. Despite lacking the ability to metastasize, they are still quite dangerous as they can invade deeply into the underlying bone.

Basal cell carcinomas are the most common skin cancers. They are caused by overexposure to the sun and are seen most commonly in fair-skinned people. People with pigmented skin are more protected from the effects of the sun's rays. Basal cell carcinomas often appear as an elevated nodule with a central depression or ulceration. This feature gives this lesion the unappealing name "rodent ulcer." Surgical resection, cryocauterization (freezing with liquid nitrogen), and, in some cases, irradiation are used to treat basal cell carcinoma.

Squamous cell carcinoma is a malignancy of stratified squamous epithelium and, as such, can occur anywhere that this epithelium normally exists, or even in places where the normal epithelium has undergone metaplasia (a change in type) to stratified squamous epithelium. Here we are only considering squamous cell carcinoma of the skin. As sunlight is the most common causative agent, it is usually seen on sun-exposed skin, and most often in those with little pigmentation. It may appear as a flat plaque, an elevated hyperkeratinized area, or as a persistent ulcer. As true malignancies, these do have the ability to metastasize, although few actually do move to distant sites. They can become life-threatening and must be treated. Often resection (surgical removal) is curative.

Squamous cell carcinoma is often preceded by a premalignant lesion called an actinic keratosis. At this stage, the epithelial cells are exhibiting aberrant growth (dysplasia), but have not yet become invasive. Having any suspect lesions examined by a dermatologist is a good way to keep actinic keratoses from progressing to squamous cell carcinoma.

Malignant melanoma develops from melanocytes, and once present can metastasize widely. Several types exist and they can occur in places other than the skin. Here we are considering those of the skin that, as you might by now suspect, are related to sun exposure. Pale skin increases risk; sunbathing or working unprotected in the sunlight greatly contributes to your chance of developing this sometimes-deadly disease. One third to one half of malignant melanomas begin in pigmented features of the skin, such as freckles or moles. These must be watched for signs of change. A familial predisposition also exists, so you should exercise caution if other members of your family have developed this disease.

How can we recognize potential melanomas from normal pigmented features? Criteria used to diagnose malignant melanoma rely on an alphabetical memory aid: <u>a</u>symmetry, <u>b</u>orders, <u>c</u>olor, and <u>d</u>iameter. You should watch for signs of <u>a</u>symmetry within pigmented features of skin, such as elevated and nonelevated areas mixed within a single lesion. If the <u>b</u>orders are irregular, especially if you see pigment "seeping" out beyond the borders, again, this calls for caution. An individual lesion in which the <u>c</u>olors are mixed, dark and light or a variety of shades in one lesion, indicates the need for caution. And lastly, any lesion larger than the <u>d</u>iameter of the eraser on a pencil (>6 millimeters) must be examined. Keep in mind, however, that a lesion of a smaller size does not indicate that all is well. Even the largest malignancies began as one cell.

Melanomas must be surgically removed. If metastases are present, radiation and/or chemotherapy may be in order. This malignancy is one for which immunotherapy holds increasing promise.

So, do we have a "take-home message" to this brief discussion about skin cancer? Yes, we do. It is this: skin cancer exists in a variety of dangerous forms, but since they arise where we can see them and we know what causes most of them, we can protect ourselves. First, cover up when you will be exposed to sunlight. Wide-brimmed hats, long sleeves, and, of course, sunscreen are all good weapons in the fight against skin cancer. Second, monitor your own skin for the signs of cancer. Be especially vigilant in examining moles and freckles in sun-exposed areas of the skin. Third, talk to your health-care provider about your risk. A regular (annual) examination by a dermatologist may be recommended. If so, stick to the schedule. It would be tragic to postpone the diagnosis and treatment of these cancers that are so easily cured early in their course, and so potentially harmful if ignored.

What You Should Know

1. Your skin, the main component of your integumentary system, is a large and important protective organ.

2. The many important functions of your skin include providing a protective barrier, vitamin D synthesis, thermoregulation, sensory reception, immune surveillance, and a minor role in excretion.

3. Your skin has three major layers: an epidermis, a dermis, and a hypodermis.

4. The epidermis, the epithelial component of your skin, is a cornified stratified squamous epithelium.

5. Your epidermis is arranged in four or five layers with distinct morphologies and functions. The main cell type is the keratinocyte.

6. Melanocytes are the cells that provide the skin with pigmentation. They produce the pigment melanin from the amino acid tyrosine.

7. Melanin has an important protective function: it shields us from harmful ultraviolet rays present in sunlight.

8. Markings on our hands and feet (i.e., fingerprints) are called dermatoglyphics and are determined by multiple genes.

9. The dermis, largely composed of connective tissue, underlies the epidermis and is composed of a papillary layer and a reticular layer.

10. The hypodermis is a layer of loose connective tissue found deep to your dermis. The adipose tissue of the hypodermis is important for protection from thermal and traumatic injury.

11. Integumentary appendages are structures associated with your skin, including hair, nails, and several types of glands.

12. A hair shaft is an organized collection of dead, cornified epithelial cells.

13. Hair follicles extend into the dermis.

14. You should be able to identify the parts of a hair follicle and shaft.

15. The nail body (what we think of as the nail) is a dead cornified plate composed largely of keratin.

16. Sebaceous glands produce an oily secretion called sebum that lubricates the epidermis and hair, and protects them from drying out. It also discourages bacterial growth.

17. Merocrine sweat (sudoriferous) glands are widely distributed across the surface of the body and release a watery secretion with excretory and thermoregulation functions.

18. Apocrine glands are found in specific locations such as the axilla and pubis. They release a cloudy, sticky secretion.

19. Cerumin (earwax) is produced by modified sweat glands for the protection of our ears.

What Did You Learn?

Multiple choice questions: choose the best answer.

1. Functions of the integumentary system include all of the following except:
   a. Protecting our internal organs from ultraviolet irradiation
   b. Thermoregulation
   c. Limiting the movement of substances into and out of our bodies
   d. Synthesis of vitamin E
   e. All of the above are functions of the integumentary system

2. After building a snowman, you and your friend come into a warm house. You notice that your friend's cheeks are red. This is because:
   a. She is sunburned
   b. She uses lots of makeup
   c. The small arteries of her skin had been dilated while she was playing in the snow
   d. The small arteries of her skin had been constricted while in the cold and are now dilating to warm her blood
   e. She always looks that way

3. The most superficial portion of your skin is the:
   a. Dermis
   b. Hypodermis
   c. Epidermis

4. The epithelial component of your skin is the:
   a. Dermis
   b. Hypodermis
   c. Epidermis
   d. All of the above are epithelial

5. Mitosis occurs in which of the following?
   a. Stratum basale
   b. Stratum corneum
   c. Both of the above
   d. Neither of the above

What Did You Learn? (continued)

6. One of your friends is moving above the Arctic Circle, and another is moving to the tropics. As a going away present, you buy one of them a bottle of vitamin D tablets. Which one?

    a. The one moving above the Arctic Circle

    b. The one moving to the tropics

    c. Either one; it shouldn't matter where they live as everyone needs to consume vitamin D

    d. Either one; vitamin D doesn't do anything anyway

7. Melanocytes produce melanin from:

    a. Glycine

    b. Tyrosine

    c. Tryptophan

    d. Glucose

    e. Melanocytes don't produce melanin

8. Melanin is passed to epidermal cells in:

    a. Melanophores

    b. Melanosomes

    c. Melanotrophs

    d. Melamine

9. Free nerve endings in the skin of your fingers are sending messages to your brain. Your brain will interpret this as:

    a. Temperature (heat or coldness)

    b. Pain

    c. Either of the above

    d. Neither of the above

10. Fingerprints are a form of:

    a. Hieroglyphics

    b. Dermatoglyphics

    c. Dermatoletters

    d. Crop circles

11. Fingerprints are determined by:

    a. Random chance

    b. One gene with multiple alleles

    c. Multiple genes with multiple alleles each

    d. None of the above

12. Your dermis is composed of:

    a. Dense irregular connective tissue

    b. Loose connective tissue

    c. Both of the above

    d. Neither of the above

13. A cosmetics company advertises a new product that improves the health of the cells of your hair shafts. Should you buy this product?

    a. Yes. Your hair shaft cells might benefit from such a product

    b. No. Your hair shaft cells are completely dead and therefore won't benefit from this product

    c. No. You are completely bald anyway (don't choose this answer)

14. Your fingernails are adherent to thickened epithelial structures called:

    a. Nail bodies

    b. Nail beds

    c. Nail roots

    d. Lunula

15. Of the following glands, which is specifically located in the axilla, pubis, circum-anal, and areola regions?

    a. Apocrine glands

    b. Merocrine glands

    c. Sebaceous glands

    d. All of the above

16. Which of the following glands secretes a watery fluid that is important in thermoregulation?

    a. Apocrine glands

    b. Merocrine glands

    c. Sebaceous glands

    d. All of the above

17. The presence of acne suggests a derangement of the function of:

    a. Apocrine glands

    b. Merocrine glands

    c. Sebaceous glands

    d. All of the above

Short answer questions: answer briefly and in your own words.

1. What functions does your integumentary system serve?

2. Describe the three major layers of your skin.

3. What is the relationship between the keratinocytes in the layers of your epidermis? Which layers contain dividing cells? What would happen to the other layers of cells if these cells stopped dividing?

4. Imagine that you have just moved to the Caribbean. Here, you take up a lifestyle that involves lots of sailing, surfing, and lying on the beach. What changes will take place in your skin? Why do these changes take place?

5. Hard times have fallen on you and you can no longer live the life of leisure described in question four. Now you begin a new job loading burlap sacks of broken shells onto a freighter, barefoot. What change will occur in the skin of your hands and feet? Why do these changes occur?

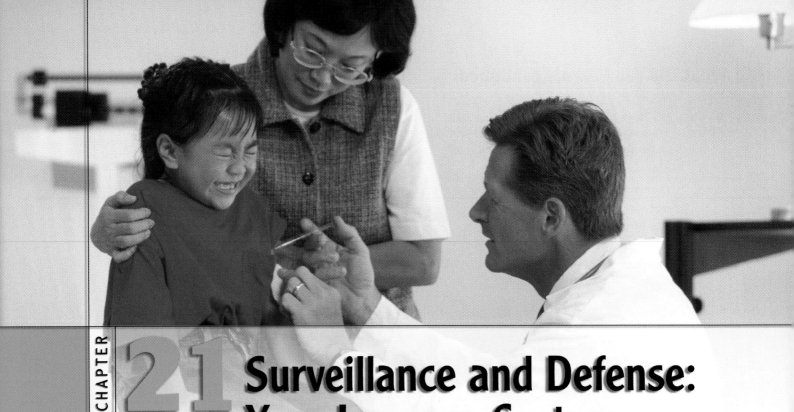

21 Surveillance and Defense: Your Immune System

What You Will Learn

- The features and activities of natural immunity and acquired immunity.
- The signs of inflammation and the cellular activities that generate this response.
- The differences between acute and chronic inflammation.
- What natural killer cells are and why they are important.
- How T and B lymphocytes develop, what they do, and how they interact with each other.
- Immunoglobulins: what they are, what they do, and what types exist.

21.1 Fences, Guard Dogs, and an Elite Security Force

We have just compared the integumentary system to a great fortress that keeps out invading enemies. But, as in any site we might try to secure, shouldn't we have back-up systems in case the enemy does breach the wall? Or what about if the enemy arises from within the fortress? Certainly, our bodies must be prepared for these possibilities; they are. In this chapter, we will have a brief overview of the immune system, the defenses our body mounts against various attackers. Despite its complexity, I refer to this discussion as a brief overview because this system is so complex that an entire course on it alone can only begin to explain its intricacies. Perhaps

you will one day take an immunology course. Here we can only start that examination.

You may notice that this discussion is based less on anatomy and rooted more in cellular activities than was the case in some of our other systems. The nature of this system largely involves wandering cells and chemicals in circulation. We will learn about the lymphoid organs, which are the organs of immunity (**FIGURE 21.1**), but they will be less central to our discussion than the roles of individual cell types.

Our immune system has two functional components. One component, called acquired immunity, is highly specific and even involves "learned" responses. We can think of acquired immunity as a highly trained elite security force that maintains a high level of surveillance for identifiable enemies. The other component,

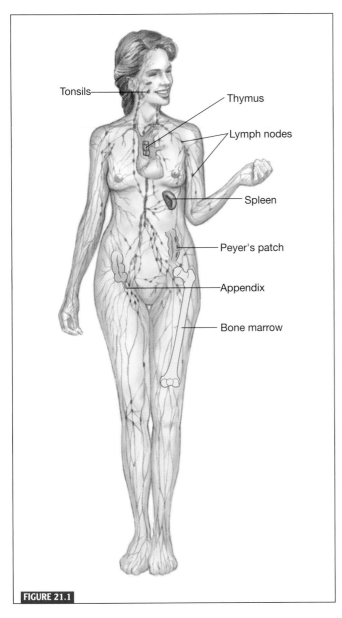

FIGURE 21.1

The immune system.

Tonsils

Thymus

Lymph nodes

Spleen

Peyer's patch

Appendix

Bone marrow

that the epithelium of the trachea and bronchi are lined with an epithelium that is effective at guarding the basement membrane even if some of the cells are killed? This certainly sounds like an effective fence.

Likewise, the saliva contains components, such as the enzyme lysozyme, that kill potentially harmful bacteria. In fact, the ongoing flow of saliva is, in itself, an effective barrier, limiting the risk of proliferation of harmful bacteria. The same can be said of the flow of lacrimal fluid across the surface of the eyes and, to some degree, of vaginal secretions, and even the flow of urine.

But what happens when these defenses are breached, as they inevitably are? Haven't we all skinned our knees, cut our fingers, developed respiratory infections, and suffered insect stings at some time? The wall of the fortress was crossed by potential pathogens in each case, but our bodies were able to mount a rapid defense and vanquish potentially harmful invaders (we survived, didn't we?). Let's examine how it did this.

Think back to when you had an injury of any sort. Didn't you see certain signs develop that were common to all injuries? The area became red, swollen, warm, and it hurt (**FIGURE 21.2**). In fact, you probably had loss of function in that area or structure as well. These are the cardinal signs of inflammation. Originally described by Celcus in the first century A.D. as rubor (redness), tumor (swelling), calor (heat), and dolor (pain); functio laesa (loss of function) was added to this description of inflammation at a later time.

Inflammation is a nonspecific response to injury that involves the blood vessels of any tissue in the body and is mounted in response to any injury. It is carried out whether the injury is a bee sting, a bullet wound, or a myocardial infarction (heart attack). The chemical and cellular mechanisms that contribute to inflammation are rather like the watchdogs of the body. Watchdogs may be very good under certain circumstances (i.e., on encountering a burglar), but may not be so good under other circumstances (i.e., on encountering the letter carrier). The same is true of inflammation. When we scrape a knee in the dirt, bacteria and debris are pushed into our bodies that must be addressed; as we are about to see, inflammation can handle that for us. When we have a myocardial infarction or a cerebrovascular accident (stroke), the injury is internal and sterile. Although there is debris that must be removed (and inflammation can do that for us), there are no invading microorganisms to be killed. In these cases, the inflammatory reaction may be excessive and do more harm than good (the letter carrier gets bitten).

So, what actually is inflammation? We know it is a nonspecific response to injury that involves blood vessels.

natural immunity, is much less refined and can be compared to a series of barriers and guard dogs that are not nearly so discriminating in their defense or specific in their response, but are valuable nonetheless. Let's begin with the more basic component.

21.2 Fences and Guard Dogs: Natural Immunity

You are already aware of many of the barriers the body uses to stop invading pathogens (the things that can cause disease). Didn't we learn that the airways leading to the lungs are lined with mucus-producing cells? And that the nose is a very effective filtering device? And also

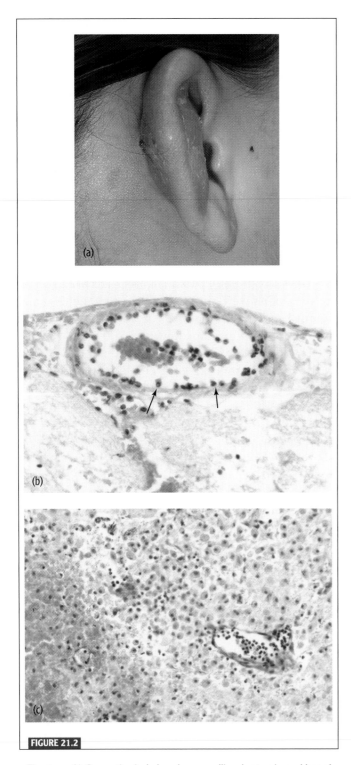

FIGURE 21.2

The signs of inflammation include redness, swelling, heat, pain, and loss of function (a). Inflammation involves changes in blood vessels that result in the movement of fluid and cells into the injured tissue. In this photomicrograph from early in the process (b), rouleaux of erythrocytes can be seen within the blood vessel. Neutrophils (*arrows*) have adhered to endothelial cells and are migrating through the vessel wall. Days later (c), macrophages are the predominant cell type.

Let's talk about what is going on exactly. There are two forms: chronic and acute. Let's start with acute inflammation. Chronic inflammation will only be mentioned briefly, as it falls more in the realm of pathology than physiology.

■ Acute Inflammation

Acute inflammation is the initial response to most injuries. It involves the activation of several control mechanisms that ultimately result in the movement of fluid and cells from the inside of blood vessels out into the interstitial space (Figure 21.2b). This movement is called exudation, and the substances that move are called exudate. Let's begin with the formation of fluid exudate.

Fluid Exudate Formation

The response of blood vessels to injury is almost immediate. We will go over the control of this response in a few moments, but first let's consider the response itself. Initially, there is a brief constriction of arterioles (a few seconds perhaps), followed by vasodilation (**FIGURE 21.3**). What happens when we dilate the arterioles? Right. The capillaries become engorged with blood. What changes might we observe grossly? Right again. There is redness and heat in the affected area. What else is going to happen? Think back to our four pressures in capillary beds (remember Starling's Hypothesis, Chapter 16?). Won't the balance of pressures be shifted to favor the movement of fluid from the vessel to the interstitial space? Think about the sudden increase in blood hydrostatic pressure pushing outward. So, fluid leaves the blood and travels into the interstitial space (we observe swelling and perhaps some pain). Now a curious thing happens. The endothelial cells contract a bit, allowing more space between them. This is called endothelial retraction and allows fluid to leave more readily and to take larger proteins with it. The presence of these proteins in the interstitial fluid further upsets the balance of pressure (it increases the interstitial osmotic pressure) and now causes more fluid to leave. Sounds like positive feedback, doesn't it?

Why is the presence of this fluid exudate a potentially good thing? Well, if any toxins are present, they will be diluted. Also, antibodies (we'll learn about these later in this chapter) and other proteins important in the immunologic defense of our bodies will be carried into the lesion (site of injury). Now, what about the cellular exudate?

Cellular Exudate Formation

How do leukocytes normally travel in the bloodstream? Think, you know this; remember axial flow (Chapter 16)?

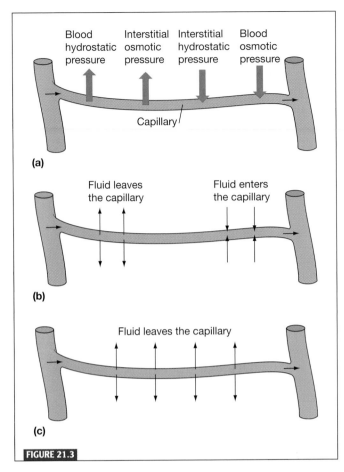

(a)

Blood hydrostatic pressure   Interstitial osmotic pressure   Interstitial hydrostatic pressure   Blood osmotic pressure

Capillary

(b)

Fluid leaves the capillary   Fluid enters the capillary

(c)

Fluid leaves the capillary

FIGURE 21.3

Starling's hypothesis explains that four pressures balance to determine whether interstitial fluid is produced or removed from the tissues surrounding capillary beds (a). During homeostasis, fluid leaves capillaries in the proximal part of the capillary bed and reenters capillaries distally (b). During inflammation, vasodilation and endothelial cell retraction alters the balance of pressures resulting in fluid exudation (c).

Being the largest objects in the stream, they are, for the most part, carried to the middle of the flow (although some sort of roll along the wall). Under normal conditions, some leukocytes do leave the blood vessels and travel in the tissues. Cells in the monocyte-macrophage lineage can leave the blood vessels and live for years in the tissues. Picture a man leaving a room full of cats without letting any cats out the door and you will be able to envision monocytes leaving capillaries, passing between endothelial cells, to travel about in the tissues without letting out erythrocytes or fluid. That is how it usually happens.

But this migration of leukocytes greatly increases during inflammation. It happens in this way (**FIGURE 21.4**). The dilation of arterioles floods the capillaries with blood; this is like a traffic jam in the capillary in which too much blood is entering and not enough is leaving the capillaries. The flow of blood (rate at which it is moving) de-

creases because of this congestion, just like a traffic jam. This results in a loss of axial flow; axial flow is speed dependent. Without axial flow, the leukocytes are no longer held in the middle of the vessel and they begin rolling along the vessel walls. Under these low-flow conditions, erythrocytes begin to clump together in stacks called rouleaux (picture a roll of Lifesavers candy with the individual candies as erythrocytes). These rouleaux of erythrocytes are now the largest bodies in the stream and take up most of the middle of the vessel, further marginalizing the leukocytes. This step is, therefore, called margination. Once the leukocytes have been pushed to the vessel margins, pavementing (the next step) begins.

Endothelial cells lining the affected capillaries insert "handles" called adhesion molecules into their cell membrane. If you can picture a man walking along a wall in a fierce windstorm, pulling himself hand over hand along the wall, you can picture the leukocytes pulling themselves along the endothelial cells, using the adhesion molecules for grip. When they reach the now-expanded gap between endothelial cells, the next step begins. Emigration is this next step. The leukocytes emigrate or leave the capillary by passing between endothelial cells into the interstitial space. Guided by chemotaxis (remember cellular "smelling"), they migrate into the injured tissue.

So, which leukocytes do this? The first cells to appear in great numbers at the site of injury do so in a matter of minutes. These are the neutrophils. If the body has watchdogs, neutrophils are the Dobermans of the group. Neutrophils (remember our granular leukocytes from Chapter 16) crawl along on pseudopodia, directed by chemotaxis, and act as first responders. They phagocytize bacteria and debris, but mainly they release hydrolytic enzymes, acids, and superoxide (oxygen-free radicals, oxygen with an unpaired electron) to kill bacteria.

Monocytes are also attracted and become activated (become macrophages) to phagocytize debris and bacteria. This starts about the same time as the neutrophil invasion, but takes longer to reach its peak. Neutrophils are the primary cells in the cellular exudate of acute inflammation; they are the hallmark of acute inflammation.

Great strategy, huh? We have fluid exudate to dilute toxins and break down bacterial and other pathogens; we have cells to subdue invaders and gobble up debris. Together these things cause the cardinal signs of inflammation already mentioned. Even the pain is a good thing (within reason). Pain informs us of our injury and causes us to stop using that structure so it can heal.

But how does all of this begin? What triggers these responses? Once triggered, what keeps them going and regulates their activity?

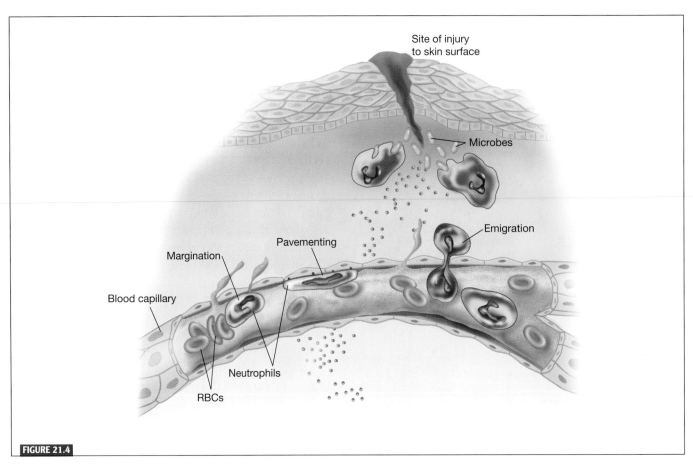

Site of injury
to skin surface

Microbes

Emigration

Pavementing

Margination

Blood capillary

Neutrophils

RBCs

FIGURE 21.4

Cellular exudation involves interplay between inflammatory cells (i.e., neutrophils) and endothelial cells. Steps in this process include margination, pavementing, and emigration.

Initiators and Mediators of Inflammation

How might you recognize a person as being injured? There are a great number of ways (there are a great variety of potential injuries), but one very common way is that you will see something leaking out of that person that only ought to be inside of that person (blood being the best example). There are many components of cells that belong in the cytoplasm, but not outside of the cell. These cytoplasmic components leak out of injured cells and can trigger inflammation. Substances that can trigger inflammation are called initiators. Other initiators of inflammation include anything that will activate mast cells and basophils (refer to Chapter 16 if you do not remember these cells). Mast cells and basophils are activated by direct trauma, cold, and a variety of molecular means (see discussion later in this chapter). When they become activated, they degranulate, releasing chemicals that mediate inflammation (mediators). Collagen is another initiator. Collagen is not normally in contact with the blood. One type of collagen in particular, collagen type IV, is part of the endothelial cell basement membrane. Endothelial cells act as a bar-

rier to keep this protein separate from the blood. When endothelial cells are injured, the blood has contact with collagen, and inflammation is triggered. Even bacterial products are inflammation initiators.

Once begun, inflammation is regulated by mediators. Mediators include substances released from the cells involved in the inflammatory response. Histamine, heparin, serotonin, and eicosanoids, such as prostaglandins and leukotreines (mentioned as lipids in Chapter 2), are all mediators of inflammation that are released from inflammatory cells. Think about the conditions that cause you to take antihistamines and aspirin, and consider what they do for you. You are using these drugs to interrupt the mediation of inflammation. Antihistamines counteract the effects of histamine, generally by inhibiting mast-cell degranulation (stopping the release of histamine). Aspirin inhibits the synthesis of prostaglandins.

Other mediators come from the plasma; they are present in circulation as potential products of four cascade mechanisms. Remember cascade mechanisms (think of the endocrine system and "mousetrap")? Cascade mechanisms are multistep processes that involve amplification to convert a small signal into a large effect. If you don't remember this concept, please review the beginning of Chapter 13 where we discussed second-messenger systems. The four cascade mechanisms of inflammation mediation are the following: the blood-clotting (coagulation) cascade, the fibrinolytic cascade, the complement cascade, and the kinin cascade.

The blood-clotting cascade is the mechanism that stops you from bleeding after injuring a vessel (**FIGURE 21.5a**; see also Figure 16.24). This cascade was presented in Chapter 16; you may want to review it now. It involves a system of molecules that are in circulation at all times and result in a delicate balance between maintaining your blood in its liquid state and causing fibrin to polymerize in the blood, making it a great deal less fluid (coagulating it). These proteins (the clotting factors) are produced by the liver. Without them, the risk of uncontrollable bleeding is a constant threat. The inherited disease hemophilia is actually a group of related diseases that, in most forms, are the result of the absence or inactivity of one of these factors. Fibrin, you will recall from Chapters 4 and 16, is the fiber component of this liquid connective tissue (blood). Its precursor, fibrinogen, is present in circulation at all times. The clotting cascade is activated by substances released from injured cells or by exposure of blood to the collagen in the endothelial basement membrane. Then fibrinogen is cleaved to fibrin, which polymerizes into fibers, forming one component of the clot. Ultimately, the fibers of fibrin bind side by side to each other (crosslink) to form a very stable clot. Platelets are the other component of this stable clot. The roles of the clotting cascade in inflammation mediation include increasing vessel permeability, and the activation of all the other inflammation mediation cascades through clotting factor XIIa, the factor common to all these cascades.

The fibrinolytic cascade is a related inflammation mediation cascade mechanism (Figure 21.5b). It results in the activation of plasminogen (which is in circulation) to its active form, plasmin. Plasmin, the product of this cascade, is a protease (protein-degrading enzyme). Through plasmin and the fibrin split products it produces, this cascade has a number of functions. It limits blood clotting, activates more clotting factor XII, which increases the activity of all four cascades (positive feedback), increases vessel permeability, and promotes chemotaxis and phagocytosis. Without an active fibrinolytic system, clotting could get out of hand. In fact, this sometimes does happen, causing clotting throughout the vasculature in a condition called disseminated intravascular coagulation (DIC).

The complement cascade is our next inflammation-mediation cascade. It has immunologic activities in addition to its inflammation mediation. This cascade also involves circulating proteins, as well as two activation pathways (Figure 21.5c). The classical pathway is triggered by antigen-antibody complexes (more about these later in this chapter). The alternate pathway is triggered by a wide variety of chemicals, such as bacterial products and plasmin. The immunologic effect of complement makes it another of our watchdogs in its own right, in addition to its role in inflammation mediation. The end product of the complement pathway is a structure called the membrane attack complex (MAC). The MAC is like a molecular doughnut, a ring with a hole in the middle, that is inserted into antibody-coated membranes. It causes lysis of undesirable cells (and sometimes, unfortunately, desirable ones) on being inserted into their membranes. This cascade's roles in inflammation mediation include promoting phagocytosis, mast-cell degranulation, neutrophil adhesion (pavementing), chemotaxis, stimulation of neutrophils and monocytes, and increased vessel permeability. Interestingly, plasmin and neutrophil lysosomal enzymes (released at the site of inflammation) are capable of activating this cascade, again eliciting positive feedback.

The fourth cascade, the kinin cascade, is perhaps the simplest (Figure 21.5d). It is triggered by the activity of factor XIIa of the clotting system. As mentioned, factor XII is the one link connecting all of our four cascades together. Factor XIIa (active factor XII) activates the precursor prekallikrein to its active form kallikrein to cleave kininogen (another plasma protein), producing bradykinin. Bradykinin has many effects in common with histamine, such as vasodilation and increasing vascular permeability. Perhaps its most notable effect, however, is its ability to induce pain, another of our cardinal signs of inflammation. This mechanism is rapidly inactivated by circulating kininases and only plays a role early in the inflammatory process.

Please study Figure 21.5 in detail to firm up your understanding of the activities of these cascade mechanisms.

■ Chronic Inflammation

Chronic inflammation is only mentioned here to distinguish it from acute inflammation. While the neutrophil is the primary cell type in acute inflammation, macrophages, along with angiogenesis (formation of new blood vessels) and fibroblast proliferation, are the hallmarks of chronic inflammation. Although macrophages are present in acute inflammation, their numbers greatly increase in chronic inflammation, and they may take on a variety of distinct morphologies.

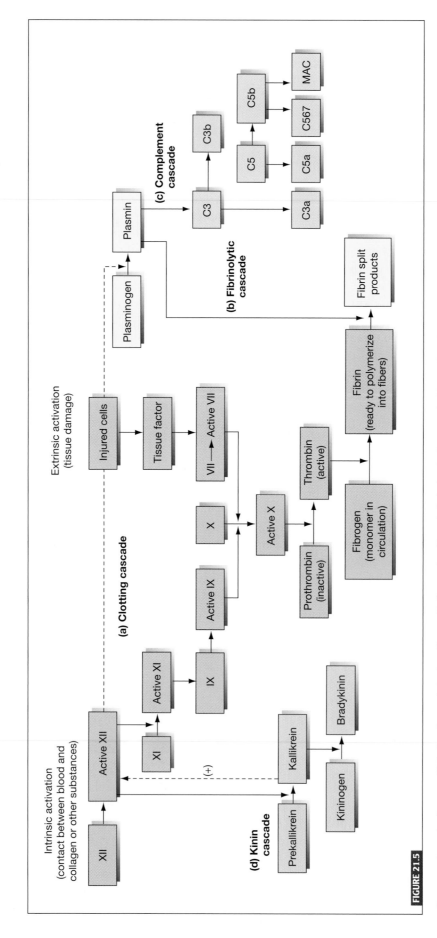

FIGURE 21.5

Four cascade mechanisms constitute the plasma-derived mediators of inflammation. These include the clotting cascade (a), the fibrinolytic cascade (b), the complement cascade (c), and the kinin cascade (d). Active factor 12 of the clotting cascade is an activator of all four cascade mechanisms.

Chronic inflammation may follow a prolonged case of acute inflammation in which the inciting pathogen (the agent causing the inflammation) has persisted. It may also occur after repeated cases of acute inflammation. Interestingly, it may also occur where no acute inflammation was present. Distinct forms of chronic inflammation play a role in a number of chronic diseases, including rheumatoid arthritis, tuberculosis, sarcoidosis, syphilis, and chronic bronchitis.

■ Natural Killer Cells

Before moving on to acquired immunity, our elite security force, I would like to mention one more "watchdog," a cell that sits on the border between the two systems. Natural killer (NK) cells are lymphoid in origin; they are a form of lymphocyte. They are most closely related to the T lymphocytes that we will learn about in our section on acquired immunity. Unlike their relatives, however, they do not rely on prior exposure to recognize and mount an effective attack against the enemy. This places them functionally nearer to natural immunity, the watchdogs and fences we have been discussing.

Natural killer cells have the unusual ability to recognize virally infected cells and neoplastic (cancer) cells, and lyse them. It is not currently known how they recognize cells as cancerous: they do not appear to use the same mechanisms used by cells participating in acquired immunity. It is easy to understand the importance of their role, however. They are on the prowl throughout our bodies looking for cells they suspect of being dangerous to our survival, and killing them when they are encountered.

They do have the ability to participate in one form of acquired immunity as well. We will soon learn that molecules that are recognized as "foreign" by our immune system are called antigens. One form of acquired immunity involves producing globular proteins called immunoglobulins, or antibodies, against these antigens. I say "against" because the role of antibodies is to bind to antigens so that they can be destroyed in a variety of ways. Natural killer cells have receptors (called Fc receptors) on their surfaces that bind the portion of the antibody molecule opposite that which binds the antigen. When antibodies bound to antigens on an invading cell's surface are encountered by NK cells, the NK cell binds to these antibodies through their Fc receptors (**FIGURE 21.6**). Then the NK cell lyses the antigen-laden cell. If you can picture this system in your mind, you are probably visualizing some form of a video game in which the invaders are coated with some special "marker," allowing the security force to recognize and destroy them. That is exactly how this works. This mechanism is called antibody-dependent cellular cytotoxicity (ADCC) and bridges the gap between natural and acquired immunity. We are now ready to study that system.

21.3 Your Elite Security Force: Acquired Immunity

Our natural immunity is very useful in defense against infectious agents, as we have been discussing, but this system has its limitations. Many bacteria and fungi have developed cell walls that are virtually impenetrable, even after phagocytosis. Also, natural immunity cannot attack agents within our cells. Some parasites, protozoa and bacteria, and all viruses can become intracellular pathogens and will never be attacked by that system (except for activities of the NK cells, as discussed).

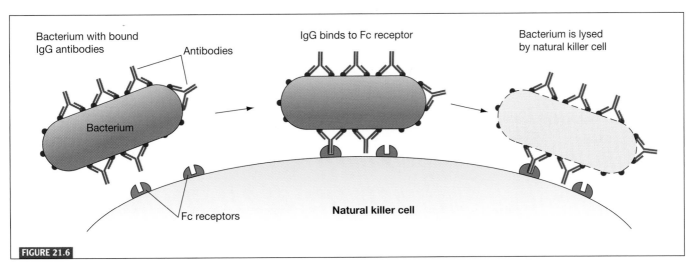

Bacterium with bound IgG antibodies

Antibodies

Bacterium

Fc receptors

IgG binds to Fc receptor

Bacterium is lysed by natural killer cell

Natural killer cell

FIGURE 21.6

Antibody-dependent cellular cytotoxicity (ADCC).

A much more sophisticated system of immunity exists to defend us from such invaders. In fact, despite amazing advances in medicine, very few drugs have been developed that are specific and effective against viruses. We continue to rely on our immune systems (and chicken soup) to keep us free of these ubiquitous and potentially deadly agents.

This complex system, our acquired immunity, is comprised of bone marrow-derived cells. Some myeloid cells (remember Chapter 16) of the monocyte-macrophage lineage participate in acquired immunity as well. Notable among these are the dendritic cells of lymphoid organs and Langerhans cells of the skin, macrophage-type cells specialized not for phagocytosis but for antigen presentation, as we will discuss shortly. Lymphoid cells give rise to T cells and B cells, as well as NK cells (already discussed). You have already been introduced to lymphoid cells in Chapter 16. Now we will discuss T and B lymphocyte functions in acquired immunity in some detail. Let's begin with an introduction to the lymphoid organs, and then follow these cells as they develop, mature, and then become activated when we are threatened with infectious agents.

■ Preparation for Defense: Lymphoid Organs and Lymphocytes

Lymphoid Organs

The lymphoid organs, or organs of immunity (Figure 21.1), can be divided into two groups: primary and sec-ondary lymphoid organs. Primary lymphoid organs include the bone marrow and the thymus. These are the sites of origin and early development of the lymphocytes. The thymus was briefly introduced in Chapter 13, but it is more aptly considered a lymphoid organ, not an endocrine gland; the hormones it produces are related to its immune functions. It lies within the mediastinum, superficial to the great vessels of the heart (**FIGURE 21.7**). Largest in infancy, it begins to involute by about age 10. Its maximal size is 20–50 grams, but after puberty it is progressively replaced with adipose and loose connective tissue.

Lymph nodes are the main secondary lymphoid organs, a category that also includes the spleen, adenoids, tonsils, appendix, and alimentary canal-associated lymphoid tissue called Peyer's patches. As shown in Figure 21.1, lymph nodes are distributed throughout the body and are interconnected by lymph vessels (Chapter 16). The spleen is an interesting organ that we have not yet discussed in any detail. You already know its location, as it is near the splenic flexure of the colon. The spleen is made up of red pulp and white pulp (**FIGURE 21.8**). Red pulp is highly vascular, composed mainly of sinusoids. It is a major site of erythrocyte recycling: worn out red blood cells are removed from circulation and broken down here. The white pulp is mainly aggregations of white blood cells.

All secondary lymphoid organs have one common purpose: they are places where lymphocytes, macrophages, and dendritic cells come into close contact to

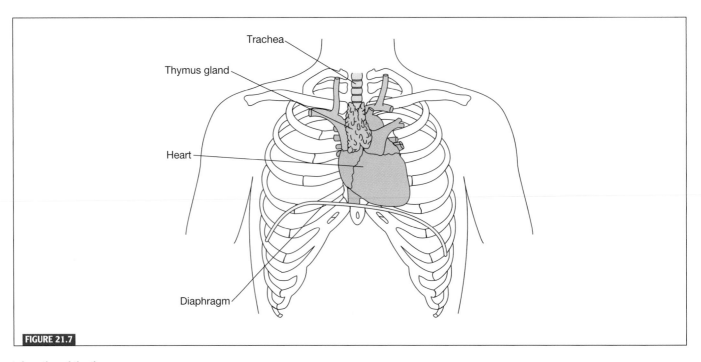

FIGURE 21.7

Location of the thymus.

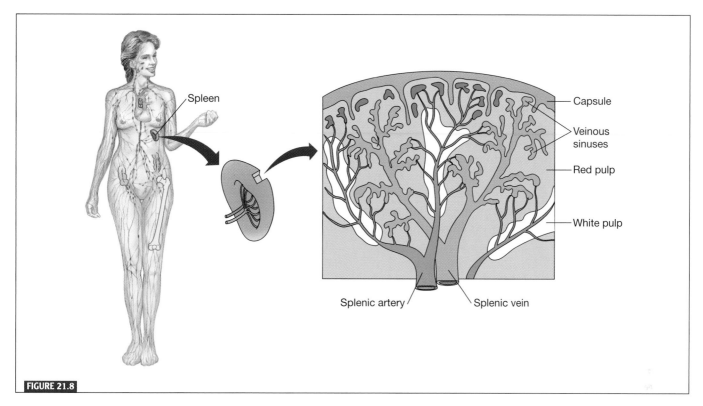

FIGURE 21.8

The spleen.

Development of T and B Lymphocytes

Both T and B cells originate in the bone marrow. B cells remain in the marrow longer as they develop; T cells begin development here, but leave the marrow early on to finish developing in the thymus. When the lymphocytes reach the proper stage of maturation, they leave the primary lymphoid organs and enter the blood vessels. They may exit the capillaries and wander about the interstitial space. Ultimately, they reenter lymph vessels and make their way to the secondary lymphoid organs (most often the lymph nodes). Alternatively, some lymphocytes may take a different route: they may stay in the vasculature and directly enter the spleen.

If lymphocytes have not been triggered to generate immunity at this time (we'll discuss that process in a moment), they continue their migration through the body. They reenter lymph vessels, and then the vasculature through the thoracic duct into the left subclavian vein, or the right lymphatic duct into the right subclavian vein (for review, return to Figure 16.20b). In this way, they can repeatedly travel through the interstitial spaces of the body, seek out an invading menace, then return to their "headquarters" (the secondary lymphoid organs) to

generate an immune response. They serve as the police stations of our immune system security force.

exchange information with other patrol officers (lymphocytes). Similar to the situation of a security force, things get interesting once a challenge arises. If, in the course of their surveillance, they encounter a microbial "enemy," acquired immunity is called into action. The endless migration through the body may seem a dull occupation for these cells. If, however, they did not follow this repetitive course, their "beat," microbial attackers might get a foothold unnoticed. Let's now examine what happens when the inevitable microbes appear.

■ A Call to Arms: Acquired Immunity in Action

Red alert, red alert! Intruders detected! It may not be quite that dramatic, but when our patrolling lymphocytes detect the presence of microbes, they jump into action. We've been focusing on lymphocytes, but let's add a little to our patrolling force. Monocytes are also on patrol, and when they encounter microbes, they differentiate into macrophages. Likewise, dendritic cells in the lymph nodes and Langerhans cells in the skin (remember, these are in the monocyte-macrophage lineage) are looking for invaders as well. All of these cells (lymphocytes included) are actually looking for molecules foreign to the body called antigens. Antigens are associated with microbes and foreign cells, anything that does not belong in the body. The immune system is able to mount a reaction against these molecules. The presence of antigen is the means by which the cells of the immune system detect invaders.

Once an antigen is encountered, the cells of the monocyte-macrophage lineage (macrophages, dendritic cells, and Langerhans cells) phagocytize and process the antigen. This "processing" involves breaking it down into manageable pieces and inserting it into their plasma membrane, associating it with their own integral membrane proteins, which are exposed on their surfaces. They then head for the nearest lymph node. Lymphocytes similarly head for the nearest lymph node on encountering an antigen.

Once in the lymph nodes, the macrophages and related cells again change their role (sort of a promotion for the patrolmen). They become antigen-presenting cells. Antigen-presenting cells do exactly what their name implies; they present the antigen to other cells to stimulate a highly specific response against the antigen. Again, think of the lymph node as the police station. The antigen-presenting cells are gathering together with lymphocytes and are showing them the "wanted poster," the antigen that will enable them to recognize the intruders. Now, to understand what the lymphocytes will do next, we need a little more information on the two types of lymphocytes.

Lymphocytes all look more or less alike (if you've seen one, you've seen them all). But as we have just learned, there are two major types: B lymphocytes and T lymphocytes. Although they look alike, we can tell them apart, and now we must be able to; otherwise, we would not understand what they were about to do. Just as security officers have badges or emblems on their uniforms so their rank and responsibilities are recog-

nizable, different types of lymphocytes have different cell-surface proteins as markers identifying their type. Let's start with B lymphocytes.

Your B Lymphocytes and Their Role in Immunity

The ultimate role of the B lymphocyte is to differentiate into a plasma cell. Plasma cells are terminally differentiated B lymphocytes; their function is the production of antibodies. Antibodies are globular proteins (immunoglobulins) that react (bind to) specific antigens. We have learned about receptor-ligand interactions before (think about neurotransmitters or hormones and their receptors). We likened these interactions to keys and locks. The same situation exists here. A small portion of an antigen, called its epitope, is the specific ligand for the antibody. A number of different antibodies may each recognize different epitopes on the same antigen, thereby covering the antigen with antibody molecules after they encounter it. Antigens can be any class of molecule: an antibody will exist that binds to each antigen even though the antigen has never been encountered before. Think about it. Your immune system is ready to attack antigens it has never even seen!

The cell-surface markers of B lymphocytes include two types (isotypes) of antibodies called IgM and IgD. Antibody isotypes and their functions are described in **TABLE 21.1**, and their form is demonstrated in **FIGURE 21.9**. Note that the immunoglobulin molecule is shaped like the letter "Y." The antigen-binding sites (called Fab) are on the two upper arms of the "Y"; these two arms are called the "variable" region. The constant region (called Fc) makes up the base of the "Y." Note also that the Fab consists of two heavy chains and two light chains, while the constant region is composed of two heavy chains.

| **Table 21.1** | Immunoglobulin Isotypes and their Functions |

Isotype	Location	Functions
IgM	B-cell surface and in serum	Can form pentameres (units of five) and thereby aggregate much antigen at once. The first antibody secreted in an immune response
IgD	B-cell surface, secreted in minute quantities	Specialized functions unknown
IgG	Serum and bound to Fc receptors on neutrophils and macrophages	Most abundant isotype, highest affinity for antigens, directs macrophages and neutrophils to antigen, and activates complement cascade
IgE	Bound to Fc receptors on mast cells, basophils, and eosinophils of mucous membranes in GI, respiratory, and urogenital tracts	Directs the activities of mast cells, basophils, and eosinophils, enabling them to recognize antigens and initiate inflammatory response
IgA	Mucous membranes and milk	Secretion of this isotype into milk enables passage of immunity temporarily from mother to infant (passive immunity)

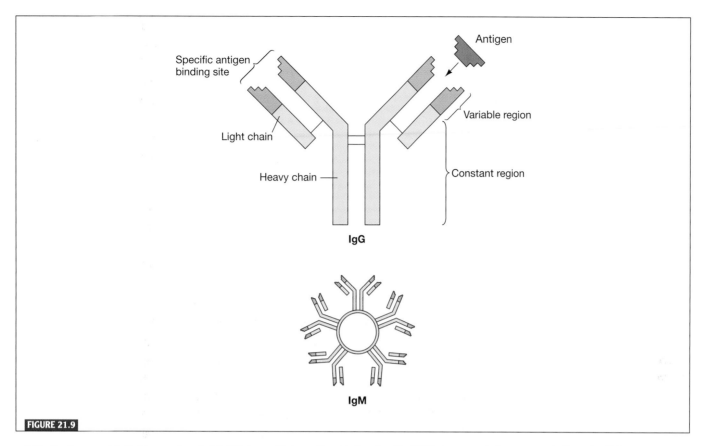

FIGURE 21.9

Antibodies (immunoglobulins) have a characteristic "Y" shape with two antigen binding sites. The IGM isotype can exist in a pentameric (five-subunit) form.

B lymphocytes start out with IgM and IgD on their surfaces. When they encounter antigen that is the specific ligand for their antibody, they begin to produce and secrete immunoglobulins specific for that antigen (just like the ones on their surface). Note that for its entire life, an individual B lymphocyte can produce immunoglobulins reactive with only a single epitope. Initially, the B lymphocyte secretes IgM. With its pentameric form (Figure 21.9), much antigen can rapidly be bound by IgM. This inactivates the antigen or prepares it (and the microbe it is on) for phagocytosis, complement-mediated lysis, or ADCC (complement-mediated lysis and ADCC were described previously).

This is, after all, the role of the B lymphocyte. On encountering the antigen it recognizes, it differentiates into a plasma cell and produces antibody. Ultimately, on signals received from other immune system cells, the lymphocyte may switch the isotype to a form that will be more effective against that specific invader, in its specific location. Typically, the switch is from IgM to IgG.

The B-lymphocyte response is rarely an independent event. You may recall that bacteria can evade natural immunity with an impenetrable coat. Although the B-cell response can be generated against this defense with no additional help (hurrah for our B cells!), usually other help is necessary. B lymphocytes internalize and process the antigens that bind their surface antibodies. They present them on their membranes and use them to activate T lymphocytes that will, in turn, help the B lymphocyte mount its response. With this, we must introduce the T cells and their surface markers.

Your T Lymphocytes Function in Several Ways

T lymphocytes possess surface antigen-binding molecules that are in many ways similar to antibodies. They are smaller molecules, however, with only two chains, one variable region, and one constant region (**FIGURE 21.10**). They are always membrane bound: they are never secreted.

T-cell antigen receptors (TCR) will bind antigen only when that antigen is bound to a cell-surface glycoprotein called the major histocompatability complex (MHC). This combination of antigen and MHC is called "antigen in the context of MHC." MHC antigens (the MHC glycoproteins) are molecules that vary greatly from one individual to the next. The major histocompatability complex is the basis for tissue rejection when organs are transplanted from one individual to another: their

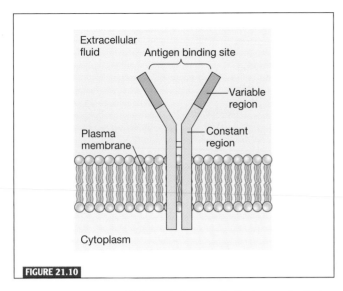

FIGURE 21.10

T-cell antigen receptors (TCR) are similar to antibodies but are simpler in form. Note that they have one antigen binding site only.

MHC must match or the recipient will recognize the tissue as foreign. The actual function of MHC under normal circumstances, however, is that T cells recognize antigen only in the context of MHC. The proper MHC (your individual MHC) must be present for your T lymphocytes to "see" the antigen.

Two major types of MHC molecules present antigen to T lymphocytes (**FIGURE 21.11**). Class I MHC antigens are glycoproteins synthesized in cells in the manner that you now know well: rough endoplasmic reticulum (RER) to golgi to plasmalemma (Chapters 3 and 14). Along the way to the cell surface, they pick up any antigens present within the cell, like a sponge picking up dirt. These commonly include viral products in infected cells or tumor-associated antigens in malignant cells. Virtually all cells make class I MHC.

The other type of MHC molecules, called class II (logical name, huh?) follows a different pathway. They are transported to vesicles, where they combine with antigens that have been internalized (by phagocytosis or pinocytosis) by the cell as part of antigen processing. Class II MHC and attached antigens are then inserted into the cell membrane. Only antigen-presenting cells (macrophages, dendritic and Langerhans cells, and B lymphocytes) express class II MHC.

So, how do T cells "see" antigen? Their antigen receptors (TCR) associate with the MHC molecules we have been discussing. As they mature in the thymus, they gain this ability. As they develop their TCR in the thymus, the TCR must recognize MHC and must not be activated by MHC alone. If these criteria are not met, apoptosis will be triggered and that premature T lymphocyte will die. This rigorous selection process (98% of all T cells entering the thymus do not survive) avoids the possibility of T cells attacking normal cells in the body (see the "When Things Go Wrong" section at the end of this chapter). This is not a problem for B lymphocytes, which rely on T cells for antigen presentation to become activated. Now let's look at the T cell-B cell interactions.

Two to Tango: T-Cell and B-Cell Interactions

Remember, B cells have class II MHC antigens; once they have pinocytosed foreign antigens, these products are inserted into their membrane bound to class II MHC. When immunoglobulins on the surface of a B cell bind antigen, a second signal can be received by the B cell, triggering it to synthesize and secrete antibody. This second signal comes in the form of molecules called cytokines, produced by a T cell that has recognized antigen bound to class II MHC on the B-cell surface. In effect, the B cell shows the antigen to the T cell and asks its opinion; it asks if it should secrete antibodies against this substance. The cytokines produced by the T cell give it this permission (**FIGURE 21.12a**). Since cytokines work only over very short distances, close contact between the cells is needed. This close contact occurs in the lymph nodes and spleen and keeps immune responses localized. There is no need for lymphocytes in nodes behind your knee to respond to a cut on your finger (let's keep things in perspective!).

Only one kind of T cell can give this permission: a helper T cell. You may have heard of these before; they are the main cell type destroyed by HIV as the disease AIDS develops. Helper T cells have a surface molecule called CD4 that helps TCR bind to class II MHC plus antigen. The HIV virus uses CD4 to enter helper T cells and, ultimately, to cause their death.

But, you ask, what about class I MHC that binds to viral and cancer-related antigens? Class I MHC is recognized by another type of T cell: cytotoxic (killer) T cells. Just as helper T cells have the CD4 molecule to aid them in their work, cytotoxic T cells have CD8 molecules on their surfaces (Figure 21.12b). Once cytotoxic T cells bind antigen in the context of class I MHC, they secrete cytokines that kill the target cell to which they are bound (the virally infected or cancerous cell).

All of these cell interactions involve signals delivered between cells that are in close proximity to each other. Again, these interactions occur in the secondary lymphoid organs, such as lymph nodes, and result in the elimination of microbes, virally infected cells, and tumor cells. The list of cytokines involved in these processes is immense and growing rapidly as immunologists (scientists who study the immune system) discover additional

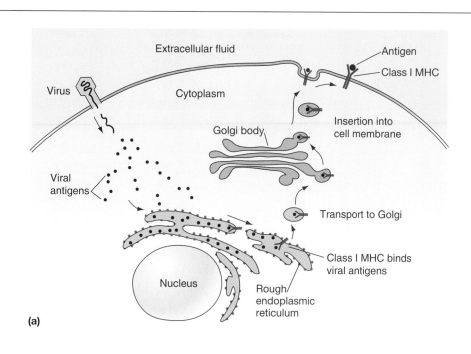

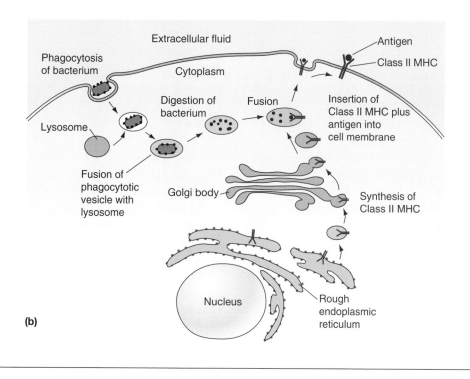

FIGURE 21.11

T cells recognize antigen only in the context of MHC. MHC exists in two forms: class I, which is present on the surface of virtually all cell types (a); and class II, which is present only on antigen-presenting cells (b).

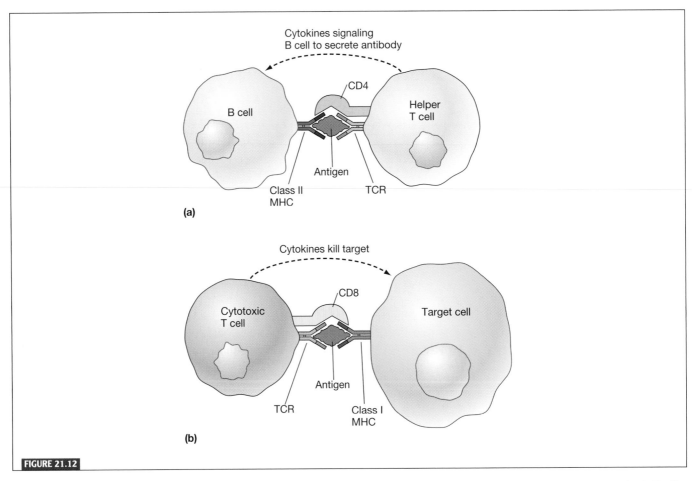

FIGURE 21.12

B cells present antigen to helper T cells in the context of class II MHC (a). This leads to cytokine release from the T cell, resulting in antibody production by the B cell. Cytotoxic T cells recognize antigen in the context of class I MHC on the surface of target cells such as virally infected cells or neoplastic cells. This leads to release of cytokines from the cytotoxic T cell that kill the target cell.

ways in which the cells of the immune system interact with each other and with other cell types.

Acquired Immunity: How Your Immune System Learns

We have been discussing only primary immune responses, the responses that are activated when T and B lymphocytes encounter an antigen for the first time. As they eliminate that antigen through the secretion of antibodies and cytokines, they also proliferate within the lymph nodes, generating daughter cells like themselves to fight the infection. Some of these daughter cells are specialized for a different function, however. These cells, called memory cells, are long lived and, as their name implies, maintain a molecular "memory" of the event in case the same antigen is encountered in the future. This is the "learned response" I alluded to earlier and is the reason this system is referred to as "acquired" immunity. In this way, a subsequent exposure to the same pathogen will cause a more specific and rapid response. Your immune system "learns" to recog-

nize the pathogen readily and to mount a highly effective response against it.

This is the principle behind vaccination (immunization); we allow our immune systems to see antigens in a nonpathogenic form (a form that does not cause disease), so if the pathogenic (disease-causing) form is encountered later on, they will remember the antigens and mount a more effective response than they would have without the vaccination. Through ongoing exposures to the microbes we encounter each day, our elite security force becomes very highly trained indeed!

Our discussion of acquired immunity has only scratched the surface of the activities of this amazing system. Despite the vast amounts of research being conducted daily, the ability of viruses such as HIV to elude our capacity for effective drug development points to our need for continued study. Much of what you have just read is relatively new knowledge: for example, less than 50 years ago, scientists only knew of the existence of lymphocytes. Their subtypes and functions were unknown. Imagine what now lies ahead!

Breaching Homeostasis . . . When Things Go Wrong

Immunodeficiency and Autoimmune Diseases

As you can imagine, a system as complex as the immune system can have a great number of things go wrong. Can't you see that defects in this system can exist in two basic "flavors," excessive immunity or insufficient immunity? We will briefly explore these two possibilities in this "Breaching Homeostasis" section.

A classic example of insufficient immunity is severe combined immunodeficiency (SCID). Children with this illness are frequently portrayed in the media, due to the dramatic features of this disease. Severe combined immunodeficiency patients must live their lives in a "bubble" so that nothing in their environment can infect them. This disease results from a mutation in the gene that encodes an enzyme involved in the generation of variability in immunoglobulins and T-cell antigen receptors. Since B and T cells can not mature and function in the absence of this enzyme activity, acquired immunity can not function. Genetic engineering holds great promise for a cure for this rare but dreaded illness.

Examples of excessive immunity abound. Many of us suffer from allergies to inhaled substances (i.e., pollen) or ingested substances (i.e., nuts). Here the culprit is IgE. Some MHC gene alleles produce MHC molecules that are overly effective at presenting specific antigens (i.e., antigens in nuts, pollen, animal dander, and dust mites). Antigens such as these are responsible for allergies and are called allergens. When allergens are encountered at mucous membranes, responding B cells switch classes to produce IgE. IgE induces mast-cell degranulation and, hence, inflammation. This leads to the responses we observe that can range from sneezing and runny nose and eyes to the potentially life-threatening anaphylaxis. Allergists desensitize allergy sufferers by introducing allergens under the skin in very small quantities. By administering the allergens in this alternate way, B cells are induced to make IgM and later IgG. The memory cells thus induced will subsequently generate a rapid and effective response and inactivate allergens encountered in the mucous membranes before an allergic response can be generated by IgE-antigen interaction.

Other conditions of excessive immunity include autoimmune diseases. Autoimmune diseases are caused by the generation of immune responses to molecules present in normal tissues. The flaws in the system that lead to this aberrant response are still poorly understood. Normally, T cells in the thymus learn not to react to potential antigens in our own tissues ("self" antigens). This is called immunologic tolerance. All of the body's potential antigens are somehow cataloged in the thymus for this purpose. The process involves triggering the T-cell receptor without activating any later signals. If tolerance breaks down (through largely unknown mechanisms), disease ensues. Examples of autoimmune diseases include multiple sclerosis, systemic lupus erythematosus, and juvenile onset diabetes (see "Breaching Homeostasis" in Chapter 13). Clearly there are many mysteries remaining to be solved before we can fully understand our immune system.

What You Should Know

1. Your immune system can be divided into two functional components: natural immunity and acquired immunity.

2. Natural immunity is the less advanced form. It is relatively nonspecific in choosing its targets and at mounting responses against those targets.

3. Inflammation is one form of natural immunity. It involves blood vessels and is a nonspecific response to any injury in any tissue.

4. The cardinal signs of inflammation are redness, swelling, heat, pain, and loss of function.

5. Inflammation may be beneficial or harmful to the surrounding tissues.

6. Acute inflammation is the initial response to most injuries in most tissues. Fluid and cellular exudate are formed in acute inflammation and the neutrophil is the principle cell of this response.

7. Initiators trigger inflammation; mediators modify the response.

8. Four important cascade mechanisms are involved in inflammation mediation. They are the blood-clotting cascade, the fibrinolytic cascade, the complement cascade, and the kinin cascade.

9. Chronic inflammation sometimes follows acute inflammation, but can occur in the absence of an acute phase. Acute inflammation may resolve without the development of chronic inflammation.

10. Macrophages, fibroblast proliferation, and angiogenesis are the hallmarks of chronic inflammation. Chronic inflammation plays a major role in the pathogenesis of a number of important diseases.

11. Natural killer cells are another component of natural immunity. They are lymphoid in origin and mount relatively nonspecific attacks against virally infected cells and neoplastic (cancer) cells.

12. Lymphocytes and cells of the monocyte-macrophage lineage are important in acquired immunity.

13. Lymphocytes begin their life in the bone marrow. T lymphocytes develop in the thymus while B lymphocytes continue developing in the bone marrow.

14. The bone marrow and thymus are primary lymphoid organs. Lymph nodes, adenoids, tonsils, the appendix, Peyer's patches, and the spleen are secondary lymphoid organs.

15. Secondary lymphoid organs are the sites in which lymphocytes, macrophages, and dendritic cells come into close contact to exchange the information necessary to mount an immune response.

16. Antigens are molecules that the immune system recognizes as foreign.

17. B lymphocytes differentiate into plasma cells, which produce immunoglobulins (antibodies).

18. Antibody diversity enables our immune system to mount a defense against any antigen our immune systems will encounter.

19. Antibodies can inactivate molecular antigens, prepare microbes for phagocytosis, trigger lysis of cells by complement, or activate ADCC.

20. T-cell antigen receptors, unlike antibodies, are never secreted and enable T cells to recognize antigen only in the context of (when bound to) MHC.

21. Two forms of MHC exist. Class I MHC is found on all cells and is used to present viral and cancer-associated antigens to T cells. Class II MHC is found only on antigen-presenting cells and is used to present a wide variety of antigens to T cells.

22. Antigen-presenting cells include macrophages, dendritic cells, Langerhans cells, and B lymphocytes.

23. Helper T cells trigger antibody secretion from differentiated B cells called plasma cells; cytotoxic T cells secrete cytokines that kill virally infected cells and cancer cells.

24. Memory cells are T and B lymphocytes that are generated in response to exposure to an antigen. They live for decades and enable us to rapidly mount an effective immune response against pathogens we have previously encountered.

25. Memory cells provide the functional basis for immunization.

What Did You Learn?

Multiple choice questions: choose the best answer.

1. Which of the following is not a part of natural immunity?
   a. Inflammation
   b. Antibody production
   c. Natural killer cell activity
   d. All of the above are part of natural immunity.

2. Cardinal signs of inflammation include all of the following except:
   a. Pain
   b. Redness and swelling
   c. Heat
   d. Loss of function
   e. All of the above are included in the cardinal signs of inflammation.

3. Which of the following is part of acute inflammation?
   a. Cellular exudate formation
   b. Fluid exudate formation
   c. Both of the above
   d. Neither of the above

4. Which of the following requires changes in blood vessels?
   a. Cellular exudate formation
   b. Fluid exudate formation
   c. Both of the above
   d. Neither of the above

5. Acute inflammation would occur in response to:
   a. A stab wound
   b. A gunshot wound
   c. A myocardial infarction
   d. A bee sting
   e. All of the above

6. The principle cell type in the exudate of acute inflammation is the:
   a. Neutrophil
   b. Macrophage
   c. Lymphocyte
   d. Erythrocyte

7. As injured endothelial cells lift off of their basement membrane, inflammation may be initiated. This is due to:
   a. Substances released by the injured cells
   b. Exposure of the blood to collagen in the basement membrane
   c. Both of the above
   d. Neither of the above

8. Your physician says that your chronic bronchitis involves chronic inflammation. What cell type do you now picture as contributing greatly to your infirmity?
   a. Neutrophils
   b. Macrophages
   c. Lymphocytes
   d. Erythrocytes

9. Which of the following is not a plasma-derived mediator of inflammation?
   a. The blood-clotting cascade
   b. The kinin cascade
   c. The fibrinolytic cascade
   d. The complement cascade
   e. All of the above are plasma-derived mediators of inflammation.

10. Natural killer cells are important in our defense against:
    a. Viral diseases
    b. Cancer
    c. Both of the above
    d. Neither of the above

11. Where do T and B lymphocytes originate?
    a. Lymph nodes
    b. Spleen
    c. Thymus
    d. Bone marrow
    e. Tonsils

12. Antigen presentation takes place in secondary lymphoid organs. Which of the following is not a secondary lymphoid organ?
    a. Lymph nodes
    b. Spleen
    c. Thymus
    d. Peyer's patches
    e. All of the above are secondary lymphoid organs.

13. Which cell type lyses antibody-coated cells in a process called ADCC?
    a. Langerhans cells
    b. Macrophages
    c. Natural killer cells
    d. Dendritic cells

14. _____ differentiate into plasma cells.
    a. T lymphocytes
    b. B lymphocytes
    c. Both of the above
    d. Neither of the above

What Did You Learn? (continued)

15. A lactating mother secretes _____ in her milk, passing important immunities to the newborn.

   a. IgM

   b. IgD

   c. IgG

   d. IgE

   e. IgA

16. Which class of immunoglobulin is the most abundant and has the highest affinity for antigen?

   a. IgM

   b. IgD

   c. IgG

   d. IgE

   e. IgA

17. Antibodies can do all of the following except:

   a. Inactivate molecular antigens

   b. Prepare microbes for phagocytosis

   c. Trigger lysis of cells by complement

   d. Activate ADCC

   e. Antibodies do all of the above.

18. Which of the following is true of the T-cell antigen receptor (TCR)?

   a. They are secreted like antibodies.

   b. They recognize antigen only in the context of (when bound to) MHC.

   c. Both of the above are true.

   d. Neither of the above is true.

19. Memory cells are derived from:

   a. T lymphocytes

   b. B lymphocytes

   c. Both of the above

   d. Neither of the above

20. Immunization against potentially dangerous diseases is effective because it enables us to generate a population of _____ that will help us to mount a rapid, effective defense if we encounter the pathogen that causes the disease.

   a. Neutrophils

   b. Macrophages

   c. Memory cells

   d. Immunocytes

   e. None of the above

Short answer questions: answer briefly and in your own words.

1. Describe how an inflammatory response is generated. Include the characteristics of inflammation in general, and the differences between acute and chronic inflammation.

2. What is the difference between mediators and initiators of inflammation? List a few examples of initiators and mediators.

3. Lymphocytes are important components of acquired immunity. Where do they originate? How do the two major classes differ? Describe the development and function of these cell types.

4. Do you suffer from allergies? Describe the cellular basis for the symptoms you develop (if you don't have any allergies, think of the symptoms experienced by someone you know). What can be done to alleviate your symptoms? Are these temporary or permanent measures? How do they work (on the cellular level)?

5. What types of T cells exist and what do they do? Does one play a role in the development of AIDS? Please explain that role.

Appendix A: The Metric System

Biomedical research relies on a great variety of highly accurate measurements. These measurements are invariably made and recorded using units of the metric system. In this appendix, the metric system is introduced, the units are presented and examples are given to show what might be measured in each unit. Please look over this information so you can understand the measurements presented in the text.

In this simple system of measurement, there are separate units used for mass, volume, and length. Its simplicity lies in the fact that, unlike the English system in which arbitrary conversions must be made between units (12 inches = 1 foot, 3 feet = 1 yard), all conversions between units in the metric system simply involve moving the decimal point. The details and examples are listed below. To use scientific notation, remember:

10^{-2} = one one-hundredth or 0.01
10^{-3} = one one-thousandth or 0.001
10^{-6} = one one-millionth or 0.000001
10^{-9} = one one-billionth or 0.000000001

Mass

The basic unit is the gram; to convert to other units, simply move the decimal point as required.

Unit	Comparison to Basic Unit	Used to Measure (Example)
Kilogram (kg)	1,000 g or 10^3 g	The mass (weight) of the body
Gram (g)		The mass of an organ
Milligram (mg)	0.001 g or 10^{-3} g	The mass of one carpal bone
Microgram (µg)	0.000001 g or 10^{-6} g	The mass of one hair
Nanogram (ng)	0.000000001 g or 10^{-9} g	The mass of an organelle

In other words,
1,000 g = 1 kg
1,000 mg = 1 g
1,000 µg = 1 mg

Volume

The basic unit is the liter. Again, you simply move the decimal point to convert to other units.

Unit	Comparison to Basic Unit	Used to Measure (Example)
Liter (l)		The volume of blood in the body
Milliliter (ml)	0.001 l or 10^{-3} l	The volume of blood drawn for a diagnostic test
Microliter (µl)	0.000001 l or 10^{-6} l	The volume of CSF produced per minute

In other words,
1,000 ml = 1 l
1,000 µl = 1 ml

Length

The basic unit is the meter. Again, conversion involves moving the decimal point.

Unit	Comparison to Basic Unit	Used to Measure (Example)
Meter (m)		The height of the body
Centimeter (cm)	0.01 m or 10^{-2} m	The length of the arm
Millimeter (mm)	0.001 m or 10^{-3} m	The length of a finger
Micrometer (µm)	0.000001 m or 10^{-6} m	The diameter of a cell
Nanometer (nm)	0.000000001 m or 10^{-9} m	The diameter of an organelle

In other words,
100 cm = 1 m
1,000 mm = 1 m
1,000 µm = 1 mm
1,000 nm = 1 µm

Please perform the following conversions:

MASS	VOLUME	LENGTH
391 g = ___ kg	873 μl = ___ ml	0.83 m = ___ cm
870 mg = ___ g	1.29 ml = ___ μl	0.83 m = ___ mm
2.39 g = ___ mg	3.79 l = ___ ml	2.87 μm = ___ nm
1,210 μg = ___ mg	250 ml = ___ l	398 nm = ___ μm
2.3 mg = ___ μg	1,287 μl = ___ ml	2.91 mm = ___ μm
324 μg = ___ mg	1,810 ml = ___ l	879 μm = ___ mm

Answers (Don't look until you have completed the above problems):

MASS	VOLUME	LENGTH
391 g = 0.391 kg	873 μl = 0.873 ml	0.83 m = 83 cm
870 mg = 0.87 g	1.29 ml = 1,290 μl	0.83 m = 830 mm
2.39 g = 2,390 mg	3.79 l = 3790 ml	2.87 μm = 2,870 nm
1,210 μg = 1.21 mg	250 ml = 0.25 l	398 nm = 0.398 μm
2.3 mg = 2,300 μg	1,287 μl = 1.287 ml	2.91 mm = 2,910 μm
324 μg = 0.324 mg	1,810 ml = 1.81 l	879 μm = 0.879 mm

Conversion Factors

It is best to select one system of measurement and stick to it throughout your work. History repeatedly teaches the lesson that when we combine measurement systems, things can go awry. If, however, you find it necessary to convert between systems, the following tables might help you.

To change	To	Multiply by
centimeters	inches	0.3937
centimeters	feet	0.03281
cubic feet	cubic meters	0.0283
cubic meters	cubic feet	35.3145
cubic meters	cubic yards	1.3079
cubic yards	cubic meters	0.7646
feet	meters	0.3048
gallons (U.S.)	liters	3.7853
grams	ounces avdp	0.0353
grams	pounds	0.002205
inches	millimeters	25.4000
inches	centimeters	2.5400
inches	meters	0.0254
kilograms	pounds	2.2046
liters	gallons (U.S.)	0.2642
liters	pints (dry)	1.8162
liters	pints (liquid)	2.1134
liters	quarts (dry)	0.9081
liters	quarts (liquid)	1.0567
meters	feet	3.2808
meters	yards	1.0936
millimeters	inches	0.0394
ounces (avdp)	grams	28.3495
ounces	pounds	0.0625
pints (dry)	liters	0.5506
pints (liquid)	liters	0.4732
pounds	kilograms	0.4536
pounds	ounces	16
quarts (dry)	liters	1.1012
quarts (liquid)	liters	0.9463

Fahrenheit and Celsius (Centigrade) Scales

°Celsius	°Fahrenheit
−273.15	−459.67
−250	−418
−200	−328
−150	−238
−100	−148
−50	−58
−40	−40
−30	−22
−20	−4
−10	14
0	32
5	41
10	50
15	59
20	68
25	77
30	86
35	95
40	104
45	113
50	122
55	131
60	140
65	149
70	158
75	167
80	176
85	185
90	194
95	203
100	212

Zero on the Fahrenheit scale represents the temperature produced by the mixing of equal weights of snow and common salt.

	°Fahrenheit	°Celsius
Boiling point of water	212°	100°
Freezing point of water	32°	0°
Normal body temperature	98.6°	37°
Comfortable room temperature	68–77°	20–25°
Absolute zero	−459.6°	−273.1°

Absolute zero is theoretically the lowest possible temperature, the point at which all molecular motion would cease.

■ To Convert Temperature Scales

To convert Fahrenheit to Celsius (Centigrade), subtract 32 and multiply by $\frac{5}{9}$.

$$°C = \tfrac{5}{9}(°F - 32)$$

To convert Celsius (Centigrade) to Fahrenheit, multiply by 9/5 and add 32.

$$°F = (\tfrac{9}{5} \times °C) + 32$$

Appendix B: Answers to Multiple Choice Questions

Chapter 1

1. c	4. d	7. d	10. d
2. a	5. b	8. c	
3. c	6. b	9. a	

Chapter 2

1. d	6. b	11. a	16. a	21. d	26. a
2. c	7. c	12. b	17. c	22. c	27. c
3. b	8. d	13. d	18. b	23. d	28. a
4. c	9. b	14. a	19. c	24. c	29. c
5. e	10. b	15. d	20. c	25. e	30. b

Chapter 3

1. c	5. d	9. b	13. a	17. b
2. d	6. d	10. b	14. c	18. a
3. b	7. e	11. b	15. a	19. b
4. a	8. a	12. c	16. b	20. e

Chapter 4

1. c	5. b	9. b	13. c	17. b
2. d	6. a	10. b	14. e	18. b
3. e	7. a	11. e	15. a	19. d
4. c	8. c	12. d	16. a	20. a

Chapter 5

1. e	5. d	9. b	13. b	17. a
2. b	6. c	10. c	14. a	18. c
3. b	7. d	11. e	15. b	19. a
4. c	8. c	12. b	16. c	20. a

Chapter 6

1. e	5. d	9. c	13. b	17. e
2. c	6. c	10. b	14. b	18. c
3. a	7. a	11. a	15. a	19. d
4. d	8. c	12. c	16. a	20. a

Chapter 7

1. a	5. c	9. b	13. b	17. d
2. b	6. a	10. d	14. e	18. c
3. d	7. a	11. b	15. a	19. e
4. a	8. e	12. b	16. c	20. b

Chapter 8

1. b	5. d	9. b	13. d	17. d
2. d	6. a	10. c	14. a	18. b
3. a	7. b	11. a	15. d	19. b
4. c	8. b	12. c	16. d	20. b

Chapter 9

1. c	5. a	9. d	13. e	17. e
2. a	6. e	10. b	14. a	18. a
3. a	7. a	11. d	15. c	19. d
4. a	8. c	12. b	16. b	20. b

Chapter 10

1. b	5. c	9. b	13. e	17. c
2. b	6. e	10. c	14. a	18. a
3. c	7. d	11. d	15. c	19. e
4. b	8. c	12. a	16. b	20. b

Chapter 11

1. a	5. b	9. d	13. a	17. b	21. c
2. c	6. b	10. b	14. b	18. a	22. e
3. c	7. b	11. a	15. c	19. d	
4. b	8. a	12. a	16. a	20. b	

Chapter 12A

1. a	4. a	7. a	10. a
2. d	5. b	8. d	
3. b	6. c	9. a	

Chapter 12B

1. b	5. c	9. a	13. c	17. a
2. d	6. d	10. a	14. a	18. b
3. c	7. a	11. b	15. b	19. c
4. c	8. b	12. b	16. b	20. a

Chapter 12C

1. d	4. a	7. c
2. a	5. d	8. b
3. a	6. a	

Chapter 12D

1. b	4. c	7. d	10. a	13. d
2. b	5. b	8. c	11. e	14. a
3. d	6. c	9. b	12. a	

Chapter 13

1. b	6. a	11. d	16. b	21. e
2. b	7. e	12. a	17. b	22. b
3. a	8. b	13. d	18. c	23. a
4. b	9. d	14. a	19. c	24. b
5. c	10. b	15. c	20. a	25. a

Chapter 14

1. b	4. c	7. b	10. c	13. a	16. a
2. d	5. b	8. a	11. e	14. d	17. b
3. b	6. b	9. b	12. c	15. b	18. a

Chapter 15

1. d	5. c	9. a	13. c	17. d	21. d
2. b	6. c	10. b	14. b	18. b	22. c
3. b	7. b	11. a	15. c	19. d	23. b
4. b	8. d	12. a	16. a	20. c	24. a

Chapter 16

1. a	6. b	11. b	16. b	21. a	26. d
2. a	7. b	12. d	17. a	22. a	27. b
3. a	8. d	13. a	18. b	23. a	
4. c	9. d	14. c	19. a	24. c	
5. a	10. c	15. c	20. e	25. c	

Chapter 17

1. c	5. c	9. c	13. c	17. d
2. d	6. c	10. d	14. b	18. d
3. c	7. c	11. c	15. c	19. b
4. d	8. a	12. b	16. e	20. c

Chapter 18

1. a	6. b	11. b	16. c	21. c	26. b
2. e	7. c	12. d	17. a	22. a	27. c
3. b	8. c	13. c	18. b	23. a	28. c
4. c	9. a	14. b	19. d	24. b	29. b
5. c	10. a	15. d	20. b	25. b	30. e

Chapter 19

1. e	6. a	11. b	16. a	21. b	26. b
2. e	7. c	12. b	17. b	22. d	
3. a	8. a	13. e	18. a	23. b	
4. d	9. a	14. a	19. b	24. c	
5. a	10. d	15. c	20. b	25. a	

Chapter 20

1. d	4. c	7. b	10. b	13. b	16. b
2. d	5. a	8. b	11. c	14. b	17. c
3. c	6. a	9. c	12. c	15. a	

Chapter 21

1. b	5. e	9. e	13. c	17. e
2. e	6. a	10. c	14. b	18. b
3. c	7. c	11. d	15. e	19. c
4. c	8. b	12. c	16. c	20. c

Appendix C: Pathologic Conditions Presented in Anatomy and Physiology: Understanding the Human Body

Although this is not a pathology textbook, some basic knowledge of pathology aids in developing an understanding of anatomy and physiology. Throughout the text, information on injury, disease, and the methods the body uses to fight them are presented. In some cases, only a passing mention is made of the condition. In other instances, the process is discussed in detail. The most extensive presentations can be found in the boxes *Breaching Homeostasis . . . When Things Go Wrong* located at the ends of some chapters.

This appendix lists the pathological conditions presented in this book and the locations where you can find them. The letters B.H. indicate that the information is presented in a *Breaching Homeostasis . . . When Things Go Wrong* feature.

Appendix D: Aerobic Cellular Metabolism/Oxidative Phosphorylation

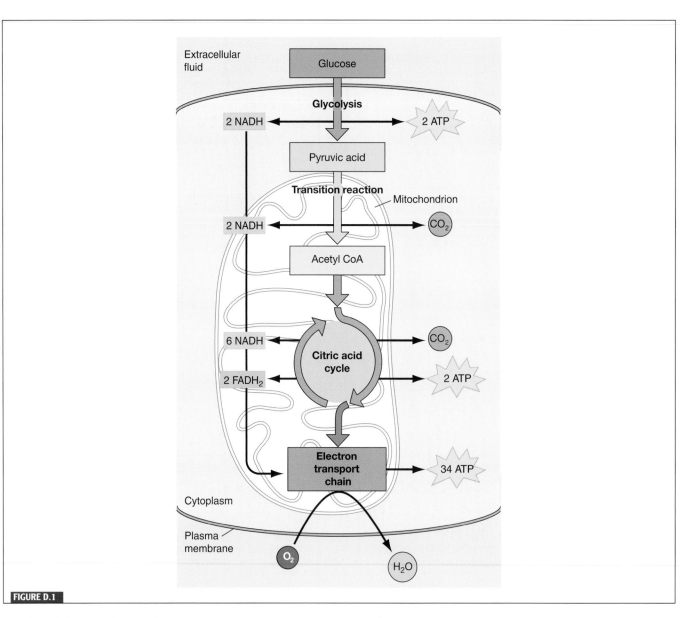

Aerobic cellular respiration overview.

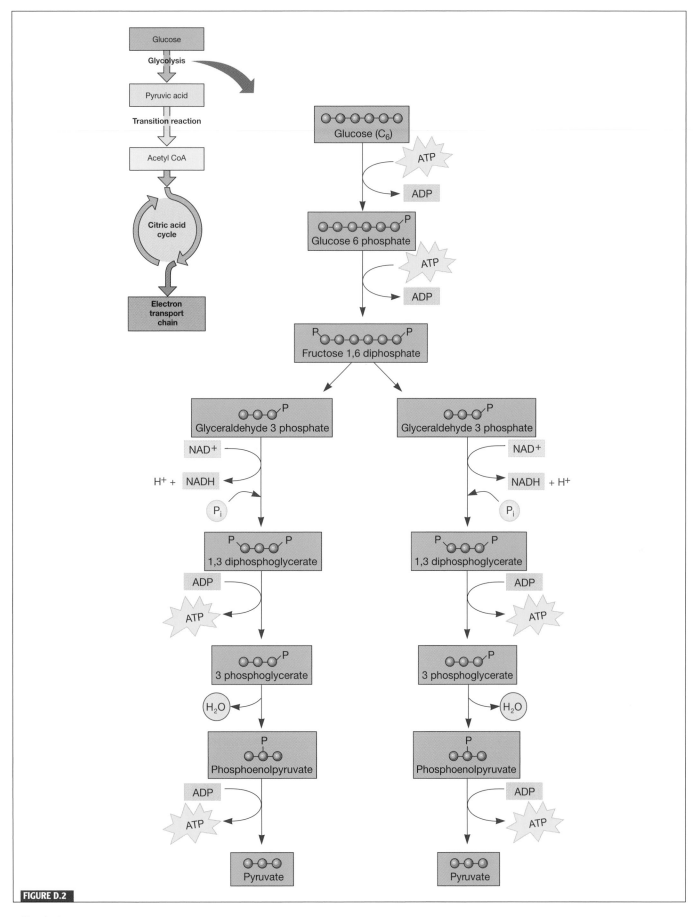

FIGURE D.2

Glycolosis.

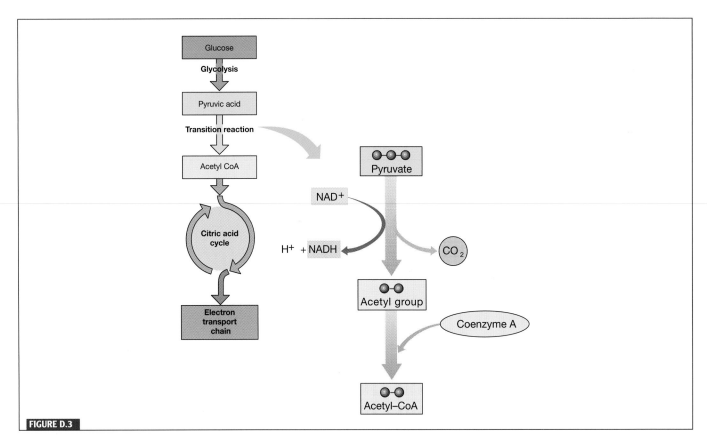

FIGURE D.3

Transition reaction.

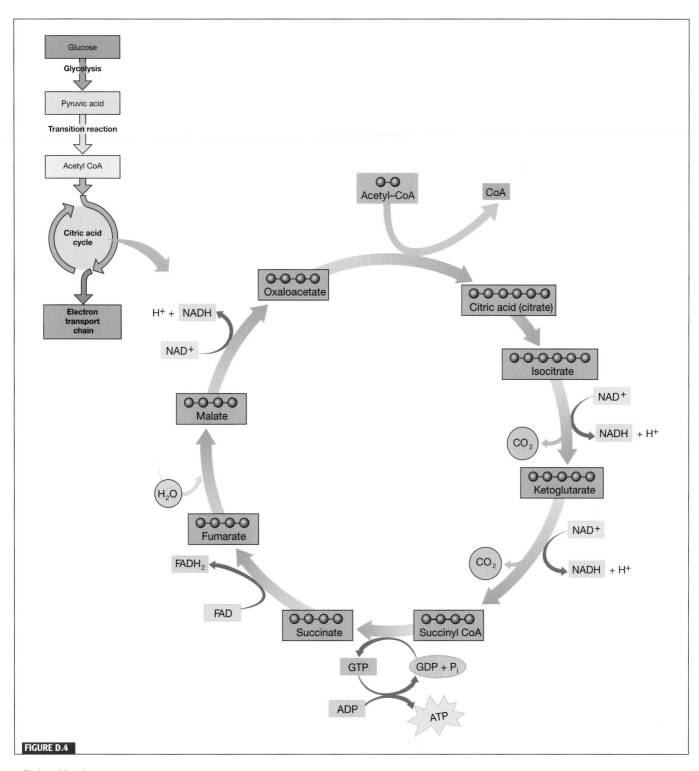

Citric acid cycle.

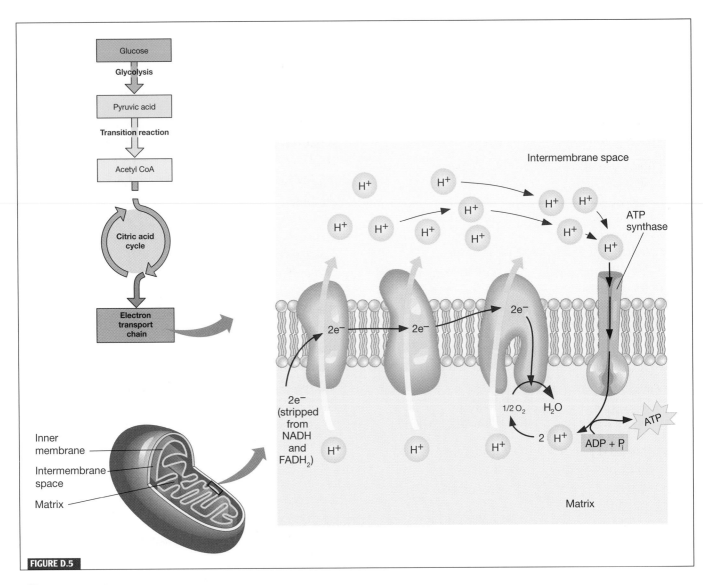

FIGURE D.5

Electron transport.

Glossary

Glossary (GLOS-ar-ē) A list of technical terms with definitions, included at the back of many textbooks.

This glossary is intended only as a quick look-up resource as you study this textbook or come across biomedical terms in your daily life. Please do not use it as your primary information resource; the actual text should be used for this purpose. The pronunciation guide is here to help you learn to use these terms verbally. This is an important aspect in the development of your understanding of anatomy and physiology. Emphasis should be placed on the capitalized syllable (it is accented). All vowels that do not have a line over them are to be pronounced with the short vowel sound as in the words *bat, bet, bit, not, nut.* All vowels with a line over them are to be pronounced with the long vowel sound, as in the words *mate, be, bite, no, glue.* As you use this guide, be sure to pronounce the words several times aloud. This will aid your pronunciation and reinforce your memory.

Abdominopelvic cavity (ab-DOM-in-ō) The organ cavity that is inferior to the diaphragm

Abduction (ab-DUK-shun) Movement of a limb away from the midline

Absorption (ab-SORB-shun) To move a substance into the body, such as the absorption of nutrients in the gastrointestinal tract

Acetabulum (a-sa-TAB-ū-lum) The socket of the coxal bones into which the head of the femur fits

Acetyl CoA (a-SĒ-til) A co-enzyme important in many metabolic processes

Acetylcholine (a-SĒ-til-KŌ-lēn) A choline-derived neurotransmitter

Acetylcholinesterase (a-SĒ-til-KŌ-lēn-EST-er-āz) An enzyme that removes acetylcholine from the synaptic cleft

Acid (a-SID) A molecule that ionizes into a hydrogen cation and some anion other than a hydroxyl

Acini, pancreatic (a-SĒN-ī) The exocrine component of the pancreas

Acquired immunity A component of the immune system comprised of lymphocytes and cells of the monocyte-macrophage lineage

Acromegaly (ak-RŌ-meg-alē) A disorder caused by the secretion of excessive growth hormone during adulthood

Acromial (ak-RŌ-mē-al) Pertaining to the shoulder

Acrosome (AK-ra-zōm) The anterior component of the head of sperm, contains modified lysosomes

ACTH Adrenocorticotropic hormone

Actin (AK-tin) A cytoskeletal protein that is important in muscle contraction

Action potential Seen in electrically active cells, a wave of depolarization and repolarization moving along the cell membrane

ADCC Antibody-dependent cellular cytotoxicity, the mechanism used by natural killer cells in immune defense

Adduction (ad-DUK-shun) Movement of a limb toward the midline

Adenine (AD-a-nēn) A nitrogenous base that is present in adenine nucleotides

Adenocarcinoma (ad-enō-KAR-sin-ōma) A malignancy of glandular epithelium

Adenohypophysis (ad-enō-HĪ-pof-a-sis) Anterior pituitary

Adenylate cyclase (ad-en-a-lāt SĪ-klās) An enzyme responsible for production of cyclic AMP

ADH Antidiuretic hormone, produced by the posterior pituitary

Adipocyte (AD-ip-ō-site) Fat cell, a mesenchymal derivative

Adipose (AD-ip-ōs) Pertaining to fat tissue

Adrenal gland (ad-RĒN-al) An endocrine gland located superior to the kidneys

Adrenocorticotropic hormone (ad-RĒN-ō-kor-tik-ō-trō-pik) A hormone produced by the anterior pituitary, stimulates secretion of some hormones from the adrenal cortex

Alanine (AL-a-nēn) An amino acid

Aldosterone (al-DOS-ta-rōn) A mineralocorticoid hormone produced by the adrenal cortex; important in the maintenance of fluid and electrolyte balance

Alimentary canal (ĀL-I-men-tery) The gastrointestinal tract, extends from the mouth to the anus

Allele (ah-LĒ-l) Alternate forms of a gene

Alveolus (al-VĒ-o-lus) The sacks in the lung in which gas exchange between the blood and the atmosphere occurs

Ameloblasts (a-MĒ-lō-blast) Tooth cells that produce enamel

Amine (AM-ēn) A class of compounds that are derivatives of the amino acid tyrosine; includes the thyroid hormones and the catecholamines

Amino acid (am-ĒN-ō) The building blocks of protein, consist of a central carbon, a hydrogen, an amino group, a carboxyl group and one of twenty side chains that provide identity and chemical characteristics

Ammonia (am-MŌN-ē-a) NH_3, a nitrogenous waste resulting from the breakdown of amino acids

Amorphous ground substance (ā-MOR-fus) A component of the extracellular matrix of mesenchymal derivatives (connective tissues)

Amphiarthrosis (am-FĒ-arth-rō-sis) A slightly movable joint

Amphipathic (am-fē-PATH-ik) Molecules having a hydrophobic moiety and a hydrophilic moiety; membrane phospholipids are examples of amphipathic molecules

Amplification (AM-PLIF-i-kā-shun) A characteristic of cascade mechanisms resulting in an increased effect at each step

Ampulla (AM-pūl-la) A widened area in a duct

Anaphase (an-NA-fāz) A phase of nuclear division (mitosis and meiosis)

Androgen (an-DRŌ-jen) Hormones that produce male characteristics, i.e., testosterone

Angiotensin (AN-gē-ō-ten-sin) Product of the renin-angiotensin system, increases blood pressure

Angiotensinogen (AN-ge-ō-ten-SIN-ō-jin) Inactive circulating precursor of angiotensin, produced by the liver

Anion (an-Ī-on) A negatively charged atom or molecule

Antebrachial (an-TĒ-brāk-ē-al) Forearm

Anterior (an-TEAR-ē-or) Toward the front surface of the body

Antibody (an-TĒ-body) Immunoglobulin, product of the immune system, specifically from plasma cells; participates in defense by binding to specific sites (epitopes) on foreign molecules (antigens)

Antidiuretic hormone (an-TĒ-dī-ūr-et-ik) ADH, hormone from posterior pituitary important in regulating the fluid volume of the body

Antigen (an-TI-jen) Molecules of foreign origin, recognized by the immune system and bound by antibodies

Aorta (ā-OR-ta) The body's largest artery, traveling from the heart through the thoracic and abdominal cavities

Apneustic center (ap-NEW-stick) Center in pons, involved in regulation of respiration

Apocrine glands (ap-Ō-krin) A form of sweat gland localized to the armpits and several other locations

Apoprotein (A-PŌ-prō-tēn) Proteins that transport lipids in the blood

Apoptosis (AP-a-TŌ-sis) Programmed cell death; a mechanism of cell death through which genes are turned on within a cell that result in its death; cell suicide

Appendicular skeleton (ap-PEN-dik-ū-lar) The component of the skeleton that includes the arms and legs and the bones that attach them to the axial skeleton

Arachnoid mater (ar-AK-noid) The central layer of the meninges

Arbor vitae (AR-bōr VĒ-tā) The white matter of the cerebellum

Arginine (AR-jen-ēn) An amino acid

Artery (AR-ter-ē) a high-pressure blood vessel, leading from the heart to the capillaries

Articulation (ar-TIK-ū-lā-shun) A joint

Asparagine (asp-AR-a-jēn) An amino acid

Aspartic acid (asp-ART-ik) An amino acid that also serves as a neurotransmitter

Astrocyte (AS-trō-sīt) A type of glial cell; stromal cell of the central nervous system

Atherogenesis (a-THER-ō-jen-is-is) Development of an atheroma

Atheroma (a-THER-ō-ma) Lesion of atherosclerosis

Atherosclerosis (a-THER-ō-skler-ō-sis) Disease characterized by lesions in the walls of arteries causing the potential for blockage

Atom (at-TOM) Basic unit of matter, consists of a nucleus containing protons and neutrons, orbited by electrons

Atomic number The number of protons in the nucleus of an atom; it provides an atoms identity (which element it represents)

ATP Adenosine triphosphate, the fuel that runs the molecular machinery of the body, product of oxidative phosphorylation

Atria (Ā-trē-ah) The superior chambers of the heart

Atrioventricular bundle (of His) (ā-TRĒ-Ō-ven-trik-ū-lar, HISS) Fibers that conduct action potentials from the atria to the ventricles, through the fibrotendinous ring

Atrioventricular node (ā-TRĒ-Ō-ven-TRIK-ū-lar) The secondary pacemaker of the heart

Atrioventricular valve (ā-TRĒ-Ō-ven-TRIK-ū-lar) The one-way valves located between the atria and ventricles of the heart; the tricuspid is on the right side, the bicuspid or mitral is on the left side

Autonomic nervous system (autō-NOM-ik) The motor component of the nervous system that innervates involuntary effectors (smooth muscle, cardiac muscle and glands)

Autophagy (autō-FAJ-ē) Means "self-eating," the process used by cells to recycle worn-out organelles

Autorhythmicity (autō-rith-MIS-itē) The hearts ability to generate its own beat

Axial flow (AKS-ē-al) The property of moving fluids that results in the flow being fastest in the middle of the stream; the largest particles tend to be pulled into this fast current

Axial skeleton (AKS-ē-al) The component of the skeleton that includes the skull, vertebral column, ribcage and sternum

Axilla (AKS-ill-a) Pertaining to the armpit

Axillary (AKS-il-ar-ē) Pertaining to the armpit

Axon (AKS-on) An extension of a neuron that carries impulses away from the cell body

Axoplasm (AKS-ō-plaz-um) The cytoplasm of the axon

Axoplasmic flow (AKS-ō-plaz-mik) The movement of the axoplasm distally in an axon; used as a transport mechanism

B lymphocytes (Lim-fō-sīts) A type of leukocyte that develops in the bone marrow and differentiates into plasma cells

Base A molecule that dissociates into a hydroxyl anion and any cation other than hydrogen; molecules that bind hydrogen ions in an aqueous (watery) solution also act as bases

Basement membrane The membrane that epithelial cells sit on

Basophils (bās-Ō-filz) One type of granular leukocyte

Bicuspid (bī-KUS-pid) The left atrioventricular valve

Bile (BĪ-el) The product of the liver; it has both secretory and excretory functions

Bilirubin (bil-ē-RU-ben) Breakdown product of hemoglobin; produced in the liver and excreted in bile

Blood brain barrier A barrier separating the contents of the blood from the extracellular fluid of the brain and spinal cord, consisting largely of modified endothelial cells acting under the influence of astrocytes

Blood clotting Coagulation of the blood, stops bleeding after an injury

Blood type A genetic trait that results in specific carbohydrates being expressed on the surface of red blood cells; determines compatability of blood for transfusions

Bowman's capsule (BŌ-manz) The glomerular capsule in renal corpuscles

Brachial (BRĀ-kē-al) Pertaining to the arm

Bradykinin (brā-dē-KĪN-in) A mediator of inflammation, product of the kinin cascade

Brain stem One component of the brain, consists of the medulla oblongata, pons, and midbrain

Bronchioles (bron-KĒ-ōlz) fine airways between the bronchi and alveolar ducts

Bronchus (bron-KUSS) Airways between the trachea and bronchioles

Buccal (BUCK-al) Cheek

Buffer (buf-FUR) A molecule that consumes a strong acid or base and produces a weak acid or base in its place

Bulbourethral gland (BUL-bō-ū-rēth-ral) Gland in the male reproductive tract that produces its secretion during sexual excitement, prior to orgasm; also called Cowper's gland

Calcaneal (KAL-kan-ēl) Heel

Calcitonin (KAL-si-tō-nan) Hormone produced by the thyroid, reduces blood calcium levels

Calcitrol (KAL-si-trol) Active vitamin D, necessary for calcium and phosphate absorption in the small intestine and resorption in the kidneys

Calmodulin (kal-MOD-ū-lin) A calcium binding protein important in the calcium second messenger system

Calvarium (KAL-AVR-ē-um) The flat bones of the skull that encase the brain

Cyclic AMP or cAMP A cyclic form of adenosine monophosphate, used as a second messenger

Canaliculi (kan-al-IK-ū-li) Small canals that interconnect the lacunae in bone

Cancellous bone (KAN-sell-us) Spongy bone; bone with trabeculae or spicules as its matrix structure

Capillary (KAP-i-lar-ē) The smallest blood vessels; the blood vessels through which exchange occurs

Carbohydrate (kar-bō-HĪD-rāt) Sugars: molecule consisting of carbon, hydrogen, and oxygen in which the hydrogen to oxygen ratio is 2:1 and which have one or more ring-shaped structures that contain three to seven carbons as well as oxygen; monosaccharides have one ring, these bind together to form polysaccharides

Carbonic anhydrase (kar-BON-ik an-HĪ-drās) An enzyme that combines carbon dioxide and water to produce carbonic acid

Carboxypeptidase (kar-BOX-Ē-pep-tĭd-ās) A protein-digesting enzyme produced in the pancreas and active in the small intestine

Carcinoma (kar-SIN-ō-ma) A malignant cancer of epithelial origin

Cardia (of stomach) (KAR-dē-a) The region of the stomach that is in the superior and medial position

Cardiac minute output (KAR-dē-ak) The amount of blood pumped per minute per ventricle

Cardiovascular (KAR-dē-ō-VASK-ū-lar) Pertaining to the heart and blood vessels

Carpal (KAR-pul) Pertaining to the wrist

Cartilage (KAR-ti-lāj) A mesemchymal derivative (connective tissue) with a firm amorphous ground substance

Cascade (KAS-kā-d) A mechanism involving multiple steps that occur in sequence once initiated

Catecholamine (kat-a-KŌL-a-mēn) A specific group of amines, derivatives of the amino acid tyrosine, with biological activities; includes epinephrine and norepinephrine

Cation (KAT-ī-on) A particle (atom or group of atoms) with a positive charge

Cauda equina (KAW-d-a ē-KWĪ-na) Spinal nerves that extend beyond the distal end of the spinal cord

Cecum (SĒ-kum) A pouch that is the most proximal structure of the large intestine

Central nervous system (CNS) The brain and spinal cord

Centriole (SENT-rē-ōl) An organelle that is important in nuclear division (mitosis and meiosis)

Centromere (SENT-rō-mēr) The point at which chromatids are joined, in a chromosome

Cephalic (se-FAL-ik) Pertaining to the head

Cerebellum (ser-a-BELL-um) The second largest structure of the human brain, located posterior and inferior to the cerebrum

Cerebrospinal fluid (CSF) (ser-Ē-brō SPĪ-n-al) The fluid that is in the ventricles, subarachnoid space and central canal of the spinal cord; floats and protects the central nervous system and serves as its interstitial fluid

Cerebrovascular accident (stroke) (ser-Ē-bro VAS-kū-lar) Injury produced by occlusion of an artery in the brain, resulting in focal neuronal death and neurologic deficit

Cerebrum (ser-Ē-brum) The largest structure of the human brain, the site of our intellectual activities and much of our integrative activity

Cerumen (sēr-RU-men) Earwax

Cervical (ser-VI-kal) Term means neck but can be applied to specific organs as well (e.g., cervix of the uterus)

Chemotaxis (KĒ-mō-TAX-iss) Attraction of cells by chemical means

Chiasma (optic) (kĭ-AZ-ma) Structure in which the optic nerves cross over

Cholecalciferol (KŌL-ē-kal-SIF-er-ol) One form of vitamin D

Cholecystokinin (CCK) (KŌL-ē-sis-tō-KĪN-in) An intestinal hormone

Cholesterol (kōl-EST-er-ol) A lipid that is important in cell membrane structure and hormone synthesis

Chondrocyte (KON-drō-sīt) Cartilage cell

Choroid plexus (KOR-oid PLEX-is) Structure of modified ependymal cells and capillaries for CSF production

Chromatid (KRŌM-a-tid) Condensed chromatin in the form that makes up one half of each chromosome

Chromatophilic substance (KRŌM-at-ō-filik) Rough endoplasmic reticulum in neurons

Chylomicron (ki-lō-MĪK-ron) Lipids combined with proteins for transport from small intestine to the liver

Chyme (KIME) Liquid mixture of food and gastric secretions

Chymotrypsin (kĭm-ō-TRIP-sin) Protein digesting enzyme produced by the pancreas for use in the small intestine

Cilia (SIL-ē-a) Structure on the surface of some epithelial cells that beat to move secretions (i.e., mucus) along the surface

Ciliary body (SIL-ē-ar-ē) Structure in the eye composed of the ciliary muscle (alters shape of lens to allow focusing) and ciliary process (produces aqueous humor)

Circumduction (sir-kum-DUK-shun) A complex rotational movement in which a limb describes a cone (abduct your arm, and, while keeping your elbow straight, move your arm so that your hand travels in a large circle)

Citric acid cycle Also called Krebs cycle, one step in aerobic cellular respiration (ATP synthesis)

Clitoris (CLIT-or-is) Small, anterior structure of erectile tissue in the vulva that is homologous to the penis of the male

Coccyx (kok-SIK-s) The vertebrae of our tail bone

Codon (KŌD-on) Three nucleotides in messenger RNA, encoding either one amino acid or stop

Collagen (KOL-a-jen) A fibrous extracellular matrix protein

Colon (KŌL-ōn) The main component of the large intestine

Column, renal Part of the medulla of the kidney

Columnar epithelium (kō-LUM-nar epi-THĒ-lē-um) Epithelial cells that are column-shaped

Commissural fibers (kom-ISH-ūr-al) Nerve fibers that interconnect the two cerebral hemispheres

Commissure, anterior and posterior (kom-ISH-ūr) Two structures composed of commissural fibers

Compact bone Dense bone, composed of microscopic osteons (Haversian units)

Complementarity (of nucleotides) (kom-ple-men-TAR-it-ē) The rules that govern which nucleotides can bind together, thereby enabling nucleotides present in one chain to determine the order of the nucleotides in another chain; used in DNA synthesis, transcription, and translation

Conchae, nasal (kon-KA) Three bony plates within each side of the inner nose

Conduction myofiber Purkinje fiber, myocardial cells specialized for rapidly conducting an action potential

Connective tissue Mesenchymal derivatives, a type of tissue consisting of cells and an extracellular matrix of fibers and amorphous ground substance

Contralateral (kon-tra-LAT-er-al) Opposite side

Conus medularis (kō-NUS med-ū-LAR-is) The tapered point at the distal end of the spinal cord

COPD Abbreviation for chronic obstructive pulmonary disease; chronic bronchitis with emphysema

Cor pulmonale (kor pul-mō-NAHL-ē) Right-sided congestive heart failure

Cornea (KOR-nē-a) The clear membrane in the anterior of the eye

Cornification (KORN-i-fi-KĀ-shun) The process of producing, or the presence of, a protective layer of dead cells on the surface of stratified squamous epithelium

Coronal section (kor-Ō-nal) Frontal section, dividing into an anterior and posterior part

Coronary artery (KOR-ō-nar-ē) Arteries that supply the heart muscle

Corpus albicans (KOR-pus al-BI-kanz) The ovarian scar tissue that remains following regression of a corpus luteum, after ovulation

Corpus callosum (KOR-pus kal-Ō-sum) A structure composed of commissural fibers that interconnects the two cerebral hemispheres

Corpus cavernosum (KOR-pus ka-ver-NŌ-sum) Erectile body composed of venous sinusoids. Two are present in the penis

Corpus luteum (KOR-pus LŪ-tē-um) Hormone secreting structure present in the ovary following ovulation

Corpus spongiosum (KOR-pus spon-JĒ-ō-sum) Erectile body in the penis through which the urethra passes

Cortex (KOR-tex) The outer portion of an organ, as opposed to the medulla

Corti, organ of (KOR-tē) A structure in the ear, involved in hearing

Corticosteroids (KOR-ti-kō-STER-oidz) Glucocorticoid hormones from the adrenal cortex, includes cortisol and cortisone

Covalent bond (kō-VĀL-ent) Bonds involving the sharing of electrons; may be polar or nonpolar

Coxal (KOKS-al) The bone of the pelvis comprising the fused ileum ischium and pubis bones

Cranial (KRĀ-nē-al) Pertaining to the skull

Crural (KRU-ral) Pertaining to the leg

Cryptorchidism (kript-ŌR-kid-is-um) Undescended testis

Cuboidal epithelium (kū-BOY-dal epi-THĒ-lē-um) Epithelial cells that are square in shape

Cysteine (SIS-tēn) An amino acid

Cytochrome (sīt-Ō-krōm) Certain molecules that are important in cellular respiration

Cytokinesis (sīt-ō-kīn-Ē-sis) Division of the cytoplasm, part of cell division

Cytoplasm (sīt-ō-PLA-zm) The component of the cell that lies between the membrane and the nucleus

Cytosine (sīt-Ō-sēn) An amino acid

Cytoskeleton (sīt-ō-SKEL-it-on) The cell's skeleton, composed of microtubules, intermediate filaments, and microfilaments

Cytosol (sīt-Ō-sol) The gel-like substance found in the cytoplasm among the organelles

Cytotoxic (sīt-ō-TOK-sik) Poisonous to cells

Dalton's law A gas law that indicates that each gas in a mixture exerts its own pressure as if the other gases were not present

Dartos (DAR-tōs) The smooth muscle of the scrotum, involved in thermoregulation for the testes

Deamination (de-am-i-NĀ-shun) Removal of amine groups from amino acids producing nitrogenous wastes

Decussation of pyramid (dē-kū-SĀ-shun) Crossing of motor fibers from one side to the other, in the medulla oblongata

Deep Away from the surface, opposite of superficial

Degranulation (dē-GRAN-ū-lā-shun) Release of inflammation mediators stored in mast cells and basophils

Dendrite (DEN-drī-t) Extensions of neurons that carry graded potentials toward the cell body, usually multiple and branched

Dendritic cells (den-DRIT-tik) Cells of the monocyte-macrophage lineage that are specialized for presenting antigens to lymphocytes

Dentin (den-TIN) The hard tissue of the tooth found deep to the enamel

Deoxyribonuclease (dē-oxē-rīb-ō-NŪ-KLĒ-ās) An enzyme that breaks down DNA

Deoxyribonucleotides (dē-oxē-rīb-ō-NŪ-KLĒ-Ō-tǐd-z) The nucleotides of DNA

Deoxyribose (dē-oxē-RĪB-ōs) The modified pentose monosaccharide (missing one oxygen) found in the nucleotides of DNA

Depression Downward movement of a structure such as the jaw or shoulders, opposite of elevation

Dermatoglyphics (derm-at-ō-GLIF-iks) Fingerprints

Dermis (DER-miss) The connective tissue of your skin found deep to the epidermis

Desmin (DEZ-min) The intermediate filament protein of muscle tissue

Diabetes insipidus (dī-a-BĒ-tēz in-SIP-i-dus) A disease characterized by excessive thirst and urine output, caused by an inability to secrete antidiuretic hormone

Diabetes mellitus (dī-a-BĒ-tēz MEL-i-tus) A disease characterized by excessive thirst and urine output caused either by the inability to secrete or to respond to insulin

Diaphysis (dī-AF-i-sis) The shaft of a long bone

Diarthrosis (dī-arth-RŌ-sis) A freely movable joint

Diastole (dī-ASS-tō-lē) The phase of cardiac relaxation or low blood pressure

Diencephalon (dī-en-SEF-a-lon) The portion of the brain consisting of the thalamus, epithalamus, and hypothalamus

Differentiation The process through which cells gain specialized structures and functions

Diffusion (dif-ŪSH-un) The passive movement of substances from a region of their higher concentration to a region of their lower concentration

Digestion (dǐ-JEST-jun) The breaking down of food by chemical and mechanical means

Diploe (DIP-plō) The core of spongy bone found between the internal and external plates of dense bone, in a flat bone such as the bones of the skull

Distal (DIS-tal) The end of a structure that is further from its beginning or site of attachment, opposite of proximal

Diuresis (dǐ-ūr-Ē-sis) Production of a high volume of dilute urine

Dopamine (DŌP-a-mēn) A neurotransmitter of the amine class

Dorsal (DŌR-sal) Toward the back surface of your body, opposite of ventral

Dorsiflexion (dōr-si-FLEK-shun) To move the foot and ankle superiorly (arch your foot)

Ductus (vas) deferens (duk-tus de-fer-ENZ) Duct in the male reproductive tract that conveys sperm from the epididymis to the ejaculatory duct

Duodenum (dū-OD-en-um) The most proximal region of the small intestine

Dura mater The most superficial layer of the meninges

Dust cell Resident cells of the monocyte-macrophage lineage in the lungs; phagocytize debris in alveoli

Dysplasia (dis-PLĀ-shē-a) Aberrant growth, one step in the development of cancer

Edema (a-DĒM-a) The presence of an excessive amount of interstitial fluid in a tissue or structure

Effector (ē-FEK-tōr) Muscle (smooth, skeletal or cardiac) and glands

Eicosanoids (ī-KŌS-an-oids) A group of bioactive lipids that includes leukotreines and prostaglandins

Ejaculatory duct (Ē-jack-ū-la-tōr-ē) A duct in the male reproductive system where sperm, from the ductus deferens mix with the secretion of the seminal vesicles

Elastin (ē-LASS-tin) An elastic (stretchy) extracellular matrix protein

Electrogenic pump (ē-LEK-trō-GEN-ik) An integral membrane protein that pumps ions (an ATPase) in such a way as to generate an electrical gradient (i.e., the $Na^+K^+ATPase$)

Electron (ē-LEK-tron) A negatively charged particle that orbits the nucleus of an atom

Electron transport One step in the production of ATP by aerobic cellular respiration

Elevation Upward movement of a structure like the jaw or shoulders (shrug), the opposite of depression

Enamel (ē-NAM-el) The hard, shiny material on the exposed surface of teeth

Endocardium (en-DŌ-CAR-dē-um) The layer of the heart that lines the chambers; composed of endothelial cells

Endochondrial ossification (en-do-KOND-rē-al oss-if-i-KĀ-shun) Production of bone in a preexisting cartilage model

Endocrine gland (END-ō-krin) Glands that secrete their products directly into the interstitial fluid for transport in the blood (ductless glands); glands that produce hormones

Endocrinocyte (end-ō-KRIN-ō-sīt) A cell that produces hormones

Endocytosis (end-ō-sīt-Ō-sis) The process of bringing substances into a cell (i.e., phagocytosis and pinocytosis)

Endometrium (en-dō-MĒ-trē-um) The lining of the uterus

Endomysium (en-dō-MĪ-sē-um) Connective tissue within a muscle that surrounds myofibers within a fascicle

Endoneurium (en-dō-NŪR-ē-um) Connective tissue within a nerve that surrounds nerve fibers within a fascicle

Endoplasmic reticulum (en-dō-PLAZ-mik ra-TIK-ūl-um) A tubular organelle composed of phospholipid bilayer; may be granular (rough), with bound ribosomes; or agranular (smooth) indicating no bound ribosomes

Endorphin (en-DŌRF-in) A neuropeptide that inhibits pain

Endosteum (end-OS-tē-um) The tissue located on the surface of bone, within the medullary cavity, consisting mainly of osteoprogenitor cells

Endothelium (en-dō-THĒ-lē-um) The cells that line blood vessels and any space through which blood flows

Enkephalin (en-KEF-a-lin) A neuropeptide that inhibits pain

Enterocyte (ENT-er-ō-sīt) Intestinal cells

Enteroendocrine (en-ter-ō-END-ō-krin-ō-sīt) Hormone producing cells of the intestine

Enzyme (EN-zīm) Proteins that catalyze (speed up) chemical reactions

Eosin (Ē-ō-sin) A histologic dye that stains the contents of the cytoplasm orange-red

Eosinophil (ē-ō-SIN-ō-fil) One class of granular leukocyte

Ependyma (a-PEN-di-ma) Epithelial cells of the central nervous system

Epicardium (ep-a-KARD-ē-um) The lining of the exterior surface of the heart, visceral pericardium

Epicuticle (ep-ē-KŪ-ti-cal) Modified epidermis along the proximal edge of the finger or toe nails

Epidermis (ep-i-DER-mis) The superficial, epithelial component of the skin

Epididymis (ep-i-DID-a-mus) Tubular structure that is the site of sperm maturation

Epimysium (ep-i-MĪS-ē-um) Connective tissue that surrounds a muscle

Epinephrine (ep-in-EF-er-in) A catecholamine that serves as a neurotransmitter and a hormone from the adrenal medulla; important in sympathetic nervous system activity; also called adrenalin

Epineurium (ep-i-NŪR-ē-em) Connective tissue that surrounds a nerve

Epiphyseal plate (ep-i-FIS-ē-al) Connective tissue between the epiphysis and diaphysis of long bones that serves as the site of lengthwise growth of long bones; replaced with bone as we age

Epiphysis (e-PIF-i-sis) The ends of a long bone

Epithelioma (ep-i-thē-lē-ŌM-a) Benign neoplasm of epithelium

Epithelium (ep-i-THĒ-lē-um) One of the five classes of tissue, tissues that line some surface

Epitope (ep-i-TŌ-p) The portion of an antigen that an antibody binds to; most antigens contain many different epitopes

Erythrocyte (ē-RITH-rō-sīt) Red blood cell

Erythropoeisis (ē-RITH-rō-pō-Ē-sis) Production of red blood cells

Esophagus (ē-SOF-a-gus) Tubular component of the alimentary canal that begins at the larynx and extends to the stomach

Estradiol (est-tra-DĪ-ōl) One form of estrogen

Estrogen (EST-rō-jen) Female sex hormones

Etiology (ē-tē-AH-lō-jē) The specific agent or mechanism that causes an illness

Euchromatin (Ū-krōm-a-tin) Light staining chromatin, that which is available for transcription

Eupnea (Ūp-nē-a) Quiet breathing

Eversion (ē-VER-shun) To rotate the soles laterally, opposite of inversion

Excitotoxicity (ex-SĪ-tō-tox-I-sit-ē) Injury-inducing excessive stimulation of a neuron

Exocrine gland (EX-ō-krin) Glands that secrete their products (e.g., sweat, saliva, digestive enzymes) through ducts

Exocytosis (ex-ō-sīt-Ō-sis) Removal of substances from a cell, opposite of endocytosis

Exon (EX-on) Expressed region of a gene, the portion that encodes a protein

Extension (ex-TEN-shun) Increasing the angle of a joint to move bones apart (i.e., straighten your elbow); opposite of flexion

Extracellular Outside of the cell

Extracellular matrix The noncellular components of mesenchymal derivatives (connective tissue) including fibers (such as collagen) and amorphous ground substance

Exudate (EX-ū-dāt) The fluid and cells that leave blood capillaries during inflammation

Fab (pronounced as individual letters) The abbreviation for the antigen binding fragment of an antibody

Facet (FA-set) A flattened area on the surface of a bone, for articulation with another bone

Facial (FĀ-shul) Pertaining to the face

Fallopian tube (fal-Ō-pē-an) Uterine tube, extends from each ovary to the uterus

Fascicle (FA-si-kl) A bundle of myofibers in a muscle or nerve fibers in a nerve

Fc (Pronounced as individual letters) The constant region of an antibody, the opposite end from the Fab

Feedback, negative The main mechanism in the maintenance of homeostasis: a change in one direction is counteracted by a change in the opposite direction

Feedback, positive A mechanism used only rarely during homeostasis but seen in a number of pathological conditions: a change in one direction leads to a further change in the same direction

Femoral (FEM-or-al) Pertaining to the thigh

Fibrin (FĪ-brin) The protein that polymerizes to form the fibrous component of a blood clot

Fibrinolytic (fī-brin-ō-LIT-ik) A cascade mechanism that activates the enzyme plasmin, which cleaves uncrosslinked fibrin, limiting a blood clot; now a related therapy used during myocardial infarction and a limited number of stroke cases

Fibroblast (FĪ-brō-blast) The main cell type in typical connective tissues

Fibrocartilage (FĪ-brō-KAR-ti-lāj) Cartilage with an increased amount of collagen fibers in the extracellular matrix, for added strength

Fibrotendinous ring (FĪB-rō-TEND-in-us) The ring of connective tissue in the heart that electrically isolates the atria from the ventricles and of which all heart valves are a part

Filum terminale (FĪ-lum ter-min-AL-ā) Filaments of connective tissue that attach the distal end of the spinal cord to the coccyx

Fimbriae (FIM-brē-ā) The finger-like extensions at the ovarian end of the uterine tubes

Fissure (FI-shur) A narrow, deep crack-like groove

Fixator (FIX-ā-tor) A muscle in a muscle group that stabilizes the origin as the prime mover contracts

Flexion (FLEK-shun) Decreasing the angle of a joint to bring bones closer together; opposite of extension

Folia (FŌ-lē-a) The gray matter of the cerebellum

Follicle stimulating hormone (FSH) A gonadotropin hormone produced by the anterior pituitary that plays a role in gamete development

Fossa (FAH-sa) A round depression on the surface of a bone

Frameshift mutation A genetic mutation that results in the displacement of the reading frame of the codons

Frenulum, lingual (LING-ū-al FREN-ū-lum) a ridge of tissue that attaches the inferior surface of the tongue to the floor of the mouth

Frontal Pertaining to the forehead

Fundus, of stomach (FUN-dis) The region of the stomach lateral to the esophagus that is used for storage during a large meal

Fusiform (FŪ-zi-form) Pointed on both ends widest in the middle

GABA, gama amino butyric acid A neurotransmitter

Gamete (GAM-ēt) Reproductive cell with 1n genetic content; human reproduction involves fusion of a female gamete (ova) with a male gamete (sperm)

Gametogenesis (gam-ĒT-ō-jen-is-is) Production of gametes

Ganglion (GAN-glē-on) A collection on neuron cell bodies outside of the CNS

Gap junction A specialized, pore-like intercellular junction through which ions can pass between cells

Gaster (GAS-ter) The belly or wide part of a muscle

Gastric inhibiting peptide (GIP) An intestinal hormone with inhibitory effects on the stomach

Gastrin (GAS-trin) A hormone produced by the stomach that increases activity of the stomach

Genetic mutation Alteration of the sequence or arrangement of nucleic acids in the genes

Genotype (JĔN-ō-tīp) An individuals genetic makeup, as opposed to his/her identifiable characteristics (phenotype) that results from that genotype

Germ cell The cells of the lineage that differentiates into gametes

GFAP, glial fibrilary acidic protein The intermediate filament protein of glia

Gingiva (JIN-ji-vah) The gums

Glans (GLANZ) The structure located on the distal end of the penis or clitoris

Glia (GLĒ-a) The stroma of the central nervous system, also one of the five tissue types, the cells of which make up much of (but not all of) the stroma of the central nervous system

Glomerulus (glō-MER-ū-lus) The tuft of capillaries found in the renal corpuscle

Glucagon (GLŪ-ka-gon) A pancreatic hormone that increases blood glucose levels

Glucocorticoid (glū-cō-COR-ti-coid) Hormones produced by the zona fasciculata of the adrenal cortex, including cortisol and cortisone; these hormones are important in resistance to stress

Gluconeogenesis (GLŪ-kō-NĒ-ō-JEN-is-is) Production of glucose using noncarbohydrate sources (protein and lipid) for materials

Glutamine (GLŪT-am-ēn) An amino acid

Glutamic acid (glū-TAM-ik) An amino acid that also serves as a neurotransmitter

Gluteal (GLŪ-tē-al) Pertaining to the buttocks

GLUTs (GLŪ-tz, or individual letters) Membrane proteins that serve as carriers during facilitated diffusion of glucose

Glycine (GLĪ-sēn) An amino acid that also serves as a neurotransmitter

Glycocalyx (glī-kō-KĀ-liks) Carbohydrates found on the surface of cells, most of which are the carbohydrate moieties of membrane glycoproteins

Glycogenesis (GLĪ-kō-jen-is-is) Production of glycogen for glucose storage

Glycogenolysis (glī-kō-jen-AH-lis-is) Breakdown of glycogen releasing glucose

Glycolipid (GLĪ-kō-LIP-id) A lipid molecule with a carbohydrate attached

Glycolysis (glī-KAHL-is-is) The breakdown of glucose to two pyruvic acids during ATP production

Glycoprotein (glī-kō-PRŌ-tēn) A protein molecule with a carbohydrate attached

Glycosyltransferase (glī-KŌS-el-TRANZ-fer-ās) An enzyme that attaches a carbohydrate to some other molecule, usually a protein or lipid

Golgi apparatus (GŌL-jē) Organelle in which proteins are modified and packaged for export from the cell

Gomphosis (gom-FŌ-sis) A fibrous joint in which a fibrous connective tissue peg fits into a hole in a bone

Gonadocorticoids (gō-NAD-ō-KŌR-ti-koid) Sex hormones produced by the adrenal cortex

Gonadotropin (gō-NAD-ō-TRŌP-in) Luteinizing hormone and follicle stimulating hormone, produced by the anterior pituitary

Graafian follicle (GRA-fē-in FOL-i-kul) Vesicular ovarian follicle, the last stage in ovarian follicle development prior to ovulation

Gray matter Component of the central nervous system composed mainly of neuron cell bodies

Growth hormone (hGH) Hormone produced by the anterior pituitary that promotes growth

Guanine (GWA-nēn) A nitrogenous base that is present in guanine nucleotides

Gyrus (JĪ-rus) An outward fold of the cerebral cortex

Haustra (HOW-stra) The sack-like bulges of the colon

Haversian unit (ha-VER-sē-an) Osteon, the layered microscopic structures that make up dense bone

HCl (hydrochloric acid) A strong acid present in gastric secretions

HDL (high density lipoprotein) Transport form of lipids in the blood, composed of lipids and an apoprotein; returns unused lipids to the liver for processing

Hematopoeisis (hē-MAT-ō-pō-ē-sis) Production of blood cells

Hematoxylin (hē-ma-TOX-a-lin) A histologic dye that stains nuclei and certain other cellular components deep blue-purple

Hemostasis (hē-mō-STĀ-sis) Cessation of the flow of blood, as in either clotting or loss of flow within a vessel

Henle, loop of (HEN-lē) The loop of the nephron

Henry's law The gas law that states that the concentration of a gas in a liquid is proportional to the concentration of that gas in the atmosphere above the liquid and dependent on the solubility of that gas in the liquid

Hepatic (he-PAT-ik) Pertaining to the liver

Hepatocyte (he-PAT-ō-sīt) Liver cell

Heptose (HEP-tōs) A monosaccharide containing six carbons

Herniation (her-nē-Ā-shun) The movement of one organ or structure through or into another (i.e., viscera through the muscle of the body wall or brain tissue into a ventricle), resulting in a hernia

Hexose (HEX-ōs) A monosaccharide containing six carbons, such as glucose

hGH Abbreviation for human growth hormone

Histidine (HIS-ta-dēn) An amino acid

Histocompatability antigen (HIS-tō-kom-pat-a-BILL-i-tē ANT-i-jen) Cell surface glycoproteins that enable T cells to identify antigens; play a role in organ graft rejection

Histology (his-TOL-ō-gē) The study of tissues or microscopic anatomy

Histones (HIS-tōn-z) Proteins that organize DNA in the nucleus

Histophysiology (HIS-tō-fiz-ē-AH-lō-gē) The study of function at the tissue level

Homeostasis (ho-me-o-STĀ-sis) The relatively constant state of conditions that must be maintained in the body to retain health

Howship's lacunae (HOW-ships la-KŪN-nā) Pit of resorption, site of bone resorption by an osteoclast

Human chorionic gonadotropin (HCG) (kor-ee-ON-ik gō-NAD-ō-trō-pin) Early embryonic and placental hormone that maintains the corpus luteum, necessary for the maintenance of pregnancy

Hydrogen bond Weak bond in which a hydrogen atom is bound to one atom in a molecule but is attracted to another; important in developing the three-dimensional structure of molecules such as proteins

Hydrogen (HĪ-drō-jen) The element in which atoms have one proton in the nucleus

Hydrolase (HĪ-drō-lās) An enzyme that cleaves some molecule through the consumption of a molecule of water

Hydrostatic pressure (HĪ-drō-STĀ-tik) Mechanical fluid pressure

Hypercalciuria (hī-per-kal-si-ŪR-ē-a) Higher than normal urine concentration of calcium

Hyperextension (hī-per ex-TEN-shun) To extend a joint past the straight position

Hyperplasia (hī-per-PLĀ-sha) Increased rate of cell division

Hyperpolarization (hī-per-pōl-er-i-SĀ-shun) Increase in the charge (beyond resting membrane potential) of a polarized membrane

Hypersecretion (hī-per-sa-KRĒ-shun) Increase beyond normal in the secretion of some substance

Hypertrophy (hī-PER-trō-fē) Increase in the size of cells, such as in muscle by increased exercise

Hypodermis (hī-pō-DER-mus) Subcutaneous tissues, the connective tissue deep to the dermis

Hypothalamus (hī-pō-THAL-i-mus) One structure of the diencephalon of the brain

Ileocecal valve (il-ē-ō-SĒK-al) Sphincter at the opening between the ileum and the cecum (the start of the large intestine)

Ileum (IL-ē-um) The distal portion of the small intestine

Immunoglobulin (IM-ū-nō-GLOB-ū-lin) Globular protein important in immunity; produced by plasma cells; also called antibodies

Immunohistochemistry (IM-ū-nō-HIS-tō-chem-is-trē) Localization of specific molecules in tissue sections through the use of antibodies; important technique in research and diagnosis

Immunosurveillance (IM-ū-nō-sur-VĀ-lan-s) The monitoring of the internal environment for the presence of infectious or "non-self" agents

Inclusion, cytoplasmic (sīt-ō-PLAZ-mik in-KLŪ-shun) Stored material within the cell

Incus (IN-kus) Anvil, one of the bones of the inner ear

Indole (IN-dōl) A simple substance that results from the digestion of proteins One of the waste products that give feces their characteristic odor

Infarction (in-FARK-shun) Localized death of cells due to ischemia (lack of blood flow)

Inferior (in-FEAR-ē-or) Below (in the anatomical position), farther away from the head than, opposite of superior

Inflammation (in-fla-MĀ-shun) Nonspecific response to injury; involves movement of cells and fluid out of blood vessels

Infundibulum (in fun-DIB-ū-lum) The fine, stalk-like attachment of the pituitary gland to the hypothalamus

Insulin (IN-sa-lin) Hormone produced by the pancreas that lowers blood glucose levels; derangement in insulin activity leads to diabetes mellitus

Integument (in-TEG-ū-ment) Pertaining to the skin

Interatrial septum (in-ter-ĀT-rē-al SEP-tum) The wall that separates the heart's two atria

Intercallated disk (in-TER-kal-āt-ed) The specialized membrane structure between cardiac muscle cells that contains gap junctions and allows ions to flow from one cell to the next

Intercostal (in-ter-KOS-tal) Between the ribs, as in intercostal muscles

Intermediate (in-ter-MĒD-ē-āt) Between

Intermediate filaments One of three major components of the cytoskeleton; composed of five classes of protein expressed in a tissue specific manner

Interneurons (in-ter-NER-onz) Association neurons; neurons that are neither sensory nor motor

Interphase (IN-TER-fā-z) One of the phases of nuclear division; the phase cells are in when they are not actively involved in mitosis or meiosis

Interstitial (in-ter-STI-shul) Lying between

Interstitial fluid (in-ter-STI-shul) The extracellular fluid that lies between and bathes the cells of our tissues

Interventricular septum (in-ter-ven-TRIK-ū-lar SEP-tum) The wall that separates the heart's two ventricles

Intrapleural (in-ter-PLUR-al) Between the visceral and parietal pleura, as in intrapleural space and pressure of the respiratory system

Intron (IN-tron) Intervening regions in the genes, must be removed from mRNA before translation

Inversion (in-VER-shun) Rotate soles medially, opposite of eversion

Involute (IN-vō-lūt) To loose parenchyma, become smaller or regress with age such as what occurs in the thymus

Ion (Ī-on) A charged atom or group of atoms

Ionic bond (ī-ON-ik) Bond between two ions of opposite charges (cation and anion)

Ipsilateral (ip-si-LAT-er-al) Same side

Ischemia (is-KĒM-ē-a) Localized lack of blood flow, generally caused by arterial obstruction

Isoleucine (īs-ō-LŪ-sēn) An amino acid

Isotype (Ī-sō-tīp) The specific subtype of an immunoglobulin (IgG, IgM, IgE, IgA, IgD)

Isovolumetric (īs-ō-vol-ū-MET-rik) No change in volume, as in isovolumetric contraction or relaxation

Jejunum (je-JŪN-um) The middle region of the small intestine

Juxtaglomerular apparatus (jux-ta-glō-MER-ū-lar) A structure in the nephron that includes the macula densa of the distal convoluted tubule and the juxtaglomerular cells of the afferent arteriole

Kallikrein (kal-i-KRĪN) An enzyme active in the kinin cascade

Keratin (KER-a-tin) The intermediate filament protein of epithelial cells

Keratinization (ker-a-TIN-i-zā-shun) The dead layer on the surface of cornified (keratinized) stratified squamous epithelium or the process of producing that layer

Keratinocyte (ker-a-TIN-ō-sīt) The epithelial cells of the skin

Kinases (KĪ-nā-s) A molecule that regulates the activity of an enzyme, usually through phosphorylation

Kinin cascade (KĪ-nin cas-KĀD) One of four cascade mechanisms important in inflammation mediation

Kreb's cycle Also called citric acid cycle, one step in aerobic cellular respiration (ATP synthesis)

Kupffer cell (KUP-fer) Resident member of the monocyte-macrophage lineage in the liver

Lacrimal (LAK-ri-mal) Pertaining to the tears, also a bone in the vicinity of the lacrimal ducts

Lactogen, human placental (LAK-tō-jen) Hormone produced by the placenta late in pregnancy that promotes lactation

Laminin (LAM-in-in) Extracellular matrix protein, component of basement membranes

Langerhans, islets of (L-AHNG-er-hanz) Pancreatic islets, endocrine tissue of the pancreas

Laryngopharynx (la-RING-ō-far-ank-z) Inferior portion of the pharynx

Larynx (LAR-ank-z) Cartilage structure where the digestive and respiratory systems diverge, inferior to the pharynx; includes the epiglottis and the vocal cords

Lateral (LAT-er-al) Away from the midline of the body, to the side

LDL, low density lipoprotein Transport form of lipids in the blood composed of lipids and apoproteins, conveys lipids from the liver to tissues throughout the body

Leucine (LŪ-sēn) An amino acid

Leukocyte (LŪK-ō-sīt) White blood cell

Leukotreines (LŪK-ō-trī-ēn-z) Eikosanoid lipids used for communication between leukocytes

Leydig cells (LĪ-dig) Interstitial endocrinocytes, hormone producing cells of the testis

Ligament (LIG-a-ment) Structure of dense regular connective tissue that interconnects two bones

Ligand (LĪ-gan-d) The molecule that binds to a receptor (i.e., a neurotransmitter is the ligand for a neurotransmitter receptor)

Ligation (lī-GĀ-shun) To tie-off, such as tubal ligation whereby the uterine tubes are tied-off, cut, and tied or otherwise obstructed

Lipase (LĪ-pā-s) A lipid-digesting enzyme

Lipid (LI-pid) An nonpolar organic molecule composed of carbon, hydrogen, and oxygen, such as triglycerides, eicosanoids, and steroids

Locus (LŌ-kus) Location, especially the location of a gene on a chromosome

Luteinizing hormone, LH (LŪT-in-īz-ing) A gonadotropin hormone produced by the anterior pituitary that triggers ovulation and stimulates release of estrogen and progesterone

Lymph node (LIM-f) Secondary lymphoid organs, site of B-cell maturation, centers of immune surveillance

Lymphatic vessel (lim-FAT-ik) A series of vessels beginning as fine vessels within tissues and ending as the thoracic duct and right lymphatic duct, which ultimately join the subclavian veins. These vessels interconnect lymph nodes and convey lymphatic fluid, which is derived from interstitial fluid

Lymphocyte (LIM-fō-sīt) A class of leukocytes, includes T and B lymphocytes

Lyse (LĪ-s) To rupture or burst, as in to burst a cell

Lysine (LĪ-sēn) An amino acid

Lysosome (LĪ-sō-sōm) An organelle composed of a phospholipid vesicle containing acids and hydrolytic enzymes; these fuse with phagocytotic and autophagocytic vesicles to degrade their contents

Lysozyme (LĪ-sō-zīm) An antibacterial enzyme present in secretions such as saliva

MAC (as individual letters) Membrane attack complex, product of the complement system that is inserted into antibody-coated membranes to lyse potentially pathogenic cells

Macrophage (MAK-rō-faj) Means "big-eater," a cell that is a differentiated member of the monocyte-macrophage lineage, usually specialized for phagocytosis

Malignant (mal-IG-nant) A characteristic of some neoplastic cells that indicates an invasive growth pattern and the ability to metastasize from one part of the body to another; malignant neoplasms typically have the ability to kill their host

Mammary (MAM-ar-ē) Pertaining to the breast

Maximus (MAX-i-mus) Muscle naming term indicating the largest muscle in a group

Meatus (mē-Ā-tus) A tube-like canal through a bone

Medial (MĒ-dē-al) Toward the midline of the body

Mediastinum (mē-dē-a-STĪN-um) Tissues in the medial aspect of the thoracic cavity, includes the esophagus and the thymus and contains the heart

Medulla (med-Ū-la) The middle, as opposed to the cortex

Medulla oblongata (med-Ū-la ob-long-AH-ta) The most inferior portion of the brain stem; the structure at which the spinal cord meets the brain

Megakaryocyte (me-ga-KAR-ē-ō-sīt) Bone marrow cell that gives rise to platelets

Meiosis (mī-Ō-sis) Nuclear division that results in daughter cells with half the genetic content of the parent cell; used in gametogenesis

Melanocyte (me-LAN-ō-sīt) Pigment cells present in the skin

Melanosome (me-LAN-ō-sōm) Packets of the pigment melanin that are produced by melanocytes and transferred to epidermal cells (keratinocytes)

Melatonin (me-la-TŌN-in) Hormone produced by the pineal gland, role in initiating sleep

Meningeal (men-IN-gē-al) Pertaining to the meninges

Meninges (me-NIN-gē-z) The membranes that surround the central nervous system, composed of three layers: dura mater, arachnoid mater, and pia mater

Menses (MEN-sēz) The bloody fluid and tissue that flows from the female reproductive tract during menstruation

Menstrual cycle (MEN-strū-al) The female reproductive cycle

Menstruation (men-strū-Ā-shun) The flow of bloody fluid and endometrial tissue that is expelled as menses during the menstrual phase of the menstrual cycle

Mental (MEN-tal) Pertaining to the chin

Merocrine (MER-ō-krin) A mechanism of secretion; here the term applies to the sweat glands that are widely distributed across the surface of the body, especially abundant on the palms and soles

Mesangial cell (mes-ANJ-ē-al) A cell located in the renal corpuscle, important in the maintenance of the glomerular basal lamina

Mesencephalon (mez-en-SEF-a-lon) The midbrain

Mesenchymal derivative (mez-EN-ki-mal dē-RIV-a-tiv) All of the tissues that develop from the embryonic tissue mesenchyme; includes typical connective tissues, cartilage, bone, and blood

Mesenchyme (MEZ-en-kīm) Embryonic connective tissue

Mesentery (MEZ-en-ta-rē) Double fold of the lining of the abdominopelvic cavity (peritoneum) that anchors the viscera and provides access for blood vessels and nerves

Mesocolon (MEZ-Ō-cōl-on) The mesentery that holds the colon in place

Mesothelium (MEZ-ō-thē-lē-um) The serous membrane that lines the body cavities

Mesovarium (MEZ-ō-var-ē-um) The mesentery that supports the ovaries

Metaphase (MET-a-fāze) The phase of nuclear division (mitosis and meiosis) in which the chromosomes line up along the equatorial plane

Metaphysis (met-A-fi-sis) The location at which the epiphyses and diaphysis of a long bone meet

Metaplasia (met-a-PLĀ-sha) Altered growth, one of the stages in the cellular response to injury, in the progression toward neoplasia

Metarteriole (met-ar-TEAR-ē-ōl) A small blood vessel that bypasses a capillary bed

Metastasis (met-AST-a-sis) The process by which malignant (cancer) cells migrate from one location in the body to another; also applies to the lesion growing in the new location (the secondary lesion)

Metastatic (met-a-STA-tik) Pertaining to metastasis

Methianine (meth-Ī-a-nēn) An amino acid

MHC (major histocompatability complex) A group of glycoproteins important in immune surveillance and in organ graft rejection (organ donors and recipients must be MHC compatible)

Microfilaments (MĪK-rō-fil-a-ments) The smallest diameter component of the three parts of the cytoskeleton

Microfractures (mīk-rō-FRAK-turz) Microscopic fractures within bone matrix, usually removed by remodeling

Microglia (mīk-rō-GLĒ-a) Members of the monocyte-macrophage lineage resident in the CNS

Microtubules (mīk-rō-TŪB-ūlz) The largest diameter component of the three parts of the cytoskeleton

Microvilli (mīk-rō-VI-lī) Modification of the apical surface of epithelial cells that increase the cell's surface area; also called brush border (i.e., in the small intestine)

Micturition (MIK-tūr-i-shun) Urination

Midbrain The most superior component of the brainstem, mesencephalon

Midpiece (of sperm) The portion of the sperm posterior to the head that contains mitochondria

Midsagittal (mid-SAJ-i-tal) A sagittal section in the middle plane of the body

Millivolt One thousandth of a volt

Mineralocorticoid (min-er-al-ō-KŌR-ti-coid) Hormone of the zona glomerulosa of the adrenal cortex (i.e., aldosterone) that regulates fluid and electrolyte balance

Minimus (MIN-i-mus) Muscle naming term indicating the smallest muscle in a group

Ministroke Transient ischemic attack, ischemic event (focal loss of blood flow) in the brain that is of brief duration and does not leave permanent damage; may precede a cerebrovascular accident (stroke) and as such, medical attention must be sought even if symptoms completely resolve

Mitochondria (mī-tō-KON-drē-a) Organelle that is the site of oxidative phosphorylation (aerobic cellular respiration)

Mitosis (mī-TŌ-sis) Nuclear division in which the two daughter nuclei are each identical to the parent nucleus

Mitral valve (MĪ-tral) Bicuspid valve, the left atrioventricular valve

Moiety (MOY-it-ē) Portion or piece; glycoproteins have a carbohydrate moiety and a protein moiety, amphipathic molecules have hydrophobic and hydrophilic moieties

Molarity (mō-LAR-it-ē) A measure of concentration based on the molecular weight of the solute, expressed in grams (a one molar solution is the molecular weight of the solute, expressed in grams, per liter)

Molecule (MOL-i-kūl) A group of atoms bound together, the smallest possible amount of a compound

Monocyte (MON-ō-sīt) A leukocyte that is a member of the monocyte-macrophage lineage

Monocyte-macrophage lineage A group of related cells that differentiate from monocytes into cells generally specialized for phagocytosis; includes osteoclasts, Kupffer cells, dust cells, and dendritic cells

Monoglyceride (mon-ō-GLI-ser-īd) A lipid consisting of a glycerol and one fatty-acid side chain

Monosaccharide (mon-ō-SAK-a-rīd) The smallest unit of carbohydrate, consisting of a single ring-shaped structure of carbon, hydrogen, and oxygen with a 2:1 hydrogen to oxygen ratio

Mucin (MŪ-sin) Glycoprotein present in mucus

Mucosa (mū-KŌS-a) The layer in the wall of a tubular organ that lines the lumen; usually consists of the epithelium and the lamina propria, the connective tissue immediately deep to the epithelium

Muscularis (mus-kū-LAR-is) A muscular layer in the wall of a tubular organ such as the alimentary canal

Mutism (MŪ-ti-sm) An inability to speak

Myelin (MĪ-a-lin) A phospholipid that surrounds an axon or dendrite as an insulating sheath

Myelination (mī-a-lin-Ā-shun) The process of applying a myelin sheath or the sheath itself

Myocardium (mī-ō-KARD-ē-um) The layer of cardiac muscle in the wall of the heart

Myoepithelial cells (mī-ō-epi-THĒ-lē-al) Epithelial cells that have the ability to contract

Myofiber (mī-ō-FĪB-er) Skeletal muscle cell

Myofibril (mī-ō-FĪB-ril) Subcellular structure seen in myofibers that contains contractile proteins arranged as myofilaments

Myofilament (mī-ō-FIL-a-ment) The organized contractile proteins of muscle; exists in two types, thick (composed of myosin) and thin (composed of tropomyosin, troponin and actin)

Myograms (MĪ-ō-gram) A graph plotting the force of contraction of a muscle or myofiber over time

Myometrium (mī-ō-MĒ-trē-um) The smooth muscle of the uterus

Myxedema (mix-a-DĒ-ma) Hyposecretion of thyroid hormones later in life than infancy

Na⁺K⁺ATPase (sodium potassium ATPase) Integral membrane protein (enzyme) that cleaves ATP to release energy used to pump sodium ions out of the cell and potassium ions into the cell

Nares (NAR-ēz) Nostrils

Nasal (NĀ-zal) Pertaining to the nose

Nasopharynx (na-zō-FAR-ankz) The most superior portion of the pharynx, posterior to the nasal cavity, superior to the oral cavity

Natural immunity Our more primitive and less specific form of immune defense consisting of barriers, inflammation, and natural killer cell activity

Natural killer cells A form of lymphocyte involved in natural immunity These cells identify and lyse virally infected cells and neoplastic (cancer) cells

Necrose, necrosis (nek-RŌS) Death of cells

Neoplastic (nē-ō-PLAZ-tik) Means new growth. Cancerous, although may be benign or malignant

Nephron (NEF-ron) The functional units of the kidney consisting of the renal corpuscle, proximal convoluted tubule, loop of the nephron, distal convoluted tubule, and related capillaries and collecting tubules

Nerve Collection of neuron (nerve) fibers (axons, dendrites, and myelin sheaths, if myelinated) outside of the CNS

Neuroeffector junction (nūr-ō-ē-FEK-tor junk-shun) The junction between an axon and an effector cell (muscle or gland cell); often considered a type of synapse

Neurofibral node (nūr-ō-FĪB-ral NŌD) The spaces between adjacent myelin sheaths in a myelinated nerve fiber; also called nodes of Ranvier

Neurofilaments (nūr-ō-FIL-a-ments) The class of intermediate filament proteins seen in nervous tissue

Neurohypophysis (nūr-ō-hī-POF-a-sis) Posterior pituitary

Neurolemma (nūr-ō-LEM-a) The cell body of a neurolemmocyte that is wrapped around the myelin sheath it provides to an axon or dendrite; neurolemma exists only in the PNS and assists in regeneration of a nerve fiber after injury

Neurolemmocyte (nūr-ō-LEM-ō-sīt) The cell responsible for myelination in the PNS

Neurotransmitter (nūr-ō-TRANZ-mit-er) A molecule (i.e., acetylcholine and glutamic acid) that is released by from the synaptic bulb in response to an action potential and diffuses across the synaptic cleft to bind to a receptor in the postsynaptic membrane

Neutron (NŪ-tron) A noncharged, subatomic particle present in the nucleus of an atom

Neutrophil (NŪ-trō-fil) One type of granular leukocyte; main cell type of acute inflammation

Nissl bodies Rough endoplasmic reticulum of a neuron; also called chromatophilic substance

Nitrogenous waste (nī-TRAH-jen-us) Nitrogen-containing waste products such as ammonia (NH_3) and urea; results mainly from deamination of amino acids

Norepinephrine (nor-epi-NEF-er-in) A catecholamine that serves as a neurotransmitter and a hormone from the adrenal medulla; important in sympathetic nervous system activity

Nucleic acid (nū-KLĀ-ik A-sid) Chains of nucleotides as in DNA and RNA

Nucleolus (nū-klē-Ō-lus) Organelle present in the nucleus; composed mainly of RNA, is the site of ribosome synthesis

Nucleotide (NŪ-klē-ō-tīd) A molecule consisting of a nitrogenous base, a pentose sugar, and one or more phosphate groups; assemble into chains called nucleic acids

Nucleus (NŪ-klē-us) The protons and neutrons at the center of an atom, or the prominent organelle in a cell that contains the cells genetic material (DNA), or a collection of neuron cell bodies in the CNS

Odontoblast (ō-DON-tō-bla-st) The cells of teeth that produce dentin

Olecranal (ō-LEK-ran-al) Pertaining to the back of the elbow

Oligodendrocyte (ol-i-gō-DEN-drō-sīt) The cells that provide myelination in the CNS

Omentum (ō-MEN-tum) Mesenteric membranes that support the stomach and proximal small intestine (lesser omentum) and that overly much of the intestine (greater omentum)

Oocyte (Ō-Ō-sīt) Female gamete

Oogenesis (ō-ō-JEN-a-sis) Production of the female gamete

Oogonia (ō-ō-GŌN-ē-a) Immature stage in oocyte development

Opposition (op-ō-ZISH-un) Movement of a digit across the palm

Opsin (OP-sin) A glycoprotein that is part of the photopigments of the retina

Oral Pertaining to the mouth

Orbit (OR-bit) The eye socket

Orbital Pertaining to the eye

Organ A collection of tissues organized to perform some function or functions

Organelle (or-gan-EL) A subcellular structure that performs some function for the cell

Oropharynx (o-rō-FAR-ānkz) The part of the pharynx that is posterior to the mouth, inferior to the nasopharynx, and superior to the laryngopharynx

Osmolarity (os-mō-LAR-i-tē) Pertaining to the concentration of a solution

Osmoreceptors (os-mō-rē-SEP-tor-z) Receptors in the hypothalamus that measure the concentration of the extracellular fluids and can trigger thirst and ADH secretion from the posterior pituitary

Osmosis (os MŌ-sis) Diffusion of water across a semipermeable membrane

Osmotic pressure (os-MAH-tik) The force (pressure) that must be applied to stop osmosis; related to the difference in the concentration of the solutions either side of the membrane

Osteoblast (OS-tē-ō-blast) Cells that produce bone matrix; related to osteoprogenitor cells and osteocytes

Osteoclast (OS-tē-ō-klast) Cells that resorb bone matrix as the first step in remodeling; are multinucleated giant cells in the monocyte-macrophage lineage

Osteocyte (OS-tē-ō-sīt) Terminally differentiated cells in the osteoblast lineage; reside in lacunae and maintain bone matrix

Osteogenesis (os-tē-ō-JEN-a-sis) Formation of bone; performed through endochondrial and intramembranous ossification

Osteomalacia (os-tē-ō-mal-Ā-sha) Bone disease caused by deficiency of vitamin D in adults

Osteon (OS-tē-on) Haversian unit, the layered microscopic structures that make up dense bone

Osteoporosis (os-tē-ō-por-Ō-sis) A disease characterized by a measurable decrease in bone mass

Osteoprogenitor cells (os-tē-ō-prō-JEN-i-tor) The stem cells of bone; daughter cells of this lineage differentiate to become osteoblasts and then osteocytes

Otic (Ō-tik) Pertaining to the ear

Ovary (Ō-var-ē) The primary sex organ of females

Ovulation (ah-vū-LĀ-shun) Release of an oocyte from the ovary; triggered by a surge of LH

Oxytocin (oks-a-TŌS-in) Protein hormone released from the posterior pituitary; stimulates contraction of uterine smooth muscle and milk let-down reflex

Palmar (PALM-ar) Pertaining to the palm of the hand

Pancreas (PAN-krē-as) An organ of both the digestive and endocrine systems; it secretes digestive enzymes as an exocrine function and the hormones insulin and glucagon, as an endocrine function

Pancreatic acini (pan-krē-AT-ik a-SĒ-nī) The exocrine component of the pancreas

Pancreatic islets (pan-krē-AT-ik Ī-letz) Islets of Langerhans, endocrine tissue of the pancreas

Parafollicular cells (pa-ra-fah-LIK-ū-lar) Cells of the thyroid that secrete the hormone calcitonin

Paranasal sinuses (pa-ra-NĀ-sal SĪN-i-sez) Air spaces lined with mucous membranes present in some skull bones

Parasagittal (pa-ra-SA-jit-al) A sagittal section that is not in the middle plane of the body

Parasympathetic nervous system, PNS (PA-ra-sim-pa-the-tik) The component of the autonomic nervous system that predominates during periods of energy conservation and restoration (rest and digest)

Parathyroid glands (pa-ra-THĪ-roid) The endocrine glands that secrete parathyroid hormone

Parenchyma (par-ENK-a-ma) The cells of an organ that do the actual work of that organ; the parenchyma is supported by the stroma

Parietal (par-Ī-et-al) Refers to the part of a serous membrane (mesothelium) that lines a cavity, as opposed to the visceral component that lines the surface of the organ residing in the cavity

Pathophysiologic (PATH-ō-fiz-ē-ō-lah-jik) Functioning that occurs outside of homeostasis

Pavementing (PĀV-ment-ing) During cellular exudate formation, the attachment of leukocytes to endothelial cells and leukocyte movement along the endothelial surface of the capillary

Pedal (PĒ-dal) Foot

Pedicels (PED-i-selz) Extensions of podocytes, present in glomeruli

Pelvis (PEL-vis) The region of the body that includes the cavity that holds the internal organs of reproduction and urinary bladder (the pelvic cavity), and the coxal bones

Pelvis, renal (RĒ-nal PEL-vis) The space in the notched side of the kidney that the calyces empty into and the ureter drains

Penis (PĒ-nis) Male copulatory organ

Pentamere (PENT-a-mer) One molecule composed of five similar parts, i.e., pentameric IgM

Pentose (PENT-ōs) A monosaccharide containing five carbons

Pepsin (PEP-sin) Proteolytic (protein digesting) enzyme present in the stomach

Pepsinogen (pep-SIN-ō-jen) Inactive form of pepsin, as it is produced and secreted, prior to activation in the stomach lumen

Pericardium (pe-ri-KAR-dē-um) Around the heart, as in the parietal and visceral pericardium (the serous membrane that lines the pericardial cavity)

Perikaryon (pe-ri-KAR-ē-on) The neuron cell body

Perimysium (pe-ri-MĪ-sē-um) The connective tissue that surrounds fascicles within a muscle

Perinatal (pe-ri-NĀ-tal) The period of time just before and after the delivery of a baby

Perineurium (pe-ri-NŪR-ē-um) The connective tissue that surrounds fascicles within a nerve

Perinuclear (pe-ri-NŪK-lē-ar) The area in the cytoplasm that is around the nucleus

Periosteum (pe-ri-OST-ē-um) The dense connective tissue and osteoprogenitor cells that are on the external surface of a bone (compare to endosteum)

Peripheral nervous system, PNS (per-IF-er-al) The nervous system components excluding the brain and spinal cord

Peristalsis (pe-ra-STAHL-sis) Rhythmic, wave-like muscle contractions that move distally in a tubular structure, propelling its contents

Phagocytosis (fā-gō-sī-TŌ-sis) Cell eating, the form of endocytosis that uses pseudopodia to bring large particles into a cell; most cells types lack this ability; it is most developed in macrophages

Pharynx (FAR-inkz) Throat, consists of three regions: nasopharynx, oropharynx, and laryngopharynx

Phenotype (FĒN-ō-tīp) The characteristics we can see and measure in an individual that are determined by his or her genotype (genetic makeup)

Phenylalanine (fēn-al-AL-a-nēn) An amino acid

Phosphagen system (FOS-fa-jen) The system that supplies energy in contracting muscle during the early seconds of contraction; includes fuel in the form of stored ATP and phosphocreatine

Phosphocreatine (fos-fō-KRĒĒ-a-tin) A high-energy molecule stored in muscle used to generate ATP, while contractions are being fueled by the phosphagen system

Phosphodiesterase (fos-fō-dī-EST-ĒR-āz) An enzyme that inactivates cAMP to limit the activity of the cAMP second messenger system

Phospholipid (fos-fō-LIP-id) A molecule that contains a polar phosphate head and two nonpolar fatty acid tails, interconnected by a glycerol; this is the major component of the cell membrane, the phospholipid bilayer

Phosphorylate (fos-FŌR-a-lāt) To add phosphate groups to a molecule

Photopigment (FŌ-tō-PIG-ment) A molecule such as rhodopsin, containing a glycoprotein called an opsin, and retinal, a vitamin-A derivative; part of the retinal light receptors used for vision

Pia mater (PĒ-a MAT-er) The deep layer of the meninges

Pineal gland (pī-NĒ-al) Endocrine gland and nervous system structure; produces the hormone melatonin

Pinna (PI-na) The flap-like structure of your external ear; composed of a core of elastic cartilage covered with skin

Pinocytosis (pē-nō-sī-TŌ-sis) The form of endocytosis practiced by most cell types; like "cell drinking"

Pituitary (pi-tū-i-TAR-ē) Endocrine gland attached to the hypothalamus, composed of an anterior and posterior lobe

Plantar (PLAN-tar) Pertaining to the sole of the foot

Plasma (PLA-z-ma) The fluid component of blood

Plasmalemma (plaz-ma-LEM-a) The cell membrane, or plasma membrane, composed mainly of phospholipid bilayer

Plasmin (PLAZ-min) The enzyme that cleaves non-crosslinked fibrin to limit blood clotting, as the product of the fibrinolytic cascade

Plasminogen (plaz-MIN-ō-jen) The inactive form of plasmin normally found in circulation

Platelet (PLĀT-let) Cell fragments produced by megakaryocytes that are important in blood clotting

Pleura (PLŪR-a) The serous membrane (mesothelium) that line the pleural cavities (parietal pleura) and the lungs, which are contained in those cavities (visceral pleura)

Plexus (PLEK-zus) Networks of nerves from the rami of adjacent spinal nerves

Pneumocyte (NŪ-mō-sīt) The epithelial cells that line the alveoli, present in two varieties: type one, which are simple squamous cells; and type two, which are cuboidal and produce surfactant

Pneumotaxic center (nū-mō-TAK-zik) Center in the pons involved in pulmonary ventilation

Podocyte (PŌ-dō-sīt) Cells that wrap processes (pedicels) around the capillaries of the glomeruli

Polar (PŌ-lar) Having opposing positively and negatively charged regions, such as in a polar molecule

Polydipsia (pah-lē-DIP-sē-a) Excessive thirst, seen in diabetes patients

Polymorphonuclear leukocyte, PMN (pah-lē-MOR-fō-nūk-lē-ar LŪK-ō-sīt) Neutrophils, a type of granular leukocyte

Polyuria (pah-lē-ŪR-ē-a) Excessive urine volume, seen in diabetes patients

Pons (PON-z) The component of the brainstem that is intermediate between the medulla oblongata and the midbrain

Popliteal (pop-lit-Ē-aL) Pertaining to the back of the knee

Portal system (POR-tl) A vascular arrangement in which one capillary bed is followed in series by a second capillary bed; used for delivery of some substance from one organ to another (i.e., hypothalamus to anterior pituitary)

Posterior (pos-TER-ē-ar) Toward the rear surface of the body, opposite of anterior

Premalignant (prē-ma-LIG-nant) A pathologic lesion that is not malignant but is considered a precursor of malignancy; a lesion in which malignancy may arise (i.e., benign polyps in the colon)

Primary sex organ The organ of either sex in which gametogenesis occurs (the testes and ovaries)

Process, of bone (PRAH-ses) Any structure protruding from the surface of a bone

Prolactin (prō-LAK-tin) A hormone produced by the anterior pituitary that stimulates lactation

Proliferative (prō-LIF-er-ā-tiv) Pertaining to proliferation, cell division

Proline (PRŌ-lēn) An amino acid

Pronation (prō-NĀ-shun) A movement of the forearm in which the palm rotates posteriorly or inferiorly; opposite of supination

Proprioception (PRŌ-prē-ō-sep-shun) The ability to sense the position of the body or a limb in three-dimensional space

Prostate (PRAH-stāt) Gland in the male reproductive tract that secretes some of the fluid content of semen

Protein (PRŌ-tēn) A molecule composed of a chain of amino acids; this is a highly diverse group of extremely important molecules

Proteolytic enzyme (prō-tē-ō-LIT-ik) Enzymes that cleave (cut) proteins; important in both the synthetic and degradative processes

Prothrombin (prō-THROM-bin) Inactive precursor of thrombin, an enzyme that cleaves fibrinogen to activate fibrin and cause blood to clot

Proton (PRŌ-ton) A positively charged particle that is one component of the atomic nucleus

Protraction (prō-TRAK-shun) Movement of a structure (such as the jaw) anteriorly, opposite of retraction

Proximal (PROK-zi-mal) The end of a structure that is closest to its beginning or site of attachment; opposite of distal

Pseudostratified (sūd-ō-STA-ti-fīd) False stratification, when an epithelium appears to be stratified, but all cells are in contact with the basement membrane

Pulmonary (PUL-mon-ar-ē) Pertaining to the lungs

Purine (PŪR-ēn) One of the two forms of nucleotides (based on the structure of the nitrogenous base) that make up our DNA and RNA (the other form being pyrimidines); adenine and guanine nucleotides are purines

Pyloris (pī-LOR-is) The most distal region of the stomach, the structure that connects to the duodenum

Pyramid, renal A structure of the medulla of the kidney that contains the collecting ducts

Pyrimidine (pūr-RIM-a-dēn) One of the two forms of nucleotides (based on the structure of the nitrogenous base) that make up our DNA and RNA (the other form being purines); thymine, cytosine, and uracil nucleotides are pyrimidines

Pyruvic acid (pī-RŪ-vik) An early breakdown product of glucose that contains three carbons

Rami, ramus (RĀ-mī, RĀ-mus) Branches of spinal nerves

Ranvier, node of (RON-vē-ā) The spaces between adjacent myelin sheaths in a myelinated nerve fiber; also called neurofibral nodes

Reflex (RĒ-flex) A function of the nervous system consisting of involuntary responses to specific stimuli; usually very similar among individuals

Reflex arc (Rē-Flex ar-k) The functional unit of the nervous system; consists of a receptor, a sensory nerve, a center (in the CNS), a motor nerve, and an effector

Refractory period (rē-FRAK-tōr-ē) The period of time after a threshold stimulus in which a second stimulus cannot initiate an additional action potential (absolute refractory period) or in which a larger than normal stimulus is required to reach threshold and stimulate an additional action potential (relative refractory period)

Renal corpuscle (KŌR-pus-el) The part of the nephron that includes the glomerular (Bowman's) capsule, glomerular space, and glomerulus

Renin (REN-in) An enzyme secreted into the blood by the juxtaglomerular apparatus in response to low blood pressure; cleaves angiotensinogen to angiotensin I

Reperfuse (rē-per-FŪZ) To reestablish blood flow after it has been stopped

Repolarize (RĒ-pō-ler-īz) To reestablish membrane polarity after depolarization; one part of an action potential

Resorption, tubular, (rē-SORB-shun) Movement of substances from filtrate within the renal tubules, into the blood during urine production

Reticular (re-TIK-ū-lar) Means network, as in reticular connective tissue and zona reticularis

Retina (RE-tin-a) Component of the nervous tunic of the eye, the structure in which light is converted into receptor potentials

Retraction (rē-TRAK-shun) Movement of a structure (such as the jaw) posteriorly, opposite of protraction

Rhodopsin (rōd-OP-sin) A photopigment that is best stimulated by blue to green light

Rhythmicity (rith-MIS-it-ē) The characteristic of a repeating beat, as in the autorhythmicity or self-generated beat of the heart

Ribonuclease (rī-bō-NŪ-klē-āz) An enzyme that cleaves ribonucleic acid (RNA)

Ribonucleotides (rī-bō-NŪ-klē-ō-tīdz) The molecules that join together in chains to produce RNA

Ribosome (RĪB-ō-zōm) The organelles that are the sites of protein synthesis; may be free (free in the cytoplasm) or bound (attached to endoplasmic reticulum)

Rotation, lateral To turn a structure away from the midline (turn your head to the side)

Rotation, medial To turn a structure toward the midline (return your head to the anatomical position from the side)

Rouleaux (rū-LŌ) Rows of erythrocytes sticking together and moving in capillaries as single units; seen during cellular exudate formation in acute inflammation

rRNA Ribosomal RNA, the RNA of which ribosomes are composed

Rugae (RŪ-gā) The folds in the mucosa of the stomach

Saccharide (SAK-a-rīd) A unit of a carbohydrate or sugar composed of carbon hydrogen and oxygen arranged in a ring structure; a single saccharide is called a monosaccharide; two bound together is a disaccharide, three a trisaccharide, and more than three is a polysaccharide

Sagittal (SAJ-i-tal) A plane of section that divides the body into left and right components; if it is in the midline it is a midsagittal section, if it is to either side of the midline it is a parasagittal section

Salt A molecule that dissociates (ionizes) into a cation other than the hydrogen ion (H^+) and an anion other than the hydroxyl ion (OH^-)

Saltatory conduction (SAL-ta-tō-rē con-DUK-t-shun) Nerve impulse conduction in a myelinated fiber

Sarcoidosis (sark-oid-Ō-sis) A disease characterized by chronic inflammation in the form of granulomas distributed widely in the body; the cause is currently unknown

Sarcolemma (SARK-ō-lem-a) The plasma membrane of a muscle cell

Sarcomere (SARK-ō-mer) The repeating units of thick and thin myofilaments in a myofibril

Sarcoplasm (SARK-ō-plazm) The cytoplasm of a muscle cell

Sarcoplasmic reticulum (sark-ō-PLAZ-mik re-TIK-ū-lum) The smooth endoplasmic reticulum of a muscle cell; terminal cisterns are part of this organelle

Schlemm, canal of See *scleral venous sinus*

Scleral venous sinus (SKLAH-ral) The canal through which aqueous humor leaves the anterior cavity of the eye; the canal of Schlemm is another name for this structure

Serine (SEAR-ēn) An amino acid

Serotonin (ser-a-TŌ-nin) An amine neurotransmitter

Sodium potassium ATPase ($Na^+K^+ATPase$) Integral membrane protein (enzyme) that cleaves ATP to release energy used to pump sodium ions out of the cell and potassium ions into the cell

Sebaceous gland (sa-BĀ-shus) Glands of the skin that produce sebum, an oily, lipid secretion that is released into hair follicles

Secretin (se-KRĒT-in) Small intestinal hormone involved in regulation of digestive activities

Sella turcica (SEL-a TŪR-si-ka) Feature of the sphenoid bone that houses the pituitary gland

Semen (SĒM-en) Secretion of the male reproductive tract consisting of sperm and fluids that transport and support the sperm

Semilunar valve (SE-mĭ-LŪN-ar) One-way valves in the proximal aorta and pulmonary trunk

Seminal vesicle (SEM-i-nal VES-i-kul) Exocrine gland in the male reproductive tract that produces much of the fluid content of semen

Seminiferous tubule (sem-in-IF-er-us) The tubules of the testes in which spermatogenesis occurs

Semipermeable membrane (SE-mē-PERM-ēa-bul) A membrane that allows some substances to cross but does not allow others to cross; the selectivity is largely based on the chemical properties of the molecules or atoms that are passing through or being excluded

Sense (SEN-s) Our ability to perceive conditions of the internal and external environment and our bodies; our ability to collect and transmit data pertaining to these conditions

Septae (SEP-ta) Walls

Sequelae (sē-KWELL-ā) That which follows; for example, bleeding and scab formation may be sequelae of falling down and scraping your knee

Serosa (ser-Ō-sa) The outer layer of a multilayered tubular structure such as the alimentary canal; composed of mesothelium (i.e., visceral peritoneum)

Sertoli cell (ser-TŌ-lē) Cells lining the seminiferous tubules that support the cells of the spermatogenic lineage; also called sustentacular cells

Serum (SEAR-um) Part of the fluid component of blood; the fluid that is left once the cells have been removed (leaving plasma), the plasma has clotted, and the components of the clot have been removed

Sesamoid bone (SE-sa-moyd) Bone present within a tendon, such as the patella. Most sesamoid bones are quite small and vary among individuals

Simple epithelium (epi-THĒ-lē-um) Epithelial cells (lining cells) that are arranged in a single layer

Sinoatrial node (sī-nō-ĀT-rē-al NŌ-d) The primary pacemaker of the heart

Skatole (SKĀ-tōl) A simple substance that results from the digestion of proteins; one of the waste products that give feces their characteristic odor

Sliding filament theory The theory that explains the molecular basis of muscle cell contraction

Solute (SŌL-ēūt) A molecule that dissolves in a solvent to produce a solution

Solution (sō-LŪ-shun) One or more solutes plus a solvent

Solvent (SOL-vent) A fluid in which a solute will dissolve

Somatic nervous system (sō-MA-tik) The motor component of the nervous system that innervates voluntary effectors (skeletal muscle)

Sperm (SPER-m) The male gamete

Spermatids (SPERM-a-tidz) Cells in the spermatogenic lineage that have a 1n genetic content but are not mature sperm

Spermatocyte (sperm-AH-tō-sīt) Cells in the spermatogenic lineage that differentiate into spermatids; these cells have a 2n genetic content

Spermatogenesis (sper-MA-tō-jen-a-sis) Production of sperm

Spermatogonium (sper-MA-tō-gō-nēum) The stem cell of the spermatogenic lineage

Sphincter (SFINK-ter) A ring of smooth muscle

Spicule (SPIK-ūl) The fine plates of bone tissue that make up spongy bone; also called trabeculae

Squamous epithelium (SKWĀ-mus epi-THĒ-lē-um) Epithelial cells that are flattened in shape

Starling's hypothesis A hypothesis that explains the movement of fluid into and out of capillaries

Statoconia (sta-tō-KŌ-nē-a) Calcium carbonate crystals in the inner ear that are involved in balance

Stellate (STEL-āt) Star-shaped, as in the shape of an astrocyte

Stem cell Undifferentiated cells that divide to produce daughter cells that can differentiate into mature cell types; if a stem cell has the ability to produce daughter cells in only one lineage (i.e., stem cells of the intestinal epithelium can produce daughter cells in the intestinal epithelial lineage only), it is a **committed stem cell**; stem cells that produce daughter cells that can differentiate along multiple lines are called **pleuripotent stem cells** (i.e., the daughter cells of some mesenchymal stem cells can differentiate into a variety of mature mesenchymal cell types); stem cells whose daughter cells can differentiate along any lineage are called **totipotent stem cells** (i.e., embryonic stem cells); it is stem cells of these last two types that are causing great excitement in the research community at this time

Strata (STRA-ta) Layers

Stratified epithelium (STRA-ti-fīd) Epithelium in which the cells are arranged in multiple layers

Stratum basalis (of endometrium) (STRA-tum bā-SAL-is) The basal (bottom) layer of the endometrium; the layer that contains the endometrial stem cells that divide to produce a new stratum functionalis after menstruation

Stratum functionalis (of endometrium) (STRA-tum funk-shun-AL-is) The upper layer of the endometrium, the layer into which the early embryo implants; this layer is sloughed off during menstruation

Stroke volume The volume of blood that is pumped by each ventricle during each ventricular systole

Stroma (STRŌM-a) The cells of any organ that support its parenchyma

Subarachnoid space (sub-ar-AK-noid) The space in the meninges that is deep to the arachnoid mater and superficial to the pia mater; this space contains cerebrospinal fluid

Subcellular (sub-SEL-ū-lar) Structures that are smaller than a cell, such as organelles and cytoplasmic inclusions

Subclinical (sub-KLIN-i-kal) Condition in which symptoms are too mild to come to clinical attention

Submucosa (sub-mū-KŌS-a) The layer in the wall of a tubular organ that is immediately deep to the mucosa; usually consists of well vascularized loose connective tissue

Substance P A neuropeptide important in the perception of pain

Subthreshold stimulus (sub-THRESH-hōld) A stimulus in an excitable membrane that is not large enough to evoke an action potential

Sudoriferous (sū-dō-RIF-er-us) Sweat glands

Sulcus (SUL-kus) A groove or trench-like depression in a bone, or a shallow groove in the surface of the brain

Superior (sū-PEAR-ē-ōr) Above, higher than, opposite of inferior

Superoxide (sū-per-OX-īd) O_2^- The oxygen free radical; important in immunologic defense of the body and for its damaging effects on cells

Supination (sup-i-NĀ-shun) A movement of the forearm in which the palm is rotated anteriorly or superiorly; opposite of pronation

Sural (SŪR-al) Pertaining to the calf

Surfactant (sūr-FAK-tant) A detergent-like phospholipid that reduces the surface tension of the alveolar membranes, thereby reducing elastic recoil in the lungs; synthesis begins late in fetal development; its absence is responsible for the respiratory distress of many premature infants

Sustentacular cell (sus-ten-TAK-ū-lar) Cells lining the seminiferous tubules that support the cells of the spermatogenic lineage; also called Sertoli cells

Sympathetic nervous system The component of the autonomic nervous system that predominates during periods of stress, it is responsible for the fight-or-flight response

Symphesis (SIM-fa-sis) A cartilaginous joint in which fibrocartilage is present between the articulating bones

Synapse (SIN-apz) The junction between two neurons, although the term may also be applied to the junction between a neuron and an effector cell (more properly called a neuroeffector junction)

Synarthrosis (sin-arth-RŌ-sis) An immovable joint

Synchondrosis (sin-kon-DRŌ-sis) A cartilaginous joint in which hyaline cartilage is present between the articulating bones

Syncytium (sin-SISH-ē-um) A cell with multiple nuclei, a giant cell; skeletal muscle fibers are one example

Syndesmosis (sin-des-MŌ-sis) A fibrous joint that is an amphiarthrosis

Synostosis (sin-os-TŌ-sis) A bony joint, such as where two bones become fused together during development

Synovial joint (sin-Ō-vē-al) A diarthrosis (freely movable joint) in which there is a space (the synovial space) between the articulating bones

Systole (SIS-tō-lē) The phase of cardiac contraction or high blood pressure

T lymphocyte (Lim-fō-sīt) Leukocytes of the lymphocytic lineage that mature in the thymus

T_3 & T_4 The thyroid hormones triiodothyronine and thyroxine

Tarsal (TAR-sal) Pertaining to the ankle

Telodendria (tel-ō-DEN-drē-a) Branches of an axon located distally, also called axon terminals

Telophase (TEL-ō-fāz) One of the phases of nuclear division

Tendon (TEN-don) A structure of dense regular connective tissue that attaches muscle to bone

Terminal cistern (SIS-tern) A special feature of sarcoplasmic reticulum in which calcium ions are held when a muscle fiber is not contracting

Testosterone (tes-TOS-ter-ōn) An androgenic hormone

Tetany (TET-an-ē) Sustained contraction of a muscle fiber; may be complete or incomplete

Tetrose (TET-rōs) A monosaccharide containing four carbons

Thalamus (THAL-a-mus) A region of the diencephalon of the brain

Thoracic cavity (thōr-A-sik) The body cavity that is located superior to the diaphragm; it is subdivided into the pleural cavities and the pericardial cavity and contains the mediastinum

Threonine (THRĒ-ō-nēn) An amino acid

Threshold stimulus A stimulus to an excitable membrane that is capable of evoking an action potential

Triose (TRĪ-ōs) A monosaccharide containing three carbons

Thromboembolus (THROM-bō-EM-bō-lus) A blood clot moving within a blood vessel

Thymine (THĪ-mēn) A nitrogenous base that is present in thymine nucleotides

Thyroglobulin (thī-rō-GLOB-ū-lin) The protein that contains the thyroid hormones during their storage as thyroid colloid in thyroid follicles

Thyroid (THĪ-roid) Endocrine gland located anterior and lateral to the trachea

Thyroid colloid (KAH-loid) The gel in which thyroid hormones are stored within the thyroid follicles; composed of thyroglobulin

Thyroid stimulating hormone, TSH A hormone produced by the anterior pituitary that stimulates release of T_3 and T_4 from the thyroid

Thyroxine (thī-ROKS-in) The thyroid hormone T_4

Tight junction An intercellular junction that holds adjacent cells tightly together

Tissue (TISH-ū) A group of similar cells working together to perform specific functions, the construction materials of the body

Trabeculae (tra-BEK-ū-lē) The fine plates of bone tissue that make up spongy bone; also called spicules

Trachea (TRA-kē-ā) Component of the respiratory system; the airway that extends from the larynx to the bronchi

Tract (TRAK-t) A collection of neuron fibers in the central nervous system

Transcription (tranz-KRIP-shun) The process in protein synthesis by which messenger RNA (mRNA) is produced by copying the gene (DNA) into RNA; involves complementarity

Translation (tranz-LĀ-shun) The process during protein synthesis in which the chain of amino acids is produced, based on the codons present in the mRNA; this step occurs in ribosomes

Transmembrane protein (tranz-MEM-brān) An integral membrane protein, one which spans the thickness of the phospholipid bilayer

Treppe (TRE-pē) The phenomenon by which an individual muscle fiber produce successively stronger contractions during the beginning of a series of contractions that is begun in a resting fiber

Tricuspid valve (trī-KUS-pid) The right atrioventricular valve

Triglyceride (trī-GLIS-er-id) A fat containing three fatty acid side chains attached to a glycerol

Triiodothyronine (TRĪ-ī-ŌDŌ-thī-rō-nēn) The thyroid hormone T_3

Trinucleotide (trī-NŪKLEŌ-tīd) Three nucleotides in a row, in a nucleic acid

Trisaccharide (trī-SAK-a-rīd) A carbohydrate composed of three monosaccharides

tRNA, transfer RNA The molecule that transports individual amino acids to ribosomes during transcription

Trochanter, greater and lesser (TRŌ-kan-ter) Features of the proximal end of the femur

Tropomyosin (trō-pō-MĪ-ō-sin) The protein that makes up the backbone of the thin myofilament

Troponin (trō-PŌ-nin) A calcium-binding protein that is attached to tropomyosin in thin myofilaments

Trypsin (TRIP-sin) A protein digesting enzyme produced by the pancreas

Tryptophan (TRIP-tō-fan) An amino acid

T-tubule, transverse tubule (tranz-VERS) A feature of the sarcolemma, tubules of the sarcolemma that extend into the sarcoplasm to carry the action potential to the terminal cisterns

Tubular resorption (TŪB-ū-lar rē-SORP-shun) Movement of substances from filtrate within the renal tubules, into the blood during urine production

Tubular secretion (TŪB-ū-lar sa-KRĒ-shun) Movement of substances from the blood into the filtrate of the renal tubules during urine production

Tubulin (TŪB-ū-lin) The protein from which microtubules and centrioles are made

Turbinates (TUR-bin-ātz) Nasal conchae; three bony plates within each side of the inner nose

Twitch A single contraction in an isolated muscle fiber, initiated by a single action potential

Tyrosine (TĪ-rō-sēn) An amino acid

Umami (ū-MOM-ē) One of the five primary tastes, also called savory

Umbilical (um-BIL-i-kal) Pertaining to the navel

Uracil (ŪR-a-sil) A nitrogenous base that is present in the uracil nucleotides of RNA

Urea (ūr-Ē-a) A nitrogenous waste produced by the liver from ammonia

Ureter (ŪR-a-tūr) A muscular duct in the urinary system that extends from the kidneys to the urinary bladder

Urethra (ū-RĒ-thra) A duct in the urinary system that extends from the urinary bladder and exits the body in the vulva (female) or through the penis (male); in the male, the urethra is also a component of the reproductive system: it also conveys semen

Urine (ŪR-in) The waste product produced by the kidneys, stored in the urinary bladder, and excreted through the urethra

Urobilinogen (ūrō-bil-IN-ōjen) The breakdown product of bilirubin (which results from hemoglobin breakdown) that gives feces their characteristic color

Urolithiasis (ūrō-lith-Ī-a-sis) Kidney stones

Uterine tube (Ū-ter-in) Fallopian tube, extends from each ovary to the uterus

Uterus (Ū-ter-us) Muscular organ in the female reproductive system that is the location of development of the embryo and fetus and the contractions of which are responsible for labor and delivery

Vagina (va-JĪN-a) Female copulatory organ and passageway through which the baby exits the body during delivery

Valence (VĀ-lens) The combining capacity of an atom, determined by the number of electrons in the outermost energy level

Valine (VĀ-lēn) An amino acid

Vasa vasorum (VĀ-sa va-SŌR-um) Small blood vessels that supply the needs of the walls of large blood vessels

Vasculature (VAS-kū-la-tur) The blood vessels

Vasoactive (VĀ-ZŌ-ak-tiv) Having an effect on the blood vessels, specifically on the muscular tone in muscular arteries, arterioles, and precapillary sphincters

Vasodilation (VĀ-ZŌ-dĭ-LĀ-shun) The degree to which muscular arteries, arterioles, and precapillary sphincters are dilated, affecting the amount of blood flowing through capillaries

Vein (VĀN) The low pressure blood vessels that extend from venules to the heart

Ventral (VENT-ral) Toward the front surface of the body, opposite of dorsal

Ventricle (VENT-ri-kul) The large, inferior chambers of the heart

Venule (VEN-ūl) The smallest of the veins, those to which the capillaries lead

Villi (VIL-ī) Mucosal projections into the lumen present in the small intestine

Vimentin (vī-MEN-tin) The intermediate filament protein of mesenchymal cells

Visceral (VIS-ser-al) Refers to the part of a serous membrane (mesothelium) that lines the surface of the organ, as opposed to the parietal component that lines the surface of the cavity

Vitamin (VĪT-a-men) Organic substances that are not proteins, carbohydrates, fats, or minerals, yet are necessary for the maintenance of homeostasis and (with exceptions) cannot be produced by our bodies

VLDL, very low density lipoprotein Transport form of lipids in the blood composed of lipids and apoproteins, conveys lipids from the liver to adipose tissue

Vulva (VUL-va) Female external genitalia

White matter Component of the central nervous system composed mainly of nerve fibers; myelin makes these tissues appear white, grossly

Index

Photo Credits

Chapter 1
Chapter opener © Custom Medical Stock Photo.

Chapter 2
Chapter opener courtesy of MIEMSS.

Chapter 3
Chapter opener courtesy of Bill Branson/National Cancer Institute. **Figure 3.4** © Photos.com. **Figure 3.13** Courtesy of Robert Clark. **Figure 3.17(a, b)** © Photos.com; **(c)** © Corbis; **(d)** Photodisc/Getty Images; **(e, f)** Courtesy of Robert Clark; **(g)** © Dr. Dennis Kunkel/Visuals Unlimited; **(h)** © Carolina Biological/Visuals Unlimited.

Chapter 4
Chapter opener © Photos.com. **Figure 4.1** © Photodisc. **Figure 4.2(a)** Courtesy of Pfizer, Inc. **Figure 4.3(top)** Courtesy of Robert Clark; **(middle)** Carolina Biological/Visuals Unlimited; **(bottom)** Dr. Fred Hossler/Visuals Unlimited. **Figure 4.4(top)** Courtesy of Robert Clark; **(top middle)** © Donald Fawcett/Visuals Unlimited; **(bottom middle)** © Visuals Unlimited; **(bottom)** Dr. Richard Kessel/Visuals Unlimited. **Figure 4.6(top left)** © Visuals Unlimited; **(top middle)** © Robert Calentine/Visuals Unlimited; **(top right)** © Carolina Biological/Visuals Unlimited; **(bottom left)** © Biodisc/Visuals Unlimited; **(bottom middle)** © Gladden Wills, MD/Visuals Unlimited; **(bottom right)** © Dr. Richard Kessel/Visuals Unlimited. **Figure 4.7(left)** © Dr. David M. Phillips/Visuals Unlimited; **(middle)** © Robert Calentine/Visuals Unlimited; **(right)** © Dr. John Cunningham/Visuals Unlimited. **Figure 4.8(left, right)** Courtesy of Robert Clark.

Chapter 5
Chapter opener © AbleStock. **Figure 5.1(upper left, middle)** ©Photos.com; **(upper right, lower left)** © Photodisc; **(lower right)** © Keith Brofsky/FogStock/Alamy Images.

Chapter 6
Chapter opener © Eyewire Images, Inc. **Figure 6.1** © Photodisc. **Figure 6.3(a,b)** Courtesy of Robert Clark. **Figure 6.4** Courtesy of Robert Clark. **Figure 6.5** Courtesy of Robert Clark. **Figure 6.7(left)** Science Vu/Visuals Unlimited. **Figure 6.9(right)** © Photos.com.

Chapter 7
Chapter opener © Phil Degginger/Alamy Images.

Chapter 8
Chapter opener © Image Shop/Phototake.

Chapter 9
Chapter opener © Ablestock. **Figure 9.1(a-c)** Science VU/Visuals Unlimited.

Chapter 10
Chapter opener © Photodisc.

Chapter 11
Chapter opener © S. O'Brien/Custom Medical Stock Photo. **Figure 11.8(b-e)** Courtesy of Robert Clark.

Chapter 12
Chapter opener © Photodisc. **Figure 12.21(photo)** © Kimberly Potvin/Jones and Bartlett Publishers.

Chapter 13
Chapter opener © Photodisc. **Figure 13.8(a,b)** Courtesy of Robert Clark. **Figure 13.12(photo)** © John D. Cunningham/Visuals Unlimited. **Figure 13.13** Courtesy of Robert Clark. **Figure 13.15(inset)** © Science VU/Visuals Unlimited.

Chapter 14
Chapter opener courtesy of Bill Branson/National Cancer Institute.

Chapter 15
Chapter opener © Photodisc. **Figure 15.6(c)** © Ed Reschke. **Figure 15.11** Courtesy of the Lance Armstrong Foundation (www.laf.org).

Chapter 16
Chapter opener courtesy of MIEMSS. **Figure 16.1(inset)** Margaret Luzier/U.S. Army Corps of Engineers. **Figure 16.6(photo)** © Kimberly Potvin/Jones and Bartlett Publishers. **Figure 16.8** © Science VU/Visuals Unlimited.

Figure 16.15 © David Sanger Photography/Alamy Images.

■ Chapter 17

Chapter opener courtesy of MIEMSS. **Figure 17.10** © Kimberly Potvin/Jones and Bartlett Publishers.

■ Chapter 18

Chapter opener © Ken Hammond/USDA. **Figure 18.7 (photo)** © Dr. Dennis Kunkel/Visuals Unlimited. **Figure 18.11** © John D. Cunningham/Visuals Unlimited.

■ Chapter 19

Chapter opener © Photos.com.

■ Chapter 20

Chapter opener © Creatas. **Figure 20.2 (photo)** © Photos.com. **Figure 20.4** © AbleStock.

■ Chapter 21

Chapter opener © Ron Chapple/Thinkstock/Creatas. **Figure 21.2(a)** © Charles Stewart & Associates 2002; **(b,c)** Courtesy of Robert Clark.